Speech Science

An Integrated Approach to Theory and Clinical Practice

THIRD EDITION

Carole T. Ferrand
Hofstra University

PEARSON

Boston Columbus Indianapolis New York San Francisco Upper Saddle River
Amsterdam Cape Town Dubai London Madrid Milan Munich Paris Montreal Toronto
Delhi Mexico City São Paulo Sydney Hong Kong Seoul Singapore Taipei Tokyo

Executive Editor and Publisher: *Stephen D. Dragin*
Editorial Assistant: *Michelle Hochberg*
Marketing Manager: *Joanna Sabella*
Production Editor: *Paula Carroll*
Editorial Production Service: *Element LLC*
Manufacturing Buyer: *Megan Cochran*
Electronic Composition: *Element LLC*
Interior Design: *Element LLC*
Cover Designer: *Laura Gardner*

Library of Congress Cataloging-in-Publication Data is on file with the Library of Congress.

10 9 8 7 6 5 4

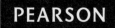

ISBN-10: 0-132-90711-9
ISBN-13: 978-0-132-90711-8

In loving memory of my parents,
Anne and Issy Friedman,
and my brother, Alan Friedman

About the Author

Carole T. Ferrand, PhD

Dr. Ferrand earned her B.A. in English Literature from the University of the Witwatersrand in Johannesburg, South Africa; and her M.S. and PhD in Communication Sciences and Disorders from the Pennsylvania State University. She teaches undergraduate and graduate level courses in Speech Science and Voice Disorders at Hofstra University in New York. Her research focuses on acoustic attributes of normal and disordered speech production. When not writing books, Dr. Ferrand enjoys reading historical fiction, hiking, and playing banjo.

Ted Ferrand researched, revised, and created the illustrations for this book. He holds a BFA from Pratt Institute in New York and has worked as a graphic designer, art educator and museum director.

Contents

CHAPTER 3

The Articulatory System 71

CHAPTER 4

*Clinical Application: Evaluation and
Treatment of Disorders Related to
Articulation* 123

CHAPTER 5

The Phonatory System   148

CHAPTER 6

Clinical Application: Evaluation and Treatment of Phonatory Disorders 190

CHAPTER 7

CHAPTER 8

CHAPTER 9

The Auditory System 284

CHAPTER 10

Clinical Application: Evaluation and Treatment of Disorders Related to Hearing Impairment 312

CHAPTER 11

The Nervous System   333

CHAPTER 12

Clinical Application: Brain Imaging in the Evaluation and Treatment of Disorders of the Nervous System   390

CHAPTER 13

Models and Theories of Speech Production and Perception　　405

Foreword

Together with the disciplines of language science and hearing science, speech science forms the theoretical framework for research and professional practice in the fields of speech–language pathology and audiology. Speech science has emerged into the forefront of the curriculum in speech–language pathology for several reasons.

First, over the past decades, an explosion of new technology has expanded the scientific knowledge base in speech–language pathology and presently influences all aspects of teaching, research, and clinical practice. Second, the study of speech science provides an opportunity to introduce students to the objective measurement of many aspects of human communication behavior and to the translation of numerical information into meaningful interpretations of this behavior. This is a critical ability for students to develop. Increasingly, speech–language pathologists and audiologists in different settings (hospitals, rehabilitation centers, early intervention centers, nursing homes, schools, etc.) are required to use and interpret information from acoustic and physiological instrumentation in order to evaluate and treat individuals with various communicative disorders. A thorough understanding of the scientific basis of the instrumentation, as well as an appreciation of the clinical relevance of the information, is therefore essential.

Third, speech science is an excellent way of helping students to understand and appreciate the scientific method and the importance of hypothesis testing, data collection, and empirical observation. Too often, however, science and clinical practice have been considered disparate subjects. This division creates the erroneous impression that clinical decision making is divorced from a scientific knowledge base.

This text is unique in its attempt to unify concepts in speech science with the clinical application to communication disorders. Students are provided with an integrated approach to speech science that emphasizes scientific concepts in relation to clinical practice. The link between theory and application is supported by current research highlighting the different diagnostic and intervention applications of the scientific material. The integration of theoretical information with clinical application makes the information more easily accessible, less intimidating, and more relevant to students.

The book also clearly guides the student to understand the relationship between acoustics, speech production, and speech perception. Concepts are integrated and explained through a thorough discussion of the speech systems of respiration, phonation, articulation, and perception. Not only do students become well acquainted with the different speech systems and how they normally function, but they are also introduced to the way these systems have been studied and measured through various instrumental means. In line with the overall goal of this book, emphasis is placed on current acoustic and physiologic measurements that are typically employed for clinical purposes as well as for research, such as fundamental frequency and intensity measures, jitter, shimmer, spectrography, electroglottography, and so on.

Scientific concepts are presented within a narrative framework that facilitates understanding the material as an integrated and coherent body of knowledge. Students thus have a firm base from which to further expand their knowledge. Consequently, depth of content is provided without sacrificing readability, and the text remains student and instructor friendly. Dr. Carole Ferrand presents the information in an unusually readable, easy-to-follow manner. Students will appreciate her lucid and accessible writing style, as well as the clear illustrations of concepts. Professors will find the material in-depth and comprehensive and the review questions and integrative case studies at the end of each chapter most helpful in stimulating classroom discussion.

Ronald L. Bloom, Ph.D.
Acting Dean
School of Health Sciences and Human Services
Hofstra University

Preface

This third edition of *Speech Science: An Integrated Approach to Theory and Clinical Practice* continues to highlight the close relationship between the scientific study of speech production and perception and the application of this material to evaluation and treatment of communication disorders. While the thrust of the book is unchanged, some additional material has been included, and the organization has been revised to enhance the flow of information. Specifically, a section on basic science concepts has been added to Chapter 1, in order to provide a more thorough grounding for students, as well as to help them appreciate how speech science relates to other branches of science. In terms of organization, the topics of resonance and the role of the vocal tract as an acoustic resonator have been combined into one chapter early in the text. This provides a seamless transition between concepts and a firm basis for understanding the source-filter theory. Discussion of the articulatory system follows, and students are led to appreciate the articulatory-acoustic relationships between vocal tract resonance characteristics and verbal output. Chapters on phonation, respiration, audition, and the nervous system follow, and the book concludes with information on classic and current models and theories of speech production and perception.

The third edition continues to follow the format of previous editions, in which each theoretical chapter is followed by a clinical chapter presenting information on evaluation and treatment of different communication disorders. All chapters have been updated with current research, and additional integrative case studies have been included with many of the clinical chapters.

A significant enhancement of the book is the inclusion of two-color illustrations to help students clearly visualize important aspects of anatomy and physiology relevant to human communicative behavior.

It is my sincere hope that instructors and students alike will continue to appreciate the book and will find the additional and revised material to be valuable.

New to This Edition

- First chapter includes additional material on basic physics concepts in narrative and tabular form which provides a more thorough grounding and review of basic concepts for students, and helps them to appreciate how speech science relates to other branches of science.

- The topics of resonance and the role of the vocal tract as an acoustic resonator have been combined into one chapter early in the text, providing students a seamless transition between concepts, and a firm basis for understanding the source-filter theory.

○ Updated research in all clinical chapters. Current research literature helps students to appreciate the ways in which instrumental techniques supplement and enhance diagnosis, evaluation, and treatment of individuals with communication disorders.

○ Additional integrative case studies facilitate student appreciation of the strong links between theory and current clinical management of patients with a wide variety of communication disorders.

○ Inclusion of two-color illustrations help students to clearly visualize important aspects of anatomy and physiology relevant to human communicative behavior.

Descriptions of current technologies such as high-speed digital imaging, electromagnetic articulography, and transcranial magnetic stimulation. Additional information regarding acoustic, aerodynamic, kinematic, and brain imaging techniques provides students with an introduction to new and innovative methods that are used to assess and treat articulatory, phonatory, respiratory, auditory, and nervous system disorders.

Carole Ferrand
Hofstra University

Acknowledgments

My husband Ted Ferrand researched, revised, expanded, recreated, and prepared for two-color printing many of the existing illustrations. He also created numerous additional illustrations, which will enable students to more fully grasp important details of structure and function of the speech systems. I appreciate his in-depth research and his ability to present complicated visual material with extraordinary clarity. I thank my colleagues Ron Bloom of Hofstra University and Janet Schoepflin of Adelphi University, who contributed their expertise in revising the chapters on the nervous system and the auditory system, respectively. My graduate students in speech science helped provide many of the new integrative case studies. Thanks to my graduate assistant, Amanda Smith, for her help preparing the spectrograms. And as always, thanks to Steve Dragin, for facilitating the revision process. I also appreciate the feedback from the users and reviewers of the second edition, whose helpful comments have been incorporated into the third edition: Rory DePaolis, James Madison University; Richard J. Morris, Florida State University; and Jayanthi Sasisekaran, University of Minnesota.

Introduction

This book arose from my experiences in teaching speech science at both undergraduate and graduate levels over the past 20 years. When I first started teaching the subject, I was surprised at how intimidated students were by the topic. It soon became clear that a key factor in alleviating their anxiety and promoting a positive learning experience was to demystify the subject by breaking the material into small, logically linked units and by making the organizational links between units of information explicit. Students are thus able to use the basic concepts as a scaffold upon which to extend their scientific knowledge. Careful structuring of the information helps students to grasp the material more easily, to retain the material beyond the next quiz or exam, and to integrate previously learned material with new concepts. However, although this scaffolding approach facilitates student understanding of the material, it does not help students to appreciate the relevance of the subject. "After all," was a frequently heard comment, "I'm going to be a clinician, not a researcher. I don't need this stuff to do therapy." It became clear, over the years, that the way to help students to appreciate the relevance of the speech science material is to explicitly connect it to clinical practice. Once students understand the connection between "science" and "clinic," the false dichotomy disappears, and students begin to appreciate the necessity of using scientific means of establishing rationales for clinical procedures, evaluating the effectiveness of treatment strategies, increasing clinical accountability, and applying the products of science and technology to clinical practice.

The explosion of technology over the past few decades has had an unprecedented effect on all areas of speech science and speech–language pathology. Due to technological advances such as electron microscopy, functional magnetic resonance imaging, ultrasound, transcranial magnetic stimulation, and electromagnetic articulography, among others, basic knowledge of the structures and functions of all systems involved in speech production and perception has expanded tremendously. The application of scientific knowledge to the diagnosis and treatment of communication disorders has resulted in dramatic changes and refinements. Acoustic, aerodynamic, and physiological technologies are rapidly becoming accepted tools in hospitals, rehabilitation centers, clinics, schools, and other settings in which human communicative behavior is of interest. This kind of information is invaluable for making finely tuned diagnoses about problems, detecting early changes in speech and voice that are not apparent perceptually, making intelligent decisions about treatment options, and assessing the outcomes of treatment.

This book takes a systems approach to the scientific study of speech production and speech perception, focusing on the physiological and acoustic generation and measurement of verbal output. Rather than study scientific concepts in isolation, concepts are explained in relation to the complex interactions of the physiological subsystems of respiration, phonation, articulation and resonance, and audition. The crucial role of the nervous system in control of voluntary movements is underscored. This approach provides a framework for discussing the articulatory-acoustic nature of speech in relation to the human capacity for producing and perceiving speech. In this way, the scientific concepts relate meaningfully to human communicative behavior.

Although a large part of the focus of this book is on information that can be obtained from instrumentation, there are four very important points that students should keep in mind. First, we cannot assume that there is a direct link between underlying anatomical and physiological factors and acoustic or other instrumental data. We make inferences from the data about the functioning of a system, but they are just that—inferences. Second, the information obtained from instrumentation may be objective, but a subjective component is always involved in the interpretation of the data. Third is the need to be aware of the validity of the information obtained. A degraded or distorted signal can yield information that is not valid. Furthermore, some kinds of analyses may not be appropriate for particular disorders. For instance, the jitter measure has been found to have decreased reliability when used with people with severe voice problems. Fourth, acoustic and other instrumental data do not replace behavioral and perceptual information but supplement it.

It is also important to keep in mind that speech production and perception, although complex processes with many levels, are, in reality, one "super system." Respiration, phonation, and articulation are so closely interwoven that they really cannot be separated. The role of audition in perception and production is crucial, and the nervous system is integral in regulating all aspects of speech. The divisions and separate discussions of these systems are purely for convenience and ease of discussion. As with any other subject, not all topics can be included in the book. The domains included under the broad rubric of speech science are numerous, varied, and complex. An author must necessarily select the topics he or she feels are most important. I have selected those that, over my 20 years of teaching speech science, have contributed most to students' understanding of speech science as a whole. The book focuses on acoustic and aerodynamic measurement and also includes discussion of techniques such as videoendoscopy, stroboscopy, ultrasound, magnetic resonance imaging, PET and SPECT scanning, and others. The book aims to tell a story—that is, to give context and shape to the narrative in a way that logically develops and furthers student understanding and retention of the material.

Overview of Chapters

The chapters are organized in accordance with the systems approach of this book and with the aim of the book, which is first to present more basic information and then to build on this information in a systematic manner. Chapter 1 presents information to help students place the study of sound in the context of a scientific framework. The first part of the chapter focuses on the physics of sound. The vibratory nature of sound is described and explained in detail, focusing on essential concepts of pressure, elasticity, and inertia. Dimensions of sound including frequency and period, pure tones and complex sounds, and intensity and amplitude are explored. The dB scale is presented, and some different applications of the scale are noted. Students are introduced to the concepts of reverberation, absorption, reflection, refraction, diffraction, and interference. An important section of Chapter 1 is the presentation of detailed information about waveforms and spectra and the different sorts of information that they provide.

Chapter 2 focuses on resonance, with an emphasis on acoustic resonators. Tube resonators and standing waves are described; and characteristics of acoustic resonators are explored, such as bandwidth, cutoff frequencies, and resonance curves. These concepts are integral to the understanding of the vocal tract as an acoustic resonator. The vocal tract resonator is shown to be a variable quarter-wave resonator with multiple resonance frequencies. An explanation follows of how the vocal tract filters the glottal sound wave, formalized in Fant's source–filter theory of vowel production.

Chapter 3 elaborates on the role of the vocal tract in articulation. Students become familiar with the structure and function of the articulators of the vocal tract. The traditional classification system of consonants and vowels is presented. Discussion of spectrography and spectrographic analysis of vowels and consonants establishes the link between articulation of a sound and its resulting acoustic structure. To put the sounds in the perspective of connected speech, the concepts of coarticulation and suprasegmental aspects of speech production are then discussed.

Chapter 4 introduces students to clinical applications of the concepts presented in Chapter 3. Kinematic measures of articulation are described, including strain gauge systems, ultrasound, electropalatography, and electromagnetic articulography, and the advantages of supplementing perceptual measures of intelligibility with instrumental measures are noted. Acoustic and kinematic measures used in evaluation and treatment of speakers with neurological disorders, hearing impairment, phonological/articulation disorders, and cleft palate are described.

Chapter 5 focuses on the phonatory system, beginning with a detailed review of the structures of the larynx and the myoelastic–aerodynamic theory of phonation. The complex, nearly periodic sound wave of the human voice is explained. This is followed by a description of acoustic variables, including speaking fundamental frequency, frequency variability, average vocal amplitude level, dynamic range, and the voice range profile. Students are led to an understanding of the physiologic and acoustic bases of vocal registers, as well as normal and abnormal voice qualities. Finally, commonly used acoustic aspects of voice—including jitter, shimmer, and harmonics-to-noise ratio—are introduced.

Chapter 6 focuses on visual methods of assessing vocal fold structure and function, including electroglottography, endoscopy with or without videostroboscopy, high-speed digital imaging, and videokymography. The clinical benefits of acoustic and visual information regarding phonatory structure and function are highlighted in contexts including identification of changes in phonatory function over the lifespan; and in areas such as neurological disorders, laryngeal cancer, hearing impairment, and transsexual voice.

Chapter 7 presents a detailed discussion of the respiratory system. Relevant information regarding anatomy and physiology helps students understand how respiration generates the power supply for speech. An important part of the chapter is the detailed discussion of respiratory volumes and capacities, which students often have difficulty visualizing but which are crucial to an understanding of the ways we use the air supply for speech and other purposes. Another important section covers the differences between vegetative and speech breathing, an understanding of which is essential in clinical intervention of many speech-related disorders. Breathing patterns for speech are highlighted, and ways that speech breathing changes over the lifespan are identified.

Chapter 8 focuses on clinical application of the principles discussed in Chapter 7. Students learn to understand how spirometric measures form the basis of pulmonary function testing; to appreciate the role of respiratory kinematic analysis in measuring lung function; and to identify measures of air pressures and flows in respiration. The difference between obstructive, restrictive, and central respiratory problems is noted, and the primary symptoms of airway obstruction, dyspnea, and stridor are discussed. Attention then turns to principles important in the clinical management of speech breathing disorders. These principles are highlighted in the evaluation and treatment of individuals with neurological disorders, those who are mechanically ventilated, and speakers with voice disorders. The chapter ends with a comparison of respiratory characteristics in individuals with asthma and those with paradoxical vocal fold motion.

The focus in Chapter 9 is on the auditory system. Information about the structure and function of the different parts of the ear is presented at the beginning of the chapter. Building on previously discussed concepts of sound transmission, the role of the middle ear in transducing air pressure vibrations into mechanical vibrations and transmitting these vibrations to the inner ear is described. The ability of the cochlea of the inner ear to perform a frequency analysis of incoming sounds is presented, followed by a comparison of conductive and sensorineural hearing loss in terms of degree and configuration. Following the description of hearing and hearing loss, the discussion turns to the perception of speech, the process of recognizing speech sounds and assigning meaning to them. Sounds are described in terms of their acoustic patterns that form the basis for phoneme recognition. Concepts central to issues in speech perception, such as categorical perception, multiple cues in perception, and trading relations between acoustic cues, are integrated into the discussion of sound recognition.

Chapter 10 begins with a description of current measures used in the diagnosis of hearing impairment, including immittance audiometry, otoacoustic emissions, and auditory brain stem testing. The importance of these measures in the screening and evaluating of middle and inner ear function, particularly in infants, young children, and hard-to-test individuals, is emphasized. In particular, otoacoustic emissions are used in neonatal screening to increase the chances of early detection of hearing problems. Discussion then turns to the components of cochlear implants and different implementation methods used to stimulate the auditory nerve. The issue of speech perception is explored with reference to hard-of-hearing and deaf individuals, as well as children with recurrent middle ear infections, language and reading disabilities, and phonological deficits.

Chapter 11 presents a discussion of neuroanatomy and neurophysiology relevant to speech production. The chapter begins with descriptions of nerve cell structure and function and continues with examination of cortical and subcortical areas of the brain. The spinal and cranial nerves are described and related to speech production, and the chapter concludes with a discussion of principles of motor control. Chapter 12 then describes brain imaging and EEG techniques, including computerized tomography, magnetic resonance imaging, functional magnetic resonance imaging, positron emission tomography, single photon emission computed tomography, transcranial magnetic stimulation, and evoked potentials. Applications of these technologies to various communication disorders are discussed, including stuttering, Parkinson's disease, multiple sclerosis, and Alzheimer's disease.

Finally, Chapter 13 presents a discussion of the nature of models and theories to help students understand the importance of conceptual and theoretical frameworks in testing ideas about systems and in predicting the behavior of systems under various conditions. Some influential models and theories of speech production and speech perception are described, such as target models, feedback and feedforward models, action theory, and motor theory.

1

The Nature of Sound

STUDENT LEARNING OBJECTIVES

After reading this chapter you will

○ Understand how human speech fits within a scientific framework.

○ Become familiar with basic science concepts and units of measure.

○ Discuss how sound is generated by changes in air pressure.

○ Describe dimensions of sound, including frequency and period, pure tones and complex sounds, and intensity and amplitude.

○ Understand the concepts of reverberation, absorption, reflection, refraction, diffraction, and interference.

○ Compare and contrast the information obtained from waveforms and spectra.

○ Understand that the decibel (dB) scale is logarithmic and is based on a comparison of target sounds to a standard reference sound.

○ Compare dB SPL, dB IL, and dB HL.

Speaking is an activity that one does effortlessly and automatically, without thinking about the physical processes involved. However, the seemingly simple act of saying "hi" to a friend involves multiple levels of perception, cognition, and neuromotor function. In order to appreciate the basic nature of speech and how humans are able to regulate and control the many processes involved, it is important to place speech in the context of a scientific framework (Table 1.1). It is, therefore, necessary to understand specifically what is meant by the term *science*. *Science* is defined as a system of knowledge covering the operation of general laws obtained and tested through the scientific method. Science can also be considered as any domain of systematized knowledge that is considered as a distinct field of investigation or object of study. Science has many different branches, including life sciences, earth sciences, and physical sciences, among others. These branches are subdivided into more specialized areas. Natural science is a domain that is concerned with the physical world and its phenomena; it includes fields such as astronomy, chemistry, biology, and physics.

Physics is the science that deals with matter, energy, motion, and force, as well as the physical processes and phenomena of a particular system. Acoustics is a branch of physics that deals with the production, control, transmission, reception, and effects of sound. Bioacoustics refers to the combination of biology and acoustics in the study of sound production and perception in animals including humans. The study of human speech thus falls into the domain of bioacoustics.

Because speech is a physical phenomenon, it is necessary to become familiar with some basic physics concepts and measurements in order to understand how humans produce and perceive speech.

Table 1.1 **Relationship of Human Speech to Science**

Term	Definition
Science	Any domain of systematized knowledge that is considered as a distinct field of investigation or object of study
Natural science	A branch of science that is concerned with the physical world and its phenomena
Physics	A branch of natural science that deals with matter, energy, motion, and force, as well as the physical processes and phenomena of a particular system
Acoustics	A branch of physics that deals with the production, control, transmission, reception, and effects of sound
Bioacoustics	A combination of biology and acoustics in the study of sound production and perception in animals including humans
Human speech	A branch of bioacoustics

International System of Units

Scientific measurement systems are based on the modernized international metric system, the **International System of Units** (abbreviated **SI** for the French name, **Système International d'Unités**). The SI uses seven base units, including length, mass, time, electric current, thermodynamic temperature, amount of substance, and luminous intensity (Taylor & Thompson, 2008). Derivatives of these units are defined in terms of the base units. Metric prefixes are used to quantify the units (Tables 1.2 and 1.3). The SI comprises two related systems: **MKS** and **CGS**. Both

Table 1.2 **Base Units and Some Derived Quantities in the MKS System**

Symbol	Unit Name	Quantity
m	meter	length (l)
kg	kilogram	mass (m)
s	second	time (t)
K	kelvin	temperature (T)
m^2	square meter	area (A)
m^3	cubic meter	volume (V)
N	newton	force (F)
J	joule	energy (E)
W	watt	power (P)
Pa	pascal	pressure (p)
Hz	hertz	frequency

Table 1.3 **Metric Prefixes Used to Quantify Metric Units**

Metric Unit	Symbol	Quantity
giga-	G	1 billion
mega-	M	1 million
kilo-	k	1 thousand
hecto-	h	1 hundred
deka-	da	1 ten
deci-	d	1 tenth
centi-	c	1 hundredth
milli-	m	1 thousandth
micro-	μ	1 millionth
nano-	n	1 billionth

systems are based on the measurement of distance, mass, and time. In the MKS system, *m* stands for meters, *k* for kilograms, and *s* for seconds. In the CGS system, *c* stands for centimeters, *g* for grams, and *s* for seconds. The CGS system uses smaller units for distance and mass than the MKS system. The ratio between the two systems is usually some power of 10. Currently, the MKS system is preferred over the CGS system, although some of the CGS units continue to be used for various applications (Rowlett, 2000).

Basic Physics Concepts

In this chapter attention will be focused on many of the basic physics concepts that are relevant to the study of speech production and perception. These include mass, force, volume, density, speed, velocity, momentum, acceleration, inertia, elasticity, stiffness, work, energy, power, intensity, and pressure. Table 1.4 displays selected physics concepts and definitions; Table 1.5 presents the formulae for some of these units.

Mass, Force, Weight, Volume, and Density

Mass (m) is a fundamental property of an object that refers to the amount of matter in the object, and it is measured in kilograms or grams.

Force (F) is defined as any influence that causes an object to undergo a change in speed, a change in direction, or a change in shape. Force is measured in **newtons** in the MKS system and **dynes** in the CGS system. 1 newton measures a force that accelerates a 1 kilogram mass at the rate of 1 meter per second squared (kg-m-s^2); 1 dyne measures a force that accelerates a 1 gram mass at 1 cm per second squared (g-cm-s^2). 1 newton equals 100,000 dynes.

Table 1.4 **Selected Basic Physics Concepts**

Concept	Definition	Measurement
Mass	Amount of matter in an object	g or kg
Force	Any influence that causes an object to undergo a change in speed, direction, or shape	newton
Weight	Force of gravity on an object	newton
Volume	Quantity of three-dimensional space occupied by a liquid, solid, or gas	liter
Density	Mass per unit of volume	g/cm^3, kg/m^3, g/mL
Speed	Distance traveled in a given unit of time	m/s
Velocity	Distance traveled in a given unit of time in a specific direction	m/s
Momentum	Mass times velocity of an object during motion	kg-m/s
Acceleration	Change in velocity as a function of time	$a = F/m$, or $F = ma$
Inertia	Resistance of any physical object to a change in its state of motion or rest	g or kg
Elasticity	Property of a material that returns it to its original shape after it has been deformed by an external force (stress)	
Deformation	Change in the shape or size of an object due to an applied force	
Strain	Relative amount of deformation undergone by an object	
Stiffness	Resistance of an elastic body to deformation by an applied force	force/meters
Work	Force exerted over a distance	joules
Energy	Ability to do work	joules
Power	Rate of work done or energy used in a period of time	watts
Pressure	Force acting on a specific surface area	pascal

Table 1.5 **Formulae for Selected Units and Derived Quantities**

Unit/Derived Quantity	Formula
Velocity	Distance/Time
Acceleration	Force/Mass
Force	Mass $\times$ Acceleration
Pressure	Force/Area
Work	Force $\times$ Distance
Power	Work/Time
Intensity	Power/Area

Weight is defined as the force of gravity on an object and is related to its mass. Weight is a force and is therefore measured by the newton. 1 kilogram of mass weighs 9.8 newtons under standard conditions on the Earth's surface. The same amount of mass would weigh less on the moon's surface due to the reduced gravitational pull. The greater the mass, the greater is the gravitational force that is exerted on the object and therefore the greater is its weight.

Volume is defined as the quantity of three-dimensional space occupied by a liquid, solid, or gas. The standard unit of volume in the metric system is the liter. 1 liter is equal to 1000 milliliters (mL) or 1000 cubic centimeters (cc) in volume.

Density is defined as mass of a substance, a material, or an object per unit of volume, or mass divided by volume. Density is measured in terms of grams per centimeters cubed (cm^3), kilograms per meter cubed (m^3), or grams per milliliter. Water has a density of 1 gram per milliliter (1.00 g/mL), or 1000 kilograms per cubic meter. The density of salt is 2.16 g/mL, and that of gold is 19.30 g/mL. Lead is about 10 times as dense as water, and Styrofoam is about one tenth as dense as water.

Speed, Velocity, Momentum, Acceleration, and Inertia

Speed is the distance traveled by an object in a given unit of time, measured in meters per second (m/s). **Velocity** has the same numerical value as speed (m/s) but also specifies the direction of the movement.

Momentum refers to the mass times velocity of an object during motion, measured by kilograms times meters per second (kg-m/s). An object with a greater mass will have a greater momentum than one with less mass. The momentum of an object is directly proportional to its velocity. Changing either (or both) mass or velocity will change an object's momentum. If an object is not in motion, its momentum is zero.

Acceleration (a) occurs when velocity changes as a function of time. The acceleration of an object is directly proportional to the force applied, and inversely proportional to the object's mass (m). This is Newton's Second Law of Motion, for which the equation is a = F/m, or F = ma (a = acceleration; F = force; m = mass). As long as force is held constant, the greater the mass of an object, the smaller its acceleration, and the smaller the mass of an object, the greater is its acceleration.

Inertia is the resistance of any physical object to a change in its state of motion or rest. This is Newton's First Law of Motion, which states that the velocity of a body remains constant unless the body is acted on by an external force. The source of the resistance is the body's mass, and inertia is therefore measured in grams or kilograms. Force must be applied to begin or change the motion of the body.

Elasticity and Stiffness

Elasticity is the property of a material that returns it to its original shape after it has been deformed by an external force. The external force is called **stress**. Conversely, **deformation** refers to a change in the shape or size of an object due to an applied force. The relative amount of deformation undergone by the object is called the **strain**. Elasticity is determined by the amount of force required to displace the object by some distance, and is measured in terms of **stiffness** (K). Stiffness thus is the resistance of an elastic body to deformation by an applied force. Force is measured in newtons, and distance is measured in meters, so stiffness can be expressed as K = Force/Meters. The greater the stiffness of an object, the greater is the force required to displace it.

Work, Energy, Power, and Intensity

Work occurs when a force is exerted over a distance and is measured in newtons times distance in meters. The measure of work is called **joules** in the MKS system or **ergs** in the CGS system. 1 joule equals a force of 1 newton through a distance of 1 meter. 1 erg equals a force of 1 dyne through a distance of 1 cm. **Energy** is defined as the ability to do work. Forms of energy include chemical energy, electrical energy, thermal energy (heat), radiant energy (light), mechanical energy (movement), sound energy, and nuclear energy. Energy is categorized as either potential energy or kinetic energy. Potential energy is stored energy that exists whenever an object that has mass has a position in a force field. For example, a cup perched on a shelf has potential energy. Kinetic energy exists whenever an object which has mass is in motion. For example, if the cup falls off the shelf, the potential energy is converted to kinetic energy as the cup falls. Because energy is based on work, it is also measured in joules. To do 100 joules of work, 100 joules of energy must be expended.

Power refers to the rate of work done or energy used in a period of time and is measured in **watts**. Thus power is a measure of how quickly work can be done. Equivalently, power equals work divided by time. 1 watt is equivalent to 1 joule/second. 100 joules of energy used in 1 second yield a power of 100 watts. This suggests that for the same amount of work, power and time are inversely proportional. Clearly, then, a more powerful engine can do the same amount of work in less time than a less powerful one. **Intensity** refers to power per unit of area and is measured in watts per square meter in the MKS system or watts per square centimeter in the CGS system.

Pressure

Pressure is defined as force acting perpendicularly on a specific surface area. The unit of measure in the MKS system is the **pascal** (Pa), which is equivalent to a force of 1 newton over 1 square meter. Multiples of the pascal are commonly used, such as decapascal or kilopascal. In the CGS system, the unit of measurement for pressure is **dynes** per square centimeter (dynes/cm^2), also called **microbar**. 1 dyne/cm^2 equals 1 microbar. Microbar and pascal are related measures, such that 1 microbar equals 0.1 Pa, and 10 microbar equal 1 Pa. 1 micropascal (μPa) is equal to one millionth of 1 Pa. Pressure is also measured in units of cm H_2O, which is the amount of pressure used to displace a column of water (Figure 1.1). Pa and cm H_2O are related: 1 kilopascal is equivalent to 10 cm H_2O. An older unit of measure is pounds per square inch (psi), which is still used in the United States. Table 1.6 displays units of pressure and the relationships among units.

With an understanding of basic science concepts and units of measurement, we are now in a position to examine the nature of sound and the process whereby sounds are generated and transmitted from speakers to listeners.

Figure 1.1 Measurement of air pressure in cm H₂O

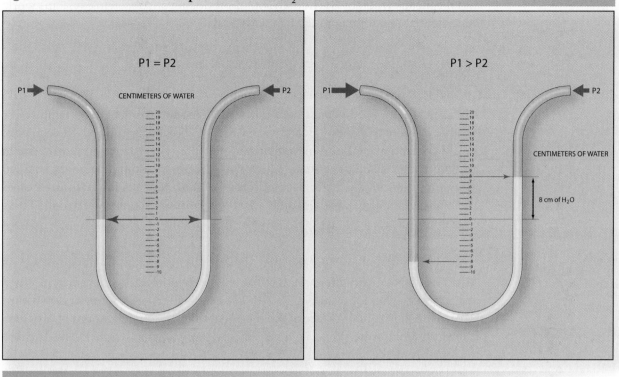

Overview of Sound

Sound occurs when a disturbance creates changes in pressure in a gas, liquid, or solid medium. Any kind of movement can create a disturbance, such as a cup being placed on a table, a book falling on the floor, a tuning fork being struck, or the human vocal folds opening and closing the glottis. The pressure changes created by the disturbance are transmitted through the medium and may end up at a listener's ear, eventually to be perceived as sound. Because the human sound production and perception systems operate primarily in air, discussion will focus on

Table 1.6 Units of Pressure

Microbar	Pascal	Kilopascal	cm H₂O
1	0.1	0.0001	0.001019744
10	1.0	0.001	0.010197443
100	10.0	0.01	0.101974429
9806.38	980.638	0.980638	10.0
4903.19	490.319	0.490319	5.0

sound in air rather than in solids and liquids. To understand the nature of sound and the means whereby the human sound producing and receiving systems work, it is essential to understand the behavior of air.

Air

Air is a gas composed primarily of nitrogen (78%) and oxygen (21%), with traces of other elements, including water vapor, carbon dioxide, and argon. Molecules of air are not stationary, but due to their thermal energy constantly move around in random patterns and at extremely high speeds. This random movement is called **Brownian motion**. As the molecules move around, they collide with each other and with whatever is in their path—walls, furniture, people, and so on. These collisions produce pressure that is relatively constant.

Air Pressure

As defined above, *pressure* is a force that acts perpendicularly on a surface. When one sits on a chair, for example, one's body exerts a certain amount of downward force on the horizontal surface of the seat, generating a certain amount of pressure. If the individual were sitting on a sofa, the pressure exerted would be less because the force would be spread out over a larger area. Pressures can be generated in different locations and areas and can increase or decrease, depending on the specific circumstances. It is necessary, therefore, to have a way of indicating the location or type of pressure. The scientific notation for pressure is P. When combined with a subscript, the location of pressure is indicated. Atmospheric pressure (P_{atmos}) at sea level is used as a basis of comparison. The absolute average pressure at sea level is 101.325 kPa. Rather than use the absolute value, scientists often use a standard measurement of P_{atmos} defined as 100 kPa. This corresponds to 1,000,000 dynes/cm^2, approximately 14.7 psi, and approximately 1019 cm H_2O at 4°C. Above sea level, P_{atmos} decreases. At 500 feet above sea level, P_{atmos} is 99.4 kPa; at 1000 feet above sea level, P_{atmos} is 97.6 kPa; and at 25,000 feet above sea level, P_{atmos} is 37.6 kPa.

Pressure in different locations can be higher or lower than P_{atmos}. For example, the pressure of the air inside a tire on a car is typically around 30 psi, considerably higher than P_{atmos}. Pressure that is higher than P_{atmos} is called **positive pressure** (P_{pos}). If the tire is punctured the air leaks out, and pressure could decrease below P_{atmos}, say to 13 psi. Pressure below P_{atmos} is called **negative pressure** (P_{neg}). Note that P_{neg} is not the same as a vacuum. A vacuum refers to a total absence of air and thus a total absence of pressure. The pressures within various locations within the body, such as the lungs ($P_{alveolar}$), trachea (P_{trach}), and oral cavity (P_{oral}), play an important role in speech production.

Airflow

Because air is a gas, it moves in predictable ways. Molecules of air have a natural tendency to spread themselves around more or less equally. To achieve this equalization, air always moves from an area of high pressure to an area of lower pressure. It is the difference in pressure, called a **pressure differential**, which causes

Figure 1.2 Laminar versus turbulent airflow

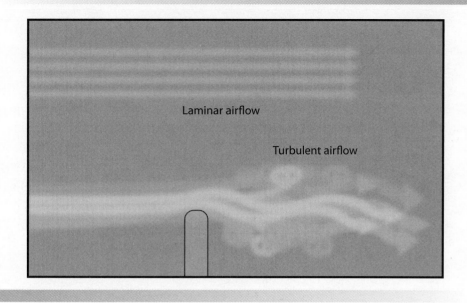

Laminar airflow

Turbulent airflow

air to flow and creates a **driving pressure**. If there is no difference in pressure between two areas, air will not flow between them, and there will be no driving pressure. The movement of air through a particular area in a certain interval of time is called **flow**. Flow is measured in liters per second (l/s), liters per minute (l/min), milliliters per second (ml/s), or milliliters per minute (ml/min). The rate of flow is known as **volume velocity**. Recall that velocity refers to speed occurring in a particular direction. Thus volume velocity refers to the speed of a volume of air traveling in a certain direction.

Air can flow with various degrees of smoothness or turbulence (Figure 1.2). Air that flows smoothly, with molecules moving in a parallel manner and at the same speed, is called **laminar flow**. **Turbulent flow** occurs when an obstacle in its way disturbs the flow. When this happens, the flow becomes less regular in its movement, resulting in little swirls, or eddies, of currents. These eddy currents create random variations in the pressure of the air. Laminar and turbulent flow can be compared to water flowing in a river. When nothing disturbs the water, the flow is smooth, with the water molecules moving at the same speed and in parallel. When rocks get in the way and the water flows around and over the rocks, the flow becomes turbulent, with little local water pressure changes. The smoothness or turbulence of airflow is an important aspect of speech production. As described in subsequent chapters, vowels are produced with a relatively laminar flow of air; fricatives are produced with a more turbulent airflow.

Air Pressure, Volume, and Density

Air pressure, volume, and density are systematically related: There is an inverse relationship between air volume and pressure and a direct relationship between air pressure and density. As the volume of a particular space increases, the pressure

Figure 1.3 Boyle's law

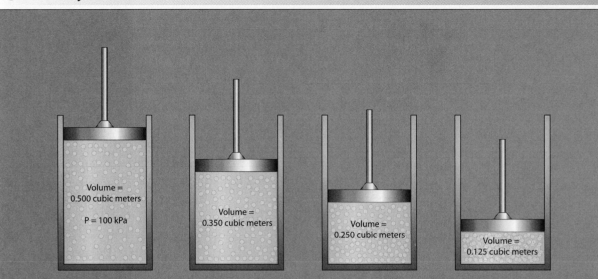

If the air pressure in the cylinder is at 100 kPa (standard atmospheric pressure at sea level) and the temperature remains constant, using Boyle's law, we can calculate the pressure in the cylinder as the piston compresses the air to a known volume. To calculate the air pressure in the cylinder when the volume has been compressed to 0.350 cubic meters, we will do the following calculations:

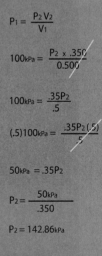

As volume increases, pressure decreases. As the graph below shows, when volume is doubled, pressure is halved.

$$P_1 = \frac{P_2 V_2}{V_1}$$

$$100_{kPa} = \frac{P_2 \times .350}{0.500}$$

$$100_{kPa} = \frac{.35P_2}{.5}$$

$$(.5)100_{kPa} = \frac{.35P_2 (.5)}{.5}$$

$$50_{kPa} = .35P_2$$

$$P_2 = \frac{50_{kPa}}{.350}$$

$$P_2 = 142.86_{kPa}$$

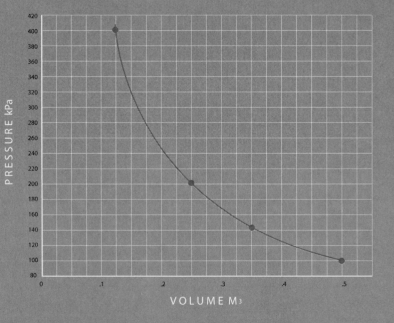

of the air within that space decreases as long as the density and temperature remain constant. As the volume of the space decreases, the pressure of the air increases, given a constant air density and temperature. This relationship is known as **Boyle's law**. Figure 1.3 shows the relationship, using the example of a container with a plunger in it. Each container has an equal density of air (i.e., an equal number of molecules), but the plungers are inserted to different depths, changing the volume. The farther a plunger is inserted, the smaller the volume of the container. However, because the amount of air within the container has not changed, the density of the air within the smaller space is increased because the same number of molecules is crowded into a smaller space. When density is increased, pressure is increased as well because the molecules collide with the surfaces and with each other more often and more forcefully. When the volume increases, the pressure decreases because the molecules are spread out over a larger space and undergo fewer and less forceful collisions. Thus when density decreases, the pressure also decreases.

Sound: Changes in Air Pressure

As discussed above, air molecules undergo Brownian motion, creating a relatively steady pressure called **ambient pressure** (P_{am}). Sound occurs when a disturbance creates alternating increases and decreases in P_{am}. A tuning fork provides an excellent example of the way in which P_{am} is changed by a disturbance and how this change results in sound (see Figure 1.4).

Figure 1.4 Compression and rarefaction

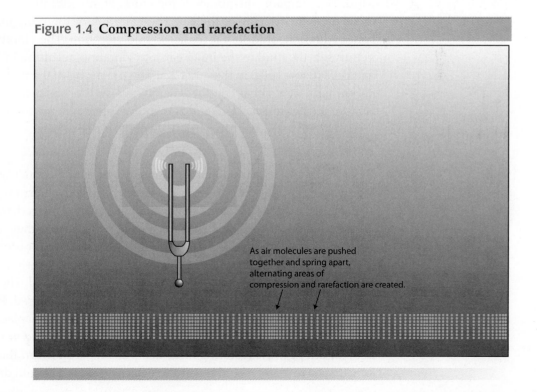

As air molecules are pushed together and spring apart, alternating areas of compression and rarefaction are created.

When a tuning fork is struck, its prongs, or tines, are set into vibration; they move back and forth (oscillate) very rapidly. As the tines vibrate, they set up a chain reaction in the air molecules in adjacent areas. As a tine moves outward, it pushes against the air molecules closest to it. These molecules are displaced from their original positions and, in turn, push against their neighboring molecules, which push against their neighbors, and so on. When molecules have been displaced in this manner and are approaching and colliding with the next group of molecules, there is an increased density of air in that area. Increased density results in an increase of pressure. Thus, when molecules approach and collide, an area of positive pressure, known as **compression**, results. The air molecules that have been displaced do not remain in their new positions but swing back toward their original positions. As molecules down the line are displaced toward their neighbors, molecules that were earlier displaced are already returning to their equilibrium positions. However, the molecules returning toward equilibrium overshoot their marks and swing farther away to the other side of their original positions. This increases the distance between the two groups of molecules involved. There is now decreased density of air in the area between the two groups of molecules, resulting in an area of lower pressure, known as **rarefaction**.

The changing distances between groups of molecules result in increasing and decreasing amounts of density and corresponding increases and decreases in air pressure. The changes in pressure continue in a wavelike motion that **propagates** (travels) from the source of the sound through the air in an ever-widening sphere (see Figure 1.4). If an ear is in the path of some of these shifting molecules, the compression of air moves the **tympanic membrane** (eardrum) inward slightly, whereas the rarefaction of air allows the tympanic membrane to move slightly outward. The tympanic membrane is therefore set into vibration through the changes in air pressure arriving at the ear. The vibration of the tympanic membrane sets bones within the middle ear (ossicles) into vibration. The vibration of the ossicles in turn sets the fluid in the inner ear into vibration, resulting in the stimulation of hair cells (nerve cells) in the inner ear. The triggering of the nerve cells generates a nerve impulse, which is conducted along the auditory pathway to the appropriate areas of the nervous system and is then interpreted by the brain as sound.

Elasticity, Inertia, and Friction

When air molecules are set into vibration by a disturbance such as a tuning fork being struck, they vibrate a tiny distance around their equilibrium positions, eventually coming to a stop. Once the molecules have been disturbed, three forces interact to keep them swinging back and forth for a while before they settle down again: elasticity, inertia, and friction (see Figure 1.5). Elasticity is a restoring force; it refers to the property of an object to be able to spring back to its original size, form, location, and shape after being stretched, displaced, or deformed. The amount of restoring force depends on the extent to which the object is displaced. **Hooke's law** states that the restoring force is proportional to the distance of displacement and acts in the opposite direction. Thus, the farther an object is displaced from its original location, the stronger the restoring force that pulls it back toward that position. All objects that have mass, including air molecules, possess a certain degree of elasticity.

Figure 1.5 Elasticity and inertia

A vibrating tuning fork sets air molecules into vibration.

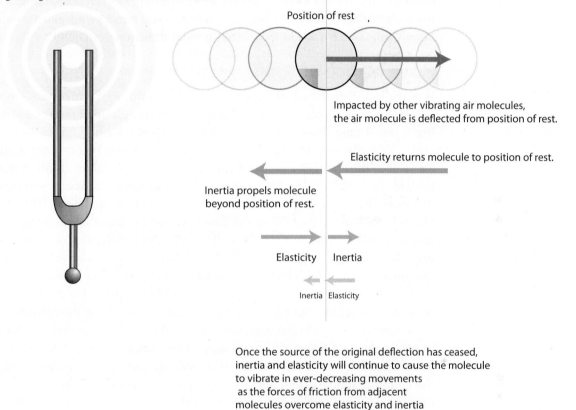

Position of rest

Impacted by other vibrating air molecules,
the air molecule is deflected from position of rest.

Elasticity returns molecule to position of rest.

Inertia propels molecule
beyond position of rest.

Elasticity   Inertia

Inertia Elasticity

Once the source of the original deflection has ceased,
inertia and elasticity will continue to cause the molecule
to vibrate in ever-decreasing movements
as the forces of friction from adjacent
molecules overcome elasticity and inertia
and the molecule returns to a position of rest.

After a tuning fork is initially struck and the molecules have been displaced, they start moving back toward their equilibrium positions due to elasticity. However, they do not immediately stop at their original positions, but due to inertia, they overshoot the mark, swinging out farther in the opposite direction. The farther the molecules travel, the stronger is the elastic recoil, which eventually overcomes the inertia and starts to pull the molecules back toward equilibrium again. Hence, the molecules swing back and forth around their original positions due to the interaction of elasticity and inertia. This means that the original disturbance that is the source of the sound (in our example, the striking of the tuning fork) does not have to be reapplied in order for the sound to continue, at least for a while.

The vibration of the air molecules does not last indefinitely. Because of the frictional resistance of the air, each time the molecules move back and forth around their equilibrium positions, they do so with slightly less amplitude. The decrease of amplitude is called **damping**. Damping finally causes the molecules to settle down once again at their equilibrium positions. At this point, no further changes in P_{am} occur, and, consequently, no further sound is generated.

It is important to realize that sources of sound cause changes in air pressure not just in one direction but in all directions. Figure 1.6 shows how increases and decreases in air pressure radiate outward from the source in all directions. You can easily appreciate this fact by walking away from a person who is talking. Although the sound of his or her voice becomes softer as you move away, you are still able to hear it, at least for a while, no matter in what direction you move.

Wave Motion of Sound

A wave is a disturbance of pressure that moves through a medium. Once molecules have been set into vibration, each molecule (or group of molecules) does not, itself, travel long distances to get to a listener's ear. Rather, the molecules travel only a tiny distance around their equilibrium positions before their motion dies away. It is the changes in air pressure caused by molecular vibration that travel toward the listener's ear. The compressions and rarefactions can propagate long distances. In the case of sound, the wave motion is longitudinal. The individual air molecules move parallel to the direction that the wave is traveling. Wave motion of water is transverse; that is, the individual molecules of water move up and down at right angles to the direction that the wave is traveling (Figure 1.6). We are all familiar with the phenomenon of water rippling outward in widening circles when a stone is dropped into a pond. These ripples are the waves, formed by water molecules moving up and down and transmitting the disturbance in all directions. In a very similar way, when a sound wave is generated by a tuning fork or other vibrating object, the air all around the fork is disturbed, so the changes in pressure radiate from the fork in all directions. The area of compression around the vibrating source is followed by an area of rarefaction, followed by another area of compression, another of rarefaction, and so on, spreading outward in a sphere. The outermost area of the sphere is called the **wave front**.

The farther the changes in air pressure travel from the source, the more damped they become because the area of the wave front is directly proportional to the square of its distance from the source (called the **inverse square law**). This means that as the sound wave propagates, the constant amount of energy in the wave is distributed over an exponentially increasing area. Stated another way, the sound's acoustic energy diminishes by a factor of $1/distance^2$. So, for example, the energy of a sound wave that is twice the distance from the source is distributed over four times the area and therefore has one fourth of the intensity compared to the source, the energy of a wave that is three times the distance of the source is distributed over nine times the area with a correspondingly decreased energy, and so on.

Mass/Spring System

Discussion to this point has focused on vibration using the example of a tuning fork. Vibration can also be described in terms of a mass/spring system (Figure 1.7).

Figure 1.6 Longitudinal versus transverse waves

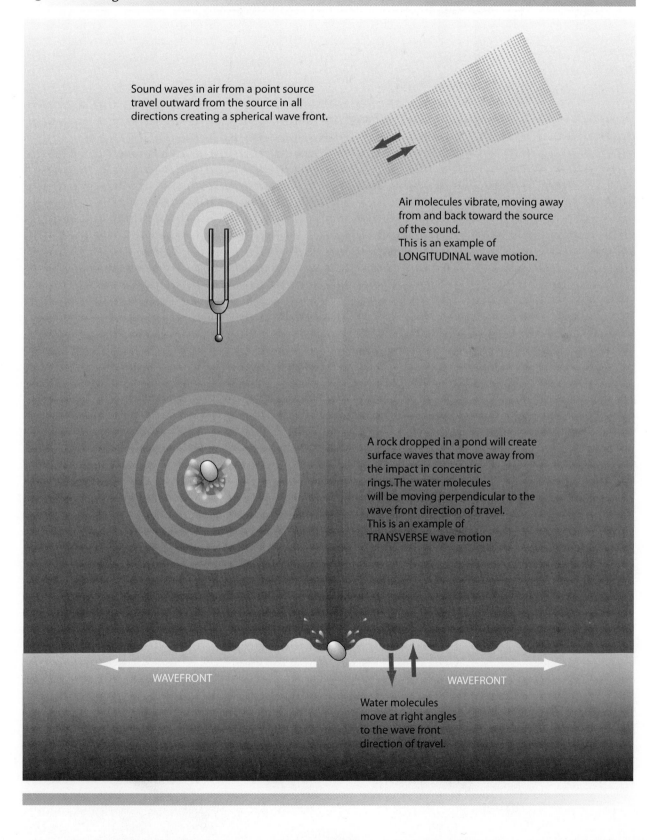

Sound waves in air from a point source travel outward from the source in all directions creating a spherical wave front.

Air molecules vibrate, moving away from and back toward the source of the sound.
This is an example of LONGITUDINAL wave motion.

A rock dropped in a pond will create surface waves that move away from the impact in concentric rings. The water molecules will be moving perpendicular to the wave front direction of travel.
This is an example of TRANSVERSE wave motion

WAVEFRONT

WAVEFRONT

Water molecules move at right angles to the wave front direction of travel.

Figure 1.7 Simple harmonic motion of a mass/spring system

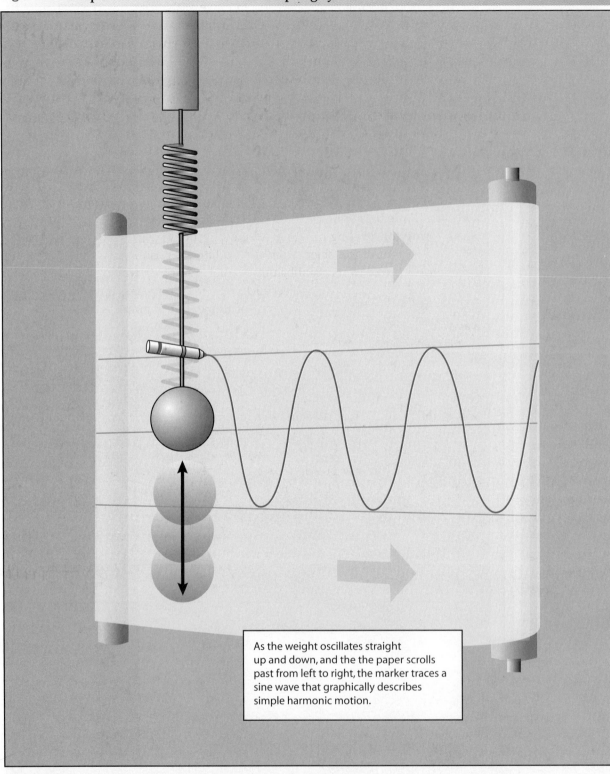

As the weight oscillates straight up and down, and the the paper scrolls past from left to right, the marker traces a sine wave that graphically describes simple harmonic motion.

Such a system is comprised of a block of a certain mass attached to a spring. The spring is fixed at one point and is free to move at the point of attachment to the block. When not disturbed, the system is in equilibrium, with no net force acting on it. If the block is pulled and then released, the spring with the attached block will recoil toward the rest position because of elasticity but will then overshoot the rest position due to inertia. As the block and spring continue to overshoot rest position, the elastic recoil forces increase and pull the block and spring back toward equilibrium. As with the example of the tuning fork, this back-and-forth motion around rest position gradually loses amplitude and dies out.

Simple Harmonic Motion

The vibration of the tuning fork and the movement of the mass/spring system occur in **simple harmonic motion** (SHM). Simple harmonic motion occurs when the restoring force acting on an object (i.e., elasticity) is directly proportional to the displacement of the object from its equilibrium position but in the opposite direction (i.e., toward its equilibrium position). Another way of thinking about SHM is in terms of a circular object such as a wheel traveling at a constant speed along a straight path. The movement of this object is graphed as a sinusoidal wave (Figure 1.8).

Simple harmonic motion is characterized by a pattern of acceleration through the equilibrium position and deceleration at the endpoints of the movement. The example of a swing illustrates this motion. When one pushes a swing, it moves away from the pusher to some maximum distance, depending on the forcefulness of the push. As it approaches this maximum point, it slows down and stops for an instant. The swing then reverses direction and starts moving back toward the pusher. As it does so, its speed increases, and it reaches its maximum speed as it passes over its rest position. As it continues to move toward the individual, its speed decreases until the swing stops for an instant, and then, once again, it reverses direction. This pattern of movement continues with decreasing amplitude until the motion dies away.

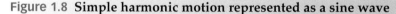

Figure 1.8 Simple harmonic motion represented as a sine wave

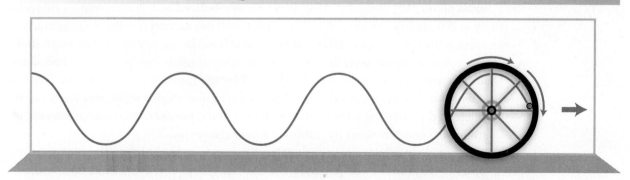

Imagine a wheel rolling along a flat surface at a constant rate of speed. Attached to the wheel is a marker that leaves a trace on a wall that runs next to the path of the rolling wheel. The trace that is generated would be a wave that describes simple harmonic motion.

Frequency, Period, Wavelength, Velocity, and Amplitude

Figure 1.9 illustrates the concepts of frequency, period, wavelength, and amplitude.

One back-and-forth movement of the tuning fork tine or molecule around the equilibrium position makes up one cycle of vibration. That is, one cycle of vibration occurs when the tine or molecule moves to a maximum distance away from its original spot, back toward rest position, moves to a maximal point in the opposite direction, and then moves back again to the equilibrium position. For sound, cycles of vibration are typically described in terms of pressure changes rather than in terms of individual movements of molecules. Acoustically, a cycle of vibration consists of an increase in pressure from P_{am} (compression), a decrease in pressure back to P_{am}, a further decrease in pressure below P_{am} (rarefaction), and a return to baseline P_{am}. Cycles of vibration are measured in terms of time in seconds. The tines of a tuning fork might vibrate at the rate of 100 **cycles per second** (cps), causing the surrounding air molecules to vibrate at a rate of 100 cps as well. If this vibration eventually reaches a listener, that person's eardrum will vibrate at 100 cycles per second. The number of cycles per second is called **frequency**, and the unit of measurement of frequency is **hertz** (abbreviated **Hz**). Thus, a tuning fork vibrating at 100 cps has a frequency of 100 Hz. The sound wave produced by the tuning fork also has a frequency of 100 Hz, and the eardrum in the path of this 100 Hz sound wave would be set into vibration at 100 Hz. Frequency can also be expressed in terms of kilohertz (kHz): 1000 Hz equals 1 kHz, and 2500 Hz equals 2.5 kHz. The perceptual counterpart of frequency is pitch. Pitch is the subjective perception of how high or low a sound is on a musical scale. The pitch of middle C on a piano has a frequency of 262 Hz; the A above middle C has a frequency of 440 Hz. An octave in music is a series of eight tones (C, D, E, F, G, A, B, C) that continue up and down on an instrument, including the voice. Doubling or halving the frequency results in a note that is one octave higher or lower. Thus, the frequency of A that is one octave higher than A above middle C is 880 Hz; the frequency one octave lower is 220 Hz. Table 1.7 shows the frequency/pitch correspondences based on a piano with 88 keys.

Period is the time it takes for one cycle of vibration to occur. For example, a wave with a frequency of 100 Hz has 100 cycles that occur in 1 second. Assuming that each cycle in the wave lasts for the same amount of time, it is clear that each must take 1/100 second (0.01 s). Period is symbolized as t. A wave with a frequency of 250 Hz has a period of 1/250 second, or 0.004 second ($t = 0.004$ s). Similarly, a wave with a period of 0.002 second (1/500 s) has a frequency of 500 Hz. From these examples, it can be seen that there is a reciprocal relationship between frequency and period. This relationship is expressed by the formula $F = 1/t$, where F is frequency, and t equals period. If one knows the frequency of a wave, its period can be calculated by putting a 1 over the frequency; if the period of the wave is known, its frequency is determined by putting a 1 over the period.

A wave in which every cycle takes the same amount of time to occur as every other cycle is said to be **periodic**. Perceptually, such a wave would have a musical tone and a specific pitch. For example, the vibrating string of a guitar or violin produces a periodic sound wave with a musical tone and pitch. However, not all sound waves have cycles lasting the same amount of time. A sound wave might

Figure 1.9 **Frequency, period, wavelength, and amplitude**

FREQUENCY = The number of cycles that occur in one second. The unit of measurment is Hertz (Hz).

PERIOD = The time it takes for one complete cycle to occur. The unit of measurement is seconds.

WAVELENGTH = The distance covered by one complete cycle. The unit of measurement is meters.

AMPLITUDE = The maximum displacement from position of rest.

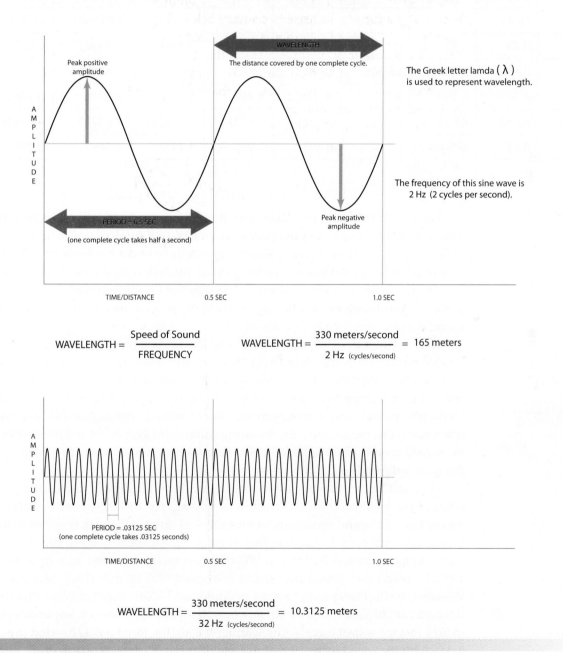

WAVELENGTH

The distance covered by one complete cycle.

Peak positive amplitude

The Greek letter lamda (λ) is used to represent wavelength.

AMPLITUDE

PERIOD = 0.5 SEC

(one complete cycle takes half a second)

Peak negative amplitude

The frequency of this sine wave is 2 Hz (2 cycles per second).

TIME/DISTANCE   0.5 SEC   1.0 SEC

$$\text{WAVELENGTH} = \frac{\text{Speed of Sound}}{\text{FREQUENCY}}$$

$$\text{WAVELENGTH} = \frac{330 \text{ meters/second}}{2 \text{ Hz (cycles/second)}} = 165 \text{ meters}$$

AMPLITUDE

PERIOD = .03125 SEC
(one complete cycle takes .03125 seconds)

TIME/DISTANCE   0.5 SEC   1.0 SEC

$$\text{WAVELENGTH} = \frac{330 \text{ meters/second}}{32 \text{ Hz (cycles/second)}} = 10.3125 \text{ meters}$$

Table 1.7 Frequency and Pitch on an Equal-Tempered Scale, Based on A4 (440 Hz)

C 16	C 33	C 65	C 131	C 262	C 523	C 1047	C 2093	C 4186
C# 17	C# 35	C# 69	C# 139	C# 278	C# 554	C# 1109	C# 2218	C# 4435
D 18	D 37	D 73	D 147	D 294	D 587	D 1175	D 2349	D 4699
D# 20	D# 39	D# 78	D# 156	D# 311	D# 622	D# 1245	D# 2489	D# 4978
E 21	E 41	E 82	E 165	E 330	E 659	E 1319	E 2637	E 5274
F 22	F 44	F 87	F 175	F 349	F 699	F 1397	F 2794	F 5588
F# 23	F# 46	F# 93	F# 185	F# 370	F# 740	F# 1475	F# 2960	F# 5920
G 25	G 49	G 98	G 196	G 392	G 784	G 1568	G 3136	G 6272
G# 26	G# 52	G# 104	G# 208	G# 415	G# 831	G# 1661	G# 3322	G# 6645
A 28	A 55	A 110	A 220	**A 440**	A 880	A 1760	A 3520	A 7040
A# 29	A# 58	A# 117	A# 233	A# 466	A# 932	A# 1865	A# 3729	A# 7459
B 31	B 62	B 124	B 247	B 494	B 988	B 1976	B 3951	B 7902

have one cycle that lasts for 0.002 second; the next might take 0.003 second, the following 0.001 second, and so on. A wave in which individual cycles do not take the same amount of time to occur is called **aperiodic** (without a period). Because this type of sound does not have a specific period, by definition it cannot have a specific frequency, or a specific pitch. Perceptually, such a wave sounds like noise. If you clap your hands or hiss through your teeth, you are producing an aperiodic sound wave.

Sound waves travel through space. The measurement of the distance traveled by a sound wave is its **wavelength** (λ). Wavelength refers to the distance in meters or centimeters covered by one complete cycle of pressure change—that is, the distance covered by the wave from any starting point to the same point on the next cycle. Frequency, period, and wavelength are closely related. The higher the frequency (the more cycles per second), the shorter in duration is the period and the shorter is the wavelength. The lower the frequency (the fewer cycles per second), the longer in duration is the period and the longer is the wavelength.

How fast a wave moves (its velocity) depends on the density and elastic properties of the medium through which it is moving. For instance, because water is denser than air, sound travels about four times as quickly through water as it does through air and even faster than that in some solids, such as steel. The speed of sound in air is around 331 m/s at 0°C (32°F), compared to 1461 m/s in water at 19°C. In a steel rod, sound may travel at a speed of 5000 m/s (Dull, Metcalfe, & Williams, 1960). The speed of sound in liquids and solids is not affected much by temperature. In gases such as air, however, temperature plays an important part in how fast the sound travels. The warmer the air, the more quickly sound propagates, with the speed increasing at the rate of about 0.6 m/s/°C (Dull et al., 1960).

For example, the speed of sound in air at 0°C is 331 m/s, whereas at 20°C (68°F) it is 343 m/s (Durrant & Lovrinic, 1995).

The relationship among the wave speed (v), the wavelength (λ), and the frequency (f) is expressed as $f = v/\lambda$ (frequency equals velocity of sound divided by wavelength) or $\lambda = v/f$ (wavelength equals velocity of sound divided by frequency).

Amplitude represents the amount of displacement from an equilibrium position over time and corresponds perceptually to the loudness of the sound. Amplitude will be discussed in greater detail in a later section of the chapter.

Pure Tones

Simple harmonic motion of a vibrating object such as a tuning fork generates a pattern of acceleration and deceleration of the molecules around the equilibrium position. This motion results in a **pure tone**. A pure tone has only one frequency and is graphed as a sinusoidal wave. Perceptually, a pure tone can be matched to a specific pitch on a musical scale and has a thin quality. An object vibrating in SHM is characterized by frequency/period, amplitude, and phase. Frequency is the number of vibrations per second, period refers to the time taken for one complete vibration back and forth, and amplitude is the maximum displacement of the object from its rest position. Phase refers to the position of the sinusoidal motion relative to some arbitrary reference position (Hixon, Weismer, & Hoit, 2008).

Visually Depicting Sound Waves: Waveforms

Sound waves are invisible and intangible; the pressure changes are miniscule and cannot be seen. This could be a problem in understanding and working with sound, which is fleeting and insubstantial. Fortunately, there are graphic ways of representing sound waves that are extremely useful in helping to visualize the nature and characteristics of sounds. A **waveform** is a graph with time on the horizontal axis and amplitude on the vertical axis. The amplitude represents the amount of whatever is being graphed. For instance, the movement of the tines of the tuning fork can be shown, as can molecular movement generated by the tuning fork. If a pen were attached to the tine of a tuning fork in such a way that as the tine oscillated back and forth, the pen moved with it and traced a line on graph paper, the vertical axis of the resulting waveform would represent the distance that the tine vibrated around its rest position, and the horizontal axis would represent the time that the tine was moving. Now imagine that a pen is attached to an individual molecule so that when the molecule vibrates around its rest position, a similar waveform results. The waveform in this instance does not depict the motion of the tine of the tuning fork but the amplitude of the motion of the molecule of air over time. When dealing with sound, what is represented on the waveform are the changes in air pressure that result from molecular motion. So an acoustic waveform shows the amplitude of air pressure changes over time. If a line is drawn at the midlevel of the graph, it would represent normal P_{am}, or baseline pressure. When the line goes above baseline, it represents an increase in pressure (compression), and the height of the line at any point represents the magnitude of pressure increase. Similarly, when the line goes below baseline, it represents a decrease in pressure (rarefaction), and the depth of the line at any point represents the magnitude of pressure decrease (Figure 1.10).

A waveform is useful in showing many different aspects of a sound. By counting the peaks in the waveform, the frequency of the wave can be calculated. By

Figure 1.10 Waveforms

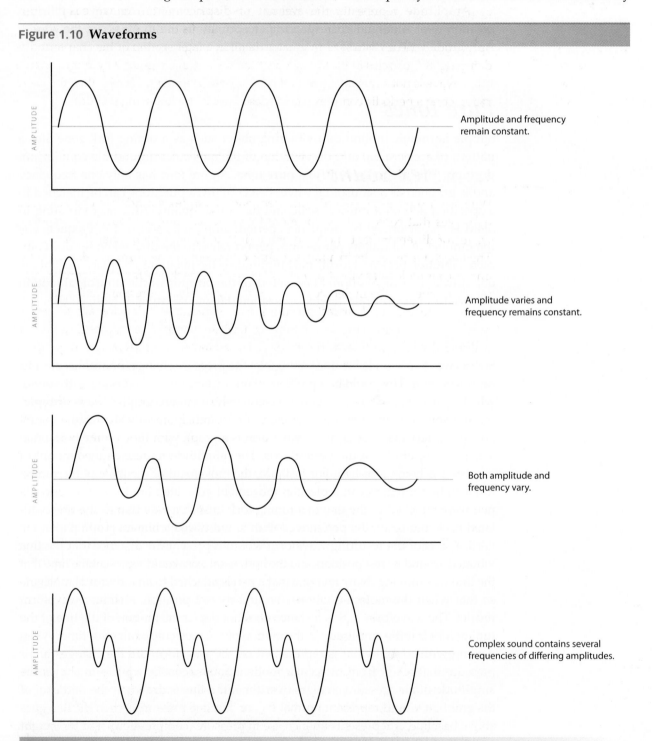

Amplitude and frequency remain constant.

Amplitude varies and frequency remains constant.

Both amplitude and frequency vary.

Complex sound contains several frequencies of differing amplitudes.

measuring the time of each cycle, the period of the wave can be determined. Also, because the vertical axis measures the magnitude of pressure changes, it is easy to visualize the relative amplitude of the wave and whether or not the wave is damping. Shape is another aspect of sound that is visible from a waveform. A smoothly varying shape, a sinusoid, indicates that the wave is a pure tone, vibrating in SHM. If all the cycles in the wave repeat themselves in a predictable fashion, the wave is periodic. If the cycles look different and take different amounts of time to occur, the wave is aperiodic. If the amplitude of the wave is decreasing over time, then the sound is damping. If the cycles in the wave repeat themselves in a regular way, but the shape of the wave is not sinusoidal (the cycles look more irregular in shape), then the wave is depicting a periodic complex sound (described in the following section).

Complex Sounds

Whereas a pure tone has only one frequency, **complex sounds** are characterized by waves that consist of two or more frequencies. Complex sounds occur when waves of different frequencies combine (interfere) with each other (Figure 1.11). The interference results in a more complex vibration of the air molecules. One can imagine air molecules vibrating in SHM as walking back and forth in a regular even manner, whereas the molecules in a complex wave do a more complex "dance" as they vibrate around their rest positions. Both walking and dancing are patterned movements, but the patterns are more complicated and varied in dancing than in walking. Corresponding to the more complex molecular movement in complex sound waves, when acted upon by the wave the tympanic membrane also vibrates in a more complex manner.

There are two types of complex sounds, periodic and aperiodic. Periodic complex sounds consist of a series of frequencies that are systematically related to each other. The lowest frequency of the sound is the **fundamental frequency** (F_0), and the frequencies above the fundamental are called **harmonic frequencies**, or just harmonics. The harmonics in a complex periodic sound are whole-number multiples of the fundamental frequency. For example, if the F_0 of a complex periodic wave is 100 Hz, the harmonics will be 200 Hz, 300 Hz, 400 Hz, 500 Hz, and so on. A complex periodic wave with an F_0 of 300 Hz will have harmonics of 600 Hz, 900 Hz, 1200 Hz, and so on. A complex periodic wave has a musical tone and a specific pitch, and it sounds richer and more resonant than a pure tone wave. In fact, the more harmonics in a sound wave, the more resonant it will sound, and vice versa. Most musical instruments, as well as the human voice, produce sounds that are periodic and complex. All vowel sounds are complex and periodic.

The harmonics in a complex periodic sound can be identified through a process called **Fourier analysis**. Jean-Baptiste Fourier (1768–1830) was a French mathematician who showed that any complex wave can be represented by the sum of its component frequencies as well as their amplitudes and phases. Fourier analysis is a highly complex mathematical procedure, which is performed these days by computer.

Aperiodic complex sounds also consist of two or more frequencies, but the frequencies are not systematically related to each other. Rather, a broad range of

Figure 1.11 Pure tones combine to create a complex periodic sound

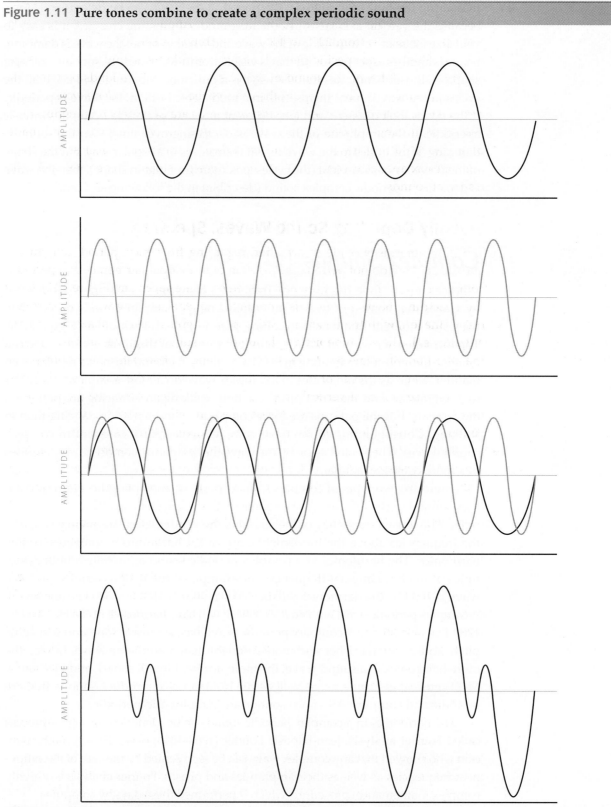

frequencies make up the sound. For example, an aperiodic complex sound could contain all frequencies between 100 and 5000 Hz. Another aperiodic sound might include frequencies from 2000 to 4000 Hz. Such waves sound like noise, with no musical tone and no specific pitch. Examples include the sound of steam escaping from a radiator or the sound of applause. There are two kinds of aperiodic complex sounds, differentiated on the basis of their duration. *Continuous* sounds are able to be prolonged, whereas *transient* sounds are extremely brief in duration. The steam hissing out from the radiator is continuous, whereas the sound made by a person hitting his or her hand on a desk is transient. Voiceless fricatives are complex aperiodic continuous sounds; voiceless stops are complex aperiodic transient sounds.

Visually Depicting Sound Waves: Spectra

While waveforms provide information regarding frequency, period, amplitude, and shape, they do not permit visualization of individual harmonics in a periodic complex sound. Harmonics can best be seen on a **line spectrum** (Figure 1.12). On a line spectrum, the horizontal axis represents frequency, starting with low frequencies to the left, with frequency increasing to the right. The vertical axis represents amplitude. Rather than depict amplitude of pressure changes, as in a waveform, the amplitude in a line spectrum shows the amount of acoustic energy present at each harmonic frequency of the sound. Each frequency in the wave, including the F_0, is represented by a vertical line, the height of which shows the amplitude of that specific frequency. Thus, what is depicted on a line spectrum is the **harmonic content** of the sound—that is, the relationship between the frequencies in the sound and their respective amplitudes. Perceptually, the harmonic content corresponds to the quality or tone of the sound. The note of middle C sounds different on a violin compared to a piano in part because each has a different harmonic content despite having the same F_0.

A line spectrum can show equally well whether a sound is a pure tone (in which case it would have just one line) or a complex sound (more than one line). What is not evident on a spectrum is time. The frequencies shown on a line spectrum are those that are present in a sound at one particular instant of time. Think of the difference between waveforms and spectra in terms of a video versus a photograph. The spectrum corresponds to a snapshot of a person at one particular instant of time; a waveform corresponds to a video, in which changes over time can be seen as the person walks around and performs different actions. Therefore, while the detailed harmonic information can be determined from a spectrum, it is not possible to judge if the sound is damping or changing in other ways over time because the overall amplitude of the sound over time is not shown.

A line spectrum is not used to represent complex aperiodic sounds, because these sounds are characterized by broad bands of frequencies. Rather than draw individual vertical lines extremely close to each other, as would be necessary to represent these sounds, the **envelope** of the wave is shown as a horizontal line that is understood to connect all the component frequencies in the sound. This kind of spectrum is known as a **continuous spectrum** (Figure 1.12). As with periodic complex sounds on a line spectrum, the height of the line at any frequency

Figure 1.12 Spectra

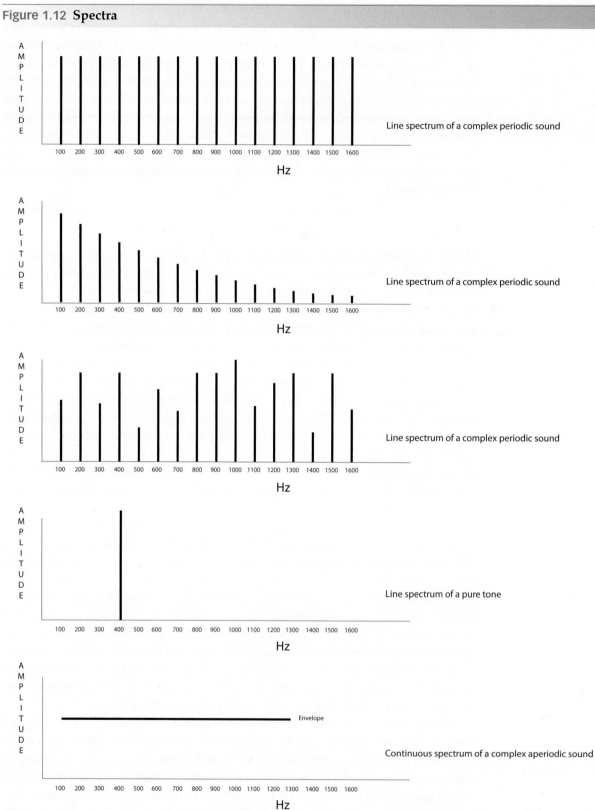

Line spectrum of a complex periodic sound

Line spectrum of a complex periodic sound

Line spectrum of a complex periodic sound

Line spectrum of a pure tone

Continuous spectrum of a complex aperiodic sound

Figure 1.13 Waveform versus spectrum

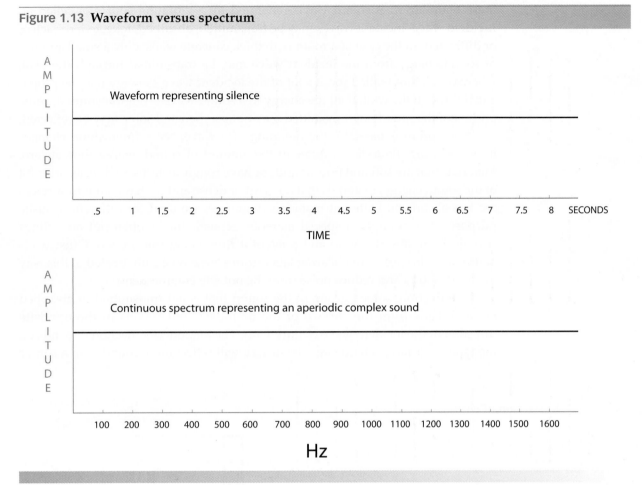

represents the amount of acoustic energy at that frequency. What cannot be seen from a continuous spectrum is the duration of the sound, so it is not possible to tell if the sound is continuous or transient.

It is important to distinguish between waveforms and spectra, because the information they provide is very different. For example, Figure 1.13 shows that a flat horizontal line on a waveform depicts silence, because the pressure is constant over time. However, a flat horizontal line on a spectrum would depict an aperiodic complex sound containing all frequencies in a certain range.

Sound Absorption, Reflection, Refraction, and Diffraction

So far, discussion has focused on sound being transmitted through the air, without taking into account any objects or boundaries that sound waves might encounter in their travels. In fact, when sound waves come into contact with walls, ceilings, floors, trees, or any other objects, they may or may not be transmitted through these boundaries. A sound wave generated by a vibrating source is called an **incident wave**. Incident waves may be transmitted, absorbed, reflected, refracted, or diffracted. In the case of a room with thick concrete walls, only a small amount of sound energy from the incident wave may be transmitted through the wall, whereas in a thin-walled room a lot of the incident wave's energy may be propagated through the wall. If all the energy in a sound wave is not transmitted, some portion of the sound not transmitted may be absorbed and some may be reflected.

Absorption is basically the damping of a wave, with diminishing changes in air pressure. Boundaries differ in the amount of sound energy they absorb. Materials that are soft and porous and/or have rough surfaces tend to absorb a lot of the sound energy; materials that are hard or dense and/or have smooth surfaces are less absorbent. Different materials, therefore, are used for different acoustic purposes. For example, a special material, acoustic tile, is often put on ceilings specifically to absorb sound and prevent it from being transmitted. Often walls and ceilings in speech and hearing laboratories are acoustically treated in this way to absorb sound and reduce noise from the outside environment.

In **reflection**, some portion of the sound that is not transmitted or absorbed bounces back from the surface of the boundary and travels in the opposite direction of the incident wave (Figure 1.14). The amount of reflection depends on the type of surface. A hard, smooth surface will reflect more sound than a soft or

Figure 1.14 Reflection of sound

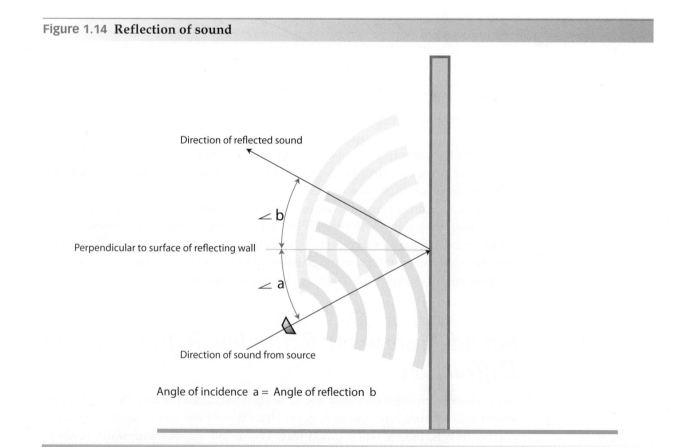

Direction of reflected sound

∠ b

Perpendicular to surface of reflecting wall

∠ a

Direction of sound from source

Angle of incidence a = Angle of reflection b

Figure 1.15 **Refraction of sound**

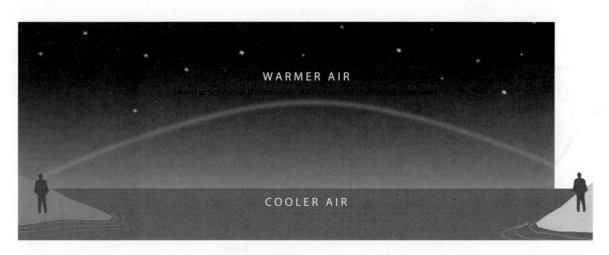

A temperature inversion, which may occur at night, traps cool air under a layer of warmer air. Sound waves closest to the surface travel more slowly through the cool air than do sound waves traveling through the warmer air above. This causes sound waves to be refracted back towards the surface.
You may have experienced this phenomenon if you have noticed that on a still night, voices may carry great distances over the surface of a lake. Cool air near the lake surface and warmer air above is causing the sound waves to bend back towards the surface.

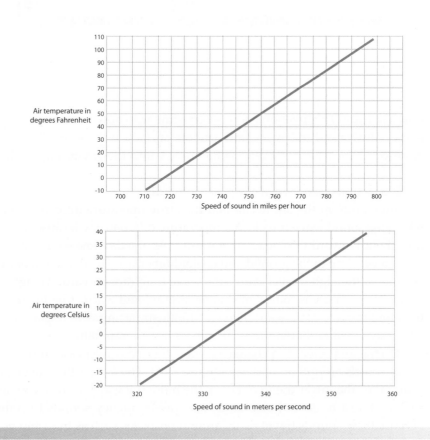

Figure 1.16 Diffraction of sound

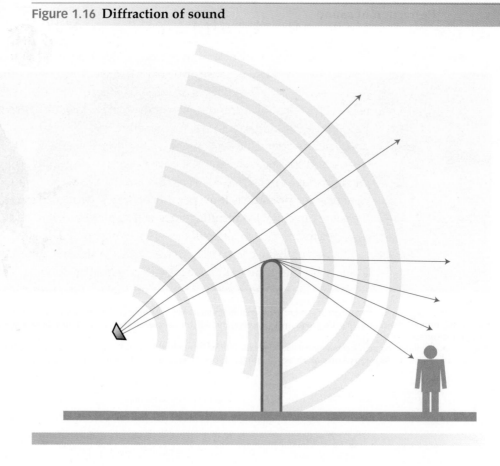

rough surface. This phenomenon is very similar to how a mirror works. A mirror is specially treated to have a hard, smooth surface. It therefore does not transmit or absorb light waves but reflects them back into the environment, allowing the image to be seen.

Refraction occurs when a wave changes direction because of a local difference of temperature in the air. Recall that the air temperature influences the speed at which the sound wave travels. A temperature difference will cause the wave to refract (bend) toward the cooler air. For example, the daytime temperature of the air is warmest close to the ground and cooler higher up. The reduction of the sound's velocity at the higher level causes the wave to refract upward. At night, however, the air temperature is coolest next to the ground and warmer higher up. The wave therefore refracts downward. Figure 1.15 illustrates refraction using the example of a body of water that induces differences in air temperature.

Diffraction refers to a change in direction as a wave passes through an opening or travels around an obstacle (Figure 1.16). The longer the wavelength of the sound (i.e., the lower the frequency), the more the wave diffracts. Some animals, such as forest birds and elephants, use low-frequency sounds to communicate because these sounds travel easily around obstacles such as trees and vegetation.

Constructive and Destructive Interference

In general, physical objects cannot occupy the same space at the same time. Sound waves, however, can, because areas of pressures can combine. Suppose that a tuning fork tuned to 100 Hz produces an incident sound wave that travels through the air, comes up against a wall, and is then reflected back toward the tuning fork. The tuning fork, in the meantime, continues to generate new incident waves 100 times per second. Thus, incident and reflected waves are combining with each other at any instant in time and space. This combining of waves is known as **interference**. The air pressure changes that form these two waves can interfere with each other in various ways. As noted earlier, pressure is force per unit of area. If two equal forces combine and act in the same direction, the resulting force will be increased; if two forces are equal but act in opposite directions, they will cancel each other out. If the areas of compression and rarefaction of the two waves combine at exactly the same time and the same moment in space, the amplitude of the resulting wave will be doubled. This happens because when two areas of high pressure combine, the resulting pressure is higher still. When two areas of low pressure combine, the pressure is further lowered at that point. This produces greater deviations from normal P_{am} and therefore increased amplitude of the wave. Interference that results in increased amplitude is called **constructive interference** (Figure 1.17). If an area of compression of one of the waves combines at exactly the same time with an area of rarefaction of the other wave, the amplitude of the resulting wave will be decreased, which is known as **destructive interference**.

Theoretically, it is possible for two sound waves with the same frequency to cancel each other out completely, resulting in an area of normal pressure (P_{am}). Because sound consists of changes in air pressure, normal P_{am}, by definition, cannot be a sound.

Figure 1.17 **Constructive and destructive interference**

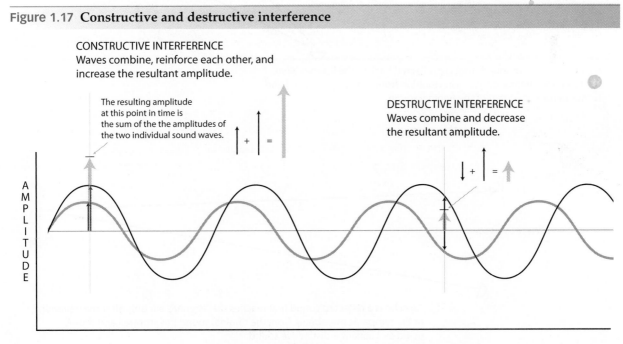

CONSTRUCTIVE INTERFERENCE
Waves combine, reinforce each other, and increase the resultant amplitude.

The resulting amplitude at this point in time is the sum of the the amplitudes of the two individual sound waves.

DESTRUCTIVE INTERFERENCE
Waves combine and decrease the resultant amplitude.

AMPLITUDE

TIME

Waves of different frequencies can also combine, and their areas of compression and rarefaction will not line up exactly. The amplitude of the resulting wave will therefore not be doubled, nor will the sound be completely eliminated. Rather, the amplitude of the sound will be changed in complex ways. This relative timing of areas of high and low pressure in waves is called **phase**.

Sound waves that combine and interfere with each other can affect the way that the sound is perceived. For example, a sound can experience **reverberation**, meaning that it lasts slightly longer because of the interference (Figure 1.18). This

Figure 1.18 Reverberation and echo

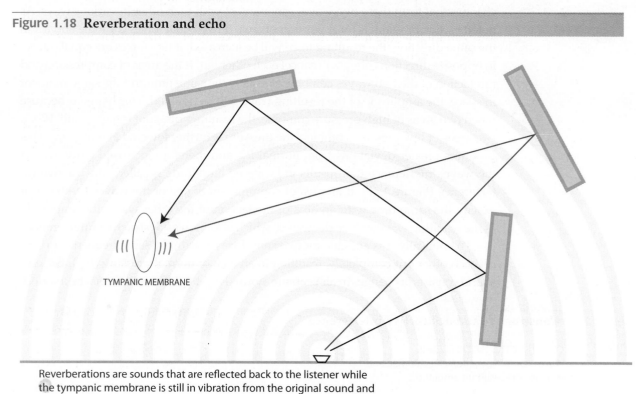

TYMPANIC MEMBRANE

Reverberations are sounds that are reflected back to the listener while the tympanic membrane is still in vibration from the original sound and is thus perceived as part of the original sound.

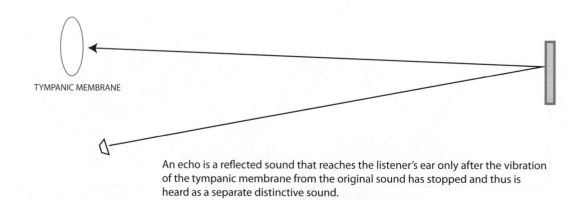

TYMPANIC MEMBRANE

An echo is a reflected sound that reaches the listener's ear only after the vibration of the tympanic membrane from the original sound has stopped and thus is heard as a separate distinctive sound.

happens when a reflected sound wave arrives at one's ear slightly delayed in time compared with the arrival of the incident wave at the same point. The duration of the delay depends on the distance between the reflective surface and the ear. The sound wave must travel to the reflective boundary and return to the ear, delaying its arrival by a fraction of a second. Only one sound is heard, but this sound is extended in duration because the reflected wave arrives in time to keep the person's eardrum vibrating longer than it would with just the incident wave vibrating it. However, if the distance between the ear and the reflective surface is substantial, then the delay will be perceptually noticeable; in this case, the reflected sound wave is heard as a separate sound—in other words, an echo. With an echo, the incident wave vibrates the eardrum, but the eardrum has time to settle down and stop vibrating before it is set into vibration once again by the reflected wave.

Reverberation can be desirable because it can increase the intensity of the sound reaching a listener. However, too much reverberation can interfere with communication by making the phonemes blend together and become garbled. This issue has become very prominent over the past few years in educational settings. Many classrooms are overly reverberant because of uncarpeted floors and bare walls that create multiple reflections of sounds. The more reflective the room, the longer the incident sound and reflections take to be absorbed and damped. This can hinder students in their understanding of the instructor's speech, which is particularly problematic for individuals with hearing disorders or other types of learning difficulties.

Attributes of Sounds

Although all sounds are generated by changes in air pressure, individual sounds are very different from one another. A high-pitched siren sounds very different from a low-pitched fog horn. A discreet whisper during class sounds different from a football cheer. The husky voice of a person with laryngitis sounds very different from that of a trained singer. We shall now explore in some detail the attributes of sounds that result in these kinds of differences, including frequency, pitch, amplitude, intensity, and loudness.

Frequency and Pitch

As described above, frequency refers to the rate at which an object vibrates and is measured in hertz (Hz). Frequency is an objective measurement of a physical phenomenon. Pitch is a psychological event relating to an individual's perception of the sound's location on a musical scale. Pitch is thus the perceptual counterpart of frequency. Frequency and pitch are related. In general, the faster the rate of vibration (the higher the frequency), the higher pitched the sound will be perceived. The slower the rate of vibration (the lower the frequency), the lower pitched the sound will be perceived. The frequency of a vibrating object depends on its physical characteristics, including its length, thickness, density, and degree of stiffness or tension. For example, on an instrument such as a guitar, thicker strings have a lower frequency, and thinner strings have a higher frequency. A string stretched between two points will have a certain degree of tension, depending on how tightly it is stretched. The more tightly the string is stretched, the higher its tension and the higher the frequency, and vice versa. Similarly, a larger tuning fork with thicker tines will vibrate more slowly than a smaller fork with thinner tines. If any one of these characteristics is changed, the frequency will change in predictable ways. Thus, increasing the length of a vibrating source without changing its density will decrease the rate of vibration. Decreasing the density of a vibrating object will increase its rate of vibration, and increasing its density will lower its frequency. Changing the tension and stiffness of an object will likewise change the frequency. As an example, consider a rubber band. If a rubber band is held loosely at either end and plucked, it will vibrate at a certain rate. If the band is stretched more tightly, it becomes stiffer and tenser, and its frequency increases when it is plucked. Note, however, that when the rubber band was stretched, it became longer, and objects that are longer generally vibrate more slowly than shorter ones. But, although the elastic band is longer when it is stretched, its density has been decreased, so it is now skinnier as well. In other words, there is the same amount of material in the rubber band, but it has been stretched out over a greater distance, and its cross-sectional area is less. The increased tension on the band and its decreased density cause it to vibrate more quickly. This interaction between length, density, and tension to determine frequency is extremely important in the production of voice, as we will see in later chapters.

Human Range of Hearing

The range of frequencies that humans are capable of perceiving is around 20 to 20,000 Hz. Frequencies below this range are called **subsonic**, and frequencies above this range are **supersonic**. This range is relatively limited. Some animals can perceive sounds well below 20 Hz, such as elephants, who make use of these subsonic sounds in their communication. Some birds, such as pigeons and chickens, can also perceive exceedingly low-pitched sounds that would be inaudible to humans (Gill, 1995). On the other hand, some dogs can hear sounds well above 20 kHz, which is why dog whistles work: The whistle emits an extremely high-frequency sound that is inaudible to humans but audible to dogs. Bats, too, are well known for their use of very high-frequency sounds to locate objects in space. Humans tend to hear best frequencies that are in the middle of their range, around 1 kHz to 4 kHz. Sounds that are above or below this midrange are not as easily perceived by the human auditory system. Conveniently, most speech sounds fall within this range.

Amplitude, Intensity, and Loudness

As described above, the term *amplitude* refers to either the distance that air molecules are displaced from their rest positions during vibration or to the measurement of the pressure changes that constitute sound. Like frequency, amplitude is a measurement of a physical phenomenon—the pressure changes that occur in the air as sound propagates through it. Because amplitude is related to pressure, it is measured in pascals in the MKS system or dynes per square centimeter (dyne/cm^2) in the CGS system. Intensity refers to power per unit of area. Recall that power is defined as the amount of energy expended in a second and is measured in watts (W).

One watt equals 1 joule per second in the MKS system or 10 million ergs per second in the CGS system. Intensity is measured in watts per square meter in the MKS system or watts per square centimeter in the CGS system. Intensity can be thought of as the amount of power required to generate a certain output, whether the output is sound or some other form of energy, such as light. For example, lightbulbs are available that produce different intensities of output (lumens). A lightbulb that uses less energy produces a less intense light than one that uses more energy. A 40 W lightbulb uses 40 W to generate a certain light output. Such a lightbulb gives off a less bright light than a 75 W lightbulb. The same is true of sound intensity. If your stereo speakers use 10 W of power, you will hear a certain loudness of sound. With 30 W, the sound output will be much greater. It is clear that there must be some kind of relationship between amplitude and intensity, which are physical measurements, and loudness, which is how one perceives the intensity generated by the degree of pressure change. The greater are the amplitude and intensity, the louder is the sound that is heard and vice versa. This relationship is logarithmic. Amplitude and intensity are related to each other: The greater the amplitude, the greater the intensity that is generated in the sound wave. However, intensity increases much more rapidly than does amplitude. Mathematically, intensity is proportional to the square of amplitude. Thus if a sound wave has a certain amplitude with a corresponding intensity level and the amplitude of that sound wave is doubled, the intensity of the wave will be quadrupled (increase of 2^2). If the amplitude is increased by a factor of 5, the intensity will be increased by a factor of 5^2 (i.e., 25). Thus, it takes only small increases in air pressure changes to generate much larger increases in sound intensity.

Decibel Scale

The **decibel (dB) scale** is designed to measure sounds in a way that takes into account their amplitudes and intensities in relation to how the sound is perceived in terms of loudness. The bel is named after Alexander Graham Bell. It is a large unit of measurement of sound intensity, based on the logarithm of a ratio. A decibel is one tenth of a bel.

The human auditory system is sensitive to an enormous range of intensity levels. From the softest sound that a person can hear to the loudest sound, which produces a feeling of pain in the ears, is a range of around 10 trillion intensities. Trying to deal with huge numbers like this on a *linear* scale would be unwieldy and confusing. The decibel scale is *logarithmic*, which has the effect of compressing the trillions of intensities into a scale with far fewer levels. The compression occurs because of the essential difference between linear and logarithmic scales. A **linear scale** is one in which units are the same distance from each other, and units can be added or subtracted (see Figure 1.19). A ruler is a linear measure. A ruler has distances marked off on it, typically in inches (in), centimeters (cm), and millimeters (mm). A distance of, say, 10 mm between two points on the ruler is 10 times greater than a distance of 1 mm. Put another way, the distance between 2 and 3 mm is exactly the same as the distance between 8 and 9 mm, which is exactly the same as the distance between 45 and 46 mm. Thus, successive units are always the same distance from each other. Temperature scales are also examples of linear

Figure 1.19   Linear versus logarithmic scale

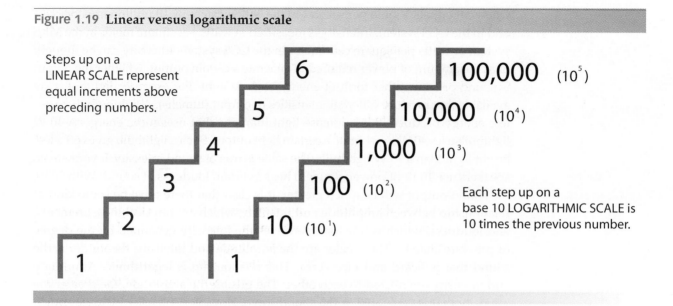

Steps up on a
LINEAR SCALE represent
equal increments above
preceding numbers.

6

5

4

3

2

1

100,000 (10^5)

10,000 (10^4)

1,000 (10^3)

100 (10^2)

10 (10^1)

1

Each step up on a
base 10 LOGARITHMIC SCALE is
10 times the previous number.

scales, with the distance between units indicating equal increments of temperature increase or decrease.

Logarithmic scales contain units that increase by greater and greater amounts going up the scale. These units cannot be added or subtracted because they are not equal. A logarithmic scale has several components. The first is a base, such as 2 or 10. A logarithmic scale with a base of 2 indicates that each successive unit increases by a factor of 2. With a base of 10, each unit increases by a factor of 10. The number of increases on a logarithmic scale is indicated by the exponent, or power (not to be confused with power as it relates to energy). A base is raised to some power. A base of 10 raised to the first power, or with an exponent of 1, is 10^1. 10 multiplied by 1 equals 10. A base of 10 raised to the second power is 10^2. In this case, the base is multiplied by itself 2 times. 10 times 10 equals 100. Similarly, 10 raised to the third power is 10^3. Multiply base 10 by itself three times, and you get 10 times 10 times 10, equaling 1000. Particularly with base 10, the exponents are often used by themselves with the understanding that this is the power to which 10 must be raised in order to equal the original number. The exponent is then called the log. For example, the log of 100 is 2, the log of 1000 is 3, the log of 10,000 is 4, and so on. Thus, whereas linear scales increase successively by some equal amount, logarithmic scales increase by successively greater amounts. Therefore, 10 trillion units of intensity on a linear scale become condensed on a logarithmic scale to around 140 units (Durrant & Lovrinic, 1995).

In addition to being a logarithmic scale, the decibel scale is also a **ratio scale**. A ratio reflects a relationship between quantities. For example, a ratio of males to females of 2:1 indicates that there are two males for every female. The ratio that the decibel scale measures is the relationship between the amplitudes or the intensities of two sounds: a target sound and a standard reference sound. Why is it necessary to establish this relationship? Amplitude and intensity are physical measures and it is possible to measure the precise amplitude or the precise intensity of any sound. However, this would not provide a particularly meaningful value. Say that a sound is measured to have amplitude of 0.045 Pa. This is not very revealing information, in terms of how loud an individual actually perceives the sound to be. It is necessary to compare this sound to a sound that has a known amplitude and intensity level in order to determine if it is higher or lower in intensity. In other words, what is needed is a standard sound that can serve as the basis of comparison for all other sounds. This is the basis for the decibel scale.

The decibel scale compares any target sound with a **standard reference sound**. The standard reference sound has a specific amplitude of 20 µPa and a specific intensity of 10^{-12} W/m². In the perceptual domain, a sound with this amplitude and intensity indicates the softest sound of a particular frequency (1000 Hz) that a pair of normal human ears can hear 50 percent of the time under ideal listening conditions. This level is known as the **threshold of hearing**. On the decibel scale, a sound of this level is indicated by 0. Keeping in mind that the decibel scale is a ratio scale, 0 dB does not mean that there is silence but that the sound in question has the same intensity and amplitude as the standard reference sound. It is also possible to have a negative number on the decibel scale; this just means that the sound in question has amplitude and intensity less than that of the standard reference sound.

The formula to derive the intensity or amplitude of a target sound (I_1 or P_1) in relation to the standard reference intensity or amplitude (I_0 or P_0) is based on the logarithm of a ratio (bel). The formula for intensity is **N(bels)=$\log_{10}$ I_1/I_0.** This means that the number of bels is equal to a logarithmic scale of base 10 on which the target intensity level (I_1) is divided by the reference intensity level (I_0). However, because the bel is a large unit, most applications in acoustics use the decibel. The formula for intensity in decibels (dB) is **N(dB)=10 $\log_{10}$ I_1/I_0.** Say, for example, the target intensity I_1 is 100 times the reference intensity I_0. We know that the log of 100 is 2. Multiplying 2 by 10 gives 20, so a sound that is 100 times as intense as the reference sound has a value of 20 dB. Using the same calculation, a sound that is 1000 times as intense as the reference sound will have a dB value of 30 (the log of 1000 is 3; multiply 3 by 10), a sound that is 10,000 times as intense as the reference will be equal to 40 dB, and so on. The standard reference for intensity is 10^{-12} W/m². Substituting this value for I_0, intensity level is expressed as the formula IL (dB) =10 $\log_{10}$ $I_1/10^{-12}$ W/m². A similar formula is used for amplitude, or sound pressure level (SPL). The only difference is that instead of multiplying the log by 10, it is multiplied by 20, because of the relationship between intensity and amplitude. (Recall that intensity is proportional to the square of amplitude.) When a number is squared its log is multiplied by two (Martin & Clark, 2012). Therefore, the formula for SPL is **SPL (dB) = 20 $\log_{10}$ P_1/P_0.** We know that the reference for amplitude is 20 µPa, so SPL (dB) = 20 log10 P1/20 µPa. To put this equation in words, dB (SPL) equals 20 times the log of the target amplitude divided by the reference amplitude. Substituting the value of the reference sound, dB (SPL) equals 20 times the log of the target amplitude divided by 20 μPa. If the target amplitude is 2000 μPa, then 2000 divided by 20 equals 100. The log of 100 is 2, and 20 times 2 equals 40. Thus, a sound with an amplitude of 2000 μPa corresponds to a dB level of 40 SPL. The equations for intensity and amplitude differ in terms of the log, but they express the same ratios.

The decibel unit is dimensionless unless it is anchored to a referent. In other words, saying that a sound has a decibel level of 30 is meaningless because the number lacks a referent or basis of comparison. By analogy, if someone told you that Sue is 4 inches taller than Mary, you still would not know how tall either of them is. By adding the information that Mary is 5 feet 5 inches, the comparison makes sense. Therefore, it is important when using the decibel scale to specify whether amplitude or intensity is being measured. When amplitude is measured, the units on the decibel scale are referenced to sound pressure level (SPL). For intensity, the units are referenced to intensity level (IL). Thus, it is clear that a sound of 30 dB SPL has an amplitude level that is 1000 times greater than the standard amplitude reference of 20 μPa; a sound of 30 dB IL has an intensity level that is 1000 times greater than the standard intensity referent of 10^{-12} W/m². Because the scale specifies a ratio, dB IL always equals dB SPL as long as equivalent reference pressures and intensities are used (Speaks, 1992). For example, 60 dB IL equals 60 dB SPL, 78.5 dB IL equals 78.5 dB SPL, and so on.

Each step in the decibel scale corresponds to a more-or-less equal increase in a person's perception of loudness, even though the actual pressure and intensity differences increase dramatically (Raphael, Borden, & Harris, 2007). Since the decibel scale is logarithmic, a 10 dB step at the threshold of hearing will be only 10 times the standard reference sound. At the intensity level for normal conversational speech, which is around 60 dB IL, intensity is 1 million times greater than the standard reference sound. See Table 1.8 for examples of sounds at various dB levels.

Since intensity is proportional to the square of amplitude, a 10-fold increase in amplitude corresponds to a 100-fold increase in intensity; a 100-fold increase in amplitude corresponds to a 10,000-fold increase in intensity (Denes & Pinson, 1993). Because of the logarithmic nature of the dB scale, doubling (or halving) the sound intensity results in an increase (or decrease) of 3 dB; increasing (or decreasing) intensity by a factor of 10 corresponds to an increase (or decrease) of 10 dB. In terms of amplitude, a doubling (or halving) of sound pressure corresponds to an increase (or decrease) of 6 dB. A 10-fold change in sound pressure corresponds to a change of 20 dB. Table 1.9 shows how these values are derived. Because of the nonlinear relationship between amplitude/ intensity and loudness, while every 6 dB SPL represents a doubling of amplitude (physical), a 10 dB increase corresponds to a doubling of loudness (perceptual).

Advantages of the Decibel Scale

One important advantage of using the decibel scale is that because of the logarithmic nature of the scale, huge ranges of intensities are condensed into around 140 units. Another advantage is that the relationship between the decibel scale and

Table 1.8 Units of dB, Approximate Loudness, and Intensity/Amplitude Increases Compared to the Standard Reference Sound

dB	Loudness	Intensity/Amplitude Increases
0	Threshold of hearing	Standard reference sound (SRS): IL: 10^{-12} W/m^2; SPL: 20 µPa
10	Normal breathing	$10^1 \times$ SRS
20	Rustle of leaves	10^2 (100) $\times$ SRS
30	Whisper	10^3 (1,000) $\times$ SRS
40	Quiet residential community	10^4 (10,000) $\times$ SRS
50	Urban residence	10^5 (100,000) $\times$ SRS
60	Normal conversation at 1 m	10^6 (1,000,000) $\times$ SRS
70	Vacuum cleaner at 3 m	10^7 (10,000,000) $\times$ SRS
80	Heavy truck	10^8 (100,000,000) $\times$ SRS
90	Power lawn mower	10^9 (1,000,000,000) $\times$ SRS
100	Bulldozer	10^{10} (10,000,000,000) $\times$ SRS
110	Disco/club	10^{11} (100,000,000,000) $\times$ SRS
120	Ambulance siren	10^{12} (1,000,000,000,000) $\times$ SRS
130	Machine gun fire at close range	10^{13} (10,000,000,000,000) $\times$ SRS
140	Jet engine at take off	10^{14} (100,000,000,000,000) $\times$ SRS
180	Rocket launch	10^{18} (1,000,000,000,000,000,000) $\times$ SRS

SOURCE: Information from Centers for Disease Control (www.cdc.gov/niosh/topics/noise/noisemeter.html); Durrant & Lovrinic (1995); and U.S. Department of Labor (www.osha.gov/SLTC/noisehearingconservation/).

absolute values of pressure and intensity is very similar to the physiological function of the human auditory system. A change in intensity that is just barely able to be perceived near the hearing threshold is produced by a 1 dB change in the stimulus. As the sound intensity level increases, the intensity change that produces a just perceivable change in loudness continues to be about 1 dB, although the absolute intensity change increases exponentially.

Table 1.9 Doubling and Halving of Amplitude and Intensity

Amplitude	Intensity
$20 \times \log10 (2/1) = 6$ dB SPL	$10 \times \log10 (2/1) = 3$ dB IL
$20 \times \log10 (0.5/1) = -6$ dB SPL	$10 \times \log10 (0.5/1) = -3$ dB IL

NOTE: 2/1 = twice original value; 0.5/1 = half original value.

Applications of the Decibel Scale

The dB scale is used in many applications. For example, it is used in conjunction with frequency to determine the limits of human hearing. The **auditory area** is a graph that represents frequency along the horizontal axis and intensity along the vertical axis (Figure 1.20). Humans can perceive frequencies from around 20–20,000 Hz and intensities from 0 to 140 dB. The human auditory system responds more easily to sounds in the midrange of frequencies (around 1 to 4 KHz) than to those that are very low or very high. Frequencies in the midrange can be perceived when they are less intense, whereas a very low- or

Figure 1.20 Human auditory area

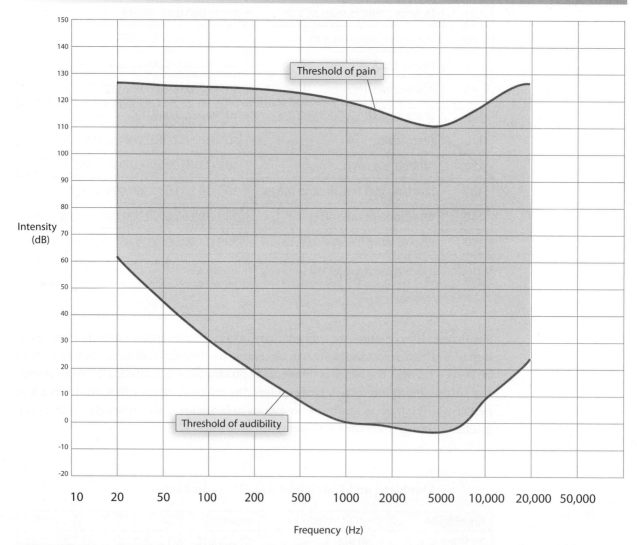

Table 1.10 **Frequencies and Intensities at the Threshold of Hearing for Normal Ears**

Frequency (Hz)	Intensity (dB)
125	47.5
250	26.5
500	13.5
1000	7.5
2000	11.0
4000	10.5
8000	13.0

NOTE: Information based on the ANSI Standard (1969) for audiometers.

very high-frequency sound needs to have much more intensity in order to be perceptible to humans. Although the threshold of hearing changes depending on the frequency of the sound, any frequency with an intensity of around 130 dB will cause a sensation of pain in the ear. This level is known as the **threshold of pain**. The graph in Figure 1.20 demonstrates that a sound in the middle of the range, say 2 kHz, requires an intensity of around 11 dB to be just audible (threshold of hearing), whereas a sound with a frequency of 125 Hz requires an intensity level of 47.5 dB. Table 1.10 shows frequencies and intensities at the threshold of hearing for normal ears based on the ANSI Standard (1969) for audiometers.

It is clear that some frequencies have a wider range of intensities at which they can be perceived, whereas others have a more limited range between the threshold of hearing and the threshold of pain. A person with normal hearing would just barely be able to perceive a 1000 Hz tone with an intensity of 7.5 dB and would feel pain in the ear when that tone had an intensity of 130 dB. However, a tone with a frequency of 125 Hz would be just barely audible at an intensity of 47.5 dB but would still cause pain at an intensity of 130 dB. Some people with hearing impairment are sensitive to smaller ranges of intensities. For example, a hearing-impaired individual may be only able to detect a 1000 Hz tone when it has an intensity of 60 dB and may find the sound painfully loud at an intensity of 90 dB.

Using an **audiogram** is a way of representing an individual's hearing by measuring his or her threshold at selected frequency levels. In this application the dB is referenced to hearing level (HL) rather than to IL or SPL. Figure 1.21 shows that in an audiogram, the threshold of hearing for different frequencies has been "straightened out," and the threshold for each frequency is set at 0 dB HL. Most audiograms only cover the range of frequencies from 125 Hz to 8 kHz,

Figure 1.21 Audiogram

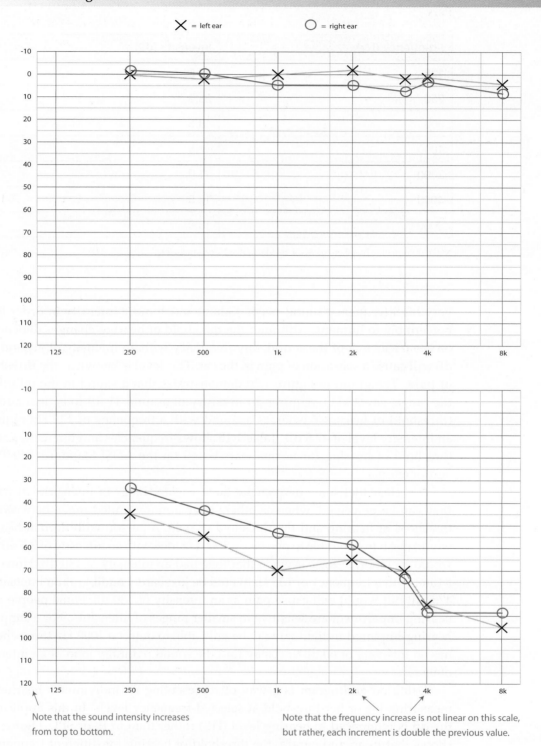

Note that the sound intensity increases from top to bottom.

Note that the frequency increase is not linear on this scale, but rather, each increment is double the previous value.

The upper audiogram represents results for a person with hearing within the normal range.
The lower one is that of a person with a hearing loss in both ears, particularly at the higher frequencies.

as these are most important for speech perception. Audiograms are plotted with frequency on the horizontal axis, usually on a logarithmic scale, and dB HL on the vertical axis on a linear scale. Normal hearing is typically better than or equal to 20 dB HL.

Summary

The study of human speech falls into the domain of bioacoustics.

Scientific measurement systems are based on the modernized international metric system, the International System of Units.

Basic physics concepts relevant to the study of speech include mass, force, volume, density, speed, velocity, momentum, acceleration, inertia, elasticity, stiffness, work, energy, power, intensity, and pressure.

Air pressure, volume, and density are systematically related: There is an inverse relationship between air volume and pressure and a direct relationship between air pressure and density.

Sound occurs when a disturbance creates alternating increases and decreases in ambient pressure.

Elasticity, inertia, and friction interact to keep molecules of air vibrating around their original positions for a while before damping.

Sound travels in a wave motion in which molecules vibrate a tiny distance around their equilibrium positions, resulting in changes in air pressure that can propagate for long distances.

Vibration of a source in simple harmonic motion results in a pure tone with only one frequency.

Periodic complex sounds consist of a series of frequencies that are systematically related to each other; aperiodic complex sounds have a broad range of unrelated frequencies and may be continuous or transient.

Sounds may be visualized on a waveform that shows pressure changes over time, or on a spectrum that shows spectral content.

Incident waves may be transmitted, absorbed, reflected, refracted, and/or diffracted.

Sound waves can interfere constructively or destructively.

Sounds differ in terms of frequency/pitch and amplitude/loudness.

The dB scale is a logarithmic ratio scale that compares the amplitude/intensity and loudness of a target sound to a standard reference sound.

REVIEW EXERCISES

1. Use an example other than a tuning fork to explain how sound is generated. Describe the forces involved in generating, maintaining, and damping vibration.

2. Define and explain the terms *reverberation, absorption, reflection, refraction,* and *diffraction.*

3. Contrast constructive and destructive interference and explain how each comes about.

4. Discuss the following statement: "Speech is a stream of periodic and aperiodic complex sounds."

5. Describe the decibel scale and identify some applications of the scale in speech and hearing.

CHAPTER

2

Resonance

STUDENT LEARNING OBJECTIVES

After reading this chapter you will

○ Understand the difference between free and forced vibration.

○ Discuss forced vibration as the basis of resonance.

○ Explain the filtering properties of acoustic resonators.

○ Describe the concepts of resonance curves, bandwidth, center frequency, and cutoff frequency.

○ Compare and contrast high-pass, low-pass, and band-pass filters.

○ Understand that the vocal tract is a variable quarter-wave resonator.

○ Describe the source-filter theory and its relationship to different vowel sounds.

○ Explain how tongue height and tongue advancement influence vowel formant frequencies.

○ Compare F_1/F_2 plots for men, women, and children.

Resonance is the tendency of a system to vibrate with greatest amplitude in response to a frequency that matches or comes close to its own natural frequency. **Natural frequency** (NF) is the frequency at which an object vibrates freely and is determined by the object's length, density, tension, and stiffness. Whenever this particular object or system is set into vibration and allowed to continue without interference, it will always vibrate at its NF. For example, the tines of a tuning fork, when struck, will oscillate back and forth at a certain frequency depending on the length and density of the fork, say 100 Hz. Its NF is thus 100 Hz, and this is the rate at which the tuning fork will always vibrate, as long as its physical characteristics remain constant.

Objects or systems can also be set into forced vibration. This occurs when the vibrations from one object set another object into vibration if the NFs of both objects match or are within a certain

distance of each other. There are many common examples of forced vibration, such as pictures hanging on walls that rattle when a car with a particularly loud stereo goes by the house. If the vibrations generated by the stereo are close to the NF of the wall, the wall will be set into vibration, causing the pictures to rattle. Another example is when a part in a car starts to rattle in sympathy with the engine noise as the ignition is turned on. Here, too, the vibration of the engine may be close in frequency to some other part of the car, which is then forced to vibrate in response to the engine noise. Another example of resonance is portrayed in cartoons in which a singer hits a particularly high note, and suddenly a wine glass shatters. The glass has a particular NF. When the singer hits a note that is close to the glass's NF, the glass is set into vibration. If the amplitude of vibration is great enough, the glass shatters as it vibrates.

The phenomenon of how the vibration generated by one object forces another object into vibration can be explained using the example of two tuning forks with identical frequencies. When one fork is struck and vibrates and is then brought close to the other fork, the pressure changes generated from fork 1 push against fork 2, eventually setting it into vibration. When tuning fork 2 begins to vibrate, the resulting sound from both tuning forks is louder than the sound generated by tuning fork 1 alone. It is also possible to use a swing as an analogy: If you push a swing very gently, the first push will hardly move the swing from its rest position. If you keep giving gentle pushes, after a time the swing will start to move, and the more pushes you give it, the greater distance back and forth the swing will move (i.e., the greater its amplitude). The timing of the pushes is very important, however. To get the swing to move, the push has to be timed with the movement of the swing toward you, when it has reached its maximum amplitude, and just before it starts swinging back to its rest position. Timed like this, the swing's amplitude will increase. If you push the swing as it is still moving toward you, its amplitude will be decreased rather than increased. If you push the swing just as it is passing over its rest position on its way toward you, it will stop. In this analogy, you are acting as tuning fork number 1, and the swing corresponds to tuning fork number 2. Why does the amplitude increase in the way just described? Essentially, what happens with the tuning forks is constructive interference of incident and reflected waves traveling between the two forks. Because the two tuning forks have the same frequency, each small vibration arrives at exactly the right moment so that areas of compression and rarefaction combine constructively and the amplitude of the resulting wave increases (Figure 2.1). Further, if you stop tuning fork 1 from vibrating, tuning fork 2 will continue to vibrate. Tuning fork 2 has not created the original sound, just as in the swing analogy the swing has not created the original movement. Instead, tuning fork 2 is vibrating in response to the vibrations of tuning fork 1. In the analogy, the swing is set into vibration in response to your pushing it.

Forced vibration is the basis of resonance. In resonance, an object is forced to vibrate in response to the vibrations of another object. In the example above, tuning fork 1 creates the original sound, and tuning fork 2 responds to the pressure wave, resulting in constructive interference and increased amplitude of vibration. Tuning fork 1 supplies the **applied** (or **driving**) **frequency**, and tuning fork 2 is the **resonator**. The frequency at which the resonance occurs is called the **resonant frequency** (RF). The RF can be thought of as the frequency at which the resonator undergoes the greatest vibratory response. The closer the applied and resonant frequencies, the greater the amplitude of the response of the resonator.

Acoustic Resonance

Acoustic resonance occurs when an air-filled container or cavity is forced to vibrate by an applied frequency or frequencies. The phenomenon of resonance was described by Hermann von Helmholtz, who used a series of spheres of different sizes to identify frequencies present in complex sounds. Each of these spheres

Figure 2.1 **Forced vibration**

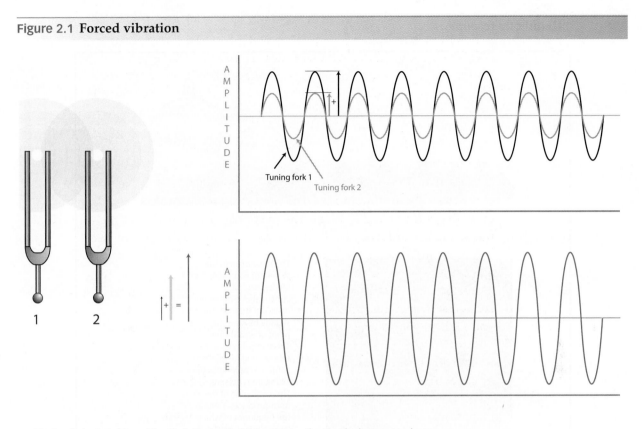

Tuning fork 1
Tuning fork 2

1   2

Tuning forks 1 and 2 are identical. Tuning fork 1 is set into vibration by being struck.
Vibration from tuning fork 1 forces tuning fork 2 into vibration.

Tuning fork 1 is said to be the "driver" and tuning fork 2 to be the "resonator".
Tuning fork 2 vibrates at the same frequency as tuning fork 1.

Incident and reflected waves traveling between the two tuning forks result in an increase in the amplitude of the sound.

consists of a body and a neck (Figure 2.2). The body contains a volume of air, and the neck contains a plug of air. The device works like a mass-spring system, with the enclosed air acting as the spring connected to the mass of the plug of air within the neck.

Helmholtz resonance occurs due to the elastic properties of air. When a sound wave is applied to the air in the container, the air is compressed and rarefied because air within the container acts as a spring that oscillates back and forth. Forcing the plug of air from the neck into the container by blowing across it compresses the air and increases the pressure within the container. Because air has elasticity, the air inside the container pushes the compressed air out again. The air flowing out passes beyond its equilibrium position, resulting in lowered pressure within the container. The air within the container continues to undergo compressions and rarefactions, with each cycle damping until the pressure changes die out. If another sound wave reaches the container at the same time that the compressed air is being pushed out, constructive interference causes increased amplitude of the sound

Figure 2.2 Helmholtz resonators

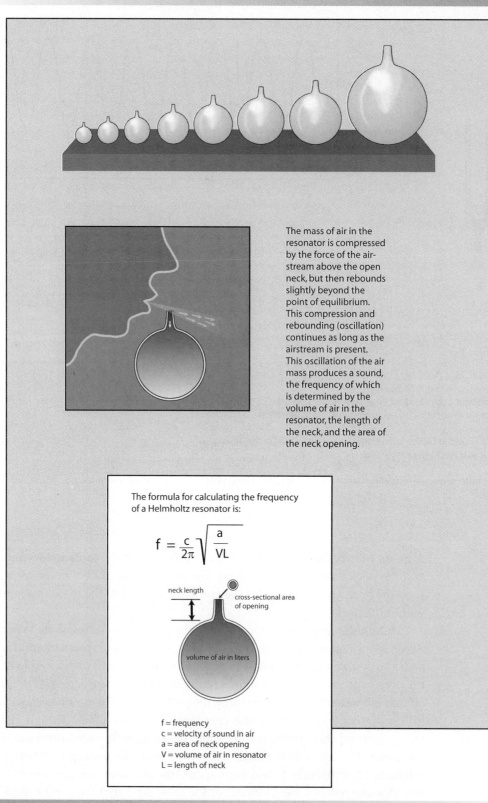

The mass of air in the resonator is compressed by the force of the airstream above the open neck, but then rebounds slightly beyond the point of equilibrium. This compression and rebounding (oscillation) continues as long as the airstream is present. This oscillation of the air mass produces a sound, the frequency of which is determined by the volume of air in the resonator, the length of the neck, and the area of the neck opening.

The formula for calculating the frequency of a Helmholtz resonator is:

$$f = \frac{c}{2\pi} \sqrt{\frac{a}{VL}}$$

neck length

cross-sectional area of opening

volume of air in liters

f = frequency
c = velocity of sound in air
a = area of neck opening
V = volume of air in resonator
L = length of neck

wave, as long as the applied frequency is close to the RF of the enclosed air. The RF of the air-filled container depends to a great extent on its volume and density. A smaller volume of air resonates more strongly to higher frequencies, whereas a larger volume of air resonates with greater amplitude to lower frequencies.

Many musical instruments are acoustic resonators in which the air is set into forced vibration. A good example is an acoustic guitar. The body of the guitar is a container with a round hole in the middle, and it is filled with air. The strings are stretched across the body of the guitar. When a string is plucked and set into vibration, a pressure wave is created. The vibration of the string sets air particles in the vicinity of the string into vibration, causing pressure changes to spread in all directions. Some of the pressure changes travel into the body of the guitar through the hole and force the air within the body, as well as the body itself, to vibrate. The air vibrates with the greatest amplitude at frequencies close to the frequency at which the string is vibrating. The string creates the driving frequency, and the air in the body resonates most strongly at this frequency. Due to constructive interference, a much louder sound is created. If the string were not stretched across the guitar, the resulting sound would be very soft. By forcing the guitar and the air inside it to vibrate with greatest amplitude at the frequency of the string, a much louder sound is created.

Tube Resonance and Standing Waves

Resonance occurs within any tube or pipe that contains air. The resonant frequency of a tube is related to the length of the tube, its geometry, and whether it has closed or open ends. Figure 2.3 illustrates how the length of a tube determines its RF.

Pressure waves within a tube create patterns that depend on how the incident and reflected waves inside the tube interfere. Resonance within the tube occurs in such a way that some points along the wave vibrate with minimum amplitude (called nodes) and others vibrate with maximum amplitude (called antinodes). In the case of a tube open at both ends, the pressure at both openings is equal to P_{atmos}. Therefore, the areas of greatest pressure always occur somewhere within the tube but never at the ends (Hixon, Weismer, & Hoit, 2008). This type of resonator is called a **half-wave resonator** because only one half of a wave fits in the resonator at any time.

In the case of a tube that is open at one end and closed at the other, the closed end acts as a fixed boundary. At the closed end of the tube is an antinode in the standing wave, while the open end creates a node in the wave because the pressure at that point is equal to the ambient pressure of the air outside the tube. The pattern of nodes and antinodes in the wave is spaced evenly throughout the tube and results in specific resonant frequencies within the tube. A tube resonator has multiple resonant frequencies, due to the fact that wavelengths of many frequencies have pressure distributions that fit the pressure requirements at the ends of the tube (Hixon et al., 2008).

A tube that is open at one end and closed at the other is known as a **quarter-wave resonator** because only one quarter of a wavelength can fit into the tube at any specific time. In a quarter-wave resonator, the lowest resonant frequency has a wavelength that is four times the length of the tube, and the higher resonant

Figure 2.3 Resonant frequency of a tube depends on its length

A hollow tube open at both ends is partially submerged in a column of water.

The column of air within the tube is set into vibration by a vibrating tuning fork held near the top of the tube.

By raising and lowering the tube into the column of water, the length of the column of air is changed and and the pitch of the sound produced is changed.

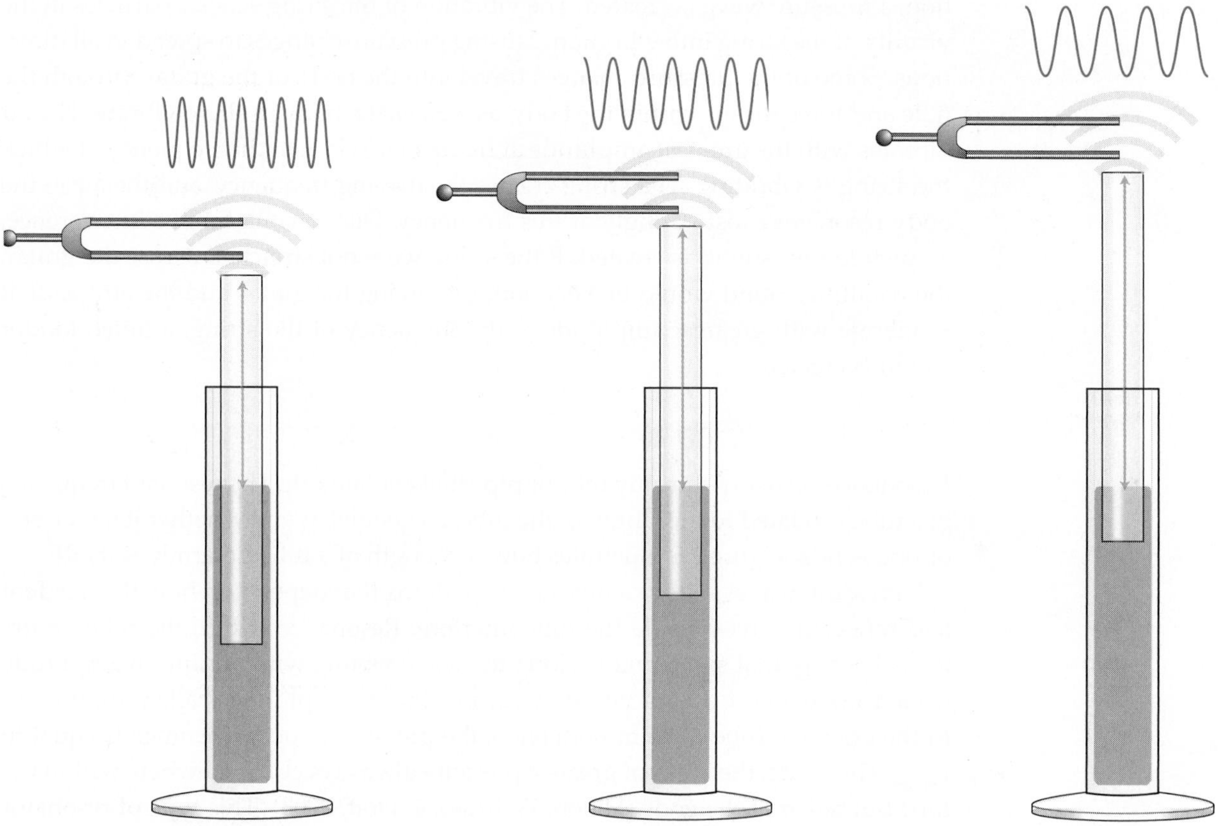

frequencies are odd number multiples of the lowest RF. When a driving frequency is introduced into the tube, incident waves travel within the tube and are reflected by the closed end of the tube. The incident and reflected waves are identical and travel in opposite directions, so their areas of positive and negative pressures occur at the same time and in the same location within the tube (Hixon et al., 2008). The wave therefore gives the appearance of being stationary rather than traveling through the medium and is called a **standing wave** (Figure 2.4).

Acoustic Resonators as Filters

Acoustic resonators are crucial in terms of speech production because of their filtering properties. The filtering can be illustrated using an example of a tube that is perfectly cylindrical along its length. This tube is an acoustic resonator because it

Figure 2.4 Standing waves

STANDING WAVES

A tightly stretched string such as a guitar string, when plucked, vibrates at its fundamental frequency and at other frequencies that are equal divisions or harmonics of that fundamental frequency. These vibrations travel back and forth between the ends of the string and reinforce each other rather than interfere with each other.

Because they are reinforcing each other, if you could watch these waves, (you can in online animations) they would not appear to be moving back and forth between the ends, but would rather appear to be stationary with maximum deflection at the antinodes and no apparent movement at the nodes (see bottom illustration).

For this reason, they are known as STANDING WAVES.

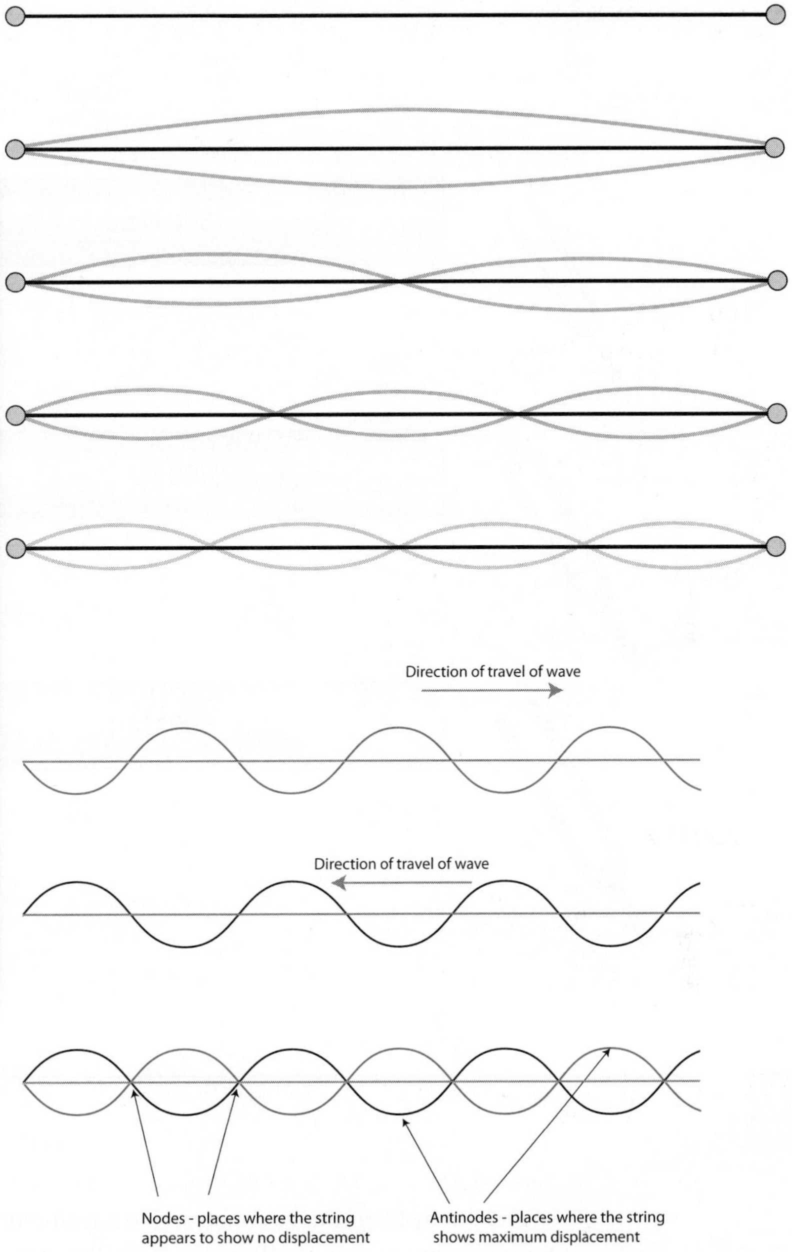

Direction of travel of wave

Direction of travel of wave

Nodes - places where the string appears to show no displacement

Antinodes - places where the string shows maximum displacement

is filled with air, and it has a RF of, say, 500 Hz. At one end of the tube is a series of tuning forks of different frequencies. If individual tuning forks were set into vibration and held up to the opening of the tube, some frequencies would be amplified, and others would be damped (Figure 2.5).

In this example, the effect of resonance is to amplify the frequencies that are closest to the tube's RF and attenuate the frequencies that are farther away from its RF. The tuning fork with a frequency of 500 Hz matches the RF of the tube, and the

Figure 2.5 Acoustic filtering

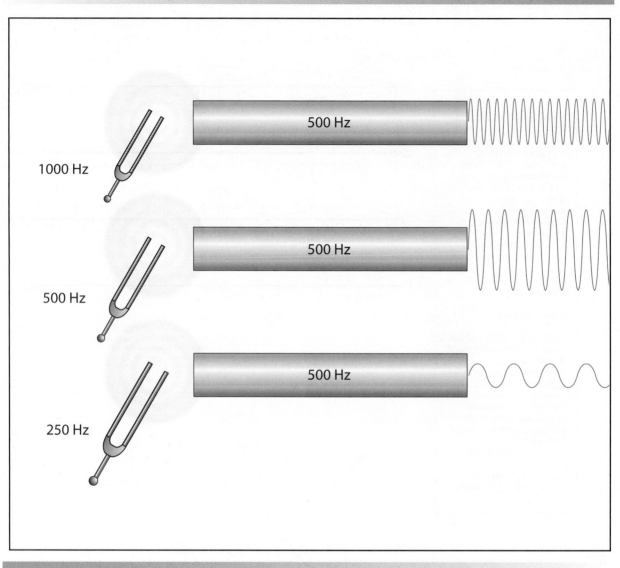

sound is amplified due to constructive interference. The farther the frequencies of the tuning fork are from the RF of the tube, the more the sound is attenuated because of destructive interference. Thus, the resonator acts as a filter by amplifying frequencies close to its own RF and attenuating frequencies farther away from its own RF. The filtering property of acoustic resonators allows humans to produce different sounds.

Bandwidth

Not all acoustic resonators are perfectly symmetrical, like the tube in the example above. Some containers are irregularly shaped or can even change their shape. The shape and other physical characteristics of the container—such as whether it is closed at both of its ends, open at both ends, or closed at one end and open at the other—determine the bandwidth of the resonator (Figure 2.6). **Bandwidth** refers to the range of frequencies that a resonator will respond to. A symmetrical tube like the one in the example will transmit only a narrow range of frequencies. The tube could have a bandwidth of 100 Hz. This means that it would respond to frequencies within 50 Hz below or 50 Hz above its RF. Frequencies between 450 and 550 Hz would be amplified, whereas frequencies below 450 Hz and above 550 Hz would be damped. This kind of resonator is said to be **sharply tuned**, or **narrowly tuned**. A narrowly tuned system responds slowly to the driving frequencies. That is, the amplitude of an applied vibration grows slowly until it reaches its greatest level. A narrowly tuned resonator is also lightly damped; once it has been forced into vibration, the vibrations take a relatively long time to fade away.

Figure 2.6 Uniform versus nonuniform resonator

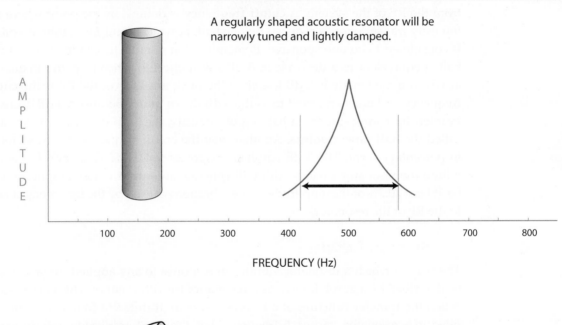

A regularly shaped acoustic resonator will be narrowly tuned and lightly damped.

AMPLITUDE

100   200   300   400   500   600   700   800

FREQUENCY (Hz)

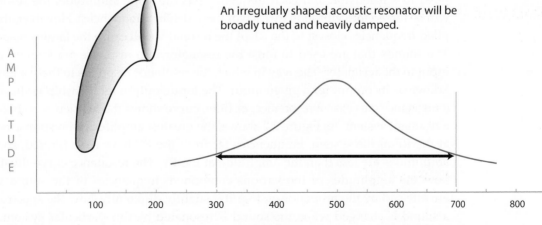

An irregularly shaped acoustic resonator will be broadly tuned and heavily damped.

AMPLITUDE

100   200   300   400   500   600   700   800

FREQUENCY (Hz)

Resonators that are more complex and irregular in shape tend to have wider bandwidths. An irregularly shaped container with an RF of 500 Hz might have a bandwidth of 400 Hz. Thus, frequencies between 300 and 700 Hz would be amplified, whereas those below 300 Hz and above 700 Hz would be attenuated. Such a resonator is more **broadly tuned**. A broadly tuned system will respond very quickly to the applied frequencies, but the vibrations will also fade more quickly. A broadly tuned resonator is heavily damped. Broadly tuned systems are common in speech and hearing applications and include the diaphragms of microphones, earphones, and loudspeakers, as well as eardrums and vocal tracts.

Cutoff Frequencies

Resonant systems seldom have a clear-cut point above which frequencies are amplified and below which they are attenuated. Instead, frequencies are transmitted with increasingly less efficiency as the driving frequency becomes farther removed from the RF of the system. A **cutoff frequency** is defined as the point where the intensity transmission is reduced by one half, at which point the resonant system is considered to be unresponsive. Remember that a reduction in intensity of one half is equivalent to a decrease of 3 dB (see Table 1.9). Therefore, the frequency at which the intensity is 3 dB less than the peak intensity of the RF is the cutoff frequency and is also referred to as the **3 dB down point**. Because a 3 dB decrease in intensity corresponds to a halving of intensity, the 3 dB down points are also called the **half-power points**. Another way the cutoff frequency can be stated is in percentage form. The 3 dB cutoff corresponds to 70.7%. Thus, any frequency within the resonator's bandwidth will generate an output whose amplitude will be at least 70.7% of the amplitude of the vibrations caused by the frequency closest to the RF of the resonator.

Resonance Curves

The way in which a resonator vibrates in response to any applied frequency can be described by a graph known as a **resonance** (or **filter**) **curve**. This curve is also called the **transfer function** of a resonant system. If different frequencies are applied to a resonator, and each frequency has the same amplitude, the resonator will be forced into vibration by each of these driving frequencies. However, the applied frequencies closest to the RF of the resonator will cause the largest response. The sounds that are used to force the resonator into response are known as the input to the resonator. The way in which the resonator responds to these sounds is known as its output for a given input. The input–output relationship is shown on a resonance curve; so a resonance, or filter, curve shows the frequency response of a resonant system. As Figure 2.7 shows, the greatest amplitude of response occurs at the RF of the system. Frequencies far from the RF have been filtered, so their amplitudes are less than the amplitude at the RF. The resonance curve illustrates how the amplitudes of the various component frequencies of the sound wave are affected by the resonator or, to put it slightly differently, how the spectrum of a sound is changed when the sound is resonated by this particular system. It is important to keep in mind that a resonance curve is not a sound wave, but describes the frequency response, or transfer function, of the resonator.

Figure 2.7 Resonance curve

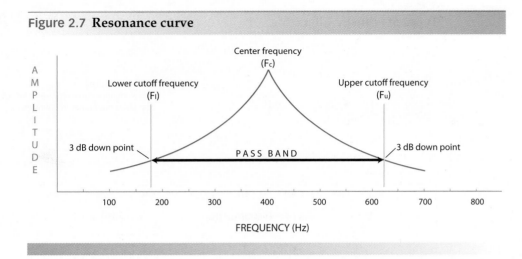

Parameters of a Filter

All resonant systems have certain characteristics. These include the resonant frequency, the upper cutoff frequency, the lower cutoff frequency, the bandwidth, and the attenuation or rejection rate. The resonant frequency is called the **center frequency** (F_c) on a resonance curve. This is the resonant frequency of the system that results in the greatest amplitude of vibration of the resonator. The center frequency depends on the physical characteristics of the resonator, such as its length and volume. In the example earlier, the center frequency of the tube was 500 Hz. The **upper cutoff frequency (F_u)** is the frequency above F_c at which there is 3 dB less intensity of response of the resonator than that at F_c. The **lower cutoff frequency** (F_l) corresponds to the frequency below F_c where the intensity is decreased by 3 dB. The bandwidth, or **passband**, refers to the frequencies between F_u and F_l, that is, the range of frequencies that the resonator will respond to. The bandwidth can be broad or narrow, depending on the physical characteristics of the resonator. The rate at which the resonator's amplitude of response is attenuated is known as the **attenuation rate**. It is also referred to as the **roll-off rate**, the **rejection rate**, or the **slope**. This parameter describes how rapidly the resonator decreases in its intensity of response to different frequencies and is measured in decibels per octave. Slopes can range from shallow to steep. A slope of less than 18 dB per octave would be considered fairly shallow. A filter with an attenuation rate between 18 and 48 dB/octave is moderately steep, while filters with cutoffs greater than 90 dB per octave are extremely steep (Rosen & Howell, 1991).

Types of Filters

Different types of filters are suitable for performing different types of functions. Four kinds of filters are commonly encountered in speech-language pathology and audiology (Figure 2.8). First is a **low-pass filter**, which responds to acoustic energy below a specific upper cutoff frequency. Acoustic energy above the F_u is attenuated at a particular rejection rate. Frequencies below the cutoff frequency are passed through the system, while those above the cutoff frequency are

Figure 2.8 **Types of acoustic filters**

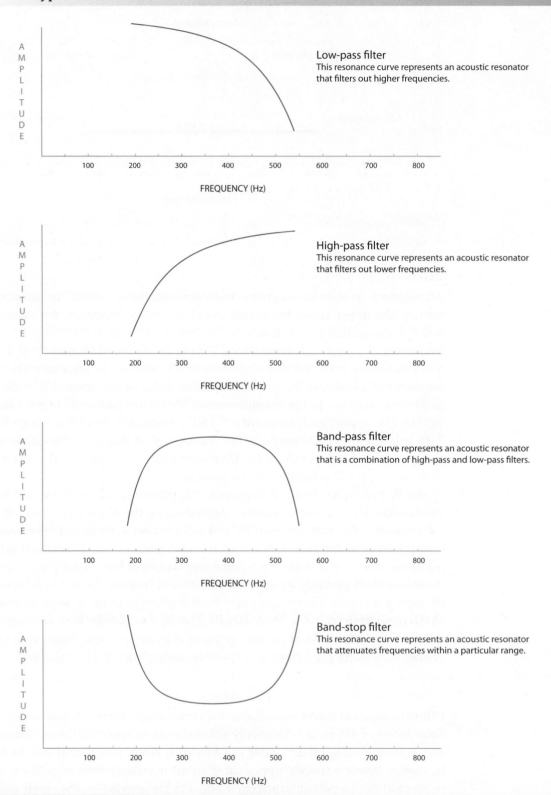

Low-pass filter
This resonance curve represents an acoustic resonator that filters out higher frequencies.

High-pass filter
This resonance curve represents an acoustic resonator that filters out lower frequencies.

Band-pass filter
This resonance curve represents an acoustic resonator that is a combination of high-pass and low-pass filters.

Band-stop filter
This resonance curve represents an acoustic resonator that attenuates frequencies within a particular range.

attenuated. Second is a **high-pass filter**, which passes energy above a designated lower cutoff frequency. Energy below F_l is rejected at a particular attenuation rate, while acoustic energy above F_l is transmitted through the system. Third, a **band-pass filter** passes energy in a particular range of frequencies between an F_l and F_u. Energy outside this range is rejected at a specific attenuation rate. A band-pass filter is a combination of low-pass and high-pass filtering. The low-pass filter transmits energy below the F_u, while the high-pass filter transmits energy above the F_l. The vocal tract is an example of a band-pass filter. Fourth, a **band-stop filter** attenuates frequencies within a particular range.

Vocal Tract Resonance

Human anatomy is uniquely suited to producing a wide variety of different sounds. The amazing capacity of our species to produce a range of sounds completely outside the scope of any other species is due to the distinct and unique evolution of the human vocal tract. Our ancestral species, such as *Homo erectus* and other species such as Neanderthals did not possess a vocal tract like ours. The vocal tracts of these species were much shorter, with the larynx positioned much higher in the neck than ours, between the first and third cervical vertebrae (Figure 2.9). Thus, such species could produce only a limited range of sounds. Only with our own species, *Homo sapiens*, do we find a larynx that is located much lower in the neck (between the fourth and seventh cervical vertebrae). This drop of the larynx resulted in a considerably longer vocal tract. An adult male's vocal tract is approximately 17 to 18 cm from the vocal folds to the lips. An adult female's is about 14 or 15 cm. A very young child's vocal tract is 6 to 8 cm in length and does not have the distinctive right-angled structure seen in adults (Vorperian & Kent, 2007).

Because the vocal tract contains the structures of the pharynx and the oral and nasal cavities, it has an extraordinary capacity to change and vary its shape. Every time one moves the tongue to a different position, or raises or lowers the velum, or opens or closes the lips and jaw, the shape of the vocal tract is changed. This ability to vary the shape of the vocal tract is what allows the wide range of different speech sounds to be generated.

Characteristics of the Vocal Tract Resonator

The vocal tract is a tube filled with air and therefore an acoustic resonator. As with all other tube resonators, it acts as a filter by selectively responding with greater or lesser amplitude to specific driving frequencies. The frequencies are produced either by vocal fold vibration or within the vocal tract itself. As an acoustic resonator, the vocal tract has certain characteristics. Four characteristics are of prime importance. First, the vocal tract can be thought of as a tube that is closed at one end (at the glottis) and open at the other end (the lips). The vocal tract is therefore a quarter-wave resonator. Second, because the vocal tract consists of the pharynx, oral cavity, and nasal cavities, it can be thought of as a series of air-filled containers that are connected to each other (Figure 2.10).

Figure 2.9 **Neanderthal versus modern human vocal tract**

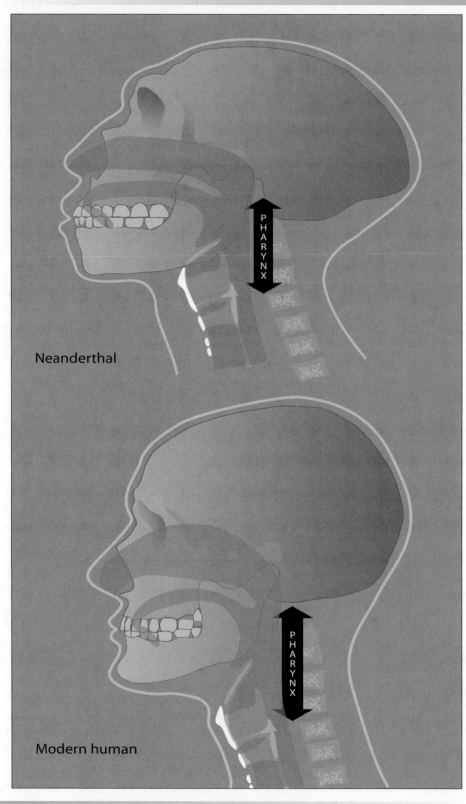

Figure 2.10 Vocal tract valves

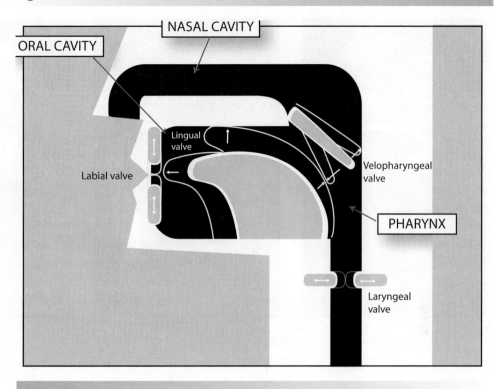

Each container has its own RF, and the overall RF of all these hooked-up containers together is different from each of the separate containers. Each cavity in the series acts as a band-pass filter to transmit certain frequencies within its bandwidth and to attenuate frequencies outside its bandwidth. Third, the irregular shape of the vocal tract makes it a broadly tuned resonator that transmits a wide range of frequencies around each RF. The fourth feature of the vocal tract is that it is a **variable resonator** whose frequency response changes depending on its shape. Each time a speaker moves his or her articulators into position for a different sound, the resonant frequencies of the vocal tract change because the cross-sectional diameter of the different cavities changes. The tube becomes more constricted in some areas and more open in other areas. The different areas of the cavities then resonate at different frequencies. Figure 2.11 shows different vocal tract constrictions and cross-sectional areas when producing the /i/ and /m/ compared with the schwa.

The resonant frequencies of the vocal tract are called **formants**. Being a tube resonator, the vocal tract resonates at numerous frequencies. Because it is a quarter-wave resonator, the higher formant frequencies are odd number multiples of the lowest formant frequency. The formant frequencies can be calculated based on the length of the vocal tract when the articulators are positioned for the mid-central schwa vowel (/ə/). In this articulatory position, the vocal tract has almost the same cross-sectional width throughout. The calculation is based on an adult male's vocal tract, which is about 17 cm long. Table 2.1 shows how the formant frequencies for the schwa vowel are derived.

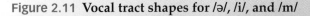

Figure 2.11 Vocal tract shapes for /ə/, /i/, and /m/

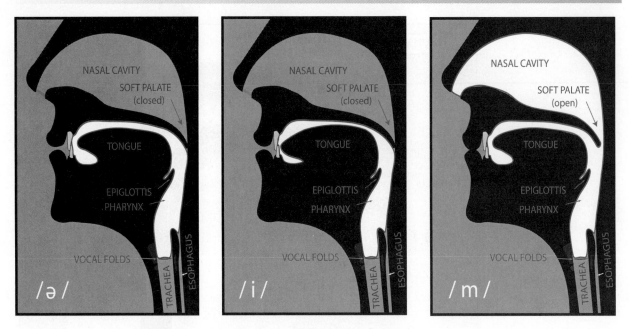

The red outline indicates the portion of the vocal tract that is acting as an acoustic resonator.

The vocal tract has very many resonant (formant) frequencies. However, because most of the acoustic energy generated by the vocal folds is at frequencies below 5000 Hz, typically only the first three formants are considered in speech production. The formants are numbered formant 1 (F_1), formant 2 (F_2), and formant 3 (F_3). F_1 is always the lowest in frequency. Changing tongue position from the neutral schwa to the position for a different vowel raises or lowers the formants from 500, 1500, and 2500 Hz to other resonant frequencies. Like any other resonator, the vocal tract will respond more strongly to driving frequencies that

Table 2.1 Calculation of Vocal Tract Resonant Frequencies for the Schwa Vowel for an Adult Male

Length of male vocal tract:	17 cm
Wavelength of lowest resonant frequency:	17 × 4 = 68 cm
Convert wavelength to frequency:	F = speed of sound divided by wavelength
	F = 34,000 cm per sec/68 cm
	F = 500 Hz
Higher RFs are odd-number multiples:	500 × 3, 500 × 5, 500 × 7, etc.
	1500 Hz, 2500 Hz, 3500 Hz, etc.

are within its bandwidth. The driving frequencies are those that are present in the complex periodic sound generated by vocal fold vibration. Like all complex periodic sounds, the glottal sound has a specific F_0 and harmonics that are whole number multiples of the fundamental. As the sound travels through the vocal tract, the F_0 and harmonic frequencies are amplified or damped by the vocal tract resonant frequencies (formants). The vocal tract is a broadly tuned resonator, so the bandwidth of each RF is relatively wide, and many harmonic frequencies that are reasonably close to an RF will be amplified. The sound that emerges from this filtering system has the same F_0 and harmonics as the glottal sound. What changes are the amplitudes of the harmonics: Some harmonics have been amplified, while others have been damped. Thus, it is the harmonic content and quality of the sound that has changed from its initial creation at the glottis to its emergence at the lips.

Source-Filter Theory of Vowel Production

The manner in which the vocal tract filters the glottal sound is formalized in the **source-filter theory** of vowel production, developed by the Swedish scientist Gunnar Fant in 1960. The theory takes the three elements involved in vowel production—the glottal sound, the vocal tract resonator, and the sound at the lips—and represents them on three graphs (Figure 2.12).

The first graph represents the glottal spectrum, showing the sound as it exists at the larynx before being modified by the filtering properties of the vocal tract. The F_0 has the greatest amplitude, with successively higher harmonics losing amplitude at a rate of 12 dB per octave. Acoustic energy up to around 5000 Hz is present. If it were possible to hear this sound, it would be perceived somewhat like a low-intensity buzz and not at all like any specific vowel sound. This first spectrum is known as the *source function* because the glottis is the source of the vowel sound. The second graph does not represent a sound but is a resonance curve representing the frequency response of the adult male vocal tract positioned for the schwa vowel, with resonances (formants) at 500, 1500, and 2500 Hz. This is known as the *transfer function.* The third spectrum represents the sound when it emerges at the lips, called the *output function.* In this spectrum, the glottal sound has been filtered according to the frequency response of the vocal tract. The same F_0 and harmonics are present in the output as in the glottal source. However, the amplitudes of the harmonics have been modified, resulting in a specific sound quality. These three graphs clearly illustrate how the sound generated by the vocal folds is modified by the resonances of the vocal tract. The theory shows graphically that when an adult male puts his articulators in position for the schwa vowel, the sound that emerges from his lips is characterized acoustically by the first three formants of 500, 1500, and 2500 Hz. Perceptually, what is heard is the schwa sound.

The source-filter theory also takes into account the effect that occurs when the sound traveling through the vocal tract is radiated beyond the mouth into the atmosphere. This effect is called the **radiation characteristic** and has to do with the lips acting like a high-pass filter when coupled to the atmosphere. This aspect of the source-filter theory is generally not emphasized to the same degree as the other elements of the theory.

Figure 2.12 **Source-filter theory**

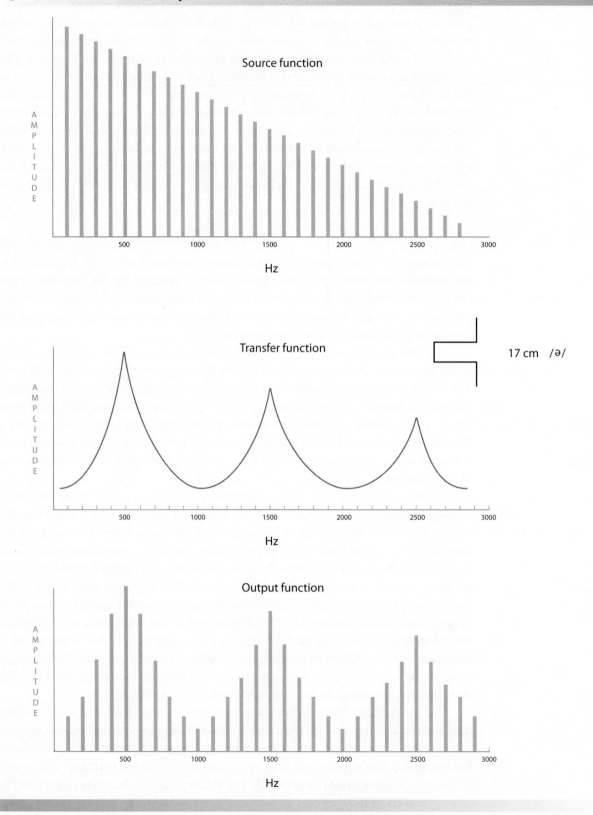

Formant Frequencies Related to Oral and Pharyngeal Volumes

As described above, the source-filter theory is based on a male's vocal tract positioned for the schwa vowel, with a relatively constant cross section. In this position, the cavities in front of and behind the constriction in the vocal tract where the sound is articulated (i.e., the oral and pharyngeal spaces) are roughly equivalent in terms of volume. For the other vowels, the vocal tract must change its shape in order to change its resonance characteristics. As the vocal tract changes in shape, the relationship between the oral and pharyngeal spaces changes as well. The formant frequencies are related to the volumes of the oral and pharyngeal spaces because containers of air will resonate at particular frequencies depending on their volume. In general, containers with a larger volume will respond most strongly to lower driving frequencies, and those with a smaller volume will respond more strongly to higher driving frequencies. The frequency of F_1 is related to the volume of the pharyngeal cavity as well as to how tightly the vocal tract is constricted. F_2 frequency is related to the length of the oral cavity. These volumes can be changed by moving the tongue to different positions. By raising the tongue toward the palate for the high front vowel /i/, the pharyngeal cavity behind the tongue constriction is enlarged and the volume of the oral cavity in front of the tongue constriction is decreased. This means that F_1 will be lower because the greater volume of the pharyngeal cavity resonates more strongly to lower harmonics in the glottal sound. F_2 will be higher due to the shorter length of the oral cavity, with resulting amplification of higher harmonics in the glottal sound (Figure 2.13). Conversely, by retracting the tongue and lowering it toward the floor of the mouth for the low back vowel /a/, the oral cavity is lengthened and the volume of the pharyngeal cavity is decreased. In addition, because back vowels are often articulated with lip rounding, the oral cavity is further lengthened. Therefore, F_1 will be higher because the smaller volume of the pharyngeal cavity will amplify the higher harmonics in the glottal sound. F_2 will be lower because the lengthened oral cavity will resonate to the lower harmonics in the glottal sound.

It should be clear from the discussion above that the F_1 and F_2 of different vowels vary systematically, depending on tongue height (vertical position of tongue) and tongue advancement (anterior–posterior position of tongue). It is important to keep in mind that formant frequencies also depend on the length of the vocal tract. The source-filter theory is based on an adult male's vocal tract. However, adult females have a shorter vocal tract than adult males, and children's vocal tracts are very much shorter than adults' (Figure 2.14). The resonances of a tube resonator such as the vocal tract are related to its length. The longer the resonator is, the lower its RFs and vice versa. Therefore, a woman's shorter vocal tract will resonate more strongly to higher frequencies than a man's, and an infant, with a vocal tract approximately half the length of an adult's, will have formants for the schwa vowel that are approximately double those of an adult male (1000, 3000, and 5000 Hz).

Each different vowel is characterized by a different pattern of formant frequencies. The output spectrum of each vowel is different because different harmonics in the glottal source have been amplified or attenuated, depending on how the vocal tract resonances have changed. Consequently, each vowel has a different quality.

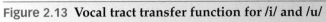

Figure 2.13 **Vocal tract transfer function for /i/ and /u/**

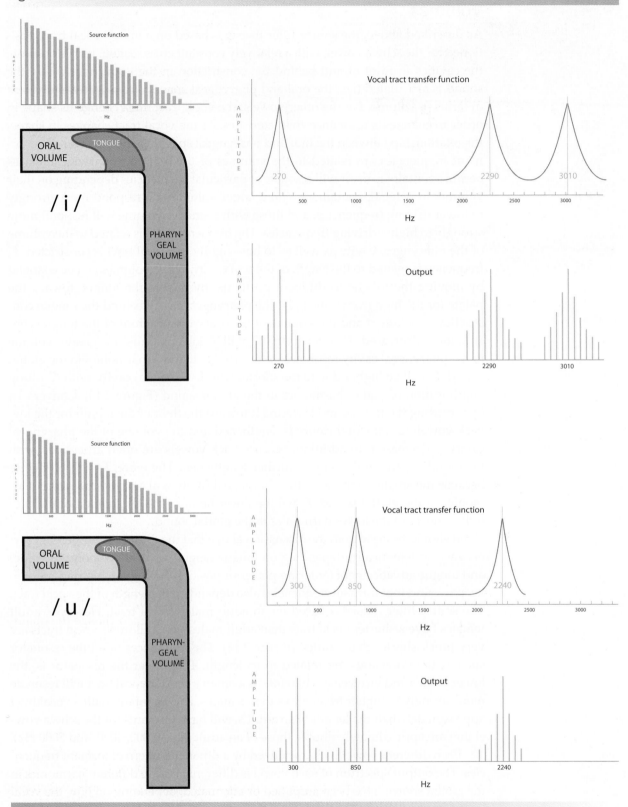

Figure 2.14 Adult versus infant vocal tract

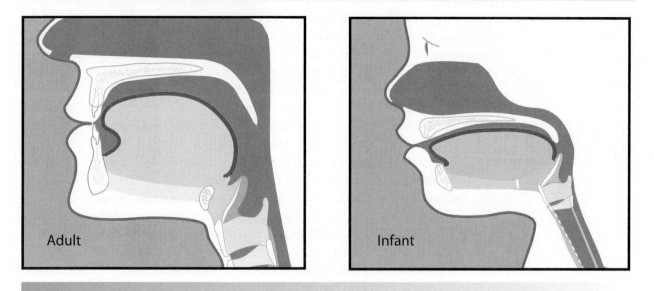

| Adult | Infant |

Every time tongue position changes for a different vowel, the filtering characteristics of the vocal tract resonator change correspondingly. Thus, there is a direct connection between articulation of vowels and the acoustic result of changing the resonant filtering properties of the vocal tract to generate different formant patterns.

An important point to keep in mind is that shaping the vocal tract in order to generate particular formants is essentially independent of vocal fold vibration. In other words, the source function and the transfer function are relatively independent. It is the rate of vocal fold vibration that gives rise to the F_0 of the periodic complex sound. The faster the rate of vocal fold vibration, the higher the F_0 that results and vice versa. In addition, the harmonic spacing of the sound wave changes according to the F_0. But this does not affect the vocal tract. When saying the /i/ vowel, no matter what the F_0, one's articulators are positioned to generate the formant patterns for /i/. These formants do not change, as long the tongue stays in the high front position. If one changes the F_0 (pitch) but keeps the tongue positioned for /i/, the filtering properties of the vocal tract remain constant, but the glottal source changes. On the other hand, a speaker can say /i/ at a particular F_0, perhaps at 150 Hz, and while keeping the F_0 constant, can change the quality of the sound by moving the tongue to a different position. In other words, tongue position can move from the /i/ to the /a/ or /u/, while maintaining the same F_0 for all three vowels. In this case, the source is constant, but the resonance and filtering properties of the vocal tract are changed.

Vowel Formant Frequencies

Vowels are characterized chiefly by the relationship among the first three formants. This relationship is the major factor in distinguishing between different vowels. In a way, vowels can be thought of as analogous to musical chords. Musical chords typically consist of three or more notes, such as C, E, and G or F, A, and C, and these notes are characteristic of that chord. Each vowel can be thought of as having a corresponding chord that is characteristic of that vowel. This analogy does not hold completely because the musical chord does not depend on the characteristics of the musician, and vowel formants do. Also, in a musical chord, the listener hears all the notes simultaneously, whereas a vowel is perceived as a single note. Nonetheless, this analogy can be a useful way of thinking about the structure of vowels.

Three elements can be manipulated to change the resonant frequencies of the vocal tract. These include the overall length of the vocal tract, the location of a constriction such as a blockage or narrowing along the length of the vocal tract, and the degree of constriction. Constrictions in the vocal tract result in a lowering of F_1. The tighter the constriction, the more F_1 is lowered. F_2 is lowered by a back tongue constriction, whereas a front tongue constriction will raise the frequency of F_2 and lower the frequency of F_1. Lip protrusion can increase the effective length of the vocal tract by about 1 cm, which will cause a decrease in the frequency of F_1 of about 26 Hz (Zemlin, 1998). In addition, the larynx may be raised or lowered by as much as 2 cm during the production of contextual speech, to increase or decrease the effective length of the vocal tract. This results in a concomitant shift in F_1 by as much as 50 Hz (Zemlin, 1998).

Keep in mind that formant frequencies depend on the length of the individual's vocal tract. Table 2.2 shows clearly that the frequencies of F_1, F_2, and F_3 increase from men's to women's to children's values.

What can also be seen in the table is the relationship between vowel height, vowel advancement, and formant frequency. Notice that for the front vowels, the highest in the series, /i/, has the lowest F_1. As the tongue decreases in height from /i/ down to /æ/, F_1 increases correspondingly. A similar relationship occurs for the back vowels. The highest vowel /u/ has the lowest F_1, and the lowest vowel /a/ has the highest F_1. Thus, there is an inverse relationship between F_1 frequency and tongue height: The higher the tongue position, the lower the F_1 frequency, and the lower the tongue position, the higher the F_1 frequency. A high tongue position increases the volume of the pharyngeal cavity, which therefore responds more strongly to lower frequencies in the glottal sound wave. Conversely, a low tongue position enlarges the volume of the oral cavity in front of the tongue constriction, decreasing the volume of the pharyngeal space, which therefore resonates to the higher frequencies in the source. The relationship can be summarized as follows: high vowels, low F_1; low vowels, high F_1.

F_2 is related to the length of the oral cavity—that is, the space in front of the tongue constriction for the vowel. The longer the oral cavity, the lower the frequencies to which it will resonate most strongly. Therefore, F_2 is associated with tongue advancement. Back vowels have a longer distance between the tongue constriction and the lips. Also, back vowels in English are typically produced with lip rounding, which further elongates the oral cavity. Because of the increased length of the oral cavity in back vowels, they are associated with a lower F_2, whereas front vowels, with shorter oral cavities, have higher F_2 values. Table 2.2 shows that the high front vowel /i/ has the highest F_2, which systematically decreases as tongue height decreases, giving the low front vowel /æ/ the lowest F_2 frequency of the front vowels. However, the lowest F_2 frequency of the front vowels is still

Table 2.2 Formant Values for Adult Men (M), Adult Women (W), and Children (C) for Front, Back, and Central Vowels

Front Vowels

	/i/			/ɪ/			/ɛ/			/æ/		
	F_1	F_2	F_3	F_1	F_2	F_3	F_1	F_2	F_3	F_1	F_2	F_3
M	270	2290	3010	390	1990	2550	530	1840	2480	660	1720	2410
W	310	2790	3310	430	2480	3070	610	2330	2990	860	2050	2850
C	370	3200	3730	530	2730	3600	690	2610	3570	1010	2320	3320

Back Vowels

	/u/			/ʊ/			/o/			/a/		
	F_1	F_2	F_3	F_1	F_2	F_3	F_1	F_2	F_3	F_1	F_2	F_3
M	300	870	2240	440	1020	2240	570	840	2410	730	1090	2440
W	370	950	2670	470	1160	2680	590	920	2710	850	1220	2810
C	430	1170	3260	560	1410	3310	680	1060	3180	1030	1370	3170

Central Vowels

	/ə/			/ɚ/		
	F_1	F_2	F_3	F_1	F_2	F_3
M	640	1190	2390	490	1350	1690
W	760	1400	2780	500	1640	1960
C	850	1590	3360	560	1820	2160

SOURCE: Information from Peterson & Barney, 1952.

higher than the highest F_2 frequency for the back vowels. For F_2 the relationship can be summarized as follows: back vowels, low F_2; front vowels, high F_2. In addition to increasing the length of the oral cavity, rounding the lips in back vowels increases the overall length of the vocal tract, resulting in generally lowered formant frequencies for back vowels.

F_1 and F_2 for the central vowels do not follow this systematic pattern relating to tongue height and advancement. Because of the centralized position of the tongue for these vowels, the formants are more evenly spaced.

F_1/F_2 Plots

F_1/F_2 *plots* are often used to graph formant information. This kind of plot, also called *vowel space*, or an *acoustic space*, is a graph with F_1 on the horizontal axis corresponding to tongue height and F_2 on the vertical axis relating to tongue advancement. One reads the F_1/F_2 chart for a vowel just the same as one would to find the coordinates on any graph: by looking at its position in relation to each axis. The plot in Figure 2.15 shows F_1/F_2 coordinates for the vowels /i/, /a/,

Figure 2.15 F_1/F_2 plots

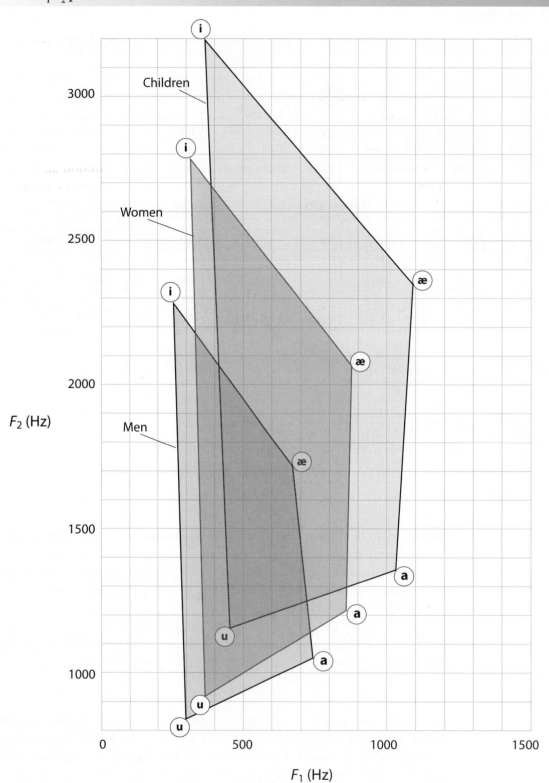

/u/, and /æ/ for men, women, and children, based on averages determined by Peterson and Barney in 1952. Looking at the /i/ for children, its F_1 can be determined by going downward and finding its value on the F_1 axis. To obtain its value for F_2, look across to the left at the F_2 axis. A plot like this can be calculated equally as well for individuals as for groups, making it a useful way of comparing individuals' and groups' formant frequency characteristics. There is considerable variability among speakers in the production of formants. One speaker's F_1/F_2 pattern for a particular vowel may be similar to a different speaker's pattern for a different vowel. In addition, the ages and genders of speakers influence their vowel formants. Reportedly, sex differences in the vowel space (lower formant frequency values for boys) start to become apparent by around age 4 years and become increasingly prominent with increasing age (Vorperian & Kent, 2007). The shape of the vowel space changes in a way that is consistent with growth patterns of the vocal tract. For example, it has been shown that between ages 14 to 15 years, males undergo a substantial lowering of the larynx, with corresponding increases in vocal tract volume. Acoustically, this is consistent with sharp drops of F_1 and F_2 frequencies for all the corner vowels (Vorperian & Kent, 2007). Girls show an increase in the vowel space only for the low vowels (Vorperian & Kent, 2007). The information presented in Table 2.2 and Figure 2.15 shows that the vowel /a/ can have a F_1 ranging from 730 to 1030 Hz, depending on whether it is produced by an adult male or a young child. F_2 ranges for this vowel from about 1090 to 1370 Hz.

Summary

An object that is vibrating freely does so without interference at a natural frequency determined by its length, density, tension, and stiffness.

Forced vibration occurs when the vibrations from one object set another object into vibration when the RFs of both objects are reasonably close to each other.

Acoustic resonance occurs when an air-filled container or cavity is forced to vibrate by an applied frequency or frequencies.

The RF of an air-filled container depends to a great extent on its volume and density: A smaller volume of air resonates more strongly to higher frequencies, and a larger volume of air resonates with greater amplitude to lower frequencies.

Standing waves are created in a tube resonator when incident and reflected waves of the same frequency interfere so that their areas of positive and negative pressures occur at the same time and in the same locations.

An acoustic resonator acts as a filter by amplifying frequencies close to its own RF and attenuating frequencies farther away from its own RF.

Narrowly tuned resonators respond slowly to driving frequencies and are lightly damped; broadly tuned resonators respond very quickly to the applied frequencies and are heavily damped.

The response of a resonating system can be graphed on a resonance curve that shows the center frequency, upper and lower cutoff frequencies, and bandwidth.

The vocal tract is a broadly tuned, variable, quarter-wave resonator with multiple resonant frequencies called formants.

The source-filter theory describes the modification of the sound produced at the larynx as it travels through the vocal tract and out the lips on three graphs: the source function, transfer function, and output function.

The frequency of F_1 is related to the volume of the pharyngeal cavity as well as to how tightly the vocal tract is constricted; F_2 frequency is related to the length of the oral cavity.

F_1/F_2 plots, also called vowel space or acoustic space, are graphs with F_1 on the horizontal axis corresponding to tongue height and F_2 on the vertical axis relating to tongue advancement.

REVIEW EXERCISES

1. Discuss the concept of resonance and explain how an acoustic resonator acts as a filter.

2. Identify the characteristics of the vocal tract in its capacity as an acoustic resonator.

3. Explain why the lowest resonant frequency of an adult male's vocal tract is approximately 500 Hz for the schwa vowel and why a young child's is approximately 1000 Hz.

4. Identify the three graphs in the source-filter theory and explain how each relates to the theory.

5. Discuss the relationship of F_1 and F_2 to the oral and pharyngeal spaces of the vocal tract.

3

The Articulatory System

STUDENT LEARNING OBJECTIVES

After reading this chapter you will

○ Become familiar with the structure and function of the articulators of the vocal tract.

○ Describe the traditional classification system of consonants and vowels.

○ Understand the link between articulation and the acoustic structure of phonemes.

○ Identify the acoustic and spectrographic characteristics of vowels and consonants.

○ Explain the role of suprasegmental factors and coarticulation in connected speech.

Articulation is the process whereby the structures within the vocal tract, such as the lips, tongue, and velum, modify exhaled air to shape specific speech sounds (phonemes). These structures move to come close to or make contact with articulators such as the teeth, alveolar ridge, and hard and soft palate. Moving the articulators to different locations and positions within the oral cavity modifies the sound wave traveling through the vocal tract, giving the sound specific characteristics that are recognized as distinctive phonemes. Much of the discussion in this chapter will focus on different phonemes, which are best transcribed using the International Phonetic Alphabet (IPA). Table 3.1 presents the IPA symbols for the consonants and vowels of English, as pronounced in many regions of the United States. Note that phonetic symbols are enclosed in slash marks to differentiate them from letters of the alphabet.

As described in Chapter 2, moving the articulators also changes the resonances of the vocal tract. To understand the processes of both articulation and resonation and the ways in which these processes can be disrupted by various problems, it is important to have a thorough understanding of the structure and function of the vocal tract and articulators.

Articulators of the Vocal Tract

The vocal tract is a hollow muscular tube around 17 cm long in adult males and somewhat shorter in adult females and children. The vocal tract consists of the cavities above the larynx—that is, the pharynx, oral cavity, and nasal cavities (Figure 3.1). The shape of the vocal tract is distinctive in several respects, which are all critical in articulation. First, the adult pharynx is shaped like a bent tube, with the oral and nasal cavities having a relatively horizontal position and the pharynx being relatively vertical. Second, the shape of the vocal tract is highly irregular and complex. Third, the vocal tract is variable in its shape. Every time one moves the tongue or lips or mandible, the shape of the vocal tract is changed.

Table 3.1 IPA Symbols for Consonants, Vowels, and Diphthongs

Consonants			
/b/	bed, cab	/s/	sun, bus
/d/	dog, red	/t/	toe, pet
/f/	fig, phone, laugh	/v/	valley, leave
/g/	girl, bag	/w/	wave, away
/h/	hat, perhaps	/z/	zoo, buzz
/j/	young, bayou	/ʃ/	ship, bush
/k/	cat, kick	/ʒ/	pleasure, beige
/l/	love, ball	/θ/	thin, bath
/m/	man, lamb	/ð/	these, weather
/n/	net, moon	/ʧ/	chime, batch
/p/	pot, top	/ʤ/	jump, giant, badge
/r/	rat, weary	/ŋ/	bang, singer

Vowels			
Front vowels		**Back vowels**	
/i/	she, legal	/u/	shoe, food
/ɪ/	hit, inside	/ʊ/	should, book
/e/	cake, ailing	/o/	photo, collate
/ɛ/	egg, federal	/ɔ/	awesome, flaw
/æ/	hat, snappy	/ɑ/	hot, argue

Central vowels	
/ə/	about, above
/ɚ/	mother, sister
/ɜ/	word, urban (minus "r" coloring)
/ɝ/	word, urban (with "r" coloring)
/ʌ/	up, under
Diphthongs	
/ɑi/	my, admire
/ɑu/	crown, shower
/ɔi/	boy, lawyer
/ei/	say, day
/ou/	show, snow

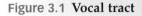

Figure 3.1 **Vocal tract**

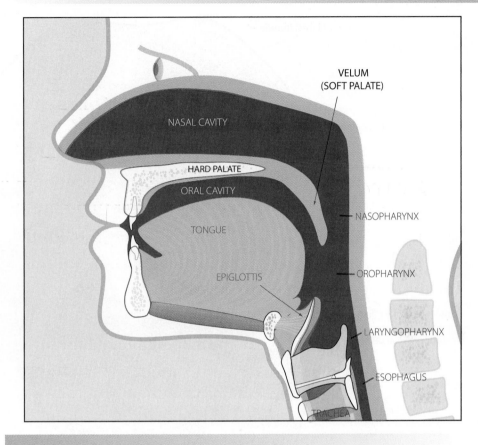

The vocal tract can be thought of as an interrelated system of movable and immovable structures that form a series of valves that can open and close either partially or completely. The upper and lower lips form a valve. The tongue can form valves at different locations by contacting the teeth, the alveolar ridge, the hard palate, or the velum. The velum forms a valve by touching the posterior pharyngeal wall. The valves channel or constrict the exhalatory airflow in certain ways to create different sounds. To understand how the valves function in speech production, the structure of the articulators that make up the valves must be appreciated.

Oral Cavity

The oral cavity (Figure 3.2) is a space, bounded by various structures. The front boundary of the oral cavity is movable, being composed of the lips. The sides of the oral cavity are formed by the cheeks, the palate acts as the roof, and the tongue makes up the movable floor of the oral cavity. The back of the oral cavity opens into the pharynx. The oral cavity is critical for many aspects of speech production. First, the opening of the oral cavity in front is the point of exit for most speech sounds. Second, the oral cavity contains important articulators, including the lips, teeth, alveolar ridge, hard palate, and soft palate (velum), as well as the tongue.

Figure 3.2 **Oral cavity**

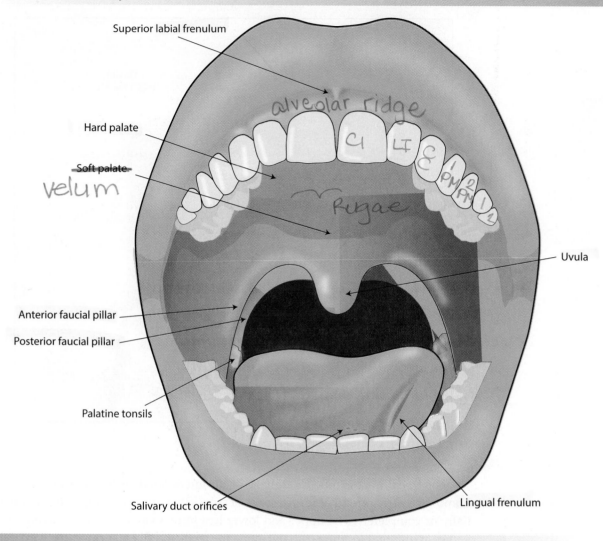

Superior labial frenulum

Hard palate

Soft palate

Anterior faucial pillar

Posterior faucial pillar

Palatine tonsils

Salivary duct orifices

Uvula

Lingual frenulum

[handwritten annotations on figure:] alveolar ridge, velum, Rugae, CI, LI, C, PM 1, PM 2, M 1, M 2

Third, the shape of the oral cavity is altered during speech, which is an integral aspect of resonance.

Lips

The two lips (adjective: labial; two lips: bilabial) are formed of muscle, mucous membrane, glandular tissues, and fat, all covered by a layer of epithelium. The underlying tissue of the lips is highly vascular, which gives the lips their characteristic red color, called vermilion. The inner surface of the upper lip connects to the midline of the alveolar region by a small flap of tissue called the **superior labial frenulum**. The lower lip is connected to the midline of the mandible by the **inferior labial frenulum**. The primary muscle making up the lips is the **orbicularis oris**. This is a circular or sphincteric muscle surrounding both the upper and lower lips. The orbicularis oris is not an isolated muscle—fibers from numerous other facial muscles insert onto it. These muscles move the skin wherever they insert. The elevators insert around the upper lip and raise it, while the depressors insert around the lower lip and lower it. Elevators include the levator labii superioris, levator anguli oris, zygomaticus major and minor, and risorius. Depressors include the depressor anguli oris, depressor labii inferioris, and mentalis. The numbers in Figure 3.3 correspond to the names of the muscles listed in Table 3.2.

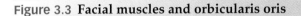

Figure 3.3 Facial muscles and orbicularis oris

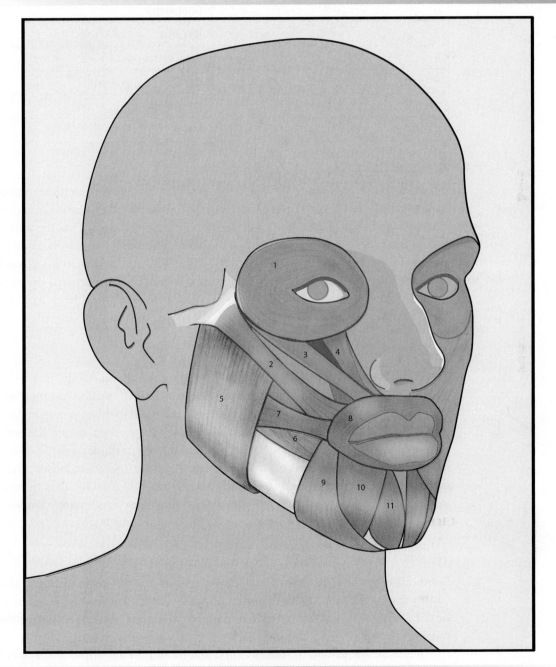

Table 3.2 Facial and Lip Muscles

1	Orbicularis oculi
2	Zygomatic major
3	Zygomatic minor
4	Levator labii superioris alaquae nasi
5	Masseter
6	Buccinator
7	Risorius
8	Orbicularis oris
9	Depressor anguli oris
10	Depressor labii inferioris
11	Mentalis

The muscles of the lips give them an enormous amount of mobility, allowing them to not only open and close very rapidly, but also to position themselves in many different ways. The lips can pucker more or less tightly, spread out to a greater or lesser extent, and assume many other positions. This flexibility and speed of motion are very important in the articulation of such sounds as /p/, /b/, /m/, and /w/. The lips are also crucial in mastication, acting to keep food and liquid within the mouth. Individuals with low muscle tone or with lip paralysis have difficulty in controlling the flow of saliva out of the mouth, as well as difficulty forming labial sounds.

Mandible

The mandible forms the lower jaw and is a large bone that has a distinctive angled shape. Figure 3.4 identifies the regions of the mandible in relation to other bones of the face and skull. The numbers in Figure 3.4 correspond to the numbers in Table 3.3.

The mandible is attached to the skull by a joint formed between the condylar process and the temporal bone. Called the temporomandibular joint, it allows the jaw to open and close—a crucial factor in both eating and articulation. The mandible can be protruded, retracted, and move from side to side. This permits the mandible to move in a rotary motion that is important in chewing. The jaw and lips often work as a unit in the production of bilabial sounds such as /p/ and /b/.

Teeth

Behind the lips are the teeth, arrayed in upper and lower sets (adjective: dental). Children have 20 teeth, 10 in the upper jaw (maxilla) and 10 in the lower jaw (mandible). Adults have 32 teeth, with 16 each in the upper and lower jaws. Humans have four types of teeth: incisors, canines, premolars, and molars.

Teeth are embedded in spaces called alveoli within the upper and lower jaws. Teeth are essential for biting, cutting, and chewing food, and they also play an

Figure 3.4 Mandible and skull

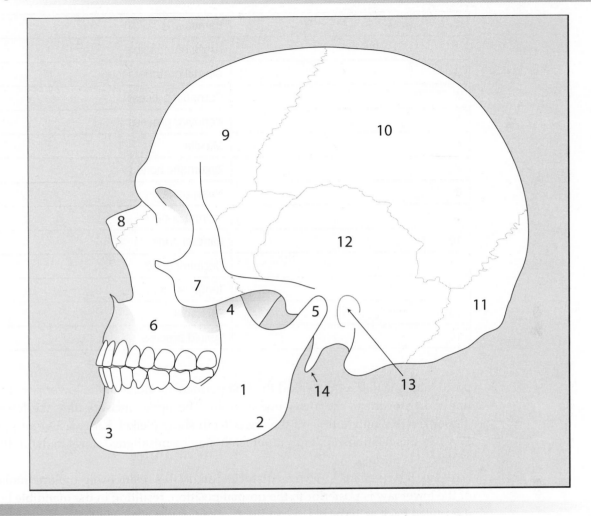

important role in speech production. They serve as an immovable articulator against which the tongue can form connections, and they also help to channel the flow of air and sound waves for some types of phonemes. The teeth are particularly important in directing the airflow for the /s/ sound and acting as an obstacle to increase the turbulence necessary for its correct production. The slushy quality of the /s/ produced by 6- and 7-year-old children with missing front teeth attests to the importance of the teeth in sound production.

Dental occlusion

The upper and lower teeth need to be in appropriate relationship to each other. If they are not, this can affect both eating and speech production. **Occlusion** refers to the relationship between the upper and lower dental arches and the positioning of individual teeth. Problems in upper and lower dental arch position and tooth relationships are referred to as **malocclusions**. There are three classes of occlusions.

Class I occlusion (see Figure 3.5) is also called **neutroclusion**. This is the normal occlusal relationship, in which the first permanent molar of the upper jaw is

Table 3.3 **Mandible and Skull**

1	Ramus
2	Angle of mandible
3	Mental protuberance
4	Coronoid process
5	Condylar process
6	Maxilla
7	Zygomatic bone
8	Nasal bone
9	Frontal bone
10	Parietal bone
11	Occipital bone
12	Temporal bone
13	Ear canal
14	Styloid process

positioned one half tooth behind the first permanent molar of the lower jaw. The upper arch overlaps the lower one in front. The upper incisors hide the lower incisors so that only a little of the lower teeth show (Seikel, King, & Drumright, 1997). In this relationship, individual teeth may be misaligned or rotated, but the occlusion is normal.

Class II occlusion is known as **distoclusion**. In this relationship the first molar of the lower jaw is posterior to the normal position, resulting in the mandible being pulled back or retracted, a condition called *overjet*. This kind of malocclusion often results from **micrognathia**, a structural problem in which the mandible is small in relation to the maxilla. *Class III occlusion* is referred to as **mesioclusion**. Here the first molar of the lower jaw is anterior to the normal position, with the mandible protruding too far forward, a condition called *prognathic jaw*. Similar to class II problems, this type of malocclusion is often found in craniofacial disorders.

Table 3.4 provides an outline of the occlusion classes.

Hard Palate

The hard palate (Figure 3.6) is a complex bony structure lined with epithelium; it makes up the roof of the oral cavity and the floor of the nasal cavity (adjective: palatal). It serves as a barrier between these two cavities, preventing food, air, and sound waves from escaping the oral cavity.

The anterior three-quarters of the hard palate are formed by the **palatine processes** of the maxilla. The maxilla is a large, complex bone, with projections called processes that articulate with other bones of the skull. The palatine processes join together at the midline and articulate at the **intermaxillary suture**. (A *suture* is an immovable

Figure 3.5 Occlusal relationships

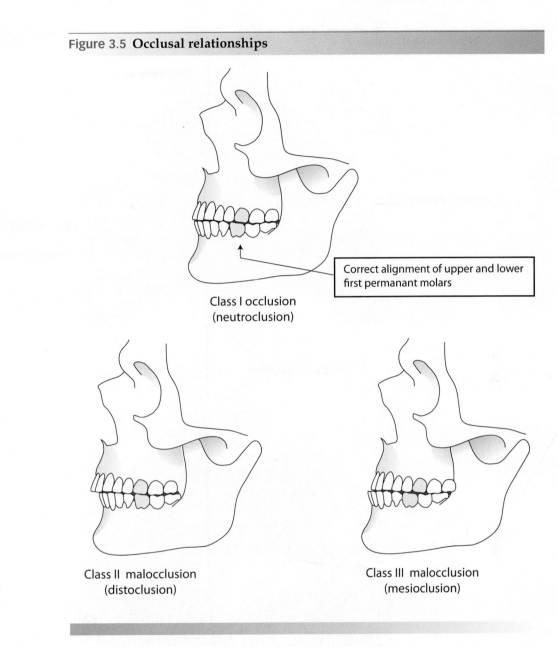

Correct alignment of upper and lower first permanant molars

Class I occlusion
(neutroclusion)

Class II malocclusion
(distoclusion)

Class III malocclusion
(mesioclusion)

Table 3.4 Occlusal Classes and Molar Relationships

Class	Occlusion	Molar Relationship
I	Neutroclusion	First molar of upper jaw is one half tooth posterior to first molar of lower jaw.
II	Distoclusion	First molar of lower jaw is posterior to normal position; mandible is retracted.
III	Mesioclusion	First molar of lower jaw is anterior to normal position; mandible is protruded.

braces *overbite*

surgery

Figure 3.6 Hard and soft palate

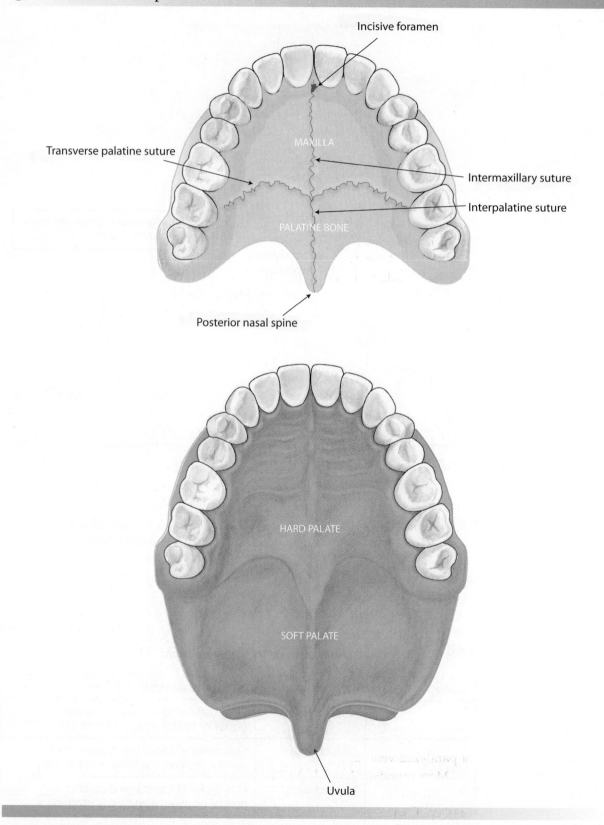

Incisive foramen

Transverse palatine suture

MAXILLA

Intermaxillary suture

Interpalatine suture

PALATINE BONE

Posterior nasal spine

HARD PALATE

SOFT PALATE

Uvula

joint.) The posterior one-quarter of the hard palate is formed by the **palatine bones** of the skull. These bones are L-shaped, and the horizontal surface of the L fuses at the midline, forming the posteriormost portion of the hard palate. The meeting of the palatine bones and palatine processes forms a suture called the **transverse palatine suture**. The palate is arched both back to front and side to side. This arch, or *vault*, differs considerably from one individual to another. In addition, the length, width, and height of the hard palate undergo considerable changes from childhood to adulthood. It has been reported that the palatal surface area is three times greater in adults than in children and that the volume of the oral cavity is six times larger (Hiki & Itoh, 1986).

The raised ridge running from side to side toward the anterior of the hard palate, a few centimeters behind the upper teeth, is called the **alveolar ridge** (adjective: alveolar). This ridge is formed by the alveolar process of the maxilla, a projection of bone containing spaces that hold the roots and nerves of the teeth. The alveolar ridge is the point of contact or approximation of the tongue for many of the speech sounds of English, including /t/, /d/, /s/, /z/, /l/, and /n/. The hard palate posterior to the alveolar ridge also serves as an immovable point of contact for the tongue in the articulation of many sounds, such as /ʃ/, /ʒ/, and /r/. Because the hard palate is instrumental in the production of many sounds, structural problems such as cleft palate can result in severe speech production difficulties.

Soft Palate

Posterior to the hard palate is the soft palate, so called because it is made of muscle and other soft tissues and contains no bone. It is also known as the **velum**. The velum (adjective: velar) consists of a number of muscles and a large flat tendon, the **aponeurosis**. This tendon attaches the velum to the posterior portion of the hard palate. Nerves, blood vessels, and glands are also located within the velum, which is covered by a mucous membrane. Being made primarily of muscle, the velum is able to move, and this movement is of prime importance in biological functions such as swallowing, as well as in speech production.

The velum at rest hangs down into the pharynx. This creates a passageway between the velum and the posterior pharyngeal wall called the **velopharyngeal passage**, or port (Figure 3.7). The velopharyngeal passage can be open or closed. Being movable, the velum is able to change its position—to raise itself up and back and make contact against the posterior pharyngeal wall. In the raised position it forms a barrier between the oral and nasal cavities so that air, sound waves, and food are prevented from entering the nasal cavities. This plays a central role in speech production, because exhaled air is forced to exit to the atmosphere through the oral cavity. When the velopharyngeal passage is open, the oral and nasal cavities are said to be coupled. When they are coupled, air is free to enter and exit the respiratory system through the nasal cavities. Sound waves are also free to travel into the nasal cavities. So is food, which can be a problem in cases of cleft palate or paralyzed velum.

Most sounds in English are *oral*—that is, they are produced with oral airflow. Only three sounds in English are formed with airflow exiting through the nasal cavities. These *nasal* sounds are /m/, /n/, and /ŋ/. Problems in velopharyngeal

Figure 3.7 Velopharyngeal passage

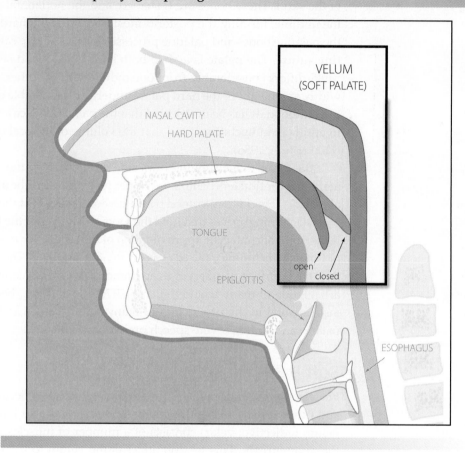

function can result in air escaping through the nasal cavities rather than through the oral cavity. This can result in **hypernasality** (excessive nasal resonance) and distortion of oral sounds. Problems can also occur when air is prevented from entering the nasal cavities for the production of nasal sounds, resulting in **hyponasality**, or insufficient nasal resonance.

The velum also forms a point of contact for the tongue in the production of the /g/, /k/, and /ŋ/ sounds.

Muscles of the velum

Five muscles make up the velum; some elevate the velum and others depress it. Table 3.5 lists the muscles of the velum and their functions, and Figure 3.8 shows these muscles.

The **levator veli palatini** muscle makes up the bulk of the velum, and its sling-like arrangement of fibers is instrumental in elevating the velum to close the velopharyngeal port. The **musculus uvuli** is located on the nasal surface of the velum. It "bunches up" the velum (Seikel et al., 1997) and also raises it. The **tensor veli palatini** used to be considered a tensor of the velum (hence its name), but it has been shown that this muscle is more involved with the function of the Eustachian tube. The fibers of the tensor veli palatini course downward and terminate in a

Table 3.5 **Muscles of the Velum**

Muscle	Attachments	Function	Notes
LVP	Temporal bone and medial wall of auditory tube cartilage to palatal aponeurosis	Raises velum	Fibers from left and right sides join; forms a sling for the velum
MU	Posterior part of palatine bones and palatal aponeurosis to mucous membrane cover of velum	Shortens and raises velum	Fibers run the length of the velum on the nasal surface
TVP	Sphenoid bone of skull and lateral wall of Eustachian tube to tendon that expands to form the palatal aponeurosis	Opens Eustachian tube	Used to be considered a tensor
PG	Front and sides of palatal aponeurosis to lateral margins of posterior tongue	Depresses velum or elevates tongue	Forms anterior faucial pillars
PP	Various origins, including anterior hard palate and midline of velum to posterior thyroid cartilage	Narrows pharyngeal cavity	Forms posterior faucial pillars

NOTE: LVP, levator veli palatini; MU, musculus uvuli; TVP, tensor veli palatini; PG, palatoglossus; PP, palatopharyngeus.

tendon. This tendon then changes direction from downward to medial, and the left and right sides of the tendon merge and expand to become the palatal aponeurosis. Contraction of the tensor veli palatini opens the Eustachian tube, which is normally closed. Opening of the Eustachian tube occurs during swallowing and allows air pressures within and outside the middle ear to equalize. The **palatoglossus** muscle depresses the velum. It forms one of the arched pillars that is visible when looking in the oral cavity toward the throat. There are two of these pillars on either side of the pharynx, called the *anterior and posterior faucial pillars*, and they mark the posterior boundary of the oral cavity (see Figure 3.2). The **palatopharyngeus** is a muscle of both the velum and the pharynx. It forms the posterior faucial pillars. The palatopharyngeus narrows the pharyngeal cavity and thus helps to guide food into the lower pharynx during swallowing.

Velopharyngeal closure

In order to close off the velopharyngeal port, the velum raises itself upward and backward and contacts the posterior pharyngeal wall. However, this movement of the velum is not a "trapdoor" motion; that is, the velum does not just swing up and down. Rather, the lateral walls of the pharynx are also involved in velopharyngeal motion. Even when the velum is fully in contact with the posterior pharyngeal

Figure 3.8 **Muscles of the velum**

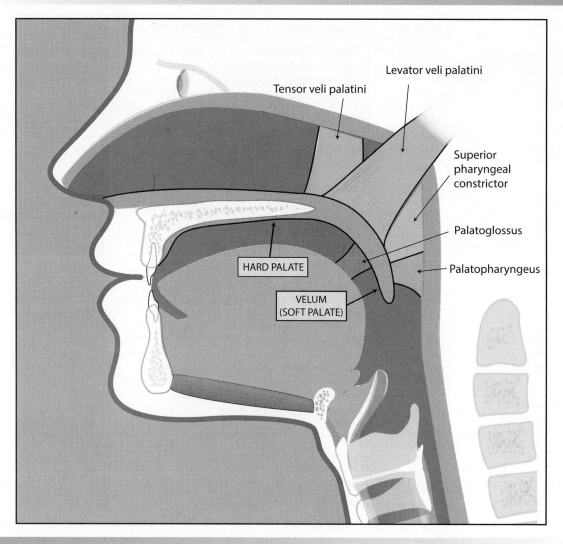

wall, if there is no movement of the lateral pharyngeal walls, air can escape around the sides of the velum and into the nasal cavities (Golding-Kushner, 1997). The velopharyngeal valve consists of the velum itself, the posterior wall of the pharynx, and the lateral walls of the pharynx. Four types of velopharyngeal closure have been observed, and they have been categorized on the basis of different contributions of velar and pharyngeal wall motion. Individuals tend to use one particular type of pattern more than the others. Table 3.6 describes these patterns of closure.

Tongue

The tongue is a large, muscular structure that occupies a good portion of the oral cavity (Figure 3.9). Because of the number of muscles making up the tongue and the way in which these muscles are intertwined with each other, the tongue has an enormous degree of flexibility and speed in its movements. The tongue is essential in many functions, including chewing, swallowing, and speaking. The tongue is,

Table 3.6 Types of Velopharyngeal Closure and Relative Contribution of Velar and Lateral Pharyngeal Wall (LPW) Movement

Type	Closure Pattern
Coronal	Mostly velar movement, with small amount of LPW movement
Sagittal	Mostly LPW movement, with small amount of velar movement
Circular	Approximately equal contribution of velar and LPW movement
Circular with Passavant's ridge	Movement of velum and LPW plus forward movement of Passavant's pad on the posterior pharyngeal wall

Figure 3.9 Tongue

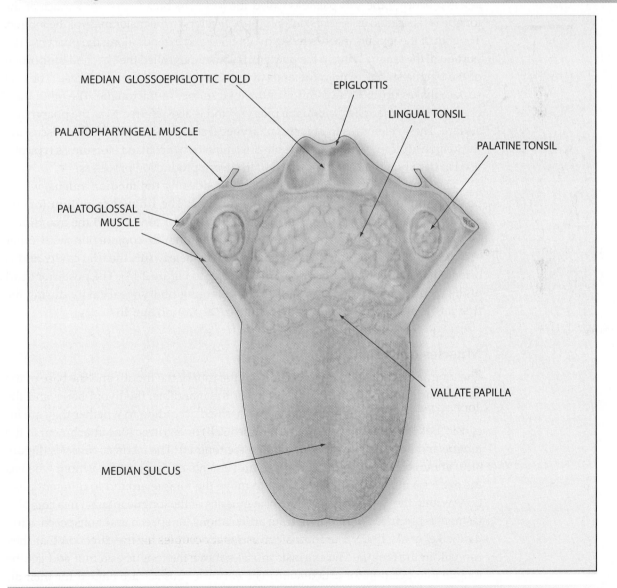

MEDIAN GLOSSOEPIGLOTTIC FOLD

EPIGLOTTIS

LINGUAL TONSIL

PALATOPHARYNGEAL MUSCLE

PALATINE TONSIL

PALATOGLOSSAL MUSCLE

VALLATE PAPILLA

MEDIAN SULCUS

without doubt, the most important and the most active of the articulators. It modifies the shape and thus the resonance characteristics of the oral cavity. It also acts as a valve by contacting or closely approximating other articulators and modifying the airstream flowing through the oral cavity.

The tongue is an example of a **muscular hydrostat** (Napadow, Chen, Wedeen, & Gilbert, 1999; Takemoto, 2001). This term is applied to muscular organs that do not have a skeleton of cartilage or bone but provide their own support through muscular contraction. By selectively contracting certain muscles, the muscular hydrostat can make a rigid support for movements of other parts of the tongue. This system allows different regions of the tongue to function semi-independently of each other. The anterior-most portion of the tongue is the *tip*, or *apex.* Just posterior to the tip is the *blade.* The blade is the part of the tongue that lies below the alveolar ridge when it is at rest. The part of the tongue lying just below the hard palate is called the *front*, and the part situated beneath the soft palate is called the *back.* The broad superior surface of the tongue is referred to as the *dorsum*, and the *body* refers to the major mass of the tongue. The root of the tongue attaches to the hyoid bone and extends along the pharynx. The portion of the tongue lying in the pharynx is sometimes called the *base,* and the portion of the tongue surface within the oral cavity is referred to as the *oral tongue.* The oral surface makes up about two-thirds of the total surface of the tongue. The other third of the tongue surface lies within the pharynx and is also referred to as the pharyngeal surface. These references to oral and pharyngeal surfaces are useful when discussing the tongue's role in swallowing; the other terminology (tip, blade, dorsum) is typically used in discussing the tongue's function in speech production processes.

The tongue is divided into right and left sides by the **median sulcus**, which provides the origination for some of the muscles. The **lingual frenulum** (or frenum) is a band of connective tissue joining the inferior tongue and the mandible.

The anatomy of the tongue develops over time, in conjunction with other structures of the vocal tract. A newborn's tongue nearly fills the oral cavity and is oriented primarily in the horizontal plane (refer to Figure 2.14). The posterior third of the tongue gradually descends into the enlarging pharyngeal cavity during the first few years of life and attains its adult size at around age 16.

Muscles of the tongue

The tongue is suspended by muscles from the roof of the mouth and the base of the skull, attaching also to the inner surface of the mandible, the hyoid bone, and the pharynx. The muscles of the tongue are classified according to whether they are intrinsic (both attachments within the tongue itself) or extrinsic (one attachment in the tongue and one in a structure external to the tongue). The intrinsic muscles (Figure 3.10) are involved in adjusting the fine movements of shape and position, whereas the extrinsic muscles (Figure 3.11) act to move the tongue around to different positions within the oral cavity. The intrinsic muscles of the tongue interact in a complex fashion to produce the rapid, delicate articulations for speech and nonspeech activity (Seikel et al., 1997). The intrinsic muscles are named for the direction that they run within the tongue. The extrinsic muscles move the tongue as a unit and get the tongue into position for articulation. The extrinsic muscles are named for their attachments. Table 3.7 lists the extrinsic and intrinsic muscles.

Figure 3.10 Intrinsic muscles of the tongue

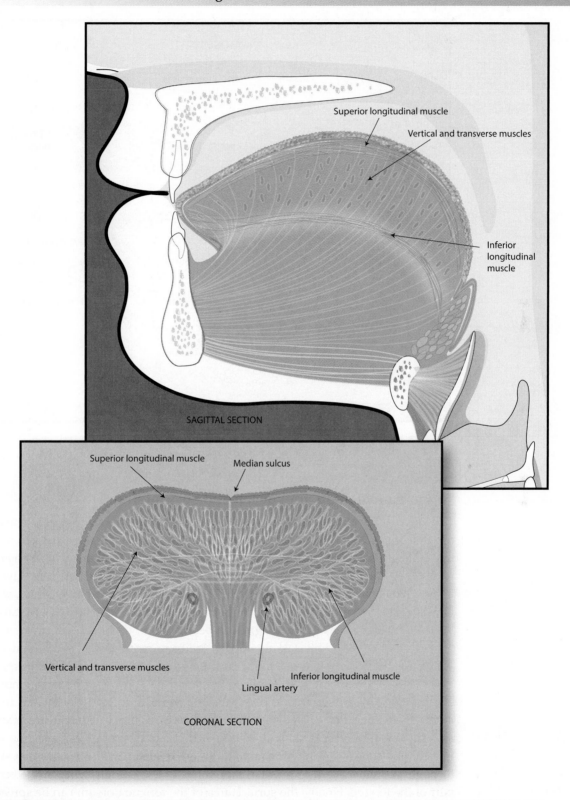

Superior longitudinal muscle

Vertical and transverse muscles

Inferior longitudinal muscle

SAGITTAL SECTION

Superior longitudinal muscle

Median sulcus

Vertical and transverse muscles

Inferior longitudinal muscle

Lingual artery

CORONAL SECTION

Figure 3.11 Extrinsic muscles of the tongue

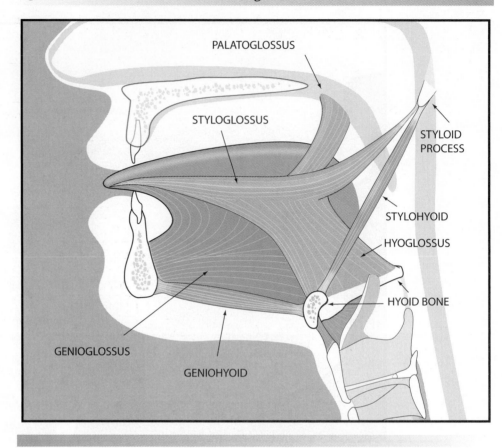

Tongue movements for speech and swallowing

The tongue is by far the most complex and the most important organ of articulation (e.g., Iskarous, 2003). Most of the tongue muscles can be activated in such a way that different segments of the tongue can be moved simultaneously and be active to different degrees (Sokoloff, 2000; Stone, Parthasarathy, Iskarous, NessAiver, & Prince, 2003). Further, neural input to the tongue muscles is extremely dense, which facilitates the fine motor control of tongue shape (Mu & Sanders, 2010). Because of this muscular complexity, the tongue can be moved around in an enormous range of ways and at incredibly fast rates. The ability to move in many different ways allows for the wide range of tongue positions and configurations during speech. Hardcastle (1976) described several movement types: The tongue body can move in a horizontal forward–backward plane and in a vertical upward–downward movement. The tip and blade can also move in a horizontal forward–backward manner, as well as vertically upward and downward. The tongue body can position itself in a convex–concave shape in relation to the palate and can also extend that shape throughout the whole length of the tongue, resulting in a grooving of the central part of the tongue. Finally, the surface area of the tongue dorsum can be spread or tapered. Green and Wang (2003) described four basic patterns of tongue movements

Table 3.7 Intrinsic and Extrinsic Muscles of the Tongue

Muscle	Attachments	Function
Intrinsic		
Superior longitudinal	Hyoid bone and median septum to lateral margins and apex	Elevates tip
Inferior longitudinal	Root of tongue and hyoid bone to apex	Pulls down tip; retracts tongue
Transverse	Median septum to lateral margins in the submucous tissue	Pulls edges toward midline to narrow tongue
Vertical	Mucous membrane of tongue dorsum to lateral and inferior surfaces of tongue	Pulls down tongue
Extrinsic		
Genioglossus	Inner surface of mandible to tip and dorsum of tongue and to hyoid bone	Contraction of anterior fibers retracts tongue; contraction of posterior fibers draws tongue forward
Hyoglossus	Hyoid bone to lateral margins of tongue	Pulls down sides of tongue
Palatoglossus	Front and sides of palatal aponeurosis to lateral margins of posterior tongue	Elevates back of tongue
Styloglossus	Styloid process of temporal bone to lateral margins of tongue	Elevates and retracts tongue

for speech: raising of the blade with simultaneous lowering of the dorsum (seen with alveolar sounds and palatal sounds), raising the body (seen with the palatal /j/ phoneme), raising the dorsum (seen with velar sounds), and raising the anterior blade with lowering of the body (seen with the lateral /l/ sound).

Speech sounds utilize a combination of different types of tongue movements. The vowels are motorically the least complex sounds, using primarily horizontal and vertical movements of the tongue body. Alveolar stops /t/ and /d/ involve much more complex movements of the tongue body and tip. Fricatives such as /s/ require even more complex interactions between the tongue muscles and movements. Understanding the motoric complexity of the /s/ and the many different muscles and movements that are involved in producing the sound helps to appreciate why so many young children have difficulty with this sound (e.g., Miccio & Ingrisano, 2000). Similarly, the /r/ sound, because of the muscular dexterity required, is difficult for young children. In fact, it is not uncommon for children to develop the muscular ability to say these sounds properly only at age 7 or 8. As the child matures, he or she gains more independence in using articulators that are in close proximity to each other (Nittrouer, Studdert-Kennedy, & Neely, 1996).

The tongue also plays a central role in swallowing; it moves food to and from the teeth for chewing, forms the chewed food into a ball (bolus), pushes the chewed food backwards to the posterior oral cavity, directs the bolus into the pharyngeal cavity, then pushes the bolus against the pharyngeal wall to move it downward, toward the esophagus (Youmans & Stierwalt, 2006). The tongue is involved in taste sensations, and also helps to detect tactile and heat stimuli. Taste buds are located between papillae on the surface of the tongue. Papillae are small elevations that help create friction between the tongue and the bolus, and may also contain taste buds. The human tongue has on average around 2000–8000 taste buds.

Pharynx

The pharynx plays a role in many functions, including swallowing, respiration, and speech. In terms of speech, it is particularly important in resonance. The pharynx is a long hollow tube made of muscle, connective tissue, and mucous lining, running behind the nasal cavities, oral cavity, and larynx. It is about 12 cm long and about 4 cm wide at the top end. It narrows, until at its bottom end it is only about 2.5 cm in width (Zemlin, 1998). The portion of the pharynx located behind the nasal cavities is called the **nasopharynx**, the section behind the oral cavity is the **oropharynx**, and the part behind the larynx is known as the **laryngopharynx** (see Figure 3.1). The laryngopharynx leads into the esophagus, posterior to the trachea. The esophagus is the part of the digestive system that leads into the stomach.

Muscles of the Pharynx

The major muscles of the pharynx (Figure 3.12) are the **pharyngeal constrictors**. These are fan-shaped muscles that overlap one another rather like roof shingles (Kent, 1997b). The inferior constrictor is the largest and strongest of the pharyngeal constrictors. It originates from the sides of the thyroid cartilage and then wraps around the lower to midregions of the pharynx (Kent, 1997b). At the lower margin of the inferior constrictor is another muscle, the **cricopharyngeus muscle**. This muscle arises from the cricoid cartilage and forms a ring around the top opening of the esophagus. It is usually referred to as the **pharyngo esophageal segment (P E segment)**. The cricopharyngeus muscle remains contracted during rest and relaxes during swallowing in order to allow food to pass into the esophagus (Tjoa, 2011). The middle constrictor extends from the hyoid bone and forms the middle portion of the pharynx. Above the middle constrictor is the superior constrictor. This muscle originates from many locations in and around the soft palate and forms the topmost section of the pharynx. The complex muscular structure of the pharynx acts to constrict the pharynx during swallowing. Other muscles of the pharynx (the stylopharyngeus and salpingopharyngeus) help to elevate and open the pharynx. An important structure located in the lateral walls of the nasopharynx is the Eustachian tube, which links the pharynx to the middle ear (Figure 3.13).

Nasal Cavities

The structure of the nasal cavities (Figure 3.14) is surprisingly complex, being formed by the fusion of many of the bones of the skull. The nose is divided into two cavities by the **nasal septum**. Three tiny structures, the inferior, middle, and superior **nasal conchae** (singular: concha, also called turbinates) form each side of the nose. The nasal cavities are lined with mucous membrane that has cilia embedded in it. This helps to warm, moisturize, and filter inhaled air. The nasal cavity is important in the resonating of the nasal sounds in English (/m/, /n/, and /ŋ/).

Figure 3.12 Muscles of the pharynx

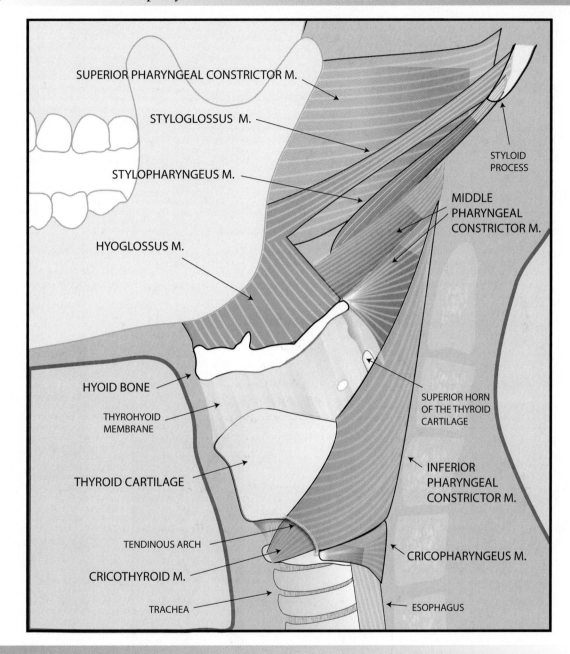

Valves of the Vocal Tract

The vocal tract can be conceptualized as a hollow tube that contains a series of valves that regulate the flow of air by opening and closing in various ways (refer to Figure 2.10). The valves are made up of the articulators, which come together in varying degrees and separate in various manners, thus constricting or obstructing the airstream in specific ways.

Figure 3.13 Eustachian tube

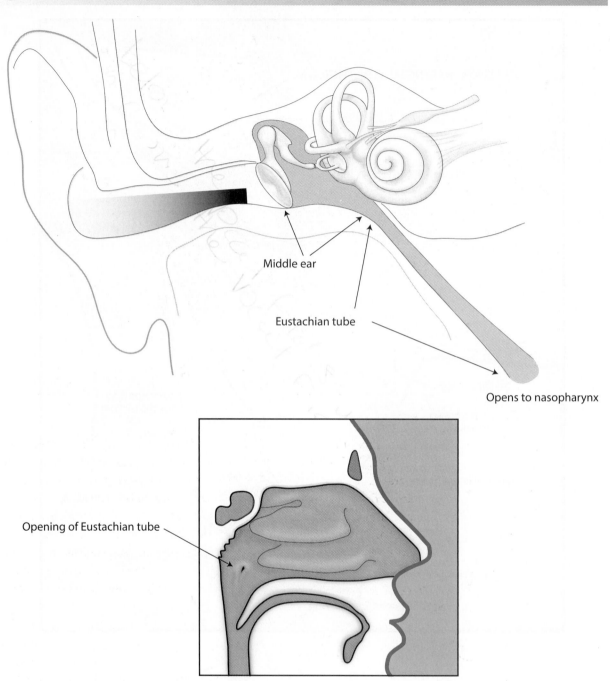

Middle ear

Eustachian tube

Opens to nasopharynx

Opening of Eustachian tube

There are four valves in the vocal tract. The first is the **labial valve**, which is formed by the lips. The lips can contact each other completely, come close to each other but not touch, or contact the teeth. The second is the **lingual valve**, formed as the tongue contacts or approaches other articulators. As discussed above, the tongue is an extremely agile and versatile organ, moving around rapidly within and out of the oral cavity, and it has the ability to contact or approximate many different structures.

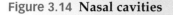

Figure 3.14 Nasal cavities

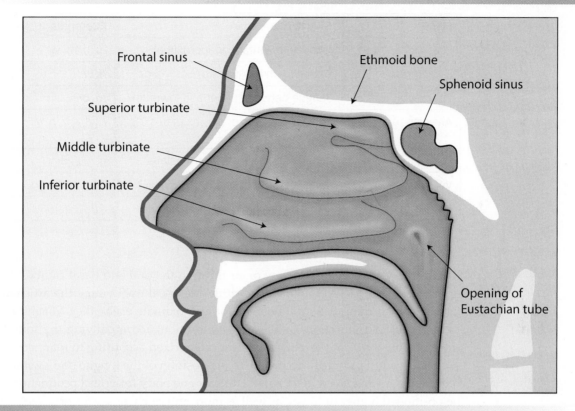

For example, the tongue can make full contact with or come very close to the teeth, the alveolar ridge, the hard palate, and the soft palate. The tongue can also protrude outside the oral cavity between the upper and lower teeth, and can change its shape.

The third is the **velopharyngeal valve**, which is made up of the velum and the posterior and lateral pharyngeal walls. This valve is of prime importance in directing the flow of air through the appropriate cavity (oral or nasal) for speech production. The fourth is the **laryngeal valve**, formed by the vocal folds. This valve plays a crucial role in the voicing of sounds. Voiced sounds are produced with vocal fold vibration. For voiceless sounds the valve must be open to allow air to flow uninterruptedly into the vocal tract.

The sounds of any language are formed by valving the airstream in specific ways to generate complex periodic and complex aperiodic sounds. The manner in which the valving occurs, and the location within the vocal tract at which the valving occurs, form the basis of a classification system for consonants and vowels.

Traditional Classification System of Consonants and Vowels

The consonants of a language are traditionally classified according to three major dimensions, the **manner of articulation**, **place of articulation**, and **voicing**. Manner of articulation refers to the specific way in which the articulators relate

Table 3.8 **Places of Articulation**

Place	Structures	Examples
Bilabial	Lips make contact or approximate	/p, b, m, w/
Labiodental	Upper teeth to lower lip	/f, v/
Interdental	Tongue between upper and lower lips	/θ, ð/
Alveolar	Tongue contacts or approximates alveolar ridge	/t, d, s, z, n, l/
Palatal	Tongue approximates hard palate	/ʃ, ʒ, tʃ, dʒ, r/
Velar	Tongue contacts velum	/k, g, ŋ/
Glottal	Vocal folds approximate slightly	/h/

to each other to regulate the flow of air through the oral and nasal cavities. Place of articulation refers to the location within the vocal tract where the articulators involved in forming the sound contact or approximate each other. Voicing refers to the vocal fold vibration, or absence of vibration, accompanying the sound. In the traditional system the vowels are not categorized according to manner, place, and voicing, but primarily according to the position of the tongue body within the oral cavity. As described in Chapter 2, the tongue body for vowel production may be positioned higher or lower, as well as more anteriorly or posteriorly, within the oral cavity.

Place of Articulation of English Consonants

There are seven primary places of articulation in English (Table 3.8). In the *bilabial* place, the lips either close completely or come close to each other in order to shape the sound wave. In the *labiodental* place, the contact occurs between the lips and teeth. In English, typically the meeting is between the upper front teeth and the lower lip. In the *interdental/linguadental* place, the tongue is positioned between the upper and lower teeth. The *lingualveolar* place (often just called alveolar) is formed by the tongue tip touching or coming close to the alveolar ridge. The *linguapalatal*, or palatal, place results from the tongue touching or coming close to the hard palate. In the *linguavelar* (velar) place, the back of the tongue touches or comes close to the velum. Finally, the *glottal* place is located between the vocal folds when they narrow slightly (but not close enough to vibrate) in the production of a sound.

Manner of Articulation of English Consonants

There are six manners of articulation in English, including stops, fricatives, affricates, nasals, glides, and liquids (Table 3.9). Stops, fricatives, and affricates are made by obstructing or constricting the flow of air through the vocal tract and are called **obstruent** sounds. Nasals, glides, and liquids are made with a less constricted vocal tract and are known as **sonorant** sounds.

Table 3.9 **Manners of Articulation**

Manner	Obstruction/constriction	Examples
Stops	Oral cavity obstructed, P_{oral} built up and released under high pressure	/p, t, k, b, d, g/
Fricatives	Vocal tract constricted, pressure released gradually	/f, v, θ, ð, s, z, ʃ, ʒ, h/
Affricates	Begins as a stop with pressure build up, pressure released gradually like a fricative	/ʧ, ʤ/
Nasals	Velopharyngeal port open, obstruction within oral cavity, air released through nasal cavities	/m, n, ŋ/
Glides	Quick tongue movement from front to back or back to front	/j, w/
Liquids	Partial obstruction of oral cavity, allowing air to move around the obstruction	/l, r/

[handwritten margin note: What happens to the airstream in the oral cavity]

Stops

Stops, or plosives, as they are also known, are made when two articulators contact each other and momentarily block the flow of air through the oral cavity. Just behind the blockage oral air pressure (P_{oral}) builds up and is then released explosively when the blockage is released (hence the term plosive). The burst of air that is released is perceived as the stop sound. To generate the high P_{oral}, the velopharyngeal valve must be closed so that air is prevented from exiting through the nasal cavities. For example, the /p/ sound is made by touching the two lips to each other, causing P_{oral} to be built up behind the lips. When the lips are opened the air is forced out in a quick rush, and only then is the sound perceived.

There are six stops in English, three voiced and three voiceless, made at three different locations within the vocal tract. Places of articulation are bilabial (/p/, /b/), alveolar (/t/, /d/), in which the tongue tip contacts the alveolar ridge, and velar (/k/, /g/), in which the back of the tongue touches the velum. See Figure 3.15.

The muscles involved in producing stops include the levator veli palatini and the pharyngeal constrictors to raise the velum, the orbicularis oris and other facial muscles for /p/ and /b/, the superior longitudinal muscle for /t/ and /d/, and the styloglossus and palatoglossus for the /k/ and /g/ (Raphael, Borden, & Harris, 2007). For the alveolar and velar stops the tongue movements are more complex, with both horizontal and vertical components (Lofqvist & Gracco, 2002). Stops require considerable motor control for their production, and acquiring the necessary neuromuscular control is a developmental process. It has been shown that adult like motor control for stops is only achieved by age 8 years, and refinement of stop production continues into the adult years (e.g., Cheng, Murdoch, Goozee, & Scott, 2007b). Some 6-year-old children have been reported to produce stop consonants without clear distinctions between movements of the tongue tip, tongue body, and lateral margins of the tongue (e.g., Cheng, Murdoch, Goozee, & Scott, 2007a). Further, the place of articulation of the alveolar and velar stops

Figure 3.15 Stops

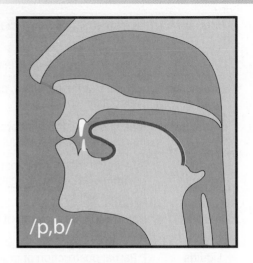

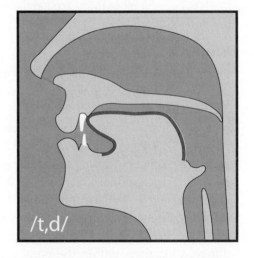

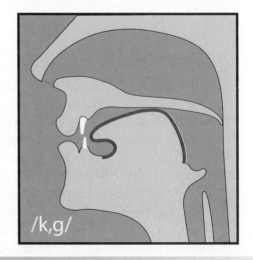

Figure 3.16 Fricatives

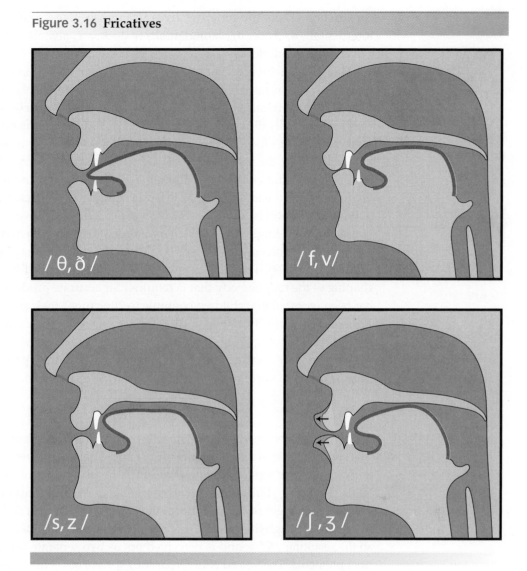

seems to shift to a more anterior position with maturation and becomes more consistent (Cheng et al., 2007a).

Fricatives

Fricatives are produced when turbulent airflow is forced under high pressure through a narrow channel somewhere within the oral cavity. The narrow channel is formed when two articulators come close to each other but do not make contact (Figure 3.16). For example, the /s/ sound is made by bringing the tongue tip and blade close to the alveolar ridge and grooving the center of the tongue by holding the sides slightly upward. Pressurized air is forced through this groove, causing a hissing sound known as frication noise to escape. For some fricatives, such as /s/, the airflow coming into contact with the teeth increases the degree of turbulence. The velopharyngeal valve is closed to prevent communication between the oral and nasal cavities, allowing high P_{oral} to be built up and released through the constriction. There are nine fricatives in English, five voiceless and four voiced: interdental /θ/ and /ð/, labiodental /f/ and /v/, alveolar /s/ and /z/, palatal /ʃ/ and /ʒ/, and glottal /h/.

The muscles involved in producing fricatives depend on the place of articulation. The velum is raised by the levator veli palatini and the pharyngeal constrictors. The labiodental fricatives require contraction of several muscles in the lower part of the face, especially the inferior orbicularis oris. Various tongue muscles are active for interdentals, with the superior longitudinal muscle playing a primary role. For alveolar fricatives, the muscles of the jaw and tongue are used, particularly the genioglossus and geniohyoid. For the glottal /h/ sound, the narrowing of the vocal folds is controlled by the intrinsic laryngeal muscles, while the vocal tract takes the shape of whatever vowel is to follow (Raphael et al., 2007). Fricatives occur less frequently than stops in English as well as in other languages, and children typically learn to produce fricatives later in the developmental process than stops (Li, Edwards, & Beckman, 2009). The later development can be explained by the more complex shaping of the tongue body that is required for accurate production of the sound. It has been reported that children continue to "fine tune" their production of fricatives throughout young childhood, until these sounds reach their adult like motoric and acoustic patterns (e.g., Nissen & Fox, 2005). There is also some evidence that starting from around age 5 years, prepubescent girls and boys may produce fricatives with slightly different vocal tract shapes (e.g., Fox & Nissen, 2005).

Affricates

The two affricates in English are made by combining features of stops and fricatives. The sound begins as a stop but changes in midstream to end up as a fricative. For the affricate /tʃ/, the tongue first positions itself in the manner of the voiceless alveolar stop /t/, and P_{oral} builds up. However, instead of releasing this pressure explosively, the tongue changes position to that of the palatal /ʃ/ fricative, and the pressurized air is released through the groove. This transition between manners occurs very rapidly, so the resulting /tʃ/ sound is perceived not as two separate sounds, but as one distinct phoneme. The voiced counterpart of / tʃ / is /dʒ /, combining the alveolar stop /d/ and the fricative /ʒ/. Affricates are considered to be palatal sounds because they are released as palatal fricatives, even though they start out as alveolar stops.

Nasals

Nasals are the only sounds in English that are made by resonating the sound wave in the nasal and oral cavities rather than the oral cavity alone (see Figure 3.17). Nasals are similar to stops, in that there is a blockage between two articulators in the vocal tract. The difference is that for nasals, the velopharyngeal valve is open. With the oral exit blocked, the outgoing sound wave is forced to exit through the nasal cavities. Oral blockage for the nasals occurs bilabially for /m/, at the alveolar place of articulation for /n/, and at the velar place for /ŋ/. Keep in mind that for the velar /ŋ/ the velum is in its open position, with the back of the tongue making contact against it to block the oral cavity. In terms of muscle activity, the palatoglossus muscle may be used in lowering the soft palate for the nasals, while the levator veli palatini muscle is least active for these nasal sounds (Raphael et al., 2007).

Figure 3.17 Nasals

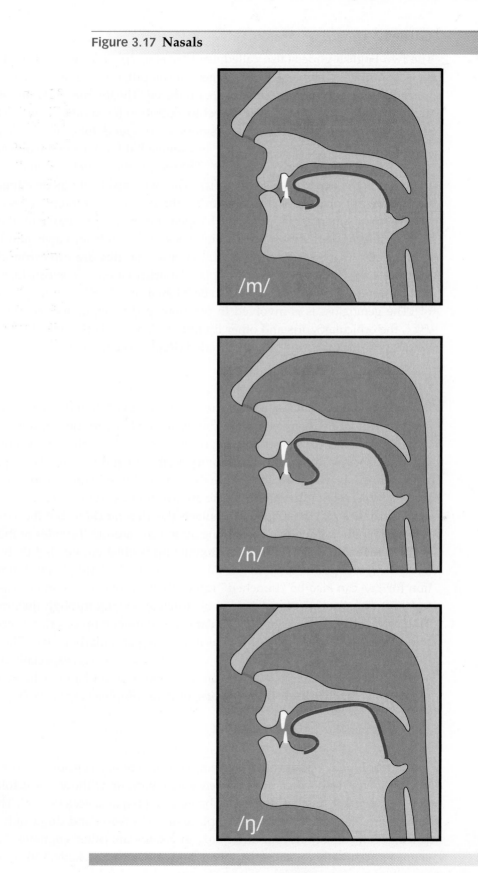

Glides

The two English glides (also called semivowels), /j/ and /w/, are made on the run, so to speak. The name glide suggests a smooth, flowing movement, and this indeed describes how these sounds are produced. The tongue shifts smoothly and rapidly from its position for one vowel to a position for another vowel. The glide sound emerges during this shift. Consider the /j/ sound, for example. To produce this sound the tongue starts out high and somewhat forward in the oral cavity, in position for a front vowel, such as /i/. The tongue then quickly shifts to the position for a high back vowel, such as /u/. The two vowel sounds on either side of the /j/ are not produced, but it is during the transition in tongue positions that the /j/ sound emerges. The opposite happens for the /w/ sound, with the tongue rapidly shifting its position from a high back to a high front vowel and the /w/ sound emerging during the quick transition. The lips are often rounded and protruded for the /w/. In terms of place of articulation, /j/ is considered to be palatal, whereas /w/ is considered to be bilabial.

The genioglossus is involved in positioning the tongue for the /j/. For the /w/, the orbicularis oris and other lip muscles are used, as is the styloglossus to elevate and back the tongue when needed (Raphael et al., 2007).

Liquids

It should be noted that some phoneticians do not place liquids in a separate category but describe them as glides. The term *liquid* is very descriptive, however. Liquids have the property of flowing, so the name of this category of sounds suggests that airflow through the oral cavity is smooth and flowing. For liquids, the tongue forms a loose blockage within the oral cavity, allowing air to flow around the blockage and out the mouth. There are two liquids, /l/ and /r/.

To produce /l/, the tongue tip contacts the alveolar ridge, but the sides of the tongue are pulled downward, allowing air to flow around the sides of the tongue and out the mouth. For the /r/, the tongue tip is often curled slightly backward (*retroflexed*) and points toward, but does not touch, the hard palate. Tongue position for /r/ can also be "bunched" rather than retroflexed. In either case, air is free to flow around the loose palatal obstruction, exiting through the oral cavity. The place of articulation for /r/ is palatal. Since tongue tip position is crucial for the liquids, the superior longitudinal muscle is particularly active. The inferior longitudinal muscle may be more active for /r/ than for /l/, especially if the /r/ is retroflexed. The shaping of the tongue dorsum is probably achieved by the interaction of the vertical and transverse muscles (Raphael et al., 2007).

Voicing

In the traditional classification system, consonants are considered to be either voiced or voiceless—that is, produced either with or without vocal fold vibration. For example, bilabial stops may be voiced, /b/, or voiceless, /p/. These two sounds are identical in manner and place of articulation and differ only in their voicing. Pairs of sounds that differ only in voicing are called **cognates**. Note that cognates occur only for stops, fricatives, and affricates. See Table 3.10.

Table 3.10 Cognates

Stops
/p, b/
/t, d/
/k, g/
Fricatives
/f, v/
/θ, ð/
/s, z/
/ʃ, ʒ/
Affricates
/ʧ, ʤ/

Any consonant can be uniquely specified by its manner and place of articulation, as well as by its voicing. A voiced alveolar stop, for example, can only refer to the /d/ phoneme, whereas a voiced alveolar fricative must be the /z/. A voiceless palatal fricative is /ʃ/. The /ð/ is described as a voiced interdental fricative. Figure 3.18 is a chart of English consonants that shows manner and place of articulation for each phoneme. For cognates, the voiceless member is placed before the voiced member.

Vowel Classification

In the traditional classification system, vowels are classified primarily according to location of the tongue body within the oral cavity. All vowels are voiced, so there is no need for a separate voicing category. All vowels are produced with a relatively open vocal tract, so there is no need for a separate manner category. Place of articulation does vary for different vowels, in terms of how high or low the tongue body is held within the oral cavity and how advanced or retracted the tongue body is within the oral cavity. *Tongue height* and *tongue advancement* are the two primary dimensions of vowel classification, but other dimensions also play a role in vowel formation, including how tense or relaxed the tongue is and how rounded the lips are; these do not carry as much weight as tongue position.

The vowels are schematized along the two major dimensions in a format called the **vowel quadrilateral** (Figure 3.19). The vowel quadrilateral loosely represents the oral cavity. The relative vertical position of any phonetic symbol in the quadrilateral represents the position of the highest point of the tongue in the articulation of the vowel. The relative horizontal position of a phonetic symbol represents the degree of tongue advancement within the oral cavity. In the vertical plane, vowels are classified as *high*, *mid*, or *low*; in the horizontal plane, vowels are considered to be *front*, *central*, or *back.* Thus, vowels are classified as high front, or high back, or mid front, or low back, or central, and so on. The highest front vowel is /i/,

Figure 3.18 Manner and place of articulation of English consonants

	STOPS	FRICATIVES	AFFRICATES	NASALS	GLIDES	LIQUIDS
BILABIAL	p/b			m	w	
LABIODENTAL		f/v				
INTERDENTAL		θ/ð				
ALVEOLAR	t/d	s/z		n		l
PALATAL		ʃ/ʒ	tʃ/dʒ		j	r
VELAR	k/g			ŋ		
GLOTTAL		h				

Figure 3.19 Vowel quadrilateral

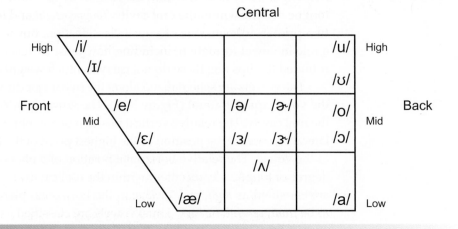

and the lowest is /æ/. If you produce each front vowel from highest to lowest, you should be able to feel your tongue progressively drop with each sound. The same is true for the back vowels, with /u/ being the highest and /a/ the lowest. The back vowels, in English, tend to be produced with lip rounding, whereas the front vowels are not. If you switch between /i/ and /u/, the highest front vowel and the highest back vowel, you should feel the body of your tongue move from a relatively anterior position for the /i/ to a more posterior position for the /u/, as well as your lips rounding for the back vowel and spreading for the front vowel. The central vowels, such as the schwa, are made with the tongue in a neutral position within the vocal tract.

Acoustic Characteristics of Vowels and Consonants

The way in which vowels and consonants are articulated, as described in the previous section, results in specific features that give each sound its characteristic acoustic structure. A well-established method of identifying the acoustic structure of sounds is through spectrographic analysis.

Spectrographic Analysis

Spectrography is a method of identifying frequency, amplitude, and duration of sounds. A spectrogram is a graph on which frequency is displayed on the vertical axis, time is represented on the horizontal axis, and intensity of acoustic energy is represented by the darkness of the trace on the screen, or by different colors. This kind of display makes it easy to look at the acoustic characteristics of sounds and to see how they change over time. As speech is characterized by rapid changes in the acoustic signal, spectrographic analysis is very handy.

The spectrograph has been around since the 1940s and has become accessible to clinicians as well as researchers thanks to advances in computer technology. Spectrographic analysis used to be a laborious, time-consuming task that was mostly done in university or industrial laboratories. These days, however, spectrographic analysis is used for diagnosis and treatment of many communication disorders in hospitals, university clinics, rehabilitation centers, and schools. Commercially available instruments are reasonably cost-effective and provide a non invasive and safe means of fine-grained acoustic analysis of speech sounds. These instruments incorporate computer systems with specialized hardware and software that allows speech to be acquired, analyzed, and displayed on a computer screen as well as auditorily by loudspeakers. Free software programs such as Praat (praat.org) that perform these types of analyses are available for downloading onto a computer, making acoustic analysis even more accessible in virtually any location or setting. The software allows the user to generate waveforms of the speech signal and to measure these waveforms instantaneously by positioning cursors on the screen of the computer monitor. The computer shows the measured values in appropriate units of frequency, amplitude, and time. Once the waveform has been captured, many different types of analyses can be performed, including spectrography.

Narrowband and Wideband Spectrograms

Spectrography is based on using a filter to scan all the frequencies in a sound and the acoustic energy present at each frequency. Different types of information about sounds may be obtained spectrographically, depending on the filter bandwidth that is used for the analysis. **Narrowband spectrograms** use a filter of 45 to 50 Hz. Most speakers' fundamental frequencies are higher than 50 Hz, so a filter with a narrow bandwidth will respond to each harmonic in the vocal signal separately. This allows the fundamental frequency and individual harmonics in the sound to be displayed. Thus narrowband spectrograms reveal the harmonic structure of a sound produced by the glottal source.

Wideband (broadband) spectrographic analysis is usually done with a bandwidth of 300 to 500 Hz. This allows acoustic energy to be detected from many harmonics in the glottal source and added together. Recall that harmonics that fall within the bandwidth of any vocal tract resonance are amplified. When the harmonics are added together, they appear on a spectrogram as broad horizontal bands of strong acoustic energy and are called formants. The center of each energy band is estimated as the center frequency of the formant, which corresponds to the resonant frequency of the vocal tract, and the range of frequencies present in the band is taken to be the bandwidth. Thus, wideband spectrograms show the formant structure of sounds such as vowels and the filtering function of the vocal tract. In addition, the speaker's fundamental frequency is indicated by the vertical lines at the bottom of the spectrogram, with each line representing one cycle of vocal fold vibration. A wideband spectrogram can also represent aperiodic sounds created within the vocal tract.

The following discussion focuses in detail on the acoustic characteristics of vowels and consonants.

Vowels

Vowel articulation is related to tongue position within the vocal tract. The four vowels at each corner of the vowel quadrilateral (/i, u, a, æ/) are called **corner vowels**. These vowels are produced with the tongue as far as possible from the neutral tongue position, and the corner vowels therefore represent the limits of vowel articulation. Vowels are periodic complex sounds characterized acoustically by their first three formants. The formants appear as wide, dark horizontal stripes on a spectrogram, reflecting the concentrations of intense acoustic energy at those harmonic frequencies that have been amplified by the vocal tract resonances. Because the vocal tract is broadly tuned, many harmonics are amplified near a vocal tract resonance, which explains why the resulting formants are so wide. Figure 3.20 shows spectrograms of front, back, and central vowels. These vowels are known as **monophthongs**, or pure vowels, and are produced with a relatively constant tongue position. Front and back vowels have characteristic formant patterns. Formants 1 and 2 in front vowels are spaced very widely apart, whereas formants 2 and 3 are close together. The high front vowel /i/ shows the greatest degree of separation between formants 1 and 2, with decreasing separation for the lower vowels. The back vowels are characterized by closely spaced first and second formants, and a much higher frequency third formant. Central vowels tend to show a more equally spaced relationship between the formants.

Figure 3.20 Front, back, and central vowels

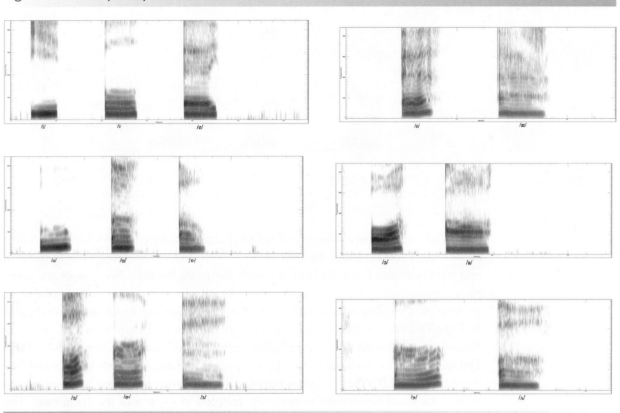

Diphthongs

A diphthong is a vowel that changes its resonance characteristics during its production. Diphthongs, like vowels, are resonant periodic complex sounds characterized by their first three formants. Diphthongs are produced by uttering two vowels as one unit. The starting point for the first vowel is called the **onglide**, and the end point of the diphthong is known as the **offglide**. For example, for the /ai/ diphthong, the tongue is in the appropriate position for /a/ and quickly shifts to the position for /i/. The acoustic result of changing tongue position is that the vocal tract filtering function changes, causing the formants to shift in frequency from the beginning to the end of the sound. These shifts in frequency are called **formant transitions**. Spectrographically a diphthong produced in isolation is characterized by a *steady-state formant* at the onglide, followed by the formant transition. Figure 3.21 shows spectrograms of the three major diphthongs in English: /ai/, /au/, and /ɔi/. The /ai/ diphthong starts out with typical formants for the /a/, with F_1 and F_2 fairly close together and a wide separation between F_2 and F_3. During the transition, the frequencies change to those typical for /i/, with a very low F_1 and considerably higher F_2 and F_3. Patterns of formant transitions for the other two diphthongs similarly show changes in frequency according to the values for the individual vowels that make up the sound. The second formant undergoes the greatest degree of frequency change for all the diphthongs. The offglide position of the tongue for all the diphthongs is always either high front (/i/) or high back (/u/).

Figure 3.21 **Diphthongs**

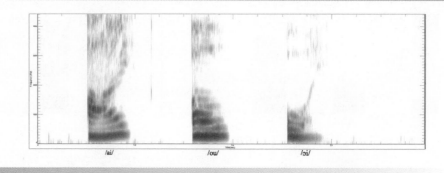

/ai/   /ou/   /ɔi/

Nasals

The nasals are the three sounds in English that are produced with a lowered velum and an obstruction within the oral cavity. The sound is resonated in both the oral and nasal cavities but exits only through the nasal cavities. Because of the complete obstruction of the oral cavity, these sounds are sometimes called *nasal stops* or *nasal plosives*. The sound exiting the nose is called the **nasal murmur** (Pruthi & Espy-Wilson, 2004) and corresponds to the interval during which the oral closure coincides with the open velopharyngeal port (Hixon, Weismer, & Hoit, 2008). The nasal murmur is characterized by the presence of **antiformants** and a **nasal formant** (Figure 3.22). When the velopharyngeal passageway is opened by lowering the velum, the nasal cavities are acoustically coupled to the rest of the vocal tract. The closed oral cavity becomes, in acoustic terms, a **side-branch resonator**, or **shunt resonator**. Air flowing through the vocal tract becomes divided, with some flowing into the nasal cavity and some into the blocked oral cavity. The divergence of the air into the oral cavity introduces antiformants into the picture, as some of the sound energy is trapped within the oral cavity and prevented from being resonated through the nasal passages. Antiformants act in a manner opposite to formants. Recall that vocal tract resonances act as pass-band filters and amplify harmonic frequencies within their bandwidths. By contrast, vocal tract antiresonances act as stop-band filters that have a damping effect on harmonic frequencies within their bandwidths. Nasals are

Figure 3.22 **Nasals**

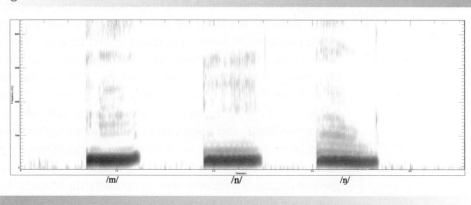

/m/   /n/   /ŋ/

therefore acoustically very complex sounds, because they have both formants and antiformants in their spectrum. On spectrograms, antiformants look like extremely weak-intensity formants. The frequencies of the antiformants depend on where in the vocal tract the blockage occurs (i.e., bilabial, alveolar, or velar). The first antiformant for /m/ (the longest side-branch resonator) occurs at around 1000 Hz, that for /n/ at around 2000 Hz, and that for /ŋ/ (the shortest side-branch resonator) at about 3000 Hz (Kent, Dembowski, & Lass, 1996).

Coupling the nasal and oral cavities also introduces an additional formant, the nasal formant, into the acoustic structure of the sound. The nasal formant is low in frequency (less than 250–300 Hz) because of the relatively large volume of the coupled pharyngeal and nasal cavities. The nasal formant is the most intense portion of the nasal murmur. Nasal murmurs also contain higher formants, but these have considerably less amplitude than the lowest nasal formant. The murmurs for each nasal sound are not exactly alike, but they are very similar. Because the nasal cavities do not change their size or shape for each sound, the resonating characteristics of the nasal cavities remain essentially the same for all the nasal sounds.

Glides

Glides are sometimes classified as semivowels and belong to a class of sounds called **sonorants**. Sonorant sounds are always voiced, and the airflow in sonorants is not completely smooth and laminar, but neither is it turbulent. The quick tongue movements that characterize glides result in rapidly changing formant frequencies. These sounds are therefore characterized by formant transitions that are much more rapid than those of diphthongs. Glides do not show the steady-state portion of the formant that is seen in diphthongs. They are extremely short in duration and often look like little more than a formant transition between two other sounds. The formant transition lasts only for about 75 msec (Pickett, 1999). See Figure 3.23. Typically, the lips are rounded for the /w/, resulting in lower frequencies for all the formants, due to the lengthening of the vocal tract. For both /w/ and /j/ in a consonant–vowel (CV) context, F_1 frequency begins at a very low value, similar to the values for high vowels /i/ and /u/ that form the starting tongue position for the glides. The formants then rise to the F_1 frequency of the following vowel.

Figure 3.23 Glides

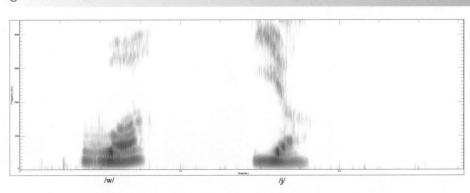

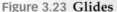

/w/   /j/

For adult males, F_2 for /w/ starts at around 800 Hz, very close to the average F_2 frequency for /u/; F_2 for /j/ starts at approximately 2200 Hz, also close to the value for /i/. F_3 for /w/ begins at approximately 2200 Hz, and that for /j/ begins at 3000 Hz (Kent et al., 1996). The frequency values for F_2 and F_3 also shift toward the F_2 and F_3 values of the following vowel.

Liquids

The liquids, /r/ and /l/, are sonorant sounds. They are characterized by steady-state formants, reflecting the fact that these sounds are not made with changing tongue motion. The /r/ sound in English is often retroflexed, with the tongue pointing backward toward the palate. This results in a characteristic lowering of F_3, bringing it close to F_2. F_3 for /r/ is around 1600 Hz, whereas F_3 for vowels ranges between approximately 2200 and 3000 Hz, depending on the specific vowel. Most /r/-colored sounds (**rhotic sounds**) show the lowering of F_3. For example, the average F_3 for adult males for the schwa (/ə/) is about 2390 Hz, whereas F_3 for the r-colored version schwar /ɚ/ is about 1690 Hz. However, the degree of F_3 lowering depends on the position of the /r/ sound within the word. Initial /r/ typically undergoes more extreme F_3 lowering; in the final position the lowering is not as much. F_1 and F_2 for /r/ are similar to those for /l/. The spectrogram in Figure 3.24 shows the steady-state nature of the liquids when they are produced as isolated sounds. The lowering of F_3 for /r/ is clearly seen in the syllables /iri/ and /ili/ (Figure 3.25).

The /l/ sound is produced by contact between the tongue tip and alveolar ridge, with enough space at the sides of the tongue allowing air to flow around the blockage. The area of the oral cavity immediately behind the blockage acts as a shunt resonator, so similar to the nasals, the /l/ sound is also characterized by both formants and antiformants. The formants for /l/ are approximately 360 Hz for F_1, 1300 Hz for F_2, and 2700 Hz for F_3. However, there is a lot of variability in the formants for /l/. F_2, in particular, is influenced by the surrounding vowels (Baken & Orlikoff, 2000).

Stops

As with all other sounds, the way in which stops are articulated determines their acoustic characteristics. There are several major differences, though, between

Figure 3.24 Liquids

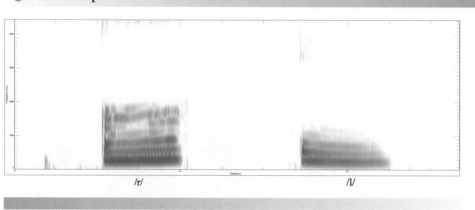

Figure 3.25 F_3 **lowering in liquids**

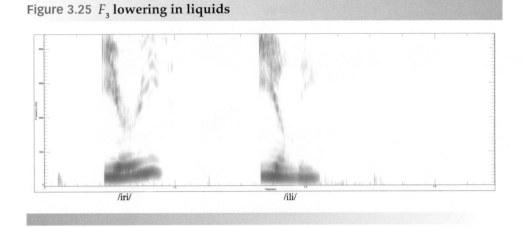

/iri/   /ili/

sonorant sounds and obstruent sounds such as stops and fricatives. Vowels and diphthongs are always produced by vocal fold vibration, and then the sound wave is filtered through the vocal tract. The vocal tract for vowels and diphthongs is relatively unconstricted, allowing the sound wave to pass through a reasonably wide channel. Glides and liquids are produced with a slightly greater degree of constriction than vowels and also have as their source the periodic glottal vibration. By contrast, the major sound source for stops is the release of the pressurized air behind the articulatory blockage, which creates a complex aperiodic transient sound. The manner in which stops are articulated results in four characteristic acoustic features: the **silent gap**, the **release burst**, **voice onset time (VOT)**, and **formant transitions.**

Silent gap

The silent gap on a spectrogram reflects the time during which the articulators are forming the blockage and P_{oral} is building up. For a voiceless stop in syllable initial position, this interval cannot be seen on the spectrogram. When the stop occurs in the medial or final position the silent gap is visible as a blank space between the preceding sound and the stop. For voiced stops, a band of low-frequency energy, the **voice bar**, is sometimes apparent during the silent gap. The voice bar is an indication that vocal fold vibration is occurring during the articulatory closure and pressure buildup.

Release burst

The release burst is a brief interval of aperiodic sound which follows the silent gap. On the spectrogram in Figure 3.26, the burst appears as a vertical line extending into the high frequencies. The line represents the broad range of frequencies characteristic of aperiodic complex sounds. The line is short in duration because the release of the stop is transient, lasting around 10 to 30 msec. Bursts are usually seen for stops in initial and medial position. They may not occur for stops in final position, which tend to be unreleased in English spoken in the United States, although they may be released in some British-English dialects. Most of the energy in the burst spectrum for /p/ and /b/ is low in frequency, between 500 and 1500 Hz, or else the acoustic energy may be spread out over a wide range of frequencies.

Figure 3.26 **Stops**

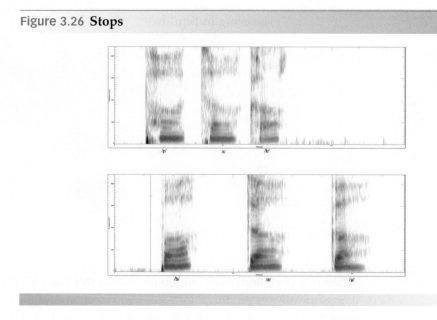

The alveolars /t/ and /d/ have a small area in front of the constriction (i.e., between the tongue tip where it contacts the alveolar ridge and the lips). This space is called the *front cavity* and acts as a high-pass filter that emphasizes the higher frequency components in the noise source (Pickett, 1999). Alveolar stops therefore have high-intensity and high-frequency energy, around 3000 to 4000 Hz (Baken, 1996; Pickett, 1999). The velar /k/ and /g/ have a larger cavity in front of the constriction. The larger volume of the front cavity resonates more strongly to lower frequencies. This has the effect of concentrating the energy in the midrange of frequencies, around 1500 to 4000 Hz, depending on the tongue position for the following vowel. The bursts of voiceless stops are longer in duration than those of voiced stops, because voiceless stops are characterized by **aspiration**. Aspiration refers to noise generated by turbulence as air moves through the glottis during the time in which the vocal folds are starting to close for the following voiced sound. The turbulent air moving through the glottis delays vocal fold closure, resulting in a longer burst. Voiced stops do not show aspiration noise, because the vocal folds are already closed and vibrating during the initial part of the stop.

Voice onset time

The difference between voiced and voiceless stops is indicated partially by voice onset time (VOT). VOT refers to the time between the release of the articulatory blockage (corresponding spectrographically to the beginning of the burst) to the beginning of vocal fold vibration for the following vowel. This interval of time is measured in milliseconds and is commonly taken as an indication of the coordination between the laryngeal and articulatory systems. VOT is usually measured in initial stops, and its values can fall into one of four categories, depending on the timing between the release of the burst and the onset of vocal fold vibration. The value can be negative, indicating that the vocal folds are vibrating before the articulatory release takes place. This is known as *prevoicing VOT lead* and sometimes occurs for voiced stops. The second category involves simultaneous voicing in which voice onset and articulatory release occur at the same time, yielding a VOT of zero. The third category includes VOT with a *short lag*, in which the onset of vocal fold vibration follows shortly after the release burst. These three categories are common for voiced stops in English. The fourth category includes voiceless stops that typically show a *long lag* time; vocal fold vibration is delayed for a relatively long period of time after the articulatory release. Categories of VOTs include voiced, voiceless unaspirated, and voiceless aspirated (Cho & Ladefoged, 1999). VOTs for voiced stops range from about –20 msec to +20 msec. Voiceless stops have longer VOTs that range from about 25 msec to 100 msec, depending on the place of articulation and the degree of aspiration.

The production of appropriate VOT is a developmental skill. Young children do not produce voiced and voiceless stops with clearly separated VOT values. Based on a body of research, Whalen, Levitt, and Goldstein (2007) reported that children's early stop productions tend to demonstrate a short lag, corresponding to voiced or voiceless unaspirated stops. This is probably because longer VOTs seen in voiceless aspirated stops require a high degree of motor coordination between the articulatory and laryngeal systems. The ability to regulate the complex muscular movements required for fine VOT distinctions continues to develop until around age 11 years (Whiteside, Dobbin, & Henry, 2003). In the elderly population, variability in VOT values is much greater than in younger speakers.

While VOT occurs for stops in all languages, there are some differences between languages. For example, English voiceless stops demonstrate a long voicing lag due to the degree of aspiration, while unaspirated voiced stops primarily show a short voicing lag. VOT values for voiced stops in French show a preponderance of voicing lead (i.e., negative values). Voiceless stops in Italian, Spanish, and Thai are unaspirated and are characterized by short voicing lags (e.g., Bortolini, Zmarich, Fior, & Bonifacio, 1995; Kessinger & Blumstein, 1997; Rosner, Lopez-Bascuas, Garcia-Albea, & Fahey, 2000). In fact, speakers of Spanish, Italian, and French often sound to English-speaking listeners as though they produce only voiced stops because none of the stops in these languages are aspirated (Raphael et al, 2007).

Formant transitions

Both voiced and voiceless stops are associated with formants as the articulators move from the constricted position of the stop to the more open position of the preceding or following vowel. In addition, voiced stops have formants superimposed on the transient noise, reflecting the contribution of voicing to the production of the sound. Formant transitions usually last around 50 msec. The slope of the formant transition—that is, whether it increases, decreases, or does not change in frequency—depends on the place of articulation of the stop and the vocal tract positioning for the following sound. In general, a very low F_1 frequency signifies that the vocal tract is constricted. The lower the F_1 frequency is, the tighter the vocal tract constriction. Because stops are constricted to the point of complete blockage, the transition for F_1 always starts off extremely low in frequency, close to zero, and therefore always increases in frequency to the appropriate frequency for the following vowel. No matter what the place of articulation of the stop, F_1

formant transitions are always rising when a stop is followed by a vowel (i.e., CV). Similarly, when moving the articulators from a vowel to a stop position, F_1 will decrease in frequency from that of the vowel to almost zero for the stop. Therefore, F_1 transitions always fall in a vowel-to-stop situation (VC). Frequency of the F_2 transition is related to the length of the oral cavity and therefore reflects the movement of the tongue in a backward–forward direction. This means that F_2 frequency transitions in stops are correlated with place of articulation of the stop. The bilabial stops show F_2 frequency transitions increasing from their starting value of approximately 600 to 800 Hz to the F_2 value for the following vowel. The starting value for F_2 for the alveolars is about 1800 Hz. A velar stop can be associated with a starting frequency of around 1300 Hz if it is followed by a back vowel or a much higher starting frequency between 2300 and 3000 Hz if it is followed by a front vowel. /k/ is articulated more posteriorly in the oral cavity when followed by a back vowel and more anteriorly when followed by a front vowel. Because F_2 is correlated with the length of the oral cavity, the position of the following vowel determines the F_2 frequency for the /k/. When followed by a back vowel, a larger front cavity is created, which therefore resonates lower frequencies; when a front vowel follows the /k/, a smaller front cavity results, which resonates the higher frequencies. F_3 transitions do not contribute as much information regarding place of articulation (Baken & Orlikoff, 2000).

Table 3.11 displays acoustic features of stop consonants.

Fricatives

Fricatives are produced when pressurized air becomes turbulent, resulting in random variations in air pressure. The acoustic result of this turbulent flow is

Table 3.11 Acoustic Features of Stop Consonants

Voiceless	Voiced
Aperiodic	Periodic + aperiodic
Longer burst	Shorter burst, with formants superimposed
Aspirated in syllable initial position	Unaspirated
/p/ Diffuse spectrum with more energy in lower frequencies	/b/ Diffuse spectrum with more energy in lower frequencies
/p/ F_2 frequency locus 600–800 Hz	/b/ F_2 frequency locus 600–800 Hz
/t/ F_2 frequency locus 1800 Hz	/d/ F_2 frequency locus 1800 Hz
/k/ F_2 frequency locus 1300 Hz (back vowel)	/g/ F_2 frequency locus 1300 Hz (back vowel)
/k/ F_2 frequency locus 2300–3000 Hz (front vowel)	/g/ F_2 frequency locus 2300–3000 Hz (front vowel)
No voice bar	Voice bar
Long VOT	Short VOT with frequent prevoicing

Figure 3.27 Fricatives

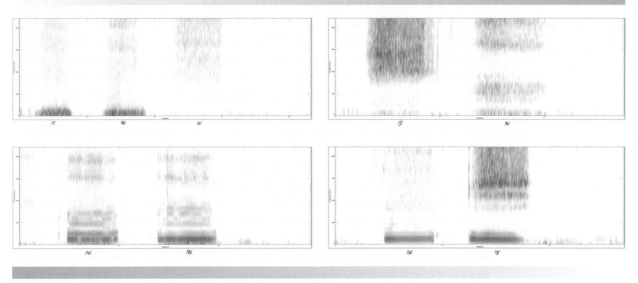

aperiodic noise, called **frication**, which sounds like hissing. Fricatives are complex aperiodic continuous sounds. On a spectrogram, a fricative looks like a wide band of acoustic energy distributed over a broad range of frequencies (Figure 3.27). The acoustic energy in fricatives is much longer in duration than stops because fricatives are continuous sounds, whereas stops are transient. The specific range of frequencies and the intensity of the aperiodic frication noise depend on the place of articulation of the fricative. In many fricatives, the airflow also collides against an obstacle, such as the teeth, that increases the amplitude of the noise produced at the constriction. The source of sound for fricatives is the vocal tract, but the sound is also resonated and shaped by the vocal tract as it travels through it. Depending on the position of the articulators for production of the fricative, certain frequency ranges in the aperiodic complex sound will be reinforced, and other frequency ranges will be attenuated. This happens because the fricative noise is resonated most strongly in the front cavity, the area in front of the location of the narrow channel that forms the articulatory constriction. The size of the front resonating cavity shapes the resulting spectrum because the smaller the size is, the higher the resonant frequency (RF) of the cavity. Fricatives that are produced most anteriorly, the /f, v, θ, and ð/, do not have much of a front resonating cavity, and so they have a very low-intensity spectrum spread out over a broad range of frequencies. The strongest resonance for /f/ ranges from about 4500 to 7000 Hz, and that for /θ/ occurs at around 5000 Hz (Pickett, 1999). For the /f/ and /θ/, the peaks of spectral energy are so high that they essentially do not play much of a part in how these sounds are perceived. For the /s/, /z/, /ʃ/, and /ʒ/, it is possible to calculate the RF of the front cavity in the same way as for the resonances of the vocal tract. The front cavity for these sounds is basically a tube that is open at one end (the lips) and closed at the other (because the constriction behind the front cavity is very small), making it a quarter-wave resonator. The front cavity for the alveolar fricative /s/ has been measured to be around 2.5 cm, so using the formula $f = v/\lambda$

(frequency = velocity/wavelength), the lowest RF of the front cavity is 3400 Hz (2.5 cm × 4 = 10 cm; 34,000/10 = 3400 Hz). There are also higher RFs that are odd-number multiples of the lowest, but it is the lowest RF that is most important for the perception of fricative sounds. Thus, the /s/ and /z/ have greatest amplitude at these very high frequencies, as can be seen in Figure 3.27. The palatal fricatives /ʃ/ and /ʒ/ have a longer resonating front cavity than the alveolars, and their major resonant region is therefore lower than that for /s/. In addition, /ʃ/ and /ʒ/ are usually made with lip rounding, which further lengthens the front resonating cavity. One can hear the effects of the lip rounding by saying "shhh," first with the lips spread out as if for the /i/ sound and then with lip rounding as if for the /u/ sound. The quality of the /ʃ/ shifts from higher in the unrounded condition to lower in the lip-rounded production. Most of the sound energy for /ʃ/ is concentrated around 2000 Hz and above. /s, z, ʃ, ʒ/ are classified as **stridents**, or **sibilants**, and have much more intense energy than the nonstridents/nonsibilants, /f, v, θ, ð/. Sibilants are also longer in duration than nonsibilants (Fox & Nissen, 2005). Fricatives can be voiced or voiceless, with voiced cognates showing a voice bar on the spectrogram. Voiced fricatives also have periodic energy from vocal fold vibration superimposed on the turbulence noise, so they are a combination of aperiodic and periodic sound. See Table 3.12.

Fricatives require a high degree of neuromuscular control of the tongue and are typically acquired by children later than stops. Nittrouer et al. (1996) reported that unlike adults, young children between ages 3 and 7 years produced articulatory constrictions for fricatives that were highly dependent on the place of articulation for the upcoming vowel. The tight coupling between fricatives and adjacent vowels decreases with advancing maturity. In addition, very young children do not acoustically contrast /s/ and /ʃ/ to the same degree as older children. The sibilant contrast continues to be developed and refined throughout the young childhood years as the child gains increasing control over his or her articulators (Nissen & Fox, 2005) and has been reported as consistently present in children at age 7 years (Mandulak, Haley, Zajac, & Ohde, 2009).

Table 3.12 **Acoustic Features of Fricatives**

Voiceless	Voiced
Aperiodic	Periodic + aperiodic
Continuous	Continuous
No voice bar	Voice bar
/s/ Intense spectral energy above 3000 Hz	/z/ Intense spectral energy above 3000 Hz
/ʃ/ Spectral energy above 2000 Hz	/ʒ/ Spectral energy above 2000 Hz
/f, θ/ Low-intensity spectrum over wide frequency range	/v, ð / Low-intensity spectrum over wide frequency range

Affricates

An affricate is made by quickly combining a stop with a fricative, so the acoustic characteristics of affricates have elements of both stops and fricatives. Affricates have a silent gap associated with the stop part of the sound, but in connected speech this interval is often not really noticeable. Frication noise follows the silent gap. Fricatives and affricates look very similar on a spectrogram, except that affricates are shorter in duration.

The Production of Speech Sounds in Context

So far, discussion has focused on the individual phonemes of speech, the segments of speech that are combined in different sequences to form syllables, words, and sentences. This process is not just a straightforward stringing together of individual speech sounds. As sounds are produced to form longer utterances, individual segments influence each other and modify the acoustic characteristics of adjacent sounds. This process is called **coarticulation**. In addition, as utterances are formed by combining segments, the pitch, intensity, and duration of specific sounds continuously change. Changes in these features are known as **suprasegmental characteristics** because these changes affect many segments over a relatively long interval of time.

Coarticulation

From the discussion of the acoustic nature of vowels and consonants, it would be easy to assume that when we speak, we produce each sound singly, moving our articulators precisely in the way described for each sound. This is not, in fact, the case. Speech is a very dynamic process. It is fast and flowing. Rather than each sound being produced in a sequence, sounds are produced in an overlapping manner; that is, they are coarticulated. Coarticulation refers to the ways in which two or more articulators move at virtually the same time to produce two or more different phonemes almost simultaneously. For example, to say the word *cat*, a speaker does not produce all the articulatory movements with their corresponding acoustic features for the /k/, moving on to the vowel only when the /k/ is completely finished, and producing the /t/ only once the vowel has been articulated. Rather, the articulatory movements overlap in time. As the speaker moves the back of his or her tongue upward to contact the velum for the /k/ sound, the blade of the tongue is simultaneously moving downward for the low front vowel /æ/. Before the vowel is complete, and possibly while the back of the tongue is still contacting the velum for the /k/ sound, the tip of the tongue moves upward to contact the alveolar ridge for the stop /t/. Because the articulatory movements overlap, the resulting acoustic features overlap as well. For this reason, it is difficult, if not impossible, to precisely specify the acoustic characteristics of individual segments in connected speech. Figure 3.28 shows some sounds made in isolation and then in a sentence.

Due to coarticulation, acoustic elements of preceding and following sounds are incorporated in any target sound in the utterance. The effects of coarticulation can be seen in numerous ways. For example, in the word *sue*, the lip rounding that

Figure 3.28 Sounds in isolation and in connected speech

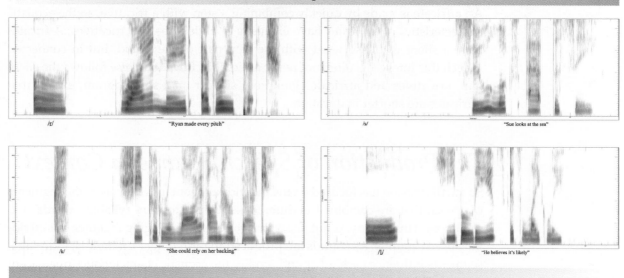

is associated with the back vowel /u/ is already present during production of the /s/. In the word *see*, the lips are already spreading on the /s/, in anticipation of the upcoming /i/ sound. Acoustically, the two /s/ sounds have their spectral peaks at slightly different frequency locations because of the influence of the following vowel (Figure 3.29).

The effects of coarticulation are also seen on vowels that either precede or follow a nasal sound. Because the velopharyngeal port is open for nasal sounds, a portion of the vowel will be nasalized. This is seen spectrographically as an additional low frequency formant (the nasal formant) and antiformants reflected as a reduction in intensity of the other formants. Thus, in the word *thumb*, the velum is already lowering during the vowel production, in anticipation of the following /m/ sound. Therefore, the /ʌ/ would likely show spectrographic evidence of nasalization, such as a nasal formant and weak F_1, F_2, and F_3. On the other hand, in the word *thud*, the vowel is not nasalized (Figure 3.30).

Figure 3.29 Effect of vowel context on spectral characteristics of /s/

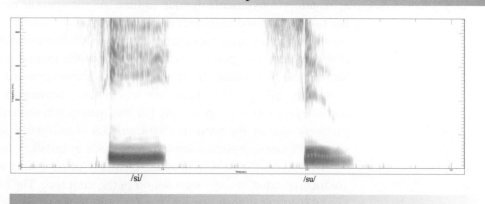

Figure 3.30 Effect of nasal context on preceding vowel

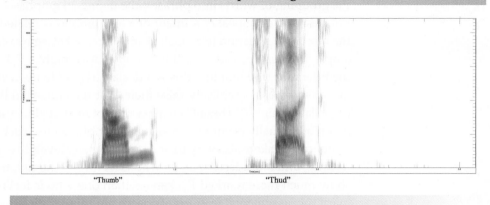

From the preceding discussion, it should be apparent that coarticulation works both ways. That is, an upcoming sound can influence the preceding sound (**anticipatory coarticulation**, or **right-to-left coarticulation**), as in the examples of the nasalized vowel and the different productions of the /s/ in *sue* and *see*. Preceding sounds can also modify ensuing sounds (**carryover coarticulation**, or **left-to-right coarticulation**). The /a/ in the word *not* would show nasalization effects because of the preceding /n/, whereas such effects would not be seen in the word *dot* (Figure 3.31).

Coarticulation is an important feature of connected speech that makes speech transmission extremely rapid and efficient. The effects of coarticulation depend on factors such as the place of the articulation of the consonant, the shape of the syllable (i.e., open or closed), the vowel context (i.e., low or high, front or back), and stress (Modarresi, Sussman, Lindblom, & Burlingame, 2004; Zharkova & Hewlett, 2009). While coarticulation is a fundamental property of speech, the degree and specific patterns of coarticulation are highly variable among individual speakers (Grosvald, 2009).

Suprasegmentals

When an individual speaks, he or she conveys a lot of information to the listener. Some of the information is carried in the actual words used, but much of the information is carried in the melody, or prosody, of speech. As one speaks, F_0 and

Figure 3.31 Effect of nasal context on following vowel

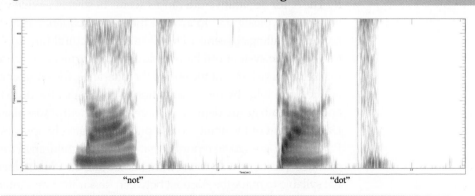

intensity levels vary continuously and these changes convey information about the grouping of words into phrases, the degree of emphasis on specific words and phrases, and the speaker's intentions and emotions related to the utterance and the discourse situation (e.g., Cole, Kim, Choi, & Hasegawa-Johnson, 2007). For example, in a sentence such as "I'll be home late tonight," F_0 is lowered at the end of the utterance to signal that this is a declarative sentence, a statement of fact. For a question, speakers typically raise their F_0 at the end, as in the question "You'll be home late tonight?" These F_0 changes are not restricted to a single phoneme or segment, but usually occur over a sequence of phonemes, such as a word, phrase, or sentence. Speakers also vary their F_0 and intensity levels to express different moods, feelings, and attitudes. A person who is feeling exuberant, for example, is likely to show much more marked F_0 changes than one who is feeling depressed. The primary suprasegmental features of speech are **intonation**, **stress**, and **duration**.

Intonation

Intonation refers to the way in which speakers vary their F_0 levels to signal linguistic aspects of speech, such as the type of utterance (declarative, question, etc.). The variation in F_0 level is often referred to as the F_0 *contour* or *pitch contour*. English is characterized by a rise–fall F_0 contour for declarative sentences, in which the F_0 starts off at a higher level at the beginning of the utterance and lowers toward the end of the sentence. So, for instance,

Harry's
going
home.

I had eggs
for
breakfast.

It has been theorized that one of the reasons speakers drop their F_0 at the ends of sentences relates to the physiology of coordinating speech breathing with phonation. The theory, developed by Lieberman (1967), is based on the mechanics of **breath groups**. A breath group refers to a phrase or sentence that is produced on one exhalation. Throughout a typical declarative breath group, subglottal pressure (P_s) stays fairly steady until the last portion of the utterance, when it drops rapidly. As P_s drops, so does F_0. The F_0 for declarative utterances seems to start at a wide variety of F_0 levels, but the endpoints typically fall to around the same frequency (Raphael et al., 2007). Thus, a pattern of falling F_0 seems to result from the natural functioning of the speech subsystems, but the system can be overridden for linguistic purposes. For a question that is marked by a rising F_0 at the end of the utterance, the speaker must increase the tension on the vocal folds by muscular action to counteract the drop in P_s. Raising pitch at the end of a breath group demands a high level of neuromuscular control (Xu & Son, 2002). Development of the ability to use pitch contrastively appears to be a gradual process. Patel and Grigos (2006) reported that 4-year-old children in their study were not able to produce questions with rising intonation but instead used increased duration of the final syllable to mark the contrast between declarative and interrogative utterances. The children were, however, able to produce declarative sentences with appropriate lowering of the pitch. The 7-year-old children in the study used pitch raising in addition

Figure 3.32 F_0 **contour for statement versus question**

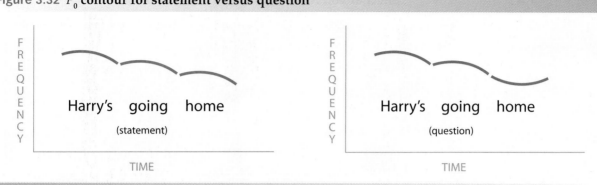

to intensity and duration cues to differentiate between statements and questions; the 11-year-olds used primarily pitch changes and relied less on intensity and duration.

Intonation patterns can be displayed on acoustic instruments and software programs that track F_0 over time and show graphically the changes in F_0 in an utterance. Figure 3.32 is a schematic representation of the F_0 contours of the utterance "Harry's going home," said as a declarative and as a question.

Stress

Stress is another important way of signaling different types of information in an utterance. Stress involves varying the frequency, intensity, and duration of a syllable or word in a way that highlights a particular portion of the utterance. A stressed syllable or word can have a higher F_0, and/or higher intensity, and/or longer duration than one that is unstressed. Some research has suggested that loudness and duration of the syllable contribute more to the prominence of the syllable than does F_0 (Kochanski, Grabe, Coleman, & Rosner, 2005).

Stress patterns differ among languages, and it can be easy to detect a foreign speaker of a language by his or her use of stress. For instance, in English, the word *HAMburger* has stress on the first syllable. Someone who stressed the second syllable, *hamBURGer* would be instantly identifiable as a nonnative speaker of English. Stress also functions on a linguistic level to signal the meaning of a word (called *lexical stress*). For example, the words *PREsent* and *preSENT* have completely different meanings. The first word, with stress on the first syllable, means either a gift or being at a particular place at a particular time. The second word, with stress on the second syllable, means to give. There are many pairs like this in English, called **heteronyms**, in which stress on the first syllable indicates a noun and stress on the second syllable indicates a verb. Some examples include *REcord–reCORD*, *ADDress–addRESS*, and *IMport–imPORT*, and there are numerous others. Another function of stress occurs at a discourse (conversational) level when emphasis is placed on the most salient information in an utterance. For example, in the sentence "He sat on a GREEN chair," it is the color of the chair that is important. This sentence could be in answer to the question "Did he sit on a red chair?" On the other hand, the question "Did he sit on a green table?" might elicit the information that "He sat on a green CHAIR." Here it is the type of furniture that is in question.

The formant patterns of vowels in stressed syllables and in speech that is clearly articulated are clear and distinct, whereas vowels in unstressed syllables often demonstrate more neutral (i.e., more like a schwa) formant frequencies, and contrasts between

Figure 3.33 **Effect of voiced versus voiceless final consonant on vowel duration**

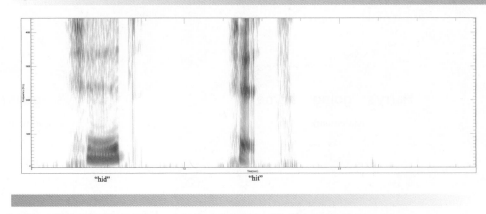

vowels become less clear (e.g., Plag, Kunter, & Schramm, 2011). Research on acoustic characteristics of vowels in regular conversational speech compared to clear speech has demonstrated that F_1 in clear speech is higher than in conversational speech, and F_2 is increased for front vowels and decreased for back vowels (e.g., Ferguson & Kewley-Port, 2002; 2007). The increased separation between formants results in a larger vowel space. The term **vowel reduction** is used when the formant patterns of a vowel become neutralized. Vowel reduction is common in the speech of individuals with communication disorders due to deafness, neurological problems, and other causes.

Duration

Duration refers to the length of time of a speech sound. Duration varies with the degree of stress on a syllable or word. However, phonemes also vary in their inherent duration just because of the way in which they are articulated. Stops, for instance, are extremely short in duration, whereas fricatives are longer. Similarly, diphthongs are longer in duration than glides. The duration of a sound can also be a cue to voicing. In English, vowels are longer when they come before a voiced consonant than when the same vowel precedes a voiceless consonant. Thus, the vowel /ɪ/ is longer in the word *hid* and shorter in the word *hit* (Figure 3.33). Likewise, the /a/ in *hard* is longer in duration than the /a/ in *heart* (Figure 3.34).

Figure 3.34 **Effect of voiced versus voiceless final consonant on vowel duration**

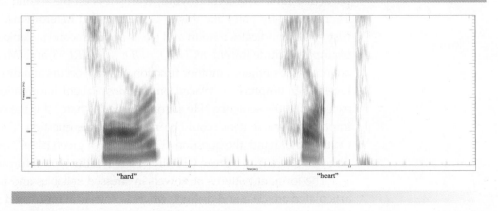

Figure 3.35 Effect of sentence length on duration of words

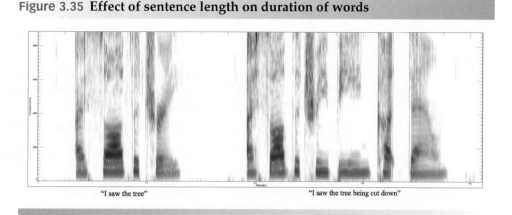

"I saw the tree"   "I saw the tree being cut down"

The duration of a syllable or word in the stream of connected speech is associated with complete units of meaning, such as a phrase or sentence. The last word in a phrase or sentence tends to be longer than it would be in other positions in a sentence, and this helps the listener to figure out the boundaries between phrases. For example, in the utterance "I saw the tree," the word *tree* is fairly long in duration. When the word *tree* occurs in the middle of a sentence, it is shorter in duration, as in the example "I saw a tree being cut down" (Figure 3.35).

These suprasegmental features are vitally important in clarifying the grammatical and cognitive/linguistic aspects of speech, in providing an emotional framework for the idea being expressed, and in enhancing the intelligibility of speech. Speech that lacks suprasegmental variation is perceived as flat and uninteresting, and speech in which the suprasegmental aspects are distorted in some way can be very difficult to understand.

Summary

The vocal tract is a hollow muscular tube that consists of the pharynx, the oral cavity, and nasal cavities.

The articulators within the vocal tract include the lips, tongue, teeth, hard palate, and velum.

The articulators valve the airstream in specific ways to generate various types of complex periodic and complex aperiodic sounds.

The traditional classification system of consonants includes place of articulation, manner of articulation, and voicing.

Vowels are categorized on the vowel quadrilateral in terms of tongue height and tongue advancement.

Spectrography is a method of identifying frequency, amplitude, and duration of sounds; a spectrogram is a graph on which frequency is displayed on the vertical axis, time is represented on the horizontal axis, and intensity of acoustic energy is represented by the darkness of the trace on the screen, or by different colors.

Vowels are characterized spectrographically by their first three formants; these appear as wide, dark horizontal stripes that reflect the concentrations of intense acoustic energy at those harmonic frequencies that have been amplified by the vocal tract resonances.

Diphthongs are characterized by a shift in frequency from the beginning to the end of the sound represented spectrographically by a steady-state formant at the onglide followed by a formant transition.

Glides are characterized by rapid formants without any steady-state portion.

Liquids are characterized by steady-state formants; rhotic sounds show a lowering of F_3; /l/ has a complex spectrum that includes formants and antiformants.

Stops are characterized by a silent gap, release burst, formant transitions, and voice onset time; voiced stops may exhibit a voice bar.

Fricatives are characterized by frication noise, which looks like a wide band of energy distributed over a broad range of frequencies; sibilants have more intense high-frequency energy and are longer in duration than nonsibilants.

Affricates contain acoustic characteristics of both stops and fricatives.

Nasal sounds are characterized by a nasal murmur, which includes antiformants and a nasal formant.

Connected speech is characterized by coarticulatory and suprasegmental factors.

REVIEW EXERCISES

1. Compare and contrast the tongue and velum in terms of their structure and function.

2. Discuss the six manners of production in English.

3. Describe the articulatory and acoustic similarities and differences in diphthongs, glides, stops, fricatives, and nasals.

4. Explain what is meant by the terms *coarticulation* and *suprasegmental*.

CHAPTER

CLINICAL APPLICATION

Evaluation and Treatment of Disorders Related to Articulation

STUDENT LEARNING OBJECTIVES

After reading this chapter you will

○ Identify kinematic measures of articulation.

○ Appreciate the advantages of supplementing perceptual measures of intelligibility with instrumental measures.

○ Discuss acoustic and kinematic measures used in evaluation and treatment of speakers with dysarthria and/or apraxia, hearing impairment, phonological/ articulation disorders, and cleft palate.

○ Explain how kinematic analysis can help to clarify underlying patterns of articulation.

○ Describe how ultrasound, EMA, and EPG information is used as feedback in clinical intervention.

Kinematic Measurement of Articulatory Variables

Problems with the resonance and filtering of the sound wave created either at the glottis or within the oral cavity can result in articulation and intelligibility problems. A patient's articulatory function can be measured with instrumental techniques that assess movement patterns (kinematics): These include cineradiography, strain gauge systems, X-ray microbeam systems, ultrasound, electropalatography, magnetic resonance imaging, and electromagnetic articulography. A patient's speech output can be assessed with acoustic analyses. The first part of this chapter describes instrumental measures of articulation. Discussion then turns to communication disorders that are often characterized by impaired articulatory production. These include neurological disorders such as dysarthria and apraxia, hearing impairment, articulation/phonological disorders, and cleft palate. For each disorder, we will look at acoustic and kinematic parameters that have been used to evaluate and treat individuals with the disorder.

Cineradiography

Cineradiography (also called cinefluorography) is a moving X-ray produced by combining radiographic and motion picture technology (Earnest & Max, 2003). The moving image is displayed on a monitor. This technology provides an excellent view of the movements of the entire vocal tract and articulators during speech but has serious safety issues due to the amount of radiation exposure (Jallon & Berthommier, 2009).

Strain Gauge

Recall from Chapter 1 that strain refers to the relative amount of deformation undergone by an object due to an applied force. A strain gauge is a device whose electrical resistance varies proportionately to the amount of strain. A strain gauge system can be affixed to articulators (usually the lips and jaw) by means of a cantilever, and any distortion (i.e., movement) of the articulator results in a corresponding distortion and change in electrical resistance of the strain gauge. The speaker is fitted with a lightweight head-mounted strain gauge, and small "beads" threaded through the cantilever beam are attached to the target articulators (e.g., Kleinow, Smith, & Ramig, 2001). The amount of change in the electrical resistance of the gauge due to the articulatory movement is measured. This type of system is non invasive, safe, and relatively low cost and has been used extensively to examine speech motor control in normal speakers as well as those with communication disorders.

X-ray Microbeam

An X-ray microbeam system uses a very narrow beam of X-rays focused on a few specific points on a speaker's articulators, usually the upper and lower lips, mandible, and tongue. Small gold pellets are attached to the articulators, and the system tracks the movement of the articulators during speech. Because of the limited amount of radiation, this type of system is safer than regular X-rays. X-ray microbeams are extremely large, complex, and expensive devices, and there are only two such systems in the world: one in Japan, and one at the University of Wisconsin–Madison. However, information obtained with these systems is available without charge to scientists, and a considerable amount of data on normal and impaired articulation has been gathered based on the data obtained from these instruments.

Ultrasound

Ultrasound refers to extremely high frequency sound waves (above 1 MHz) that have correspondingly extremely short wavelengths. Ultrasound technology is based on the principle of reflection. Sound waves are reflected when they encounter changes in the density of the medium through which they are traveling. High frequency waves generated by a transducer are directed at a specific body part. The reflected waves from the body part are received by the transducer and converted into moving images that are displayed on the ultrasound screen. For speech production purposes, the transducer is held underneath the speaker's chin. Because of the short wavelengths, very small objects can be resolved, so the spatial resolution of the images is high (Stone, 2005). Ultrasound can show either midsagittal or coronal views of the tongue.

The sagittal view displays a side view of the tongue showing tongue height, tongue advancement, and tongue slope; the coronal view visualizes a cross section of the tongue from one side to the other, providing information regarding midline grooving or depression/elevation of the sides of the tongue (Bernhardt, Gick, Bacsfalvi, & Adler-Bock, 2005; Bernhardt, Bacsfalvi, Gick, Radanov, & Williams, 2005). Depending on the specific instrument, either two-dimensional or three-dimensional images can be obtained. Ultrasound is safe and non invasive, and it provides images in real-time. The image on the screen can be frozen at any point for review. In particular, differences between alveolar, palatal, and velar places of articulation are highly visible (Bernhardt, Gick, et al., 2005). Portable ultrasound instruments are available, making it possible to use this technology in a clinical situation. Ultrasound has been used to obtain information regarding tongue shape and movement during speech production in a variety of populations (Earnest & Max, 2003).

Electropalatography and Glossometry

Electropalatography (EPG) uses a system consisting of electrodes that are mounted on a thin acrylic plate called a **pseudopalate**. A pseudopalate is custom-made to cover a speaker's hard palate and upper teeth. A surface electrode is attached to the person's wrist. This electrode generates a small, safe charge that the speaker does not feel. A current flows to the pseudopalate electrodes when the speaker's tongue makes contact with them. The palatometric contacts can be relayed to a monitor to provide visual feedback of the patterns of contact between the tongue and palate (Figure 4.1). Contact patterns are visualized in real time so this technology provides instantaneous feedback regarding the speaker's articulatory positions. For example, alveolar consonants demonstrate a horseshoe-shaped pattern, and the palatal

Figure 4.1 Electropalatography

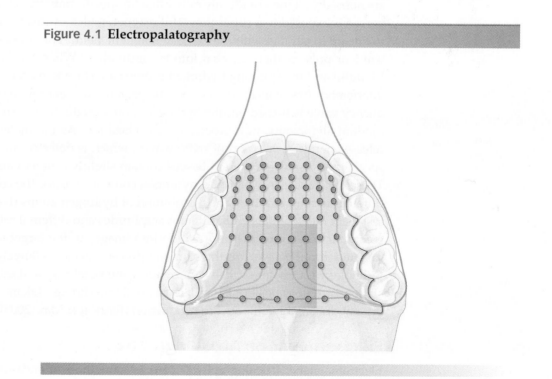

sounds exhibit a pattern of contact behind the alveolar ridge (Bernhardt, Bacsfalvi, et al., 2005). The device is safe and non invasive, and it is highly appropriate for evaluation and treatment purposes. EPG is suitable to train consonants by displaying contact patterns between the tongue and palate, and high vowels such as /i/ and /u/. However, for mid and low vowels, the tongue does not make contact against another articulator, so these sounds are not well visualized with EPG. The major advantage of EPG is that it provides a dynamic, real-time visual display of tongue-to-palate movements that are difficult to see by using other methods (Dagenais, 1995).

Glossometry is another technique used to visualize tongue positions and shapes anywhere within the oral cavity and can therefore provide images of vowel patterns. As with EPG, the speaker is fitted with a pseudopalate, which is customized to fit his or her hard palate and upper teeth. Mounted on the pseudopalate are four pairs of light-emitting diode (LED) photosensors. Hardware and software outside the speaker's mouth are used to calculate the distance between the sensors and the tongue at 10-msec intervals. These distance values are stored on a computer and are also displayed on a monitor. A more recent version of glossometry is called **optopalatography (OPG)**. OPG measures the intensity of light reflected from the surface of the tongue, as well as the location and the amount of pressure of the contact (Earnest & Max, 2003).

Magnetic Resonance Imaging

Magnetic resonance imaging (MRI) is a technique that takes advantage of the cellular basis of human tissue. One of the major components of tissue is water, and hydrogen atoms constitute one element of water molecules (H_2O). Hydrogen atoms behave like miniature magnets spinning around an axis at a certain frequency. They are normally aligned randomly rather than in specific patterns. During an MRI, the person is exposed to a super-powerful magnet, which causes the hydrogen atoms to line up in parallel with the external magnetic field. A brief radiofrequency (RF) wave or pulse is then directed into the individual. When the frequencies of the RF pulse and the spinning hydrogen protons are close to each other, constructive interference (resonance) occurs, and the proton gains energy. When the radiofrequency wave is turned off, the hydrogen atoms gradually return to their original random alignments, in a process called relaxation. As the molecules relax, they release energy in the form of radio waves, which is detected and amplified by a specialized receiver. Different tissues contain slightly different amounts of water. These differences in water and hydrogen content produce the contrasts between different tissues, based on the distribution of hydrogen atoms (Lauter, 1997). This results in radio signals with different amplitudes and different relaxation times. A computer transforms the information into images of the target structure. MRI is safe and non invasive, but the scanning process takes a relatively long time. The technology is therefore suitable for imaging the vocal tract and articulators during static articulatory positions such as sustained vowels (e.g., Takano & Honda, 2007), but not during dynamic speech production (Earnest & Max, 2003).

Electromagnetic Articulography

Electromagnetic articulography (EMA) is a method of measuring articulatory movement of the tongue, lips, jaw, and velum. Speakers wear a helmet that holds three transmitter coils. The transmitters produce alternating magnetic fields, which generate currents in tiny receiver coils (sensors) fixed to the specific articulator(s) of interest. The sensors are connected to a computer by thin, flexible wires. As the sensors move through the magnetic fields, the computer tracks them and determines the coordinates of each sensor (Al Bawab, Turicchia, Stern, & Raj, 2009). The movement patterns of the articulator are displayed on a graph on a computer screen. Up to 10 sensors may be used, and they are attached at various locations on the tongue and lips, using a dental adhesive. The newest version of the articulograph (AG500) uses six coils that are attached to a plexiglass cube around the speaker's head rather than to a helmet. The speaker is therefore able to move his or her head freely within the cube (Figure 4.2). The use of additional coils allows articulatory movements to be seen in different planes and provides a 3D image of articulators.

Figure 4.2 Electromagnetic articulography

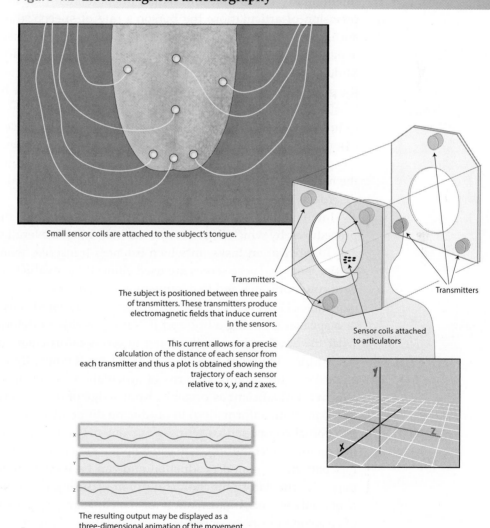

Small sensor coils are attached to the subject's tongue.

Transmitters

The subject is positioned between three pairs of transmitters. These transmitters produce electromagnetic fields that induce current in the sensors.

This current allows for a precise calculation of the distance of each sensor from each transmitter and thus a plot is obtained showing the trajectory of each sensor relative to x, y, and z axes.

Transmitters

Sensor coils attached to articulators

The resulting output may be displayed as a three-dimensional animation of the movement of the sensors or as a two-dimensional plot of their locations over time relative to x, y, and z axes.

Articulography is safe and non invasive, and it allows detailed examination of movements of articulators including the tongue and velum. The equipment has been shown to be safe even for people who wear pacemakers or implantable defibrillators (e.g., Joglar, Nguyen, Garst, & Katz, 2009). While it has some limitations in terms of its accuracy and possible sensor-related loss of intelligibility for some individuals with neurological disorders (e.g., Yunusova, Green, & Mefferd, 2009), this technology, particularly the 3D version, allows unprecedented access to movements of hard-to-see articulators such as the tongue and velum.

Articulation and Intelligibility

Correct articulation is a fundamental basis of intelligible speech. *Intelligibility* refers to the ease with which a listener is able to understand a speaker. Intelligibility is a multidimensional phenomenon that involves the degree of precision of articulation, the person's rate of speech, the length of the utterance, the familiarity and predictability of the words used, and the listener's experience with the speaker's speech patterns (e.g., Hustad, 2006; Van Nuffelen, Middag, De Bodt, & Martens, 2009). The speaker's loudness, pitch, voice quality, prosody, and degree of nasal resonance also influence his or her intelligibility (De Bodt, Huici, & Van De Heyning, 2002; Weismer & Laures, 2002). Poor or reduced intelligibility due to interference with any of these aspects can result in communicative breakdowns. Reduced intelligibility can be socially, professionally, and educationally devastating, so improving intelligibility is often one of the most important goals of clinical management for speakers with articulatory disorders.

Intelligibility is measured perceptually by two kinds of techniques: **scaling procedures**, by which listeners rate the individual's overall speech intelligibility; and **identification tasks**, in which listeners transcribe words or sentences said by the speaker. These scores are used clinically to evaluate how effectively a patient communicates and to document any changes in the speaker's intelligibility over time. However, perceptual ratings usually yield only an overall estimate of a speaker's intelligibility, and it is not possible to determine from this score what the speaker is actually doing in terms of articulation. This makes it difficult to use the score as a starting point for therapy. By contrast, determining a speaker's underlying patterns of articulation can ensure that treatment is as effective and efficient as possible. Knowledge of the movements of the articulators (kinematic information) in producing different sounds and the acoustic and perceptual consequences of these movements is therefore highly useful clinical information. Such information can help the patient to visualize and produce correct patterns of sound production and can be used to monitor changes in the person's articulatory function and progress during the course of treatment. This is not only essential information for the clinician and patient, but, in these days of cost consciousness, objective documentation of progress is an important way of assuring treatment effectiveness for third-party payers.

Dysarthria/Apraxia

Dysarthria and/or apraxia of speech result from neurological disorders such as stroke, Parkinson's disease, amyotrophic lateral sclerosis, multiple sclerosis, traumatic brain injury, and others. **Dysarthria** is an umbrella term for a group of speech production disorders in which the speech musculature is weak, paralyzed, or uncoordinated. **Apraxia** is a condition in which the patient has difficulty sequencing the articulatory movements for speech. Much research has been done on the acoustic and kinematic characteristics of neurological speech motor disorders. Acoustic measures such as duration of vowels and consonants, formant frequency information, and spectral analysis of phonemes, as well as kinematic information regarding the patient's underlying articulatory patterns, help to supplement and complement perceptual judgments about the intelligibility of an individual's speech. In addition, such measures can show how a person may be compensating for the impairment. This is clinically vital information because two people who sound similarly and who score similarly on an intelligibility test can have very different articulatory movements and compensatory strategies. Clearly, the treatment plan for each individual should target the specific underlying problem.

Acoustic Measures

Many speakers who have dysarthria exhibit difficulty with the timing of their articulatory movements. Duration of both vowels and consonants has been reported to be longer and more variable in speakers with dysarthria compared to speakers who do not have neurological problems. Caruso and Klasner Burton (1987) examined duration of vowels in speakers with amyotrophic lateral sclerosis (ALS) who were perceptually rated 80 to 85 percent intelligible during conversation. The ALS speakers' vowel durations were significantly longer than normal, indicating that these individuals may have weak, slowly moving tongue gestures. The fact that these speakers were highly intelligible suggests that changes in the speed of tongue movement may be an early indication of ALS, before speech is perceived to be distorted. Therefore, acoustic measurements that reveal timing abnormalities in articulatory function may help in the early detection of this disease. Decreased speed of articulatory movement has also been reported for speakers with other types of neurological problems (Seddoh et al., 1996; Skodda, Visser, & Schlegel, 2010). Longer durations of vowels and consonants can be evident as an overall slowing of the rate of speech. Healthy individuals typically speak at a rate around 5 syllables per second. LeDorze, Ouellette, and Ryalls (1994) reported that their nondisordered speakers had an average rate of 4.7 syllables per second, while the rate for the dysarthric speakers was considerably slower, at an average of 3.1 syllables per second.

Vowel formant analysis

F_1/F_2 plots have been used to construct vowel spaces in order to make inferences about a speaker's tongue movements (see Figure 2.15). Many speakers who have dysarthria have been shown to have a reduced vowel space, in which formant values for corner vowels /i/, /a/, /æ/, and /u/ shift to a more neutralized pattern (e.g., Bunton & Weismer, 2001; Goberman & Elmer, 2005; Weismer, Yunusova, & Westbury, 2003); or cluster in a specific area of the vowel space (e.g., Whiteside, Grobler, Windsor, & Varley, 2010). Compression of the vowel space indicates a reduced range of F_1 and F_2 frequencies. At the articulatory level, the reduced vowel space indicates that the speaker is not reaching appropriate tongue positions for the corner vowels. An F_1 that is higher or lower in frequency than normal means that the tongue is not achieving the appropriate height for that particular vowel; a higher or lower than normal F_2 frequency indicates that the tongue is too far forward (in the case of a back vowel) or too far back (in the case of a front vowel). This kind of vowel distortion can have a dramatic impact on speech intelligibility. Using formant analysis, Ziegler and von Cramon (1983) demonstrated changes in articulatory function over time for speakers with closed head injury and resulting dysarthria. Many of the patients started out being completely mute. In the period immediately following the mutism (first 8 weeks), some patients showed a marked shift of formants toward the center of the formant chart, particularly for F_2. From 8 weeks to 6 months post-injury, patients showed a gradual widening of the vowel space, and after 6 months, there was an appreciable increase in vowel space. Acoustic evidence thus demonstrated the gradual recovery of articulatory function. Specifically, it could be inferred that the patients regained some tongue mobility over time and were better able to reach vowel targets. This information provides not only objective evidence of progress in speech production but also the specific degree of progress can be documented. In a similar study, Turner, Tjaden, and Weismer (1995) constructed vowel spaces for speakers with and without ALS. Not only did the speakers with ALS have a reduced vowel space compared to the non-dysarthric speakers, but there were also differences in vowel space between the groups when the researchers manipulated rate of speech. When the normal speakers slowed their rate of speech, their vowel spaces increased, showing that their tongue movements became even more precise in reaching vowel targets. Perceptually, their intelligibility also increased. This relationship did not hold for the speakers with ALS, whose vowel spaces did not enlarge, and who did not consistently improve intelligibility when they used a slower than normal rate of speech. This is important information to know because teaching dysarthric speakers to slow their rate of speech is a popular technique for increasing intelligibility. Information about vowel space can be helpful in deciding whether a clinical strategy such as slowing rate is effective for a particular individual.

Recently, several articulatory measures have been developed based on the ratios between F_1 and F_2 of the corner vowels. Both healthy and impaired speakers produce highly variable formant patterns due to differences in the size and shape of the vocal tract, the way that the articulators are positioned, the amount of lip rounding, the type of speech task, and the vowel context (Sapir, Ramig, Spielman, & Fox, 2010). Formant ratios are helpful because they reduce the effects of variability between and within individuals so that the ratio is similar across speakers. Formant ratios are therefore more sensitive to the effects of articulatory impairment on vowel production. One formant ratio measure is called the Vowel Articulation Index (VAI) (e.g., Roy, Nissen, Dromey, & Sapir, 2009; Sapir, 2007; Skodda, Visser,

& Schlegel, 2011; Spielman et al., 2011). The VAI divides the high formant frequencies by the low frequencies to derive the ratio between them. A higher ratio indicates a larger vowel space, and a lower ratio reflects a smaller vowel space. This index seems to be sensitive to even mild degrees of dysarthria. For example, Skodda et al. (2011) reported that speakers with mild dysarthria but perceptually intelligible speech demonstrated lower VAI values compared to healthy speakers. Spielman et al. (2011) reported that speakers with Parkinson's disease increased their VAI values following treatment with the Lee Silverman Voice Therapy (LSVT), a systematic protocol that teaches patients to use a healthy louder voice. A similar ratio, called the Formant Centralization Ratio (FCR) was described by Sapir et al. (2010). The FCR increases as vowels become more centralized and the vowel space is compressed, and decreases as the vowel space expands. Sapir et al. (2010) reported that the FCR was highly sensitive in discriminating between healthy and dysarthric speakers and, furthermore, accurately reflected improvements in vowel production following LSVT treatment for the dysarthric speakers.

Another way that formant information has been used to infer articulatory function in people with dysarthria is by measuring F_2 transitions. Recall that F_2 is related to place of articulation, because it is linked to the degree of forward or backward movement of the tongue. The portion of the formant that contains a transition is measured in terms of its slope. The duration of the transition is measured in milliseconds (msec), and the extent of the transition is measured in Hz. This yields a **slope index** measured in Hz per millisecond (Hz/msec). A slope is defined as a change that is equal to or greater than 20 to 30 Hz over 20 msec (e.g., Kim, Weismer, Kent, & Duffy, 2009; Rosen, Kent, Delaney, & Duffy, 2006). A flatter slope indicates an articulatory movement that is made over a greater period of time. This reflects tongue movement that is slower with less of a range. Shallower slopes are commonly reported for speakers with dysarthria (e.g., Kim et al., 2009).

The slope index provides diagnostic information regarding whether tongue movement is close to or far from normal and also provides ongoing information regarding the course of the disease and its effect on speech. F_2 slope index has been correlated to degree of speech intelligibility and has been shown to be a sensitive index of vocal tract function for speech (e.g., Kim, Kent, & Weismer, 2011). As with measures of vowel space, information about a patient's formant transitions may also help to detect early signs of the disease, before a decrease in intelligibility can be heard perceptually. For example, Kent et al. (1991) reported that women without any neurological problems have a slope index of 3.76 to 5.4 Hz/msec. The steepness of the slope indicates that F_2 frequency changes rapidly within a short period of time as the tongue makes quick adjustments for the particular sound. A slope of 3.0 Hz/msec seems to be a dividing point between normal speakers and those with ALS, and a slope index of 2.5 Hz/msec appears to distinguish dysarthric patients with good intelligibility from those with poor intelligibility (Kent et al., 1989). To illustrate how a slope index provides information about underlying articulatory factors, Kent et al. (1991) reported on a woman with ALS who showed a much less steep slope than normal, which became even shallower as her disease progressed. At the beginning of a 2-year interval during which the woman's speech was analyzed, her average slope was 3.17 Hz/msec. By the end of

2 years, the slope declined by about 40 percent, to 1.32 Hz/msec. The reduced slope reflected the patient's weaker and slower tongue movements and her reduced range of articulatory motion. During the same period, her speech deteriorated perceptually in intelligibility, dropping on an intelligibility word test by about 50 percent. Weismer, Martin, Kent, and Kent (1992) examined F_2 slope data in normally speaking individuals and in two groups of speakers with ALS: those whose speech intelligibility scores exceeded 70 percent and those whose scores were below 70 percent. The speakers with ALS had longer transition durations than normal and shallower slopes. In both groups with ALS, formant trajectories (i.e., the paths of the formant transitions) tended to cluster around 500 and 1500 Hz for many of the words, reflecting vowel centralization. Shallow slopes have also been documented in speakers with multiple sclerosis and Parkinson's disease (e.g., Rosen, Goozee, & Murdoch, 2008; Rosen et al., 2006; Tjaden & Wilding, 2004).

Analysis of formant trajectories has been used clinically to document treatment effectiveness. For example, Dromey, Ramig, and Johnson (1995) designed a treatment approach to increase vocal loudness in a man with Parkinson's disease and examined his articulatory movements as his intensity increased throughout treatment. For all the vowels studied, the degree of the frequency change of the F_2 transitions increased, particularly for words containing high front vowels. The authors used this acoustic information to highlight the fact that their vocal intensity treatment was effective in increasing articulatory movement, even though articulation was not a focus of the treatment.

Spectral analysis of consonants

Distortion of consonants can contribute to poor intelligibility. Many people with dysarthria have particular difficulty producing stops, fricatives, and affricates, which require a high degree of tongue movement precision for accurate production. Distinguishing between alveolar and palatal fricatives also tends to be problematic because the lack of precise tongue control makes it hard to maintain the narrow and more anterior grooved tongue position for the /s/. Researchers have reported that the spectrum of the /s/ produced by dysarthric speakers may show lower frequency peaks than normal, indicating a more posterior constriction, a wider or longer constriction, reduced flow through the constriction, or some combination of these factors (e.g., Harmes et al., 1984; Tjaden & Turner, 1997). On the other hand, some dysarthric speakers may not be able to keep the tongue positioned more posteriorly for the /ʃ/, resulting in a spectrum with higher frequency peaks similar to those for /s/.

Spectral analysis of stop consonants has shown similar articulatory problems in the speech of individuals with dysarthria. Shinn and Blumstein (1983) found changed spectral characteristics in the alveolar stop /t/ in individuals with Broca's aphasia. If the closure for a stop is not complete due to a lack of articulatory control, there will be a continuous release of pressure, similar to a fricative. Spectrographically, the silent gap that is characteristic of stops is obliterated. Shinn and Blumstein observed a gradual buildup of noise, with no burst corresponding to the release of the blockage. This suggests that the patient with Broca's aphasia never completely closed off his vocal tract for the stop. Some individuals with multiple sclerosis (MS) show similar inadequate closure for stops, reflected in continuous frication. Speakers with MS in a study by Hartelius, Nord, and Buder (1995) also showed continuous voicing throughout the voiceless stops /p/ and /k/. In addition the stops were nasalized, with a nasal formant occurring during the occlusion of the voiced stop /d/.

The importance of determining the precise articulatory movements that contribute to reduced intelligibility becomes very clear from a study of speech rate in individuals with Parkinson's disease (PD). In most types of dysarthria, speech rate is slowed, but in PD the speech rate is often perceived as faster than normal. This is known as **accelerated speech**. The increased rate of speech is particularly damaging to intelligibility, and reducing speech rate is often used as a clinical tool. Ziegler, Hoole, Hartmann, and von Cramon (1988) examined speech rate in patients with PD and found that most of the patients with perceived accelerated speech actually had average rates within or close to the normal range. However, other aspects of their articulation were affected. For instance, the speakers had difficulty completely stopping sound production during stop closures, demonstrated by the presence of frication noise during the articulatory closures for voiceless stops. They also took a shorter-than-normal time to switch from an opening movement for a vowel to a closing movement for a consonant, suggesting that the articulators began to close for the consonant before the vowel target had been satisfactorily achieved. However, the vowels themselves were normal in duration. Thus, these patients demonstrated **articulatory undershoot** despite normal movement times. The authors argued that the perceptual impression of faster-than-normal speech rate must have been based on acoustic cues aside from the actual rate of speech itself, such as the articulatory undershoot. They noted that when healthy speakers increase their speech rate, the articulators do not reach their target positions with as much accuracy as they do at slower rates. Therefore, it is likely that articulatory undershoot by a dysarthric speaker with a normal or near normal rate of speech may lead to the impression of an accelerated speech rate. With this kind of information, a clinician can plan treatment to teach the patient with Parkinson's disease to be more precise in reaching articulatory targets. This kind of treatment may be more efficient than teaching the patient to slow down speech that is actually within normal limits for rate. It is clear that inferring the articulatory basis for the unintelligible speech helps to understand precisely which aspects of articulation should be targeted in therapy.

Kinematic Measures

Many different analysis systems have been used to measure and manage articulatory movement patterns in individuals with dysarthria and apraxia, including cineradiography, strain gauge systems, electropalatography, and electromagnetic articulography.

Cineradiography

Cineradiography has not been used extensively with dysarthric or apraxic individuals because of the safety issues associated with radiation. However, in an early study, Kent and Netsell (1975) used cineradiography in conjunction with spectrography to examine speech production in an individual with dysarthria.

They reported marked abnormalities in the speaker's articulatory placements for vowels and consonants, as well as lower velocities of articulatory movements and overall reduced rate of speech.

Strain gauge

Strain gauge systems do not have safety concerns and have been used to document movement patterns in many different groups of speakers. Kleinow et al. (2001) used a strain gauge to measure movements of the lip and jaw of individuals with PD under different loudness and speech rate conditions. They reported that under the loud conditions speakers with PD showed more stable articulatory movements than when they were instructed to speak more slowly than usual. The authors highlighted the clinical importance of this finding, as some therapy approaches focus on slowing down the rate of speech of patients with motor speech disorders such as PD. Langmore and Lehman (1994) noted that speakers with ALS demonstrated reduced strength and speed of movement of the articulators, particularly the tongue. The strain gauge system allowed the authors to discover that the perceived severity of the dysarthria correlated more strongly with reduced speed of articulator movement rather than with reduced tongue strength.

Electropalatography

Numerous EPG studies have demonstrated the presence of three characteristic tongue-palate configurations in adults with dysarthria: too little tongue contact (articulatory undershoot), too much contact (**articulatory overshoot**), and excessively posterior placement of the tongue (e.g., Hartinger, Tripoliti, Hardcastle, & Limousin, 2011; McAuliffe & Ward, 2006). These patterns contribute to the impression of articulatory imprecision that is common in speakers with dysarthria. EPG can be very helpful in determining the specific degree of articulatory undershoot or overshoot by counting the number of electrodes contacted by the speaker's tongue during articulation of specific sounds. McAuliffe, Ward, and Murdoch (2006) compared perceptual and EPG patterns for speakers with PD, healthy elderly speakers, and healthy younger speakers. The speakers with PD were perceptually rated as demonstrating consonant imprecision characterized by articulatory undershoot and a marked number of articulation errors. However, the EPG analysis did not show deviant tongue–palate contact patterns for this group. The researchers speculated that two articulatory factors may have contributed to the perceptual impression of consonant imprecision: reduction of tongue force and difficulty coordinating the timing of the articulatory movements. In speakers with apraxia, EPG has demonstrated speech production difficulties such as a reduction in functional independence of tongue movements, overshoot of tongue movements, distorted tongue-to-palate patterns for the /s/ sound, and impaired coarticulation (Bartle-Meyer, Murdoch, & Goozee, 2009; McAuliffe & Ward, 2006).

Another common finding in speakers with dysarthria is lengthened duration of segments (phonemes) within utterances. EPG can provide detailed information regarding aspects of segment duration such as the duration of the tongue's approach to closure or constriction of the vocal tract and the duration of the tongue's movement away from the palate (McAuliffe & Ward, 2006). However,

EPG does not provide information regarding which section of the tongue makes contact against the palate or how the tongue moves toward or away from the palate (McAuliffe & Ward, 2006).

Electromagnetic articulography

Electromagnetic articulography (EMA) has been used in assessment and treatment of dysarthria and apraxia in adults and children. For example, Goozee, Murdoch, Theodoros, and Stokes (2000) described articulatory information obtained with EMA for an adult patient with dysarthria. The authors reported that the speaker was unable to control his tongue-to-palate contact for the phonemes /t/, /s/, and /k/, resulting in the perceptual impression of consonant imprecision. Bartle, Goozee, Scott, Murdoch, and Kuruvilla (2006) investigated the coordination of tongue tip, tongue back, and jaw movements in adult speakers with dysarthria. Analysis of the articulatory patterns of each individual showed disturbances in the timing and positioning of the articulators in the production of the /t/ sound. Murdoch and Goozee (2003) used the same technology to examine the underlying articulatory patterns in children with dysarthria. Each of the four children demonstrated consonant distortions as well as increased word durations and reduced rates of speech. However, each was associated with different articulatory patterns. Kuruvilla, Murdoch, and Goozee (2007) described disturbed articulatory movements in speakers with dysarthria resulting from severe traumatic brain injury (TBI), but not in individuals with mild TBI. Taken together, these studies highlight the fact that clinical intervention approaches need to be specifically targeted to individual speakers' articulatory movements in order to maximize the chances for successful therapy outcomes.

EMA technology has been used successfully as visual feedback for speakers with dysarthria and apraxia. In a series of studies, Katz and colleagues provided visual feedback for patients with apraxia (Katz, Bharadwaj, & Carstens, 1999; Katz et al., 2007; McNeil et al., 2007; McNeil et al., 2010). Sensors were attached to the speaker's tongue tip, tongue dorsum, and lower lip. The patient sat in front of a computer monitor that displayed target areas for tongue tip contact and a real time image of the position of the individual's tongue tip. When the patient was successful in achieving the target, visual and auditory feedback were provided via the computer as well as perceptual feedback from the clinician. The authors reported that speakers improved their articulatory movements for most of the training words. In addition, the individuals demonstrated considerable generalization of accurate movement patterns to words that had not been trained, and maintained these patterns over a period of time.

Hearing Impairment

Hearing impairment is an area that has benefited greatly from knowledge of the relationships between articulatory movement patterns and acoustic output. Deaf or hearing-impaired (HI) individuals typically have a great deal of difficulty with articulation, because development of normal articulation depends on hearing the sounds of the language, as well as the output of the articulatory system while speaking. The articulatory difficulties result in reduced intelligibility, ranging from mild to severe. The kind of distortion in speech that is perceived is often labeled *deaf speech*, and it can be very easy to recognize a deaf or hearing-impaired speaker by the sound of his or her speech. Speakers may have difficulty producing vowels and consonants and may also be unable to control the suprasegmental aspects of speech. Some speakers may not be able to coarticulate the speech sounds appropriately and may produce speech as a series of separate phonemes (Tye-Murray, 1987; Waldstein & Baum, 1991). Coarticulatory difficulty may account for many of the intelligibility deficits of some deaf talkers. Acoustic and kinematic analysis (cineradiography and X-ray microbeam) have been helpful in clarifying hearing-impaired speakers' problems at the segmental and suprasegmental levels. The most frequent segmental errors in deaf speech are vowel problems, particularly neutralization of vowels. F_1/F_2 charts show marked limitations in both horizontal and vertical degree of tongue movements for vowels in deaf speakers, even those who are intelligible or semi-intelligible. Cineradiographic and X-ray microbeam data have confirmed that at least some hearing-impaired/deaf speakers move the tongue in an undifferentiated manner for all vowels (e.g., Tye-Murray, 1991). Consonant errors are also common, such as omissions and substitutions involving voicing, manner, and place of articulation. Place of articulation may be particularly difficult for many individuals with hearing impairment because of their imprecise tongue position and reduced articulatory movement. Suprasegmental problems include inappropriate, excessive, or insufficient variations in F_0 and intensity.

Acoustic Measures

Acoustic analysis of the spectra of profoundly hearing-impaired speakers' stop consonants indicates that alveolar and velar stops are often produced with the constriction farther back in the vocal tract than normal. This information is clinically helpful because it suggests a physiologically based starting place for achieving more precise articulatory targets. If a hearing-impaired child is distorting consonants by producing them too far back in the vocal tract, treatment can focus on helping the child to bring the articulators to a more forward position for the sound. Also, the effectiveness of this strategy can be checked perceptually and acoustically during the course of treatment. Acoustic analysis is also helpful in visualizing the speaker's suprasegmental patterns. Monsen (1979) tested 3- to 6-year-old severely and profoundly hearing-impaired children imitating words. He examined the duration and intonation patterns of words (also called F_0 contour). The children's task was to imitate a word with a smoothly falling, declarative contour. A falling contour should be easy to produce, since F_0 typically decreases as subglottal air pressure falls at the end of the word. However, most of the deaf children did not produce the smoothly falling F_0 contour. Some of the children produced a *flat contour*, and others showed a *changing contour*. In the changing contour pattern, the direction of the frequency change appeared to be uncontrolled: One pattern showed the F_0 first rising, then falling, then leveling, and then rising again, all over the course of a single syllable. Another suprasegmental problem is that hearing-impaired talkers often do not produce enough variation in F_0 to differentiate between declarative versus interrogative utterances. Speakers with hearing impairment have been reported as demonstrating excessive, equal, and/or misplaced stress (e.g., Lenden & Flipsen, 2007). Such atypical contour patterns can seriously degrade a speaker's intelligibility.

A major focus of many programs for deaf and hearing-impaired speakers is improving speech intelligibility. An important question is how much emphasis should be placed on different aspects of speech production to achieve optimal intelligibility. Some programs may focus more on segmental aspects of speech, while others may devote more time to suprasegmental aspects. Acoustic analysis has been used to try to determine whether segmental or suprasegmental aspects of speech production contribute most to improved intelligibility. In an interesting experiment, Maassen and Povel (1985) took speech samples of deaf children and resynthesized them acoustically with correctly produced vowels and consonants. They played the original speech and the resynthesized speech samples to listeners who evaluated the intelligibility of the utterances. Correcting the segments (phonemes) caused a dramatic 50 percent increase in intelligibility, with a major part of the increase resulting from correcting the vowels. The investigators used the same protocol to change the suprasegmental aspects of the speech samples. This also increased intelligibility scores, but only by about 10 percent. The authors advocated focusing on vowel articulation training. They proposed that once the segmental aspects have been improved, children can work on the suprasegmental aspects to fine-tune their intelligibility and naturalness of speech. Metz, Schiavetti, Samar, and Sitler (1990) also emphasized training children in the segmental aspects of speech production to improve intelligibility. They examined acoustic measures representing both segmental and suprasegmental aspects of speech production. Segmental aspects included VOT, F_2 transitions, difference between F_1 of /i/ and /a/, difference between F_2 of /i/ and /u/, and F_2 change associated with the diphthong /ai/. The suprasegmental aspects included change in F_0 associated with statements and questions, differences in vowel F_0, vowel duration, vowel intensity between stressed and unstressed syllables, and overall duration of sentences. The deaf speakers' intelligibility was rated by normally hearing listeners. The authors found that the acoustic events related to segmental control were the most important factors in how intelligible the speakers were rated, whereas suprasegmental aspects were secondary.

Speech training programs often emphasize the combination of residual hearing and visual cues to compensate for the individual's hearing loss. Although this kind of training can be helpful in improving speech sounds that are easy to see such as bilabials, interdentals, and labiodentals, less improvement tends to occur for speech sounds that are produced in the middle or back of the oral cavity. Another disadvantage of relying solely on residual hearing and speechreading cues is that the child does not receive instant feedback about his or her articulatory movements as they occur. This makes it more difficult for the child to associate the articulatory movement with the tactile feedback from the tongue and other articulators, which is an important aspect of learning speech sound production. Spectrographic analysis has the advantage of providing instantaneous visual feedback as the child produces the target sound. Ertmer, Stark, and Karlan (1996) used spectrographic displays to train two 9-year-old children with profound hearing loss to produce vowels. The children were taught to recognize the formants of different vowels and were then shown how to position their tongues to achieve the target. Analysis of the children's formants after treatment demonstrated that they improved their vowel productions. Similarly, Ertmer and Stark (1995) used spectrographic analysis with a 3-year-old boy who used mainly gestures and signs to communicate. When he did attempt to communicate orally, his utterances usually consisted of isolated vowels or isolated consonant–vowel sequences. The child produced spontaneous utterances in only three contexts: to gain attention, to label objects, and during games and puzzles. However, when he was provided with spectrographic feedback, he vocalized more to see how his sounds changed the visual display. It was apparent that the visual feedback stimulated his interest in exploring different sounds. Normally hearing babies and young children use vocal play in learning to associate the tactile and auditory connections between sounds. Because treatment using acoustic visual feedback encourages this kind of self-stimulatory vocal behavior, it allows treatment activities to be spontaneous, play oriented, and child directed. The instrumentation provides the child opportunities to discover the relationship between acoustic output and tactile feedback within the vocal tract and therefore affords much greater opportunity for internalizing the sounds of speech.

Kinematic Measures

While spectrography provides deaf and hearing-impaired individuals with visual displays of acoustic–articulatory relationships, it does not directly correlate with articulatory function. Kinematic analysis can be extremely helpful in allowing speakers to change specific articulatory patterns.

Electropalatography and glossometry

Electropalatography (EPG) and glossometry provide direct information about the movements of the articulators. This can be extremely valuable for speakers with intelligibility difficulties, since the instrumentation provides biofeedback and evidence of even small changes in articulatory performance (Kelly, Main, Manley, & McLean, 2000). For example, Fletcher, Dagenais, and Crotz-Crosby (1991a) used EPG with girls ages 10 to 16 years who were profoundly hearing impaired, with unintelligible speech. They taught the girls the place and manner of articulation for various stops and fricatives. Through the palatometric display on the monitor, the girls could see exactly where their tongues were making contact on the alveolar ridge and palate and were able to modify their positions as appropriate. The instantaneous visual feedback regarding tongue position was effective in helping the girls become more accurate in reaching articulatory positions, and their intelligibility increased correspondingly. Fletcher, Dagenais, and Crotz-Crosby (1991b) used glossometry to train 4- to 16-year-old profoundly hearing-impaired girls to produce less centralized vowels. The glossometric display provided immediate visual feedback of the vertical location of the girls' tongues in the oral cavity. Using this technology, some of the girls learned to produce more intelligible vowels and expanded their use of the oral space. They showed greater differentiation between vowels, with marked normalization in tongue positions and shapes. Bernhardt, Gick, Bacsfalvi, and Ashdown (2003) used EPG as well as ultrasound to train four adolescent hard-of-hearing speakers ages 16 to 18. All the participants had received many years of traditional speech therapy focusing on articulation without achieving correct production of specific phonemes including /s/, /ʃ/, /l/, and /r/. Incorporating visual feedback regarding tongue contact, movement, and shape was very successful in helping the speakers to achieve accurate productions of these sounds in a short period of time. Improved patterns of articulation included narrowing of the constriction for the /s/ phoneme; increased symmetry of contact for /r/; more posterior tongue placement for the back vowel /u/; and increased height of the tongue body for the high vowel /i/ (Bernhardt et al., 2005).

Cochlear Implantation

Cochlear implantation (CI) is widely used to facilitate speech perception and speech production in hard-of-hearing and deaf children and adults by providing the auditory feedback that is lacking through normal channels. (See Chapter 9 for a detailed description of CI.) However, improved access to auditory feedback does not automatically result in improvements in articulatory function (Pantelemidou, Herman, & Thomas, 2003). Speech therapy after CI is an important component of the intervention process in order to establish correct motor patterns for speech sounds (Poissant, Peters, & Robb, 2006). Acoustic and kinematic measures are helpful in implementing and evaluating the individual's speech production capabilities before and after CI.

Acoustic measures

Measures of formants and vowel spaces in children and adults have demonstrated large variability between individuals after implantation. For example, Evans and Deliyski (2007) reported vowel neutralization in two of the three adult CI users in their study, which did not change before and after implantation, while the third speaker showed a difference in only one vowel. Seifert et al. (2002) found that age at implantation had an effect on vowel articulation: Children who were implanted before their fourth birthday demonstrated essentially normal vowel space, as opposed to children implanted at older ages. Ertmer (2001) followed the vowel development in one child who was implanted at age 19 months. Her vowel inventory more than doubled after 2 months of implant experience. After 1 year, the child demonstrated an almost normal vowel space, compared to many deaf children who show an unchanging F_2 for most vowels. Horga and Liker (2006) compared vowel spaces in groups of profoundly hearing-impaired children using traditional hearing aids, children with cochlear implants, and normally hearing children. The profoundly hearing-impaired children showed a significantly reduced vowel space compared with the normally hearing and implanted children. The children with cochlear implants had better vowel differentiation than the hearing aid users. Liker, Mildner, and Sindija (2007) examined vowel spaces and fricative production in children with cochlear implants and normally hearing/speaking children. They reported that the implanted children demonstrated a smaller vowel space with higher F_2 frequencies showing fronting of vowels, particularly for the back vowels

/u/ and /o/. However, the shape of the vowel space was comparable in the two groups, suggesting that the cochlear implant users were aware of the tongue positions and relationships for the corner vowels. The implanted children showed an overlap in the frequency of their frication noise for the /s/ and /ʃ/ phonemes; unlike the hearing children who produced a clear separation of the frication noises, with that for /s/ being considerably higher than that for /ʃ/. Kunisue, Fukushima, Nagayasu, Kawasaki, and Nishizaki (2006) compared vowel spaces in school-aged children who used cochlear implants, normally hearing adults, and hearing-impaired children who used traditional hearing aids. Analysis of F_1 and F_2 over time showed that the earliest improvement in vowel production for the CI users occurred around 6 months after implantation. The improvement continued up to 12 months and then stabilized. The shape of the vowel space also normalized and was consistent with perceived improvements in vowel intelligibility for the children. By contrast, the vowel space did not improve over time for the children who used hearing aids.

Kinematic measures

Kinematic feedback has been used to help children with cochlear implants to improve their intelligibility. Pantelemidou et al. (2003) used EPG with an 8-year-old girl who had persisting difficulties with velar stops despite having made some progress with other sounds during traditional articulation therapy. During EPG therapy sessions the first half of each session focused on establishing correct tongue positions for velar stops and the remainder of the session targeted the maintenance of the correct position without the EPG. Evaluation following the course of the intervention showed that the child's productions of /k/ and /g/ improved significantly and had generalized to untaught words. Furthermore, the improvement was maintained 5 weeks following the cessation of EPG therapy. The authors noted that EPG encourages children to take an active role in discovering the relationship between tongue movements and the resulting acoustic output, and that this can be highly motivating.

Phonological/Articulation Disorders

Speech intelligibility is the prime focus in the remediation of phonological and/or articulation disorders. When very young children start learning to produce the phonemes of their language, they do not have the sophisticated perception or the fine motor control necessary to produce the sounds in the adult manner. It is very common for young children to use simpler articulatory gestures, known as **phonological processes**, in place of the adult model. The phoneme /k/, for example, requires a high degree of neuromuscular control of the articulators, and many young children find the /t/ sound easier to produce in its place. Substituting a sound with a more anterior place of articulation (e.g., /t/) for one with a more posterior place of articulation (e.g., /k/) is called **fronting**; so, for example, the /k/ in *candy* is fronted to /tændi/. Another common phonological process is for the child to omit the final consonant in a word, known as **final consonant deletion**. Thus, *cat* might become /kæ/, or *seat* might turn into /si/.

Children use numerous phonological processes, some more typical of normally developing children and others less so. The use of phonological processes tends to have an effect on children's intelligibility to varying degrees. Most children decrease and eventually eliminate these types of phonological processes as they develop more refined neuromuscular control of speech production. Some children, however, continue to use phonological processes beyond the usual age of around 3 years and require remediation to develop more intelligible speech. In this case, it is important to find out the extent of the child's knowledge of the sound system of the language. For example, if a child fronts the /k/ sound to a /t/, is it because he or she does not perceive the /k/ as a unique phoneme distinct from /t/ and therefore does not differentiate between the productions of these two sounds? Or does the child actually perceive the contrast between /k/ and /t/, but uses a different way of marking the /k/ sound to differentiate it from the /t/, a way that is not audible to listeners? If this is the case, then the child has what is called *productive knowledge* of the contrast between the sounds. Another example of productive knowledge is a child who seems to omit a final consonant but who may actually be producing the consonant in a way that is not perceptible to adults. A different child, on the other hand, may indeed completely omit the consonant.

Acoustic Measures

Acoustic measurement has been very helpful in differentiating between productive and nonproductive patterns of speech difficulty. This information is important, because treatment strategies differ for a child who has productive knowledge of a contrast and one who does not. Such information can also help to predict how quickly a child will acquire the sound. Forrest, Weismer, Hodge, Dinnsen, and Elbert (1990) tested four phonologically disordered children who all fronted /k/, producing /t/ for /k/ in all word positions. Three of the four showed no distinction between the spectra for /k/ and /t/. The remaining child (KR) showed significant distinctions between /t/ and /k/ spectra. However, the distinction was not the same one made by normally articulating children and did not result in an audible contrast between the sounds. In other words, even though it was different acoustically, KR's /k/ still sounded perceptually like a /t/. What was interesting was that treatment for all four of the children focused on sounds other than /k/. However, even though the /k/ sound had not been worked on directly, KR produced it correctly after therapy. This child, who had some knowledge of the velar–alveolar contrast as measured acoustically, acquired /k/ without treatment, whereas the other children did not. These kinds of inaudible acoustic differences suggest that the child may have a more sophisticated knowledge of the sound system than would be assumed by just doing a phonetic transcription of his or her speech (Tyler, Figurski, & Langsdale, 1993). Similar findings have been reported for other phonetic contrasts, such as /s/ and /ʃ/ (Li, Edwards, & Beckman, 2009) and voiced versus voiceless stops. Using VOT as an indication of voicing, Tyler et al. (1993) showed that of four boys with voicing difficulties, three had no significant differences in VOT between voiced and voiceless stops. One boy, however, produced significantly different VOTs for voiced and voiceless sounds, although this distinction could not be detected perceptually. This child required the shortest treatment period to acquire the voicing contrast, whereas the other three boys took much longer.

It is clear that acoustic displays of speech sounds are extremely helpful in determining underlying patterns of articulation. Visual displays of such patterns are also useful in clinical management by helping the child to perceive the differences between sounds that they may have difficulty in perceiving auditorily. Visual displays of articulatory/acoustic relationships can serve as a model against which the child can compare his or her own productions and can be very motivating. This type of information is additionally important in terms of checking the child's progress throughout the course of therapy.

Kinematic Measures

Kinematic measures have been used effectively in detecting and remediating underlying articulatory patterns in children with phonological/articulation disorders. Ultrasound and EPG have been the primary technologies employed.

Ultrasound

Adler-Bock, Bernhardt, Gick, and Bacsfalvi (2007) described the use of ultrasound as a visual feedback intervention strategy with two adolescent speakers who persistently misarticulated the /r/ sound. The participants' parents and the speech clinicians modeled the /r/ on the ultrasound, and the boys were oriented to the tongue positions and shapes used in the articulation of the sound. During the treatment sessions, the clinician and participants took turns using the transducer. Markers were set on the ultrasound display to provide the client with reference points and targets to reach when practicing articulatory positions. Acoustic information was also obtained regarding formant frequencies of the /r/ sounds. Post-therapy the boys showed marked improvement in their /r/ productions, as judged perceptually as well as in terms of acoustic analysis. Recall that the /r/ sound is characterized by a noticeably lowered F_3. Pre-therapy the lowering was not evident, while F_3 lowering for the /r/ was clearly visible following the course of treatment. In a similar study Bernhardt et al. (2008) used a portable ultrasound device to treat school-age children who demonstrated persistent difficulties with the /r/ sound despite years of traditional speech therapy. Techniques included modeling the correct phoneme, having the participants draw pictures of the tongue movements and positions, silent gestures involved in the production of /r/, and finally vocalizations with and without the visual feedback from the ultrasound. The majority of the children showed rapid improvement after only 1 to 3 hours of practice with the equipment. The authors emphasized that traditional treatment methods are still necessary to facilitate generalization of the correct production to words, sentences, and conversation.

Electropalatography

EPG has been shown to be effective in remediating children's and adolescents' articulation difficulties. Carter and Edwards (2004) used EPG with children aged 7 to 14 years who had persisting articulation problems despite years of traditional speech therapy. All the participants made significant gains after 10 therapy sessions. Gibbon and Wood (2003) used EPG with a 9-year-old boy who fronted velar sounds (i.e., produced /t/ sounds in place of /k/ sounds). Traditional speech therapy was not successful in remediating this problem. Following 15 sessions of EPG treatment, the boy was able to produce velar sounds and generalized the correct articulatory patterns to everyday environments. The authors suggested that EPG is most useful in helping children to learn how to produce new articulations that are not in their phonetic inventory and that traditional therapy techniques are helpful to generalize the newly learned patterns to connected speech.

Cleft Palate

Individuals with cleft palate form another group of speakers who very commonly have articulation problems. It is not uncommon for speakers with repaired clefts to demonstrate persisting velopharyngeal problems that contribute to both distortions of resonance and to misarticulations. Consonants that require a buildup of oral pressure, such as stops, fricatives, and affricates, are particularly challenging for many speakers with cleft palate, since intact velopharyngeal function is essential to prevent air from escaping through the nasal cavities. Speakers with clefts often have compensatory patterns of misarticulations that are unique, such as glottal stops and pharyngeal fricatives. Gibbon (2004) described abnormal patterns of articulation often present in speakers with cleft palates. These included increased tongue–palate contact; retraction of anterior consonants to more posterior tongue positions; overuse of the tongue dorsum; fronting of velar sounds; reduced separation between alveolar and velar tongue placements; complete closure which prevents a central groove for sibilant fricatives; double articulations in which a single sound is produced with two distinct places of articulation; and abnormal timing of articulation. EPG has revealed that double articulations are rather common, particularly for alveolar stops (Gibbon, Ellis, & Crampin, 2004). Double articulations may result from speakers with cleft palate using undifferentiated tongue gestures in which movement of the tongue tip and blade do not occur independently from movement of the tongue body. These kinds of abnormal patterns are often very difficult to eliminate or reduce using traditional auditory stimulation types of intervention procedures. Rather, visual feedback has been found to be beneficial for some speakers with cleft palates. For example, Michi, Yamashita, Imai, Suzuki, and Yoshida (1993) compared the use of visual feedback using EPG versus purely auditory training with children who had had their palates repaired before age 2 years but who had not received speech treatment. The EPG provided feedback regarding tongue and palate contact and the degree of frication produced by the child for the production of fricatives. The children who received this feedback improved very rapidly, to almost the 100 percent correct level. The authors noted that although there are some disadvantages of this system, including its cost and the necessity of customizing a pseudopalate, the numerous advantages outweigh the disadvantages. The advantages include the visual feedback for the child regarding his or her articulatory movements, the objective documentation of progress, the ease with which even young children can understand the feedback, and the speed and effectiveness with which articulatory gains can be achieved. A further benefit of EPG is that it allows speech–language therapists to identify unusual patterns of articulation in individuals with cleft palate who demonstrate persisting difficulties, which provides the basis for the very focused and specific intervention necessary to overcome these atypical articulatory patterns (Howard, 2004). With the use of EPG, many individuals with cleft palate have demonstrated substantial improvements in articulation (Gibbon & Paterson, 2006).

Summary

Correct articulation is a fundamental basis of intelligible speech.

Perceptual ratings yield an overall estimate of a speaker's intelligibility; utilizing acoustic and kinematic analysis allows determination of a speaker's underlying patterns of articulation.

Acoustic measures that have been used to analyze speech production include duration of vowels and consonants, vowel formant analysis, and spectral analysis of consonants.

Charts of vowel space can show changes in a speaker's articulatory patterns before and after treatment or over the course of time.

The slope index reflects tongue movement and can reveal differences between speakers with and without dysarthria.

Spectral analysis of stops and fricatives can reveal distinctions in a speaker's articulatory gestures.

Kinematic measures of articulatory patterns include cineradiography, strain gauge, electropalatometry, electroglossometry, ultrasound, and electromagnetic articulography.

Electropalatometry and electroglossometry can be valuable aids in achieving more precise articulatory targets for speakers with hearing impairment or cleft palate.

Electromagnetic articulography has been used successfully as visual biofeedback for speakers with disordered patterns of articulation.

REVIEW EXERCISES

1. Describe advantages and disadvantages of cineradiography, strain gauge, electropalatometry, electroglossometry, ultrasound, and electromagnetic articulography in the evaluation and treatment of articulation and/or phonological disorders.

2. Compare the kinds of information obtained from acoustic analysis of vowels and consonants.

3. Describe the slope index and explain how it can help to understand a speaker's articulation patterns.

4. Compare the type of information obtained from spectrography, electropalatography, and electroglossography, and comment on the types of disorders each would be most useful for.

5 Explain the usefulness of kinematic measures of articulatory function in the evaluation and treatment of articulation disorders resulting from different etiologies.

INTEGRATIVE CASE STUDIES

① Melissa

Background

Melissa is an 11-year-old girl with ataxic cerebral palsy. She is ambulatory but uses crutches to increase her sense of stability. Cognitively, Melissa is functioning within the normal range of intelligence and is attending a regular school, where she is performing at grade level. Even though Melissa does have a small group of good friends, she is frustrated because her friends and teachers often ask her to repeat herself. As Melissa will soon be entering middle school, she is concerned that the older children will make fun of her speech.

Clinical Observations

Upon reevaluation at the start of fifth grade, Melissa expressed her concerns to you, the school speech–language pathologist. Melissa has been receiving speech therapy services since kindergarten, and her speech intelligibility is fairly good. However, she still tends to slur some words due to vowel distortion and consonant imprecision, and her prosody in connected speech is noticeably monotone. Consequently, her speech sounds slow and labored. As part of a thorough diagnostic workup, you think it important to establish baselines for vowel duration, overall articulatory rate, and intonation as reflected by pitch variability. You will obtain these measures using the free downloadable acoustic program Praat.

Acoustic Measures

You tested Melissa's speech patterns in single words, sentences, and structured conversation. On the word level, spectrographic analysis showed that target formant frequencies were within the normal range. Vowel durations fell at the low end of the normal range. At the sentence level, distortions of all articulatory movements became more evident, with slow transitions between sounds and neutralized formant frequencies for all corner vowels. Consonant durations were also longer than normal, and stops were intermittently fricated. In addition, the pitch analysis program demonstrated that Melissa's average F_0 in connected speech was 248 Hz, but her F_0 range in sentences and in connected speech was limited to an average of 22 Hz, considerably lower than the expected range for her age.

Clinical Questions

a. Based on these findings, generate an age-appropriate F_1/F_2 plot for Melissa that will serve as a baseline against which to measure her progress.

b. Develop three goals related to Melissa's speech intelligibility/prosody and provide a rationale for each goal.

c. How might acoustic instrumentation be used to verify that Melissa is achieving the therapeutic objectives?

d. What other types of instrumentation could be helpful in establishing an intervention plan for Melissa?

② Aidan

Background

Aidan is an 8-year-old boy with a moderate bilateral sensorineural hearing loss. Aidan's hearing loss is congenital, and he has received amplification since age 2 years. Currently Aidan is in third grade and is functioning within normal limits within the academic setting; however, his speech intelligibility is poor. Aidan's teacher has noted that the poor intelligibility has affected his ability to communicate with his peers, which has resulted in withdrawal within the classroom and social situations. Due to increased awareness of his lack of communication skills, Aidan often displays signs of frustration and embarrassment when he is not understood. You have recently been hired as a speech–language pathologist in Aidan's school and have taken him on your caseload. Aidan is scheduled for his triennial review, and you will be evaluating his speech and language.

Clinical Observations

Aidan has received speech therapy in his current school since kindergarten. His hearing loss has progressed from mild to moderate over the past 3 years, which has greatly compromised his speech intelligibility. In addition, results from Aidan's recent audiological evaluation revealed that he is no longer receiving optimal benefit from his hearing aids, indicating worsening of his hearing loss. Informally, you observed Aidan interacting within the classroom and with peers and noted errors across the following parameters: omission and substitution of consonants, decreased intonation contours, slow rate of speech, inappropriate stress, and insufficient variation in loudness. To support your informal observations, you conducted a thorough acoustic analysis using Praat.

Acoustic Observations

Spectrographic analysis indicated a reduced vowel space and increased vowel durations with a rate of speech of 3.1 syllables per second. Alveolar and palatal fricatives were produced more posteriorly as demonstrated by lower frequency frication noise. A lack of overlap in acoustic features of adjacent sounds suggested difficulty with coarticulation. Finally, limited variation of F_0, intensity, and duration indicated decreased use of stress and intonational patterns.

Clinical Questions

a. Given the information from this evaluation, would your primary target of treatment be segmental or suprasegmental features? Provide a rationale for your answer.

b. What is the advantage of using acoustic analysis with a pediatric client? How could this instrumentation also be used as a therapeutic tool?

c. What would you expect an F_1/F_2 plot for Aidan to look like at the time of assessment and 3 months post-intervention?

d. How can the acoustic information be used to guide your treatment to assist Aidan with his place of articulation for fricatives?

❸ Mr. Frost

Background

Mr. Frost is a 45-year-old man who recently suffered a stroke. He was discharged from the hospital a week ago and referred to a university speech and hearing clinic for a speech–language evaluation. From the information you have received through the evaluation conducted by the speech–language pathologist at the hospital, you learn that Mr. Frost's speech is characterized as slow and labored, with a low degree of intelligibility. It is also indicated in the evaluation that Mr. Frost's lingual range of motion and strength are markedly decreased. Upon meeting Mr. Frost and his wife, you learn that the couple runs a large charity foundation and premorbidly had a very active social life. Mr. Frost explains that his tongue often feels "heavy," and speaking has become an extremely fatiguing activity. He and his wife express to you that their main goal is improving Mr. Frost's intelligibility so that he is better understood by his family and friends and those in his community.

Clinical Observations

Upon meeting Mr. Frost, you observe that his speech is slow and sounds slurred during conversation. His intelligibility is poor, and you detect vowel distortions and uncoordinated articulatory movements in single words as well as in connected speech. After performing an oral–motor examination, it appears that his lingual and labial movements both intra- and extra-orally are slow and uncoordinated, and lingual strength is significantly decreased.

Acoustic measures

In order to get a better clinical understanding of Mr. Frost's speech patterns as well as to establish a baseline for therapy, you use the spectrographic feature of the Praat program to collect data regarding the client's vowel and consonant duration in single words and connected speech, formant frequencies of the corner vowels, and F_2 transitions. Vowel and consonant durations were found to be significantly longer than normal. An F_1/F_2 plot showed a high degree of vowel neutralization. Stop consonants were often fricated and nasalized. Mr. Frost obtained a slope index of 1.43 Hz/msec.

Electropalatography

The university clinic is fortunate to have an EPG system. Mr. Frost is custom fit with a pseudopalate and returns 1 week following the initial evaluation to undergo further EPG assessment.

Clinical Questions

a. How would you use the above acoustic information to document for the insurance company the need for speech therapy for this client?

b. Based on the perceptual and acoustic information, what kind of EPG patterns would you expect to see?

c. What treatment goals would be appropriate given the acoustic and kinematic findings?

5

The Phonatory System

STUDENT LEARNING OBJECTIVES

After reading this chapter you will

○ Become familiar with the structures of the larynx and the myoelastic–aerodynamic theory of phonation.

○ Understand the complex, nearly periodic sound wave of the human voice.

○ Identify acoustic variables associated with vocal frequency and amplitude.

○ Appreciate the physiologic and acoustic bases of vocal registers.

○ Be able to describe differences between normal and abnormal voice qualities.

○ Describe acoustic aspects of voice including jitter, shimmer, and harmonics-to-noise ratio.

The phonatory system comprises the larynx. The vocal mechanism includes the laryngeal skeleton, laryngeal joints, three pairs of soft tissue folds, intrinsic and extrinsic membranes, and extrinsic and intrinsic muscles. Laryngeal function is controlled and regulated by the nervous system. The larynx is the means by which air is converted into sound through an extraordinarily complex process. The process involves air pressures and flows generated by the respiratory system and the muscular and elastic properties of the vocal folds that are housed in the larynx. To gain an appreciation of the process of the air-to-sound conversion, it is imperative to be familiar with the structure of the larynx and vocal folds and the way in which the structures operate.

Laryngeal Skeleton

The laryngeal skeleton is made up of one bone and nine cartilages. Three of the cartilages are unpaired, and six are paired. The unpaired cartilages are the thyroid, cricoid, and epiglottis; the paired cartilages include arytenoids, corniculates, and cuneiforms. The cartilaginous framework of the larynx is suspended from the hyoid bone. Membranes and ligaments attach the cartilages to each other. See Figures 5.1, 5.2, and 5.3.

Bones and Cartilages

The **hyoid bone** is a small U-shaped bone that forms the attachment for the tongue. The larynx is suspended from this bone by a sheet of membrane, the **hyothyroid membrane**. The hyoid bone consists of the body in the front and the major horns forming the long sides of the U. Projecting slightly upward from each major horn

Figure 5.1 Laryngeal framework

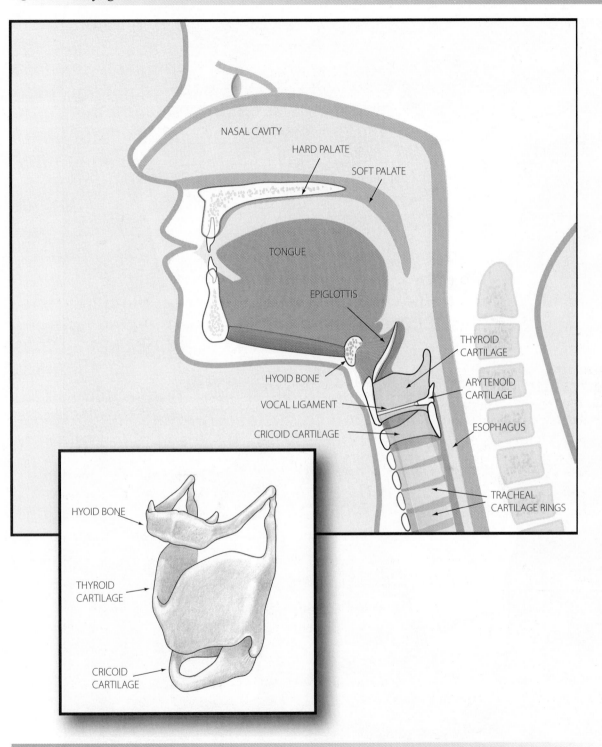

NASAL CAVITY

HARD PALATE

SOFT PALATE

TONGUE

EPIGLOTTIS

THYROID CARTILAGE

ARYTENOID CARTILAGE

HYOID BONE

VOCAL LIGAMENT

ESOPHAGUS

CRICOID CARTILAGE

TRACHEAL CARTILAGE RINGS

HYOID BONE

THYROID CARTILAGE

CRICOID CARTILAGE

Figure 5.2 Cartilages of the larynx

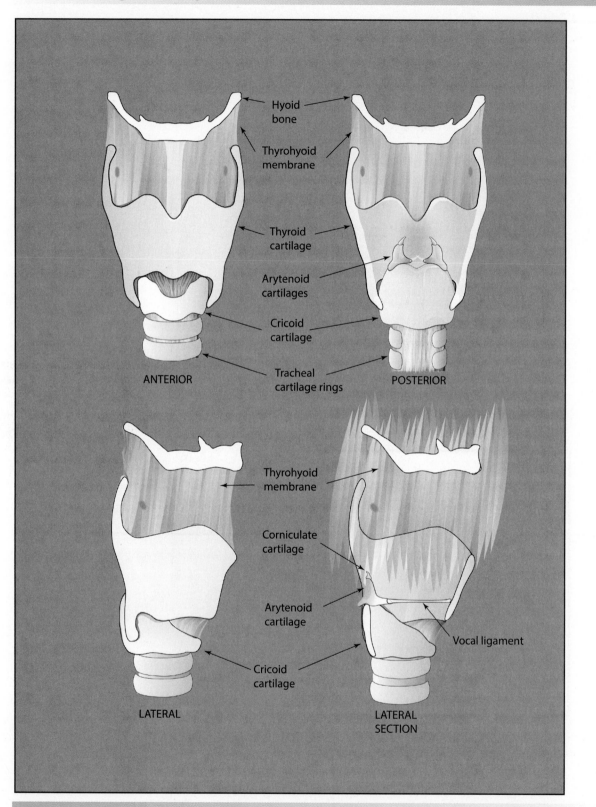

Figure 5.3 **Membranes of the larynx**

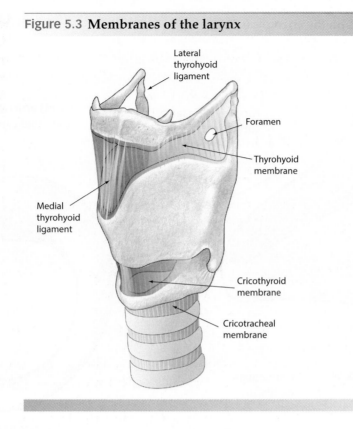

is a small protrusion, the minor horn. Inferior to the hyoid bone is the **thyroid cartilage** (Latin for *shield*), which is the largest cartilage of the larynx. This structure is formed by two laminae (plates) of cartilage that are fused in the front. The fusion of these plates occurs at an angle, which is more acute in men than in women. This protrusion is known as the Adam's apple and, because of the different angles, it is generally more prominent in men than in women. A small, V-shaped notch, the *thyroid notch*, is apparent at the top surface of the laryngeal protrusion. Two long projections, the *superior horns*, one at either side of the thyroid, extend upward and connect by means of ligaments to the hyoid bone. Two shorter projections, the *inferior horns*, extend downward and articulate with the sides of the cricoid cartilage. The posterior portion of the thyroid is open. The vocal folds are attached to the inner surface of the thyroid, just below the thyroid notch, at a fibrous structure called the **anterior commissure**.

The second unpaired cartilage, the **cricoid** (Latin for *signet ring*) **cartilage**, is so called because of its shape, being narrow in the front (the arch) and flaring to a larger, squarish plate in the back. The shape of this posterior plate explains its name, the *quadrate* (four-cornered) *lamina*. The cricoid is a complete ring of cartilage located inferior to the thyroid, just above the first ring of the trachea. A sheet of membrane, the **cricotracheal membrane**, runs between the inferior margin of the cricoid and the superior margin of the first tracheal ring.

Figure 5.4 Articular facets on the cricoid cartilage

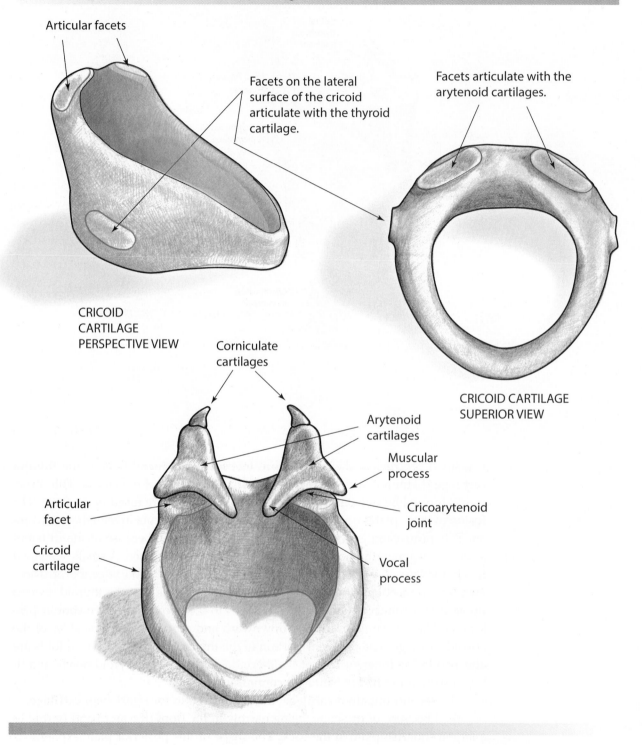

Articular facets

Facets on the lateral surface of the cricoid articulate with the thyroid cartilage.

Facets articulate with the arytenoid cartilages.

CRICOID CARTILAGE PERSPECTIVE VIEW

CRICOID CARTILAGE SUPERIOR VIEW

Corniculate cartilages

Arytenoid cartilages

Muscular process

Articular facet

Cricoarytenoid joint

Cricoid cartilage

Vocal process

The third unpaired cartilage, the **epiglottis**, is a broad cartilage shaped rather like an oak leaf. It is attached to the inner surface of the thyroid cartilage just below the thyroid notch, by the *thyroepiglottic ligament,* and attaches to the body of the hyoid bone by way of the *hyoepiglottic ligament.* The epiglottis performs an important function during swallowing by folding downward over the entrance to the larynx and acting as a bridge to direct food and liquids to the esophagus. It is less important, however, in the production of voice.

The paired **arytenoid cartilages** are small structures located on the superior surface of the quadrate lamina of the cricoid. They are pyramidal in shape, being broad and flattish at their base and extending upward to more of a point at their apex. Two projections extend from their base. The first, the elastic **vocal process**, projects anteriorly toward the thyroid cartilage. The second projection, the **muscular process**, projects laterally and posteriorly. The arytenoids play a crucial role in phonation, because the vocal folds are attached to the vocal processes. Various muscles of the larynx attach to the muscular processes and move the arytenoids, allowing the attached vocal folds to be positioned in different ways.

There are several cartilages that do not appear to play an important role in voice production. The paired **corniculate cartilages** are located at the apex of the arytenoids but may not be present in all individuals. The paired **cuneiform cartilages** are small, elastic rods of cartilage, embedded within the **aryepiglottic folds** (described below). Their primary function may be to stiffen these folds.

Joints of the Larynx

There are two pairs of joints in the larynx, both of which play important roles in the production of a normal voice. See Figures 5.5–5.7. The **cricoarytenoid joints** are formed by the articulation between the base of each arytenoid and the superior surface of the quadrate lamina of the cricoid. The joints are *diarthrodial.* This allows a wide range of motion of the arytenoids, which can glide medially and laterally, as well as tilt backward and forward in a rocking motion. Since the vocal folds are connected to the vocal processes of the arytenoids, any movement of the arytenoids affects the positioning of the vocal folds. When certain laryngeal muscles contract, the muscular processes are moved anterolaterally, bringing the vocal processes to the midline. The attached vocal folds are therefore adducted. Conversely, when the muscular processes are pulled posteriorly, the vocal processes and the attached vocal folds are separated (abducted). Thus, the cricoarytenoid joints are instrumental in vocal fold adduction and abduction.

The **cricothyroid joints** are located between each inferior horn of the thyroid and the sides of the cricoid cartilage. These joints allow the thyroid cartilage to tilt downward toward the arch of the cricoid or the cricoid cartilage to tilt upward so that the arch comes closer to the thyroid. When either the cricoid or thyroid moves in this way, the distance between the arytenoid cartilages in the back and the thyroid cartilage in front increases. Because the vocal folds are attached to the vocal processes of the arytenoids posteriorly and to the anterior commissure of the thyroid anteriorly, increasing the distance between these two points has the effect of stretching the vocal folds, making them more

Figure 5.5 Cricoarytenoid joints

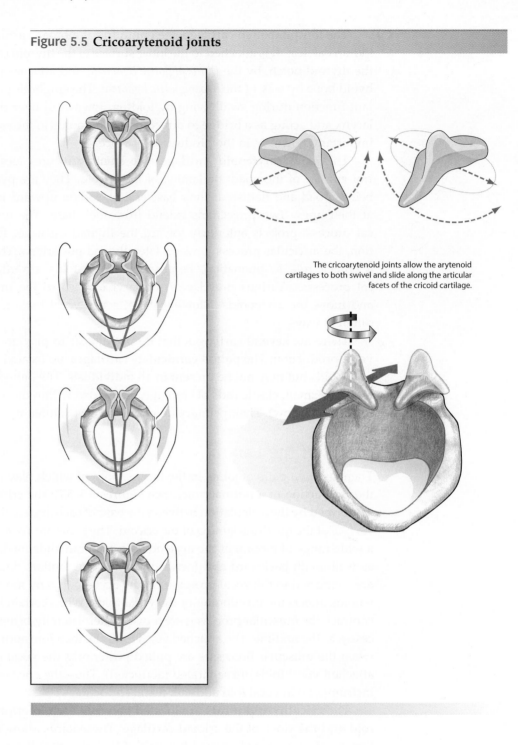

The cricoarytenoid joints allow the arytenoid cartilages to both swivel and slide along the articular facets of the cricoid cartilage.

tense and thin. When the vocal folds are elongated, stretched, and tense, they vibrate more rapidly, resulting in a higher F_0 and in the perception of a higher pitch. The cricothyroid joints, then, are the main agents of F_0 regulation in the human voice.

The structures of the laryngeal skeleton are listed in Table 5.1.

Figure 5.6 Cricothyroid joints

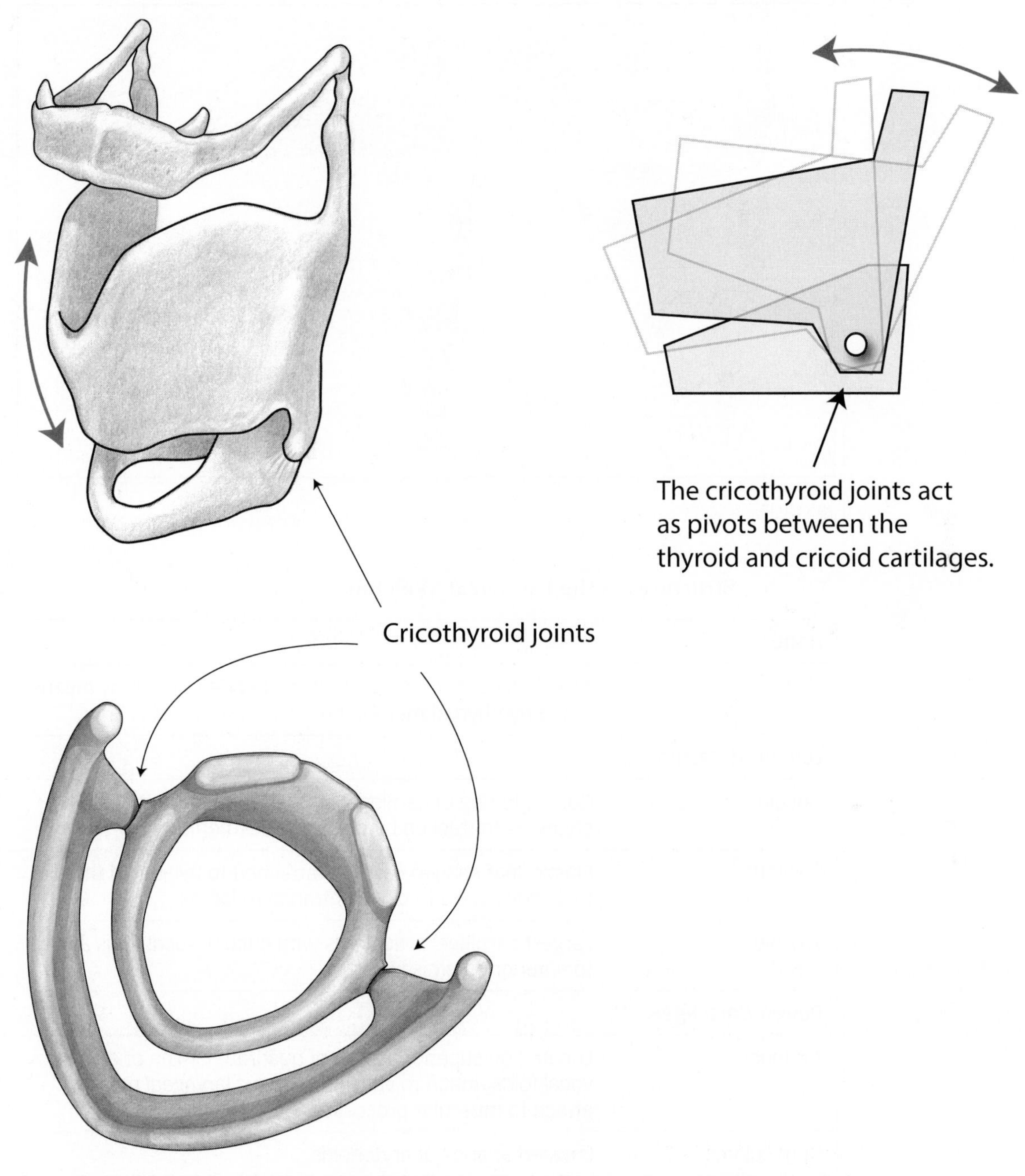

The cricothyroid joints act as pivots between the thyroid and cricoid cartilages.

Cricothyroid joints

Figure 5.7 Elongation of the vocal folds due to the cricothyroid joint

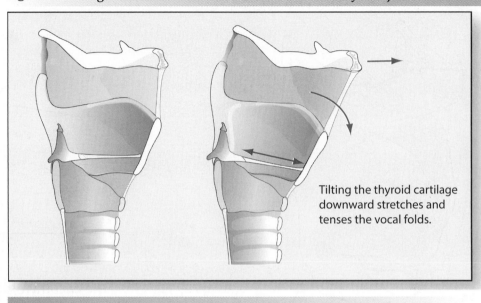

Tilting the thyroid cartilage downward stretches and tenses the vocal folds.

Table 5.1 Structures of the Laryngeal Skeleton

Bone	
Hyoid	Attachment for tongue; larynx suspended from it by means of the hyothyroid membrane.
Unpaired Cartilages	
Cricoid	Complete ring of cartilage; most inferior portion of larynx; connects to trachea by cricotracheal membrane.
Epiglottis	Elastic, leaf-shaped cartilage attached to hyoid and thyroid; folds downward to close entrance to larynx.
Thyroid	Largest cartilage; articulates with cricoid; vocal folds attach to anterior commissure.
Paired Cartilages	
Arytenoids	Located on superior aspect of quadrate lamina of cricoid; vocal folds attach to vocal processes; laryngeal muscles attach to muscular processes.
Corniculates	Located at apex of arytenoids.
Cuneiforms	Elastic rods of cartilage embedded within the aryepiglottic folds.
Joints	
Cricoarytenoid	Between base of arytenoids and superior surface of quadrate lamina; involved in adduction and abduction of vocal folds.
Cricothyroid	Between inferior horns of thyroid and lateral aspect of cricoid; involved in F_0 regulation by elongating and shortening vocal folds.

Valves within the Larynx

The inside of the larynx is essentially a hollow tube (**lumen**) with three sets of valves inside it that open and close to perform various functions. The valves are made of bundles of connective tissues and muscle fibers called folds and are arranged from superior to inferior within the larynx. They include the *aryepiglottic folds*, the **false** (ventricular) **vocal folds**, and the **true vocal folds**. See Figure 5.8.

Figure 5.8 Valves within the larynx

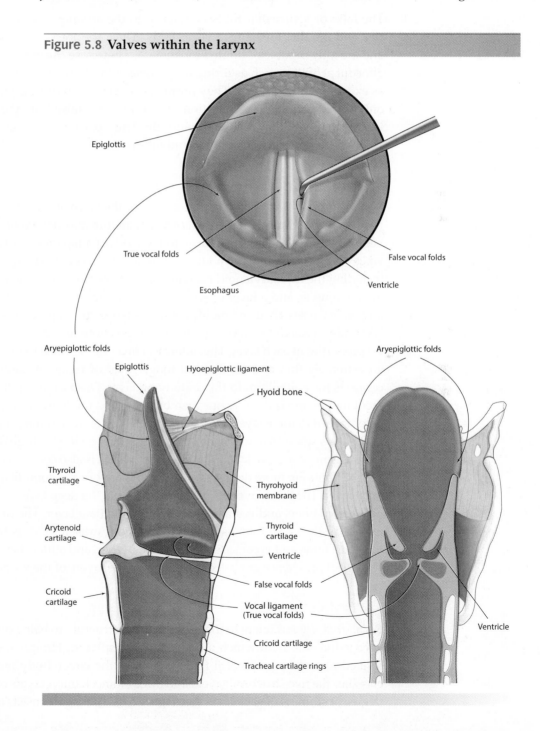

Aryepiglottic Folds

The most superior of the folds, the aryepiglottic folds, run from the sides of the epiglottis to the apex of each arytenoid cartilage. They are sheets of connective tissue and some muscle fibers that contract in a circular or sphincteric action to pull the epiglottis backward and to close the entrance of the larynx during swallowing.

False Vocal Folds

The false or ventricular folds lie inferior to the aryepiglottic folds and just superior and parallel to the true vocal folds. They are not very muscular structures and are only capable of limited movement. They close during swallowing, during effortful activities such as lifting heavy objects, and during natural functions such as excretion or childbirth. They normally remain open during phonation, closing only under pathological conditions. Separating the false from the true vocal folds is a small space, the **laryngeal ventricle**. This space contains glands that secrete mucus, keeping the larynx moist and lubricated.

True Vocal Folds

The true vocal folds are the most complex of the laryngeal valves. Only within the past several decades has the extraordinary nature and degree of their complexity been determined, thanks primarily to the work of a Japanese otolaryngologist and voice scientist, M. Hirano, and his colleagues. The vocal folds consist of five layers, including the thyroarytenoid muscle, three layers of mucous membrane surrounding the muscle, and a layer of epithelium covering the mucous membrane. Hirano and others' research, using highly sophisticated technology such as electron microscopy, has revealed the differing cellular compositions and the different biomechanical properties of each layer. The outermost layer of the vocal folds is the epithelium, an extremely thin and flexible but tough layer of tissue. A basement membrane connects the epithelium to the underlying layer. Deep to the epithelium and basement membrane is the mucous membrane, called the **lamina propria**, which itself is composed of three layers. The superficial layer of the lamina propria, also known as Reinke's space, is made mostly of elastic fibers, giving it a high degree of compliance. The intermediate layer of the lamina propria is also composed of elastic fibers, but the fibers are more densely packed and therefore less compliant than the superficial layer. The third layer of the lamina propria, the deep layer, is made up chiefly of collagen fibers and is stiffer than the intermediate layer. The final structure that makes up the vocal folds is the **thyroarytenoid muscle**. This is the main mass of the vocal folds and is considerably thicker, denser, and stiffer than the other layers. Figure 5.9 provides a cross-sectional view of the layers of the vocal folds.

Cover–Body Model

Recall that *stiffness* refers to the resistance of a structure to being displaced; compliance is the ease with which a body can be displaced. Hirano and colleagues described a model of the vocal folds known as the **cover–body model**. The model classifies the five structural layers into three biomechanical layers on the basis of the degree of stiffness of each layer (see Figure 5.9). The *cover* consists of the epithelium

Figure 5.9 Layers of the true vocal folds

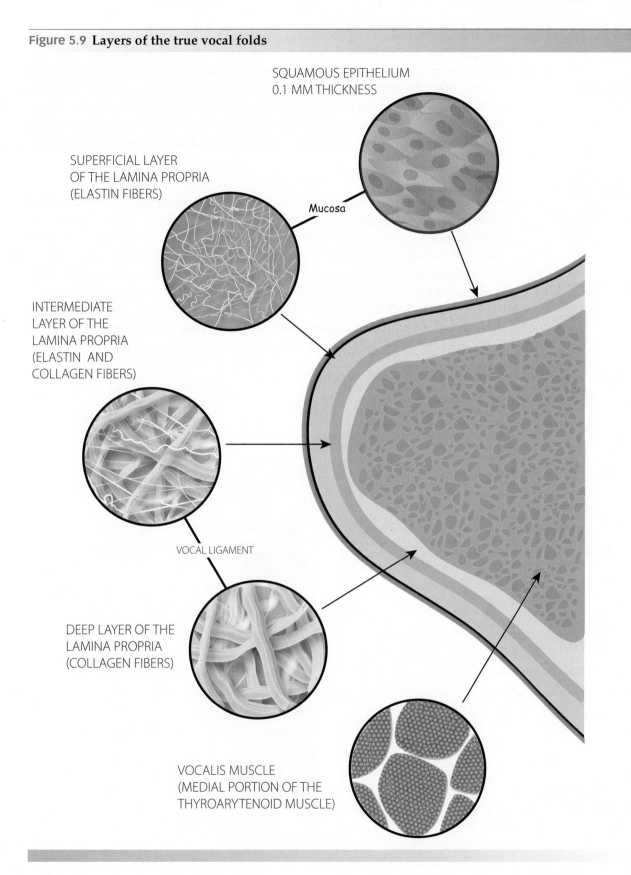

SQUAMOUS EPITHELIUM
0.1 MM THICKNESS

SUPERFICIAL LAYER
OF THE LAMINA PROPRIA
(ELASTIN FIBERS)

Mucosa

INTERMEDIATE
LAYER OF THE
LAMINA PROPRIA
(ELASTIN AND
COLLAGEN FIBERS)

VOCAL LIGAMENT

DEEP LAYER OF THE
LAMINA PROPRIA
(COLLAGEN FIBERS)

VOCALIS MUSCLE
(MEDIAL PORTION OF THE
THYROARYTENOID MUSCLE)

and the superficial layer of the lamina propria. These structures are highly compliant. The transition, or **vocal ligament**, encompasses the intermediate and deep layers of the lamina propria and is less compliant than the cover. The thyroarytenoid muscle forms the *body* of the vocal folds and is the least compliant layer of the vocal folds. The vocal folds, thus, form a multilayered and extremely complex vibrator. The structural and biomechanical complexity gives rise to a complex periodic sound wave with many harmonics that results in a rich and resonant human voice.

Glottis

The space between the true vocal folds is the **glottis**, divided into the **membranous glottis** and the **cartilaginous glottis**. The membranous glottis, which in the adult forms the anterior three-fifths of the entire length of the glottis, is bounded by the vocal ligament on either side. The vocal processes form the lateral edges of the cartilaginous glottis, which accounts for the posterior two-fifths of the glottis. The membranous glottis is around 15 mm in adult males and 12 mm in adult females. The cartilaginous glottis varies from about 4 to 8 mm in length, depending on the person's sex, age, and build. Children's vocal folds are much shorter. The shape of the glottis varies, depending on the positioning of the vocal folds (Figure 5.10).

Figure 5.10 Glottal shapes

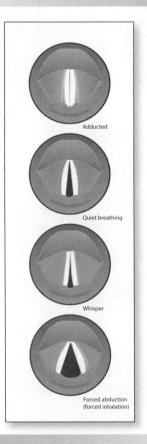

For quiet breathing, the glottis is open but not to its greatest extent. The vocal folds are in a paramedian position. The glottis opens more widely when one needs to inhale greater amounts of air, for example, during vigorous exercise. This position is known as forced abduction. For phonation the glottis is closed, with the vocal folds in the median position. Whispering is produced with the membranous glottis closed and the cartilaginous glottis open.

Muscles of the Larynx

The muscles of the larynx are divided into extrinsic and intrinsic groups. Extrinsic muscles have one point of attachment within the larynx and the other point outside of the larynx. Intrinsic muscles have both points of attachment within the larynx.

Extrinsic Muscles

The **extrinsic muscles**, also known as the *strap muscles*, are those that have one point of attachment to the larynx, either at the hyoid bone or another laryngeal cartilage, and the other point of attachment to a structure outside the larynx, such as the sternum or the cranium. The extrinsic muscles form a network that surrounds the larynx and anchors it in position within the neck. The extrinsic muscles are subdivided into the **infrahyoid muscles** and the **suprahyoid muscles**.

The infrahyoids have their external point of attachment at structures below the hyoid bone, including the sternum and scapula; the suprahyoids have one point of attachment to structures located above the hyoid bone, including the mandible and temporal bone. The infrahyoids, when they contract, pull the entire larynx downward. Contraction of the suprahyoids pulls the entire larynx upward in the neck. These large up-and-down movements of the larynx occur mainly during swallowing. Figure 5.11 shows the extrinsic muscles of the larynx. The muscles are listed in Table 5.2.

Intrinsic Muscles

There are five major intrinsic muscles of the larynx. These muscles have both their origin and insertion within the larynx itself. Two of the five muscles function to adduct the vocal folds, one muscle is the vocal fold abductor, one elongates and tenses the folds, and one forms the main body of the vocal folds. The intrinsic muscles of the larynx are shown in Figures 5.12 and 5.13 and listed in Table 5.3.

The first adductor is a paired muscle, the **lateral cricoarytenoid (LCA)**. This muscle arises from the lateral border of the cricoid and inserts into the muscular process of the arytenoids. When it contracts, it pulls the muscular process in an anterior and medial direction. This has the effect of pulling the vocal processes toward each other in an inward and downward movement. The vocal folds, attached to the vocal processes, are also brought toward each other, closing the membranous glottis. The **interarytenoid (IA)** muscle is the second adductor. This is an unpaired muscle consisting of two bundles of muscle fibers: the *transverse* portion, which runs horizontally across the posterior portions of the two arytenoid

Figure 5.11 Extrinsic laryngeal muscles

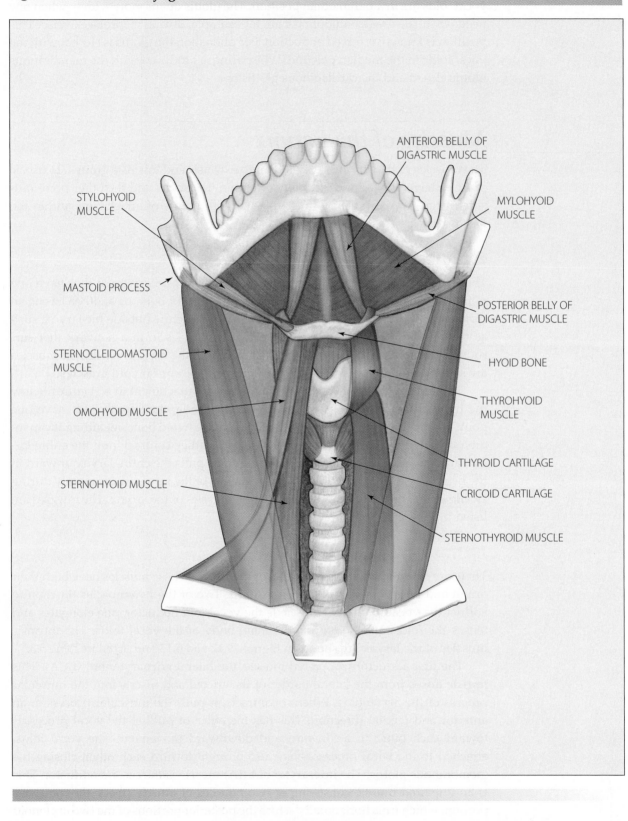

Table 5.2 Extrinsic Muscles of the Larynx

Muscle	Attachments	Function
Infrahyoids		
Sternohyoid	Clavicle and sternum to body of hyoid	Depresses hyoid bone and larynx
Sternothyroid	First costal cartilage and sternum to oblique line of thyroid lamina	Depresses hyoid bone and larynx
Omohyoid	Scapula to inferior border of hyoid	Depresses and retracts hyoid bone
Thyrohyoid	Oblique line of thyroid lamina to major horn of hyoid	Draws hyoid and thyroid closer to each other
Suprahyoids		
Digastric	Posterior belly: mastoid process of temporal bone to hyoid bone	Elevates hyoid bone
	Anterior belly: mandible to intermediate tendon of digastric muscle	Elevates hyoid bone
Stylohyoid	Styloid process of temporal bone to body of hyoid bone	Elevates and retracts hyoid
Mylohyoid	Body of mandible to hyoid	Elevates hyoid bone
Geniohyoid	Mental symphysis of mandible to body of hyoid bone	Pulls hyoid bone anteriorly and superiorly

cartilages, and the *oblique* portion, whose fibers run from the base of one arytenoid to the apex of the other arytenoid and vice versa. This arrangement of fibers forms a cross between the posterior surfaces of the arytenoids. When the interarytenoid muscle contracts, it glides the arytenoid cartilages medially toward each other, closing the posterior portion of the glottis.

The paired **posterior cricoarytenoid (PCA)** muscle is the only one that abducts the vocal folds to open the glottis. The PCA is a large, fan-shaped muscle that originates on the posterior aspect of the cricoid cartilage and inserts into the muscular process of each arytenoid cartilage. Upon contraction, the muscular processes are rotated posteriorly, which has the effect of pulling the vocal processes and vocal folds away from each other and opening the glottis.

The paired **cricothyroid (CT)** muscle is also composed of two sets of muscle fibers. The *pars recta* portion originates at the lateral surface of the cricoid cartilage. Its fibers run at an almost upright angle to insert into the inferior border of the thyroid cartilage. The *pars oblique* portion originates at the same place as the pars recta, but its fibers run in a more angled direction and insert at the anterior surface of the inferior horn of the thyroid cartilage. This muscle functions as a pitch changer. When it contracts, the thyroid cartilage is tilted downward toward the cricoid,

Figure 5.12 **Intrinsic laryngeal muscles**

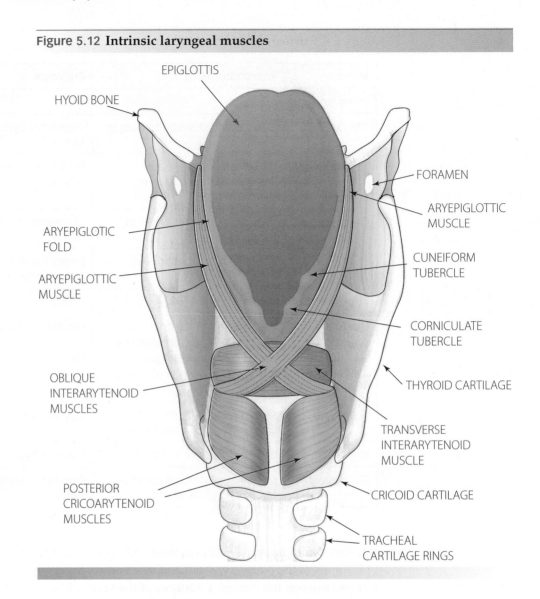

EPIGLOTTIS

HYOID BONE

FORAMEN

ARYEPIGLOTTIC MUSCLE

ARYEPIGLOTIC FOLD

ARYEPIGLOTTIC MUSCLE

CUNEIFORM TUBERCLE

CORNICULATE TUBERCLE

OBLIQUE INTERARYTENOID MUSCLES

THYROID CARTILAGE

TRANSVERSE INTERARYTENOID MUSCLE

POSTERIOR CRICOARYTENOID MUSCLES

CRICOID CARTILAGE

TRACHEAL CARTILAGE RINGS

thus increasing the distance between the anterior commissure of the thyroid and the arytenoid cartilages. Because the vocal folds are attached anteriorly at the anterior commissure and posteriorly at the arytenoids, increasing the distance between these points stretches and elongates the vocal folds, decreasing their mass per unit of area and increasing the longitudinal tension placed on them. This increases their rate of vibration, resulting in a higher frequency, perceived as a higher pitch.

The fifth muscle, the thyroarytenoid (TA), forms the main mass of the true vocal folds. This part of the vocal folds comprises the body in the cover–body model. The TA is a paired muscle, coursing from the anterior commissure to the arytenoids. The more lateral fibers, sometimes known as the *thyromuscularis*, insert into the muscular process of each arytenoid. The more medial fibers, sometimes referred to as the *thyrovocalis*, insert into each vocal process. In addition to forming the bulk of the vocal folds, the TA can exert internal tension that stiffens it and helps to increase the rate of vibration of the vocal folds.

Figure 5.13 **Actions of the intrinsic muscles**

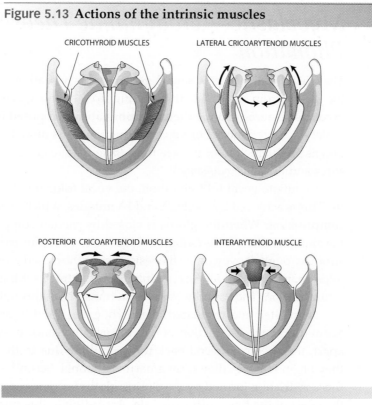

CRICOTHYROID MUSCLES

LATERAL CRICOARYTENOID MUSCLES

POSTERIOR CRICOARYTENOID MUSCLES

INTERARYTENOID MUSCLE

Table 5.3 **Intrinsic Muscles of the Larynx**

Muscle	Attachments	Function
Lateral cricoarytenoid	Lateral cricoid to muscular process of arytenoid	Adduct vocal folds
Interarytenoid		
Transverse	Lateral margin of one arytenoid to lateral margin of other arytenoid posteriorly	Adduct vocal folds
Oblique	Base of one arytenoid to apex of other arytenoid posteriorly	Adduct vocal folds
Posterior cricoarytenoid	Posterior cricoid to muscular process of arytenoid	Abduct vocal folds
Cricothyroid		
Pars recta	Anterior cricoid to inferior border of thyroid	Elongate and tense vocal folds
Pars oblique	Anterior cricoid to anterior surface of inferior horn of thyroid	Elongate and tense vocal folds
Thyroarytenoid		
Muscularis	Anterior commissure to muscular process	Body of vocal folds; shorten and relax folds
Vocalis	Anterior commissure to vocal process	Body of vocal folds; tense folds

Myoelastic–Aerodynamic Theory of Phonation

The vocal folds act as a sound generator by vibrating the air coming through the larynx from the lungs, thus setting up a sound wave in the vocal tract. The **myoelastic–aerodynamic theory of phonation**, proposed in the 1950s, is the most widely accepted model of voice production. This model describes voice production as an interaction of muscle force (*myo*), tissue elasticity (*elastic*), and air pressures and flows (*aerodynamic*).

To initiate vocal fold vibration, the vocal folds must adduct to close the glottis. This is achieved by the LCA and IA muscles, which exert a force called **medial compression**. When the glottis is closed by medial compression the pressure of the air beneath the folds (subglottal pressure, P_s) begins to increase. When the P_s is strong enough, it overcomes the resistance of the closed glottis and forces the vocal folds apart. A puff of air escapes into the vocal tract, setting the air within the tract into vibration. The sound wave is then transmitted through the vocal tract, where it is articulated and resonated. Meanwhile, the vocal folds have begun to adduct again due to the interaction of two forces. First, once the folds have been forced apart, they begin to recoil back to the midline due to their natural elasticity. As they begin to close, they form a narrow channel. Second, the air passing through this constriction formed by the closing glottis becomes negative in pressure due to the effect of the **Bernoulli principle**. According to this principle, a gas such as air passing through a narrow channel increases in velocity and decreases in pressure. The P_{neg} between the folds further helps to close them completely by pulling them toward each other. Pressures within the vocal tract immediately above the glottis (supraglottal pressures) also facilitate opening and closing of the glottis during vibration. The air that has already passed through the glottis travels up the vocal tract. The distance between the traveling body of air and the glottis increases, resulting in a negative pressure directly above the glottis. The supraglottal negative pressure reinforces the negative pressure within the glottis, which facilitates a greater closing force. As the glottis opens due to positive pressure, the air flowing through the glottis meets the mass of air directly above it, creating compression of the air and increased positive air pressure. The positive supraglottal air pressure further raises the air pressure within the glottis, creating a stronger opening force.

Once the glottis is closed by elasticity and P_{neg}, P_s begins to build up and the whole process repeats itself. One opening and closing of the glottis constitutes one cycle of vocal fold vibration. The cycle of vibration can be thought of as consisting of four phases of vocal fold movement: opening, open, closing, and closed. This is called the **duty cycle**.

During speech the vocal folds vibrate hundreds of times per second, depending on the age and gender of the individual. Vibration continues for as long as medial compression continues to be exerted, and the interaction between positive and negative air pressures maintains the alternating opening and closing of the glottis. Because vibration continues due to differences in transglottal pressures (i.e., pressures below and above the glottis) without an external force needing to be applied for each cycle, the vocal folds are considered to be a **self-sustaining oscillator**.

Note that for phonation to occur the vocal folds do not have to be completely closed but cannot be farther apart than around 3 mm. The vocal folds vibrate for as long as the individual is producing a voiced sound. For a voiceless sound or to inhale, the glottis is opened by the PCA.

Mucosal Wave

The vocal folds vibrate in an extremely complex fashion due to their layered structure, with each layer differing in its biomechanical properties. Rather than opening and closing as a whole, the folds open from bottom to top and close from bottom to top in an undulating way. This complex vibration is due to timing differences in the way that the vocal folds abduct and adduct along both their vertical and horizontal dimensions. Vertically, as the inferior edges of the folds are beginning to approximate, the superior margins are still separated. As the air flows upward through the glottis, creating negative pressure, the closing movement also progresses upward. While the superior margins of the folds are approximating and then making contact, the inferior edges are already beginning to separate as P_s builds up and forces them apart. This slight time lag between the opening and closing of the inferior and superior portions of the vocal folds is known as the **vertical phase difference**. There is a similar timing lag between the opening and closing of the vocal folds from back to front. They open from their posterior attachment at the vocal processes to the anterior portion at the anterior commissure. They close, however, in an anterior to posterior direction. This lag in closure is called the **longitudinal phase difference**. The timing differences give the vibration of the vocal folds an undulating, wave-like motion, which is particularly evident in the loose and pliable cover layer of the folds; this has been termed the **mucosal wave**. Figure 5.14 provides a schematic representation of the approximation and separation of the vocal folds during vibration.

Phonation Threshold Pressure

In order for the vocal folds to vibrate, the pressure below the vocal folds must be higher than that above so that air will flow through the glottis. The pressure differential between the subglottal pressure and supraglottal pressure (transglottal pressure) creates the driving pressure forcing air to flow through the glottis as long as the vocal folds are in an appropriate adducted position. The minimum amount of P_s needed to set the vocal folds into vibration is known as the **phonation threshold pressure (PTP)**. For conversational speech at normal loudness levels, PTP ranges from about 3 cm H_2O at low fundamental frequencies to around 6 cm H_2O at high fundamental frequencies (Kent, 1997b). At higher F_0 levels the vocal folds are thinner and stiffer, so more pressure is needed to set them into vibration. For a low F_0, a PTP of around 3 to 4 cm H_2O corresponds to a voice amplitude level of around 45 to 65 dB SPL (Kent, 1997b). Higher pressures are needed for louder speech. Pressure for a loud yell, for example, needs to be around 50 cm H_2O.

Glottal Spectrum

The F_0 and harmonics of the human voice can be well visualized on a line spectrum. The spectrum of the human voice is known as the **glottal spectrum** (Figure 5.15). The glottal spectrum corresponds to the source function in the source–filter theory.

Figure 5.14 Cycle of vocal fold vibration showing the mucosal wave

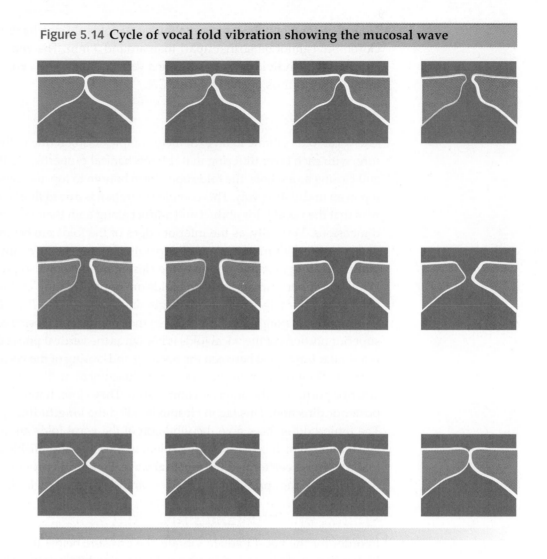

Figure 5.15 Glottal spectrum

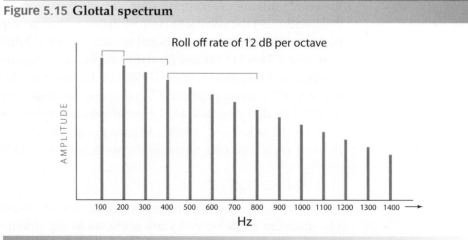

The glottal spectrum does not represent the sound of the voice one actually hears, because the sound is resonated and modified as it travels through the vocal tract and out the mouth or nose. Rather, the glottal spectrum represents the sound that one would hear if a microphone could somehow be placed within the larynx, before the sound travels through the rest of the vocal tract. The glottal spectrum shows that the F_0 is the lowest frequency and has the greatest amplitude. As the harmonic frequencies increase, their amplitudes decrease at a rate of 12 dB per octave. Thus, the glottal spectrum shows a loss of 12 dB from 100 to 200 Hz, another loss of 12 dB from 200 to 400 Hz, another loss of 12 dB from 400 to 800 Hz, and so on. Because of this decrease of acoustic energy as frequency increases, there is more acoustic energy in the lower frequencies of the voice and less in the higher frequencies. At the very highest frequencies, acoustic energy is miniscule. Acoustic energy in the human voice has been shown to be significant up to around 4000 to 5000 Hz.

Harmonic Spacing

When a speaker alters the pitch of his or her voice in conversational speech, it is the F_0 that is manipulated by adjusting the rate of vocal fold vibration. Changing the F_0 also changes the **harmonic spacing**, which refers to the distance between the harmonic frequencies in a complex sound (Figure 5.16).

It is clear that harmonic spacing must change with each different F_0 because harmonics are whole-number multiples of the F_0. Thus, if an individual has an F_0 of 100 Hz, the harmonics would be 200, 300, 400 Hz, and so on, up to around 4000 or 5000 Hz. If this individual raises his or her pitch by increasing F_0 to 200 Hz, the harmonics are now 400, 600, 800 Hz, and so on, up to around 4000 or 5000 Hz. The spacing between the harmonic frequencies has increased from 100 to 200 Hz, and there are now fewer harmonics in the person's voice. Thus, at an F_0 of 200 Hz not only does the person's pitch sound higher, but the degree of acoustic complexity of the voice has also changed. The higher the person's F_0, the wider the harmonic spacing is. This helps to explain why children's voices sound so different from adults' voices. Prepubertal children have an F_0 that is considerably higher than adults' (around 300 Hz, compared to approximately 100 Hz for adult males and 200 Hz for adult females). Not only is their pitch much higher, but, because of the wider harmonic spacing, their voices do not have the rich, resonant quality of adult voices. The fewer harmonics in the child's voice result in a quality that is thinner than an adult's. This quality has historically been an advantage for child singers in church and concert choirs, such as the Vienna Boys Choir. In previous centuries, this purity of voice was so prized in boys that some were castrated (known as castrati) in order to prevent the voice from changing at puberty.

Nearly Periodic Nature of the Human Voice

Because of their tissue and biomechanical characteristics, the vocal folds do not vibrate in a completely even, periodic manner. There are always small fluctuations in frequency and amplitude, resulting in an almost but not quite periodic sound. Consider the example of an individual attempting to produce the vowel /a/ as steadily as possible at an F_0 of 200 Hz. The goal for the speaker is to maintain the

Figure 5.16 Harmonic spacing

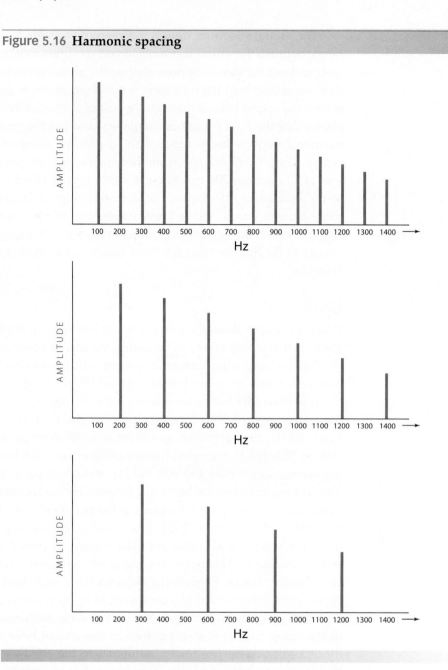

vocal folds at the precise degree of tension and stiffness that will allow them to vibrate 200 times per second. If vocal fold vibration was completely periodic, each cycle of vibration would take exactly 1/200 second (0.005 s). Because vocal fold vibration is not completely but nearly periodic, one cycle may last 0.005 s, the following cycle may last 0.004 s, the next cycle may last 0.006 s, and so on. The timing variability between cycles of vibration is called **frequency perturbation** or, more commonly, **jitter**. A similar variability between cycles is also true of amplitude. If the person sustaining the /a/ sound tries to keep the loudness level as steady as possible, the vocal folds will nonetheless vibrate with slightly different amplitudes for each cycle. This variability is known as **amplitude perturbation**, or **shimmer**.

Cycle-to-cycle variations in frequency and amplitude have been shown to result from neurologic, biomechanic, and aerodynamic factors. The larynx is especially susceptible to small fluctuations in neural, vascular, respiratory, and lymphatic transport systems; which can be detected in the vibratory patterns of the vocal folds (Titze, 1994). The left and right vocal folds may not be exactly symmetrical but may differ slightly in their tissue density and tension. Or there may be more mucus on one fold than another, causing one to have slightly increased density than the other. Variations in lung pressure can also cause perturbations in vocal fold amplitude and frequency, because P_s fluctuates slightly during the build up and release of pressure through the glottis. The articulators also have an influence on vocal fold vibration. Whenever the tongue moves forward, for example, it pulls the hyoid bone forward and upward, which in turn raises the larynx. Raising the larynx can change the stiffness of the vocal folds, thereby perturbing the F_0 (Titze, 1994). Aerodynamic events also produce fluctuations in vocal fold cycles of vibration. As the air is forced through the glottis, it can become unstable and turbulent, resulting in rapid pressure fluctuations in the vocal output (Titze, 1994).

Vocal Quality

The laryngeal tone has a fundamental frequency and harmonics, just like other periodic complex sounds. The F_0 corresponds to the perceived pitch of the voice, while the harmonics contribute to the quality of the voice. People's voices can usually be distinguished by quality. For example, if two people both say /a/ with the same F_0, others will still be able to distinguish between the voices. Voices sound different, even when the pitch is perceived as the same, because the harmonic content of the voices differs. The same is true with musical instruments. Middle C on a piano and middle C on a violin have the same F_0 (approximately 262 Hz). However, unless an individual is totally tone deaf (which very few people are), one can easily tell the difference between the two instruments; each has a uniqueness of tone, which is related to the acoustic quality of the instrument and the spectrum of the resulting sound.

Although a large amount of research has been devoted to investigating vocal quality, there is as yet no generally accepted definition of the term. One reason for this is that the concept of vocal quality has been used in different contexts by different professionals. For example, a phonetician might use quality to distinguish between phonemes; a singer might refer to the quality of different registers; and quality might be used to describe voice types such as breathy, hoarse, and harsh (Childers, 1991). Another reason is that voice quality is a multidimensional entity and is linked to numerous aspects of voice production, including F_0, amplitude, resonance characteristics, and rate of speech. The quality of a person's voice is determined by how the vocal folds vibrate as well as by the shape and configuration of the vocal tract, including length, degree of arching of the hard palate, and size of the oral cavity in relation to size of the pharynx. Women have slightly different vocal tract configurations than men, so even if men and women produce a sound with the same F_0, it is still usually easy to recognize the voice as male or female by its quality.

The way that the vocal folds vibrate plays an important role in shaping an individual's voice quality. Vocal folds that are adducted too tightly, with too much medial compression, are said to be **hyperadducted**. This can be caused by many different types of problems, ranging from habitual vocally damaging behaviors to neurological diseases. When the folds are hyperadducted, the balance between muscular tension and P_s is upset. With the folds adducted too tightly, it takes more P_s to overcome the resistance of the adducted vocal folds. The resulting voice is perceived as tense and pressed. Vocal folds that do not adduct as tightly as they should are said to be **hypoadducted**. This condition, too, can be caused by numerous factors, ranging from inappropriate usage to neurological problems such as vocal fold paralysis. As with hyperadduction, the balance between muscular and aerodynamic forces is upset. In this case, there is too little muscle force, so the vocal folds do not offer enough resistance to the flow of air. Air escapes between the vocal folds without being converted into acoustic energy. The loss of air creates turbulence as it passes through the vocal folds and adds a noisy, breathy quality to the vocal tone.

Velopharyngeal valving also contributes to voice quality. Inadequate velopharyngeal closure during the production of oral sounds results in excessive nasal resonance (hypernasality); conditions that prevent the flow of air through the nasal cavities (e.g., large adenoids in a child) result in insufficient nasal resonance on nasal sounds (hyponasality).

In the perceptual domain, dozens of adjectives have been used to describe voice quality. Just a few are pleasant, strident, rough, raspy, shrill, clear, unpleasant, harsh, hoarse, tinny, and strained. This abundance of terminology is a problem in the clinical management of voice disorders because these terms are highly subjective. What one individual perceives as rough may be perceived by another person as hoarse or strident. Professionals using these terms have no standard frame of reference for voice quality, which makes communication between them difficult. Another problem with subjective terms is that they do not indicate the underlying patterns of vocal fold vibration that are contributing to the resulting quality. There is no agreed on physiological basis for most of these terms. Even defining what constitutes a normal voice quality is difficult.

Normal Voice Quality

In order to define normal voice quality, it is important to understand that normal voices differ, depending on factors such as sex, age, build, culture, region, personality, degree of voice use, vocal sensations, and health of the speaker. Any definition of normal voice quality must take all these factors into account. The voice can be broadly defined as normal when the quality is clear; pitch and loudness are appropriate for age, sex, and situation; the voice is produced without undue effort, pain, strain, or fatigue; and the voice is satisfactory to the speaker in terms of fulfilling his or her occupational, social, and emotional vocal needs (Ferrand, 2012).

In order to provide a more objective description of normal voice, researchers and clinicians have tried to specify the acoustic and physiological bases that form the foundation of normal voice. Zemlin (1998) listed six specifiable acoustic parameters of voice production that contribute to a normal, clear vocal quality (Table 5.4).

Table 5.4 **Parameters of Normal Vocal Quality**

Maximum frequency range
Speaking F_0
Maximum phonation time
Minimum–maximum intensity at various F_0 levels
Periodicity of vibration
Noise generated by turbulent airflow

SOURCE: Information from Zemlin (1998).

These six parameters clearly demonstrate the multidimensional nature of voice quality and the interdependence of F_0, intensity, and quality. The parameters are maximum frequency range, habitual pitch, maximum phonation time, minimum–maximum intensity at different F_0 levels, periodicity of vibration, and amount of spectral noise:

Maximum frequency range: The normal voice is flexible in pitch during conversation. Speech that lacks this flexibility sounds very monotonous. Adults have a maximum frequency range of around two-and-one-half to three octaves.

Average rate of vocal fold vibration during conversation (speaking fundamental frequency [- SFF]): Children, adult women, and adult men demonstrate fairly characteristic F_0 levels during speech. F_0 levels that are much higher or lower than those expected for a person's age and sex do not sound normal.

Maximum phonation time (air cost): This refers to the longest period of time that an individual can sustain a vowel on one breath. An adult speaker should be able to sustain comfortable phonation for about 15 to 25 seconds. Children are expected to be able to sustain phonation for at least 10 seconds. A lack of ability to sustain phonation for the expected amount of time indicates a problem in adequately valving the airstream for speech.

Minimum–maximum amplitude at various F_0 levels: A healthy speaker should be able to vary his or her amplitude level by a minimum of 20 to 30 dB in the midrange of frequency. A person who shows a restricted range of amplitude variation may sound monotone.

Periodicity of vocal fold vibration: This parameter is reflected acoustically in jitter. With mass, length, tension, and P_s held constant, normal vocal fold vibration will still be nearly, and not completely, periodic. However, vibration which is excessively aperiodic may be perceived as a rough or hoarse-sounding voice.

Noise: Noise results from turbulent airflow, with a random distribution of acoustic energy. Turbulent airflow is generated when an obstacle interferes with vocal fold vibration, causing air to flow in a less laminar manner through the glottis. In a normal voice, the harmonic energy generated by the nearly periodic vibration should be much higher than any noise energy. Noise in the voice, acoustically called **additive noise** or **spectral noise**, can be heard as breathiness, hoarseness, roughness, or any combination of these perceptual attributes. A small amount of noise in the glottal source may contribute to a slightly breathy quality. More turbulence might be heard as huskiness, whereas a great deal of turbulence is usually perceived as a hoarse voice. The normal voice has a steep spectral slope, so it should have most energy at the lower frequencies and much less energy at the higher frequencies. A spectrum that shows increased energy at higher harmonics may indicate that there is additive noise in the signal contributing to the increased energy. Some noise in the spectrum, though, seems to be normal, particularly in women's voices, which lends a breathier quality to women's voices (Klatt & Klatt, 1990; Mendoza, Valencia, Munot, & Trujillo, 1996; Sodersten & Lindestad, 1990).

Abnormal Voice Qualities

Dysphonia is a generic term for any voice that sounds deviant in terms of quality, pitch, and/or loudness. Because voice quality is a multidimensional phenomenon, perceived problems in pitch and loudness often contribute to the perception of dysphonia, and vice versa. Research by Wolfe and Ratusnik (1988) has shown that moderately to severely dysphonic vowels are perceived by listeners to be significantly lower in pitch than clear or mildly dysphonic vowels. The authors reported that listeners matched dysphonic vowels with a perceived pitch that was on the average six semitones lower than the actual F_0 of the vowel. Thus, the relationship between the perception of pitch and the actual vocal F_0 varies depending on voice quality. It has also been shown that the lower the pitch of the voice and the louder the voice, the greater is the likelihood of the voice being rated more severely dysphonic (Kempster, Kistler, & Hillenbrand, 1991).

Although professionals use many different terms to describe different voice qualities, the most currently accepted terms are breathiness, roughness, and hoarseness. A breathy quality refers to a vocal tone that sounds aspirated, with audible air escape during phonation. Roughness refers to a raspy sound in the voice, with the perception of a low pitch. Hoarseness refers to a combination of breathy and rough qualities in the voice (Eskenazi, Childers, & Hicks, 1990). The terms breathiness, roughness, and hoarseness have become popular because these are the vocal qualities that are the most amenable to acoustic analysis. Researchers have therefore tried to measure these qualities in order to generate some kind of objective method of relating the perception of abnormal voice to the relevant acoustic factors in the vocal signal. Numerous acoustic measurements have been made of both normal and disordered voices in an attempt to find a cluster of measures that successfully separates normal from disordered voice.

Breathy voice

When the vocal folds do not adduct completely, the result is a continuous flow of air during the entire vibratory cycle. The air leaking out generates frication noise along with the tone generated by the vibrating vocal folds (Zemlin, 1998). The vocal folds are close enough to be vibrated, but the sound of air being continuously released accompanies the sound wave. The turbulent airflow pattern results in a less periodic acoustic signal. Because the periodic component of the voice source is weaker in the middle and high frequencies, noise tends to be especially noticeable above about 2 to 3 kHz (Hillebrand & Houde, 1996). A breathy voice signal has more high-frequency energy than a nonbreathy signal. Some researchers have reported that breathiness is associated with a relative loss of acoustic energy between 2 and 5 kHz and with an increase in noise at frequencies higher than 5 kHz (Rihkanen, Leinonen, Hiltunen, & Kangas, 1994).

Breathiness is an inefficient form of phonation, with a limited dynamic range because less subglottal pressure builds up when the vocal folds do not adduct properly. In addition, a person with a breathy voice often uses three to four times the normal amount of air per second during phonation. Breathy voice is not always abnormal, however. Breathy or aspirated voice serves to distinguish between some phonemes in several languages. For example, Zulu is a Bantu language spoken in South Africa that differentiates between aspirated and unaspirated voiceless stops, such as /k/ and /kʰ/. In Zulu, these would be heard as two distinct phonemes, based on the degree of breathiness accompanying each. On the other hand, breathiness is also a very common symptom of both organic and functional voice disorders (e.g., vocal fold paralysis), and increased breathiness may be associated with aging.

Rough/hoarse voice

A rough or hoarse voice is a very common symptom of many laryngeal disorders. It can be the first indication of some kind of voice problem, ranging from a minor bout of laryngitis to a life-threatening cancerous tumor. Hoarseness is partially determined by the amount of spectral noise resulting from the flow of turbulent air through the glottis. Hoarseness is also related to how periodically the vocal folds are vibrating. For example, when the vocal folds are irritated or swollen, they vibrate in a less periodic fashion. This occurs because the inflammation prevents the cover of the vocal folds from vibrating as freely as normal, which interferes with the mucosal wave. Since aperiodic sound is noise, the more aperiodic the vibration is, the more noise that is imposed on the vocal tone. The noise that results in the perception of a hoarse voice tends to be more prevalent at lower frequencies, between 100 and 2600 Hz.

In sum, breathiness and roughness are both characterized by additive noise, but in breathiness the noise is located at the higher frequencies, and in roughness the noise occurs at the lower frequencies. A combination of these factors is also possible and does indeed occur frequently.

Vocal Registers

The entire range of F_0 in the human voice is enormous, from under 60 Hz in the bass voice to over 1568 Hz in the soprano voice (Zemlin, 1998). The term *register* is used in both singing and speech production contexts to denote specific portions of the total F_0 range. In the singing context, the term is used extremely loosely and can refer to a particular part of a singer's vocal range, a resonance area (e.g., head voice, chest voice), a particular vocal quality, or a region of the voice defined by vocal breaks (Echternach, Dippold, et al., 2010; McKinney, 1994). In singing, *chest register* indicates a midrange of pitches, while *falsetto* refers to a much higher range of pitches. *Head register* is sometimes described as a mixture between chest and

Table 5.5 **Average Ranges in Hz for Males and Females in Pulse, Modal, and Falsetto Registers**

	Males	Females
Pulse	43–82[a] 25–80[b]	87–165[a] 25–45[b]
Modal	98–147[a] 75–450[b]	175–294[a] 130–520[b]
Falsetto	349–494[a] 275–620[b]	659–988[a] 490–1130[b]

SOURCES: [a]Zemlin (1998); [b]Baken (1996).

falsetto (Titze, 1994). In the context of speech production, the term is more clearly defined in relation to voice physiology, acoustic and aerodynamic parameters of voice production, and perceptual vocal characteristics.

In terms of voice production, the range of F_0 is usually divided into three registers: **pulse register**, **modal register**, and **falsetto register**. These are perceptually distinct regions of vocal quality that can be maintained over some ranges of F_0 and intensity. Pulse register refers to a range of very low F_0, which perceptually creates a creaky, popping sort of sound. Pulse is also called *vocal fry*, *glottal fry*, or *creaky voice*. Falsetto refers to a very high range of F_0, and is sometimes called *loft register*. Modal is the register most commonly used in normal conversational speech. Some studies have found that there is little or no overlap between fundamental frequencies in different registers (e.g., Baken, 2005; Blomgren, Chen, Ng, & Gilbert, 1998; Hollien, 1974), while other researchers have reported that despite the differences in vocal quality, overlap can occur between fundamental frequencies across different registers (e.g., Riede & Zuberbuhle, 2003; Roubeau, Henrich, & Castellengo, 2009). Table 5.5 shows the F_0 ranges associated with the three primary registers.

A key characteristic that distinguishes registers is that each is produced by a different manner of vocal fold vibration. A particular pattern of vibration is usually confined to a certain F_0 range. In normal conversational speech, when the speaker reaches the upper limits of the modal range, the manner of vocal fold vibration suddenly changes and the sound shifts to the falsetto or loft register. Similarly, at the lower limits of the modal range, these adjustments in vocal fold vibration result in glottal fry or pulse register. The change in vibration results in a corresponding change in voice quality. Often, the change in voice quality is abrupt and noticeable to the speaker and to his or her listeners. Acoustically, the transition to the register change may be characterized by increased jitter and shimmer (Echternach, Sundberg, Zander, & Richter, 2010).

Physiologic and Acoustic Characteristics of Modal, Pulse, and Falsetto Registers

Modal register is characterized by full participation of the cover and body during vibration. Individuals are able to generate the greatest range of amplitudes in this register. In modal register, the vocal folds are somewhat shorter in length compared to their nonvibrating position, the cover is slack, and the body is fully involved in vibration (Titze, 1994). The duty cycle is characterized by relatively rapid onset, with a brief open phase followed by a longer closing phase and a short closed phase (Hollien, 1974). In this register, PTP has been reported as around 2 to 7.5 cm H_2O (Blomgren et al., 1998; Jiang, Ng, & Hanson, 1999). The complete range of fundamental frequencies in modal register is around 75 to 450 Hz in men and around 130 to 520 Hz in women (Baken, 2005). Average speaking frequencies used in modal register have been reported as 211 Hz (range 175–266 Hz) for adult women and 117 Hz (range 86–170 Hz) for adult men (Blomgren et al., 1998).

Pulse register refers to the lowest range of F_0 that speakers can produce. Males and females generate similar F_0s, averaging around 48 Hz (Blomgren et al., 1998). This is approximately one octave below the frequencies for the normal modal register for a male (Blomgren et al., 1998). To achieve this extremely low frequency, the vocal folds are short and thick. In addition, the false vocal folds may come into contact with the true folds, thus increasing the vibrating mass and further decreasing the fundamental frequency (Blomgren et al., 1998; Hollien, 1974). The medial edges of the folds are loosely adducted. PTP is therefore low, with reported values ranging from approximately 2 cm H_2O (Zemlin, 1998) to 5.5 cm H_2O (Blomgren et al., 1998). The vocal folds are adducted for 90 percent of the cycle, with glottal opening and closing movements together only accounting for about 10 percent of the cycle. In addition, the vocal folds vibrate in a different manner than they do in modal register. Instead of opening and closing the glottis once per cycle, they may approximate and separate partially once, twice, or three times before completely adducting (Blomgren et al., 1998). This phenomenon is known as **multiphasic closure**. After each partial vocal fold closing, there is a burst of acoustic energy. The energy dies out, leaving a temporary interval (**temporal gap**) during which there is no acoustic energy (Titze, 1994). Below about 70 Hz, the human ear seems to be able to detect these bursts of acoustic energy and temporal gaps within each glottal cycle. This is what is heard as the creaky, popping sound of pulse register. Above 70 Hz or so, a continuous sound is perceived rather than the individual acoustic pulses and temporal gaps. The spectral slope of pulse register is shallow due to its low F_0 and many harmonics. Pulse is a perfectly normal register, and many people use it, especially at the ends of phrases and sentences (e.g., Wolk, Abdelli-Beruh, & Slavin, 2011). This register is an extension of the lower limits of the modal pitch range. Clinically, though, the use of pulse register becomes a problem when it is used habitually instead of just at the end of sentences.

Loft, or falsetto, register includes the highest frequency ranges and has been reported as 275–620 Hz in men and 490–1130 Hz in women (Baken, 2005). To achieve this very high frequency, the cricothyroid muscle exerts a great deal of longitudinal tension. High-speed photography has shown that the folds appear very long and stiff and thin and sharp along the edges, with a tight and narrow glottis (Hollien, 1974; Van den Berg, 1958). The cover of the folds is lax, while the vocal ligament is tensed (Titze, 1994). The extreme tension on the vocal ligaments prevents the folds from adducting completely during vibration, resulting in reduced amplitude of vibration and a somewhat breathy quality. The extreme stiffness also results in a higher PTP of around 6 to 8 cm H_2O (Solomon & Di Mattia, 2000). In addition, because of the extreme tension on the vocal ligaments, the vocal ligament and body of the folds do not vibrate as fully as they do in modal and pulse registers, resulting in a less complex vibration and a thinner quality to the sound. Because of both the high speed of vibration and the less complex manner of vibration of the vocal folds the quality of the tone is almost flutelike (Zemlin, 1998). When the F_0 is very high, the harmonics are widely spaced, giving the sound a thinner quality compared to the richer quality of a lower pitched sound. The spectral slope is steeper for the high-pitched voice of falsetto, with its high F_0 and few harmonics. Another factor that contributes to the distinctive quality of falsetto voice is the slightly breathy component that results from the vocal folds never quite closing during vibration.

Use of Different Registers in Singing and Speaking

Even though modal and falsetto registers are characterized by different vibratory patterns, there is actually a considerable amount of overlap between the upper limits of the modal range and the lower limits of the falsetto range. Most trained singers can produce a high note that is perceived as being within the modal register and can produce a note with exactly the same F_0 that is heard as the lower portion of the falsetto register. Also, some trained singers can push the modal register up to very high limits, around 500 Hz (Titze, 1994). Abrupt changes in register are used in some kinds of singing, such as yodeling, country/western, folk singing, soul, and gospel. In electronically amplified singing, the falsetto register is becoming more and more the acceptable register for high pitches. However, in classical Western styles of singing, such as opera, art song, and oratorio, noticeable register changes are generally unacceptable. Singers of these styles spend much time and effort learning to switch smoothly between registers with no perceivable changes in quality.

For speech purposes, modal is the most typically used register, although it is common for individuals to drop to pulse register at the ends of phrases and sentences. Use of falsetto in conversational speech is less common. However, all three registers are normal modes of vocal fold vibration. In fact, switching between registers is sometimes necessary for linguistic, esthetic, or physiologic reasons. For instance, some African and Asian languages use abrupt changes in register to distinguish between phonemes (Titze, 1994). However, if a speaker uses primarily pulse or primarily falsetto for conversational speech, this is considered by speech–language pathologists to be a voice problem requiring therapy.

Acoustic Measurement of Phonatory Variables

The most popular acoustic measures are variables related to frequency and intensity; perturbation measures including jitter and shimmer; and measures of noise in the voice such as harmonics-to-noise ratio, noise-to-harmonics ratio, and normalized noise energy.

Frequency and Intensity Variables

As described above, the vibration of the vocal folds generates a nearly periodic, complex sound wave with a fundamental frequency (F_0) and harmonics. The F_0 is the rate at which the vocal folds vibrate and corresponds to the perceived pitch of the voice. The vocal folds also generate a certain degree of amplitude during vibration, corresponding to the loudness of the speaker's voice. Measurements of vocal frequency and amplitude are commonly used in clinical practice including average F_0, frequency variability, maximum phonational frequency range, average amplitude level, amplitude variability, and dynamic range.

Average fundamental frequency

The rate of vibration of the vocal folds depends on their length, tissue density, and tension. The greater the length and tissue density and the less the tension and stiffness, the slower the vocal folds will vibrate and the lower the person's pitch. Vocal folds that are shorter, less dense, and more stiff will vibrate more quickly and give rise to the perception of a higher pitch. Vocal F_0 is determined primarily by the tension of the vocal fold cover rather than by the actual length of the vocal folds (Kent, 1997b). Children, with their small and thin vocal folds, tend to have a high frequency of vibration (around 250 to 300 Hz for boys and girls prior to puberty). Adult females have an average F_0 of 180 to 250 Hz, and adult males, with their generally longer and denser vocal folds, range in F_0 between approximately 80 and 150 Hz. Average F_0 is derived by measuring F_0 in a particular task, such as sustaining a vowel, reading aloud, or conversational speech, and averaging over the speaking time of that task. When average F_0 is measured in an oral reading or conversational speech task, it is often referred to as the person's speaking fundamental frequency (SFF). Many researchers have examined the average F_0 in different age groups and races and across both sexes. Table 5.6 lists average F_0 for different age groups and races reported in the literature.

Looking at the table, one sees a systematic pattern of F_0 values that vary according to age level and sex. Infants in the first several years of life have a very high F_0, from around 350 to almost 500 Hz. In musical terms, this is from around the F an octave above middle C to the B almost two octaves above middle C. The high F_0 is the result of the infant's very short and thin vocal folds, which have a correspondingly rapid rate of vibration. As the baby grows, his or her vocal folds lengthen and thicken, with a resulting decrease in F_0. From around age 3 to 10 years, both males and females have an average F_0 of approximately 270 to 300 Hz. After puberty, the average F_0 for males drops markedly, while that for females remains essentially the same or may decrease slightly. Again, these F_0 patterns are related to growth factors. At puberty, the male larynx enlarges considerably, and the vocal folds become longer, thicker, and denser, with a corresponding dramatic drop in F_0. A girl's larynx and vocal folds also enlarge somewhat during puberty, but not to the same extent as a boy's. By age 20, the average F_0 for males is around 120 Hz, while for females the average F_0 is approximately 100 Hz higher than males, at 220 Hz.

Average F_0 remains fairly stable for adult males and females until the sixth and seventh decades of life. At this time males' average F_0 may increase due to

Table 5.6 Average F_0 in Hz for Different Age Groups for Males (M) and Females (F) Reported in the Literature

Author(s)	Age Group	M	F	Race
Wermke & Robb (2010)	Neonates	362–394	362–394	
Robb & Saxman (1985)	11–25 months	357	357	
McGlone & Shipp (1971)	13–23 months	443	443	
Eguchi & Hirsh (1969)	3 4 5	298 286 289	298 286 289	
Awan & Mueller (1996)	5–6 5–6 5–6	240 241 249	243 231 248	W AA H
Weinberg & Bennett (1971)	5 6	252 247	248 247	
Wheat & Hudson (1988)	6	219	211	AA
Ferrand & Bloom (1996)	3–6 7–10	256 237	246 253	
Sorenson (1989)	6 7 8 9 10	251 288 229 221 220	296 258 251 266 229	
Pederson et al. (1990)	8.6–12.9 13–15.9 16–19.8		256 248 241	
Bennett (1983)	8.2 9.2 10.2 11.2	234 226 224 216	235 222 228 221	
Fitch (1990)	21–26	109	210	
Kent (1994)	20.3 47.9 73.3 85	120 123 119 136		
Hollien & Shipp (1972)	20–29 30–39 40–49 50–59 60–69 70–79 80–89	120 112 107 118 112 132 146		
De Pinto & Hollien (1982)	18–25		229	
Morgan & Rastatter (1986)	20–24		228	

Table 5.6 (*Continued*)

Author(s)	Age Group	M	F	Race
Pegoraro-Krook (1988)	20–29 30–39 40–49 50–59 60–69 70–79 80–89		195 195 191 182 181 188 188	
Russell et al. (1995)	65–68		181	
Brown et al. (1996)	21–33 20–22 40–54 42–50 69–87 65–89	136 128 135 	 189 186 175	
D'haeseleer et al. (2011)	20–28 46–52		200 184	
Honjo & Isshiki (1980)	69–85	162	177	

Values for postlingual children and adults are for conversational speech or oral reading. Some studies included race as a factor: White (W), African-American (AA), Hispanic (H). Unless otherwise stated, ages are in years. Some values have been rounded to the nearest whole number.

age-related degenerative changes that occur within the larynx, such as thinning of the vocal folds. Because objects that are thinner and less dense vibrate more quickly than those that are denser, the thinning of the male's vocal folds produces an increase in vocal F_0. Older women, on the other hand, tend to develop denser vocal folds due to hormonal changes. Thus, the F_0 of older women tends to decrease with age.

Frequency variability

People constantly change their F_0 levels as they speak to reflect different emotions, different types of accenting and stress of syllables, and different grammatical constructions. The F_0 changes contribute to the overall melody, or prosody, of speech. For instance, the sentence "Peter's going home" can be said either as a declarative statement or as a question. As a declarative, the F_0 level drops at the end of the utterance, whereas for a question the F_0 level rises at the end of the utterance. The prosody of a sentence also is influenced by the mood of the speaker. There are likely to be many more F_0 changes, and more extensive changes, when the individual is excited that Peter's going home than when the speaker is depressed by Peter's plans. Acoustically, these F_0 changes correspond to frequency variability. A certain amount of frequency variability is desirable in a speaker's voice, depending on the individual's age, sex, culture, social context, and mood. The variability is something that speakers of a particular language in a particular culture intuitively recognize. Too much or too little frequency variability sounds wrong and can indicate a functional, organic, or neurogenic voice problem.

F_0 variability is measured in terms of standard deviation (SD) from the average F_0. Standard deviation is a statistical measure that reflects the spread of scores around the average score; thus standard deviation of F_0 reflects the spread of F_0 values around the average F_0. When the variability is measured in hertz, it is called F_0SD. F_0SD in normal conversational speech is around 20 to 35 Hz or higher. F_0SD is likely to increase when the speaker is excited or agitated. In an isolated vowel F_0SD is typically much smaller. Sometimes F_0SD is converted to semitones. When the frequency variability is measured in semitones rather than hertz, it is called **pitch sigma**. Pitch sigma for normal speakers during conversation should be around 2 to 4 semitones for both males and females (Colton & Casper, 1996).

Another measure of F_0 variability is the range, which is the difference between the highest and lowest F_0 in a particular sample of speech. The range can be expressed in hertz or it can be converted to semitones and octaves. Table 5.7 displays F_0 range information for different age groups.

An interesting trend emerges from the numbers in Table 5.7. The infants (11 to 25 months) have by far the greatest range of frequencies. This is not surprising because their vocalizations include a wide variety of nonwords, such as squeaks and squeals and cries. From around age 3 years, when children have mastered speech, to just before puberty, the range of F_0 used in normal conversational speech is around 150 to 200 Hz. The range decreases further in the adult years. From approximately age 7 years on, females tend to use a wider range of F_0 than males. This may be a sociocultural rather than a physical phenomenon. Ferrand and Bloom (1996) compared F_0 ranges in various age groups of boys and girls. The 7- to 10-year-old boys in their study had a narrower range than the 3- to 6-year-old boys. The range of the 7- to 10-year-old girls, however, was as wide as for younger girls. The authors suggested that boys, a few years before puberty, start to imitate

Table 5.7 F_0 **Ranges in Hz for Spontaneous Speech for Males (M) and Females (F) in Selected Age Groups Reported in the Literature**

Authors(s)	Age Group	M	F	Race
Robb & Saxman (1985)	11–25 months	1202	1202	
Ferrand & Bloom (1996)	3–4 5–6 7–8 9–10	202 214 158 151	190 199 203 180	
Awan & Mueller (1996)	5–6 5–6 5–6	186 204 185	214 190 164	W AA H
Benjamin (1981)	Young adults Older adults	64 78	95 101	
Fitch (1990)	21–26	46	77	

Some authors provide race information for White (W), African-American (AA), and Hispanic (H) groups. Age is in years, unless otherwise stated. Some values were derived by subtracting minimum from maximum frequencies. Some values have been rounded to the nearest whole number.

the prosodic patterns of adult males, who tend to use fewer pitch levels than females, and who also, in general, avoid dramatic pitch shifts.

Maximum phonational frequency range

Maximum phonational frequency range (MPFR) refers to the complete range of frequencies that an individual can generate. This differs from the F_0 variability measure, which reflects the range of F_0 a person typically uses in connected speech. MPFR has been defined as the range of frequencies from the lowest tone that the person can sustain excluding pulse register to the highest, including falsetto. MPFR is often measured in semitones or octaves. A range of around 3 octaves is normal for young adults (e.g., Lamarche, Ternström, & Pabon, 2010), while older adults may show a decrease in range. In terms of hertz, the lowest frequency that adult males are able to produce is around 80 Hz, and the highest is in the 700 Hz range (Colton & Casper, 1996). Adult females produce a low F_0 of approximately 135 Hz, with a high level that can reach over 1000 Hz. Trained singers are able to produce an even higher F_0 than this. Kent (1994) provided normative MPFRs in semitones for individuals from age 8 years to late adulthood. The lowest value of 24.3 semitones was demonstrated by older men in poor health; the greatest range of 41.4 semitones was shown by teenaged boys. Most values fell between these extremes, in the range of 30 semitones, or 2.5 octaves.

The MPFR is a useful measure because it reflects both the physiological limits of a speaker's voice (Colton & Casper, 1996) and the physical condition of the person's vocal mechanism and basic vocal ability (Baken, 1996). It has been shown that for normally speaking adults, neither age nor sex greatly affects MPFR. What does affect this value is physical condition. Older subjects in good health tend to have larger MPFRs than younger subjects in poor physical condition.

Voice Amplitude/Intensity

The terms *amplitude* and *intensity* are often used interchangeably in the context of vocal loudness. Amplitude is controlled by regulating subglottal pressure, primarily through increasing and decreasing medial compression. When medial compression is increased, the vocal folds press together more tightly and for a longer period of time, causing the P_s to build up more strongly. Therefore, when the folds are separated by the P_s, they are pushed apart more forcefully. Due to their elastic recoil, the vocal folds also come together again more forcefully, creating a stronger excitation of the air in the vocal tract. The sound wave that is generated, therefore, has a greater amplitude and intensity.

Average amplitude level

Average amplitude refers to the overall level of amplitude during a speech task such as oral reading, conversation, or sustaining a vowel. Perceptually, this corresponds to the loudness that the individual generates during the speech activity. Amplitude level varies depending on the speaker's situation. A person's average amplitude level is likely to be much lower during a soft conversation in a classroom and much higher when cheering at a football game. Amplitudes for normal conversational speech usually range between 65 and 80 dB SPL, with an average SPL in the general range of

70 dB for adult males, females, and children (Baken, 1996; Lamarche et al., 2010). Amplitude levels do not depend on age as much as do frequency levels, although there is some evidence that amplitude may be decreased slightly in older individuals.

Amplitude variability

During any conversation, amplitude varies depending on the speaker's mood and feelings, the message he or she is conveying, the stress and accenting of syllables and words, and the social context. Amplitude variability is expressed as a standard deviation, measured in dB SPL. Standard deviation of amplitude for a neutral, unemotional sentence is around 10 dB SPL. The greater the speaker's level of excitement or enthusiasm, the greater the variability is likely to be. The ability to vary amplitude is what imparts dynamism and interest to a speaker's voice. Individuals who lack this ability tend to sound flat and monotonous. Because amplitude variability is such an important marker of emphasis and emotion, a reduced ability to vary loudness can be highly upsetting to the speaker and can seriously impact the individual's communication effectiveness.

Many neurological disorders such as Parkinson's disease are characterized by reductions in both frequency and amplitude variability.

Dynamic range

Dynamic range is similar to maximum phonational frequency range. It relates to the physiological range of vocal amplitudes that a speaker can generate, from the softest phonation that is not a whisper to the loudest shout. A healthy adult female should be able to produce a minimum level of around 50 dB and a maximum of approximately 115 dB SPL; the figures for healthy adult males should be slightly higher (Coleman, Mabis, & Hinson, 1977). A restricted dynamic range may prevent a person from using stress and emphasis patterns appropriately, reducing the flexibility of spoken language. Although amplitudes above and below the 60 to 80 dB range are not normally used for conversational speech, the ability to raise one's voice is important for special occasions that demand higher levels of loudness (Sulter, Schutte, & Miller, 1995). The dynamic range depends on the F_0 produced and tends to be greatest for F_0 in the midrange and less for F_0 that is much lower or much higher.

Voice range profile

The voice range profile (VRP, also called a *phonetogram*, or an F_0 *SPL profile*) is a graph that plots a person's maximum phonational range against his or her dynamic range. Dynamic range is plotted on the vertical axis in dB SPL, and F_0 is plotted on the horizontal axis in hertz. See Figure 5.17.

To generate the profile, the speaker sustains a vowel at various F_0 levels. At each F_0 level, the individual produces the softest and loudest sounds that he or she can. This results in two contours on the graph. The upper contour shows maximum intensity at each selected frequency, and the lower contour shows minimum intensity at each frequency. The resulting profile gives a good indication of normal frequency and amplitude relationships in the human voice. Parameters that are derived from the VRP include minimum and maximum frequency, frequency range, minimum and maximum amplitude (SPL), SPL range, average SPL, and area encompassed within the profile (e.g., Lamarche et al., 2010).

Figure 5.17 Voice range profile

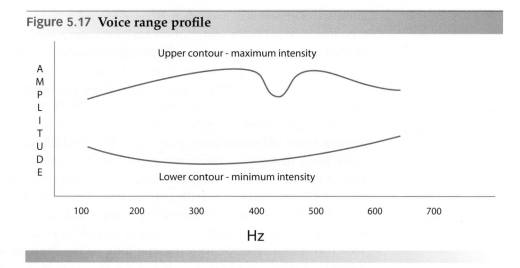

VRPs have a characteristic shape, reflecting some physiological quirks of the human voice production system. The shape is roughly similar to an oval, with narrower endpoints and a more expanded midportion. This shape results from the typical relationship between the range of frequencies and amplitudes that one can generate. Humans have a far greater dynamic range in the middle of the frequency range, whereas the dynamic range shrinks considerably at very high or very low frequencies. In the middle of the frequency range, an individual can generally vary the intensity by 20 to 30 dB, whereas at the ends of the frequency range the person might only be able to vary intensity by a few decibels (Titze, 1994).

Another feature of the shape is the dip that is often seen in the maximum intensity upper contour at around 390 Hz for men and 440 Hz for women (Sulter et al., 1995). This dip reflects a drop in maximum intensity that occurs when speakers without any voice training go from their usual conversational speech frequency range to the much higher falsetto range. Trained singers show a considerably reduced dip, indicating a smoother transition between these ranges.

The VRP can be thought of as a snapshot of vocal fold behavior at one moment in time (Aerainer & Klingholz, 1993). This picture gives very useful information for several reasons. First, a VRP can help to determine the physiological limits of any individual's voice because the dynamic and phonational frequency ranges are directly related to the person's ability to control the vocal folds (Sulter et al., 1995). A person who has difficulty achieving normal frequency and amplitude ranges will demonstrate a constricted or compressed VRP, with the upper and lower contours closer together than normal. Second, this kind of graph can show the impact of behavioral treatment or surgical intervention on an individual's voice. An expanded VRT after treatment would show graphically that the patient's phonational and/or dynamic range has increased.

Perturbation Measures

Frequency and amplitude perturbation (jitter and shimmer) are measured in terms of cycle-to-cycle differences in the period and amplitude of each cycle of vocal fold vibration. Current computer technology allows what used to be an incredibly complex mathematical procedure to be achieved at the click of the mouse. Many commercially available instruments and software programs allow measurement of jitter and shimmer, including the Multidimensional Voice Program (MDVP) by Kay Pentax, TF32 (supersedes CSpeech), Dr. Speech (Tiger Electronics), and Praat. The MDVP, TF32, and Praat programs are used worldwide for both clinical and research applications (Deliyski, Shaw, & Evans, 2005).

The slight degree of cycle-to-cycle variability in vocal fold vibration is such a natural part of human voice production that too little jitter and shimmer in the voice result in a perception of unnaturalness. The work of many researchers has shown that jitter levels of around 1 percent or less are normal in the human voice. Titze (1991) worked out a mathematical model of jitter by manipulating various aspects of the neuromuscular function of the vocal folds. He found that the very lowest level of jitter in the human voice is around 0.2 percent. These figures accord well with much research showing that jitter values in normal voices range from around 0.2 to 1 percent. Jitter values above this level indicate that the vocal folds are vibrating in a way that is not as periodic as it should be. High jitter levels suggest that something is interfering with normal vocal fold vibration and the mucosal wave. Shimmer has not been as thoroughly explored as jitter, but researchers estimate that shimmer values below 0.5 dB are normal in the human voice.

Jitter measures are extremely popular evaluation tools and are widely used in clinical practice. There are many advantages to these acoustic measures, including their easy accessibility, relatively inexpensive (or even free) costs, patient safety and lack of invasiveness, and quantifiable data that can be used to measure clinical progress and therapy outcomes (Table 5.8). Jitter has also been used as an index of vocal maturation in children and as an index of vocal aging. Children have been shown to have higher jitter values than adults; elderly adults demonstrate higher jitter values than younger adults.

Perturbation measures do pose some disadvantages (see Table 5.8). First, different acoustic programs use different mathematical algorithms to calculate jitter and shimmer, making it difficult to compare results from different instruments and programs. Also, the units of measurement of jitter and shimmer differ between programs. Some programs measure jitter in percentages and some use milliseconds. Some measure shimmer in percentages and some use decibels. Problems exist with jitter measurement because cycle-to-cycle frequency variability is affected by F_0, with higher F_0 being more difficult to measure. Some algorithms that are

Table 5.8 **Advantages and Disadvantages of Perturbation Measures**

Advantages	Disadvantages
Easy accessibility	Different calculation algorithms
Inexpensive	Not useful for moderately to severely dysphonic voices
Safe and non invasive	Validity and reliability issues due to internal and external factors
Provide quantifiable data	

used to calculate jitter take this factor into account and some do not. Because of all these uncontrolled variables it is difficult to compare perturbation measures across systems and software programs (Maryn, Corthals, De Bodt, Van Cauwenberge, & Deliyski, 2009). A serious disadvantage exists because the measurement of jitter depends on a precise determination of the period of the voice signal, so it may not be valid to calculate jitter for a voice that is aperiodic (e.g., Manfredi, Giordano, et al., 2011). Measures obtained for moderately to severely dysphonic voices may not be valid or reliable. Vocal loudness also exerts considerable influence on jitter and shimmer, with increases in both measures when speakers phonate below a level of 75 to 80 dB (Brockmann, Drinnan, Storck, & Carding, 2011; Brockmann, Storck, Carding, & Drinnan, 2008). In addition, the reliability and validity of acoustic measurements are affected by the quality of the recording device, type and placement of the microphone, computer hardware, analysis software, and amount of noise in the recording environment, as well as by individual factors such as gender and age (Deliyski, Shaw, & Evans, 2005; Deliyski, Evans, & Shaw, 2005). Finally, desktop microphones and general-purpose soundcards used in personal computers, as well as the lack of adequate sound level meters, can be problematic for accurate acoustic voice assessment (Deliyski, Evans, & Shaw, 2005; Vogel & Maruff, 2008). Since the recording environment has a strong influence on the obtained acoustic values, recording should be done in a sound-treated room with ambient noise less than 50 dB (Titze, 1995).

Because of the effects of internal and external factors on the acoustic signal, the National Center for Voice and Speech (NCVS) recommended that voice signals be classified in terms of their degree of periodicity (Titze, 1995). Three classifications are suggested (Table 5.9). Type 1 signals are nearly periodic (i.e., the healthy human voice). For these types of signals, perturbation values less than 5 percent are reported to be reliable (Titze & Liang, 1993). Type 2 signals are less periodic and contain subharmonics (fractions of the fundamental frequency) and/or frequency modulations. Type 3 signals are aperiodic and are not suitable for perturbation analysis.

Noise Measures

Noise measures provide a ratio of the proportion of harmonic sound (periodic) to noise (aperiodic) in the voice, measured in decibels. These measures are useful to quantify the relative amount of additive noise in the voice signal (Awan & Frenkel, 1994). Noise measures include harmonics-to-noise ratio (HNR), noise-to-harmonics

Table 5.9 **Suitability of Types of Signals for Perturbation Analysis**

Perturbation Type	Degree of Periodicity	Suitability for Analysis
Type 1	Nearly periodic	Values less than 5% are reliable
Type 2	Contain subharmonics and/or frequency modulations	May not be reliable
Type 3	Aperiodic	Not suitable

SOURCE: Information from Titze & Liang (1993).

ratio (NHR), and normalized noise energy (NNE). The most commonly used measures are HNR and NHR. In terms of HNR, the higher the value is, the more the harmonic components of the voice predominate over the noise. The lower the HNR is, the more noise that exists in the voice. An HNR of 0 dB reflects equal energy in the periodic and aperiodic components of the vocal signal (Verdonck-de Leeuw, Festen, & Mahieu, 2001). In terms of NHR, a low value corresponds to less noise and a stronger harmonic component in the voice and vice versa. NHR data can be converted to HNR data by means of a formula reported by Smits, Ceuppens, and De Bodt (2005):

$$HNR = 20 \times LOG\ (1/NHR)$$

For example, a value of 0.12 dB NHR would be converted in the following manner: $20 \times LOG\ (1/.12)$. $1/.12 = 8.33$. The log of 8.33 is 0.920645001. Multiply this number by 20, and the result is an HNR value of 18.4129 dB.

HNRs show a high correlation with perceptual judgments of voice quality, so this measure can be useful for making objective, quantitative assessments of breathiness, roughness, or hoarseness. HNRs for normally speaking individuals have been reported by various researchers as shown in Table 5.10. HNRs for children and for elderly adults have been reported to be lower than for young and middle-aged adults (Ferrand, 2000; 2002).

Additive noise generated by aperiodic vocal fold vibration and/or glottal turbulence results in lower-than-normal HNR or higher-than-normal NHR values. For example, if a person has some kind of problem in vocal fold vibration resulting from a growth (e.g., polyp, nodule), paralysis of one or both vocal folds, or other kind of laryngeal problem, a larger amount of air than normal escapes during vibration, creating turbulent noise (Pabon & Plomp, 1988).

Table 5.10 **Average Values for Harmonics-to-Noise Ratios (HNRs) Reported for Normally Speaking Adults (A) and Children (C)**

Authors	A/C	HNR (dB)
Awan & Frenkel (1994)	A	15.63 (males) 15.38 (females)
Bertino et al. (1996)	A	7.23
Dehqan et al. (2010)	A	18.42 (males) 18.81 (females)
Ferrand (2000)	C	2.346 (girls) 2.368 (boys)
Ferrand (2002)	A	7.82 (young women) 7.86 (middle-aged women) 5.54 (elderly women)
Horii & Fuller (1990)	A	17.3 (males) 19.1 (females)
Yumoto et al. (1982)	A	7.3

Summary

The larynx comprises one bone, nine cartilages, two pairs of joints, three sets of folds, and extrinsic and intrinsic muscles; these structures are connected by membranes and ligaments.

The myoelastic–aerodynamic theory of phonation describes one cycle of vocal fold vibration in terms of muscular, elastic recoil, and aerodynamic forces.

The sound generated by the larynx is complex and nearly periodic and is characterized by a certain amount of jitter and shimmer.

The vocal folds vibrate differently in different frequency ranges, giving rise to modal, pulse, and falsetto registers.

Voice quality is a multidimensional entity that is influenced by the degree of adduction of the vocal folds during vibration, by F_0 and intensity, and by the vocal tract structures above the larynx.

Breathiness and hoarseness can be characterized acoustically as additive noise in different frequency regions of the voice spectrum.

Measures of jitter, shimmer, and harmonics-to-noise ratios are widely used for both clinical and research purposes.

REVIEW EXERCISES

1. Explain how the vocal folds adduct and abduct. Describe all the relevant structures involved (cartilages, joints, muscles).

2. Discuss all the structures involved in the regulation of vocal F_0 and intensity.

3. Explain the relationship between voice quality and vocal registers, including a discussion of the physiological and acoustic parameters of pulse, modal, and falsetto.

4. Compare jitter, shimmer, and harmonics-to-noise ratio in terms of the types of information that each provides.

5. Identify advantages and disadvantages of acoustic measures of vocal function.

CHAPTER

6

Evaluation and Treatment of Phonatory Disorders

STUDENT LEARNING OBJECTIVES

After reading this chapter you will

○ Compare and contrast laryngeal measurement methods, including electroglottography, endoscopy with or without videostroboscopy, high-speed digital imaging, and videokymography.

○ Appreciate the clinical benefits of acoustic and visual information regarding phonatory structure and function.

○ Describe how acoustic and instrumental information is used to identify changes in phonatory function over the lifespan.

○ Discuss the uses of acoustic and visual information with regard to neurological disorders.

○ Understand why electroglottography is particularly suitable for evaluating the effectiveness of Botox injections for spasmodic dysphonia.

○ Explain how acoustic and visual instrumentation can serve as outcomes measures for benign and cancerous lesions of the vocal folds.

○ Explain the usefulness of acoustic and electroglottographic data in the clinical management of individuals with hearing impairment.

○ Appreciate the advantages of acoustic instrumentation in the evaluation and treatment of voice in transsexual individuals.

In addition to acoustic measures of phonatory function, techniques to visualize the larynx have become valuable tools in the assessment and treatment of vocal fold function and laryngeal pathologies. The chapter begins with a discussion of indirect and direct laryngeal visualization techniques, including electroglottography, endoscopy and videostroboscopy, high-speed digital imaging, and videokymography. Attention is then focused on how acoustic and visual instrumental measures have been used to investigate the effects of aging on voice. This is followed by presentation of several communication disorders that are often characterized by impaired laryngeal structure and/or function including neurological disorders, hearing impairment, laryngeal cancer, benign tumors of the vocal folds/muscle tension dysphonia/GERD/LPR, and transsexual speech. Acoustic, electroglottographic, and endoscopic parameters that have been used to evaluate and treat individuals with the disorder will be presented.

Electroglottography

Electroglottography (EGG), also sometimes called **laryngography**, has become a popular tool for evaluating vocal fold function noninvasively. Originally developed in the 1950s and refined in the 1970s by Adrian Fourcin in Britain, EGG works on the principles of conduction of electricity. Human tissues are good conductors of electricity, whereas air is a poor conductor. The EGG was developed to take advantage of this difference in conductivity between tissue and air. A high-frequency signal of very low current is generated and passed through two surface electrodes held in place with a Velcro band at either side of the person's thyroid cartilage. The individual feels nothing, and the procedure is completely safe. Because tissue conducts electricity well, when the vocal folds are closed, the resistance is low and the current passes easily from one electrode to the other. However, when the vocal folds are open, there is a relatively large body of air between them, creating more resistance to the flow of current from one electrode to the other. The changing of resistance as the glottis opens and closes is displayed on a screen as a waveform, with time along the horizontal axis and amplitude of electrical voltage along the vertical axis. The waveform is called the **Lx wave**; it reflects the surface area of contact of the vocal folds (Figure 6.1). As the vocal folds close during vibration, the resistance to the electrical current decreases and the amplitude of the waveform increases. As the vocal folds separate during vibration, the resistance to the electrical current increases and the amplitude of the waveform decreases. Thus, the Lx waveform produces a record of vocal fold vibration during phonation. For voiceless sounds, there is no Lx waveform, because voiceless sounds are not produced with vocal fold vibration.

The Lx waveform looks similar to acoustic waveforms, but what is being measured is very different. An acoustic waveform represents increases and decreases in air pressure. The Lx waveform shows increases and decreases of electrical activity, which corresponds to the opening and closing of the glottis. The Lx waveform reflects the duty cycle of vocal fold vibration. Recall from Chapter 5 that *duty cycle* refers to the phases of a vocal fold vibratory cycle, including the interval during which the vocal folds begin to close, the interval during which they are maximally closed, the interval during which they begin to open, and the interval during which they are maximally open. Baken (1992) provided a detailed interpretation of points along the Lx waveform and how they correspond to vocal fold vibration. See Figure 6.1. At point **a**, the inferior margins of the vocal folds make their initial contact, signaling the start of the closing phase. Between points **a** and **b**, the lower margins continue to close. At point **b**, the superior margins of the folds make initial contact. Between points **b** and **c**, the superior margins continue to close. At point **c**, maximal contact between the vocal folds is achieved, signaling the end of the closing phase and the beginning of the closed phase. The interval between points **c** and **d** reflects the closed phase of the cycle. At point **d**, the inferior margins of the vocal folds begin to separate, initiating the opening phase. The inferior margins continue to separate between points **d** and **e**. At point **e**, the separation of the inferior margins is complete, and the superior edges begin to open. This point, with its abrupt change in slope, is referred to as a *knee* in the opening phase. During the

Figure 6.1 Lx wave

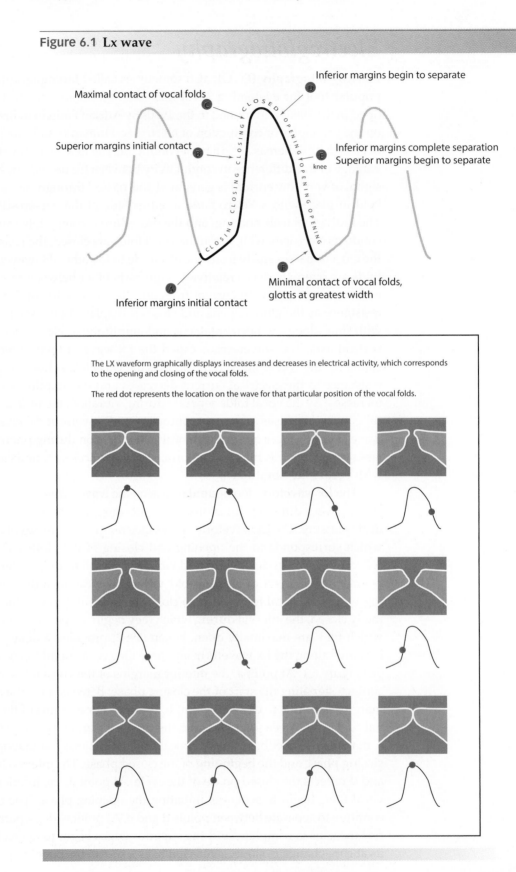

interval between points **e** and **f**, the superior margins of the vocal folds continue to open. At point **f**, contact between the vocal folds reaches its minimum, and during the interval between points **f** and **a**, the width of the glottis is at its greatest. The cycle then begins again.

It is important to keep in mind that the EGG represents relative rather than absolute contact area. The maximum peak on the Lx waveform does not necessarily mean that there is complete glottal closure. It is possible during vocal fold vibration for complete glottal closure to not occur at all. The vocal folds may be as much as 3 mm apart and vibration will still occur. In falsetto register, for example, the glottis may not completely close during vibration. Just by looking at the Lx waveform, one would not be able to tell whether complete closure was occurring. It is also not possible to specify the precise time at which glottal opening or closing is initially achieved.

By counting the peaks in a specific interval of time in the Lx waveform, it is possible to determine the speaker's F_0 very precisely. A greater number of cycles per second can indicate that the person is using falsetto. A reduced number of cycles per second can indicate pulse register. Also, by evaluating the shape of the waveform, one can make judgments about the way in which the vocal folds are opening and closing. A longer-than-normal separation time between the folds may indicate breathiness resulting from a greater volume of air passing through the glottis. A longer-than-normal closed time may indicate a hyperfunctional, pressed quality resulting from excessive medial compression. An even, regular pattern of the cycles in the waveform reflects periodic opening and closing of the folds, whereas an irregular pattern shows less periodic vibration, which may sound perceptually like hoarseness. Sample Lx waves are illustrated in Figure 6.2.

EGG and Register

Because the Lx signal matches the vocal F_0, it is easy to assess register with the EGG. Each register is associated with a characteristic Lx wave. Modal register is characterized by the description of the phases described previously. Note that the closing phase in modal register has a steeper slope than the opening phase. This reflects the fact that vocal fold closing is quick and abrupt, whereas vocal fold opening is slower and more gradual. The difference occurs because with the vocal folds closed P_s has to build up to the point at which it is stronger than medial compression, a relatively gradual process. On the other hand, once the vocal folds are open, their elastic recoil and the increasing P_{neg} between them act very quickly to close the folds.

Lx waveforms of pulse register often show more than one peak per cycle, reflecting the biphasic or multiphasic closure pattern (Blomgren, Chen, Ng, & Gilbert, 1997). The opening phase of vibration in pulse register may have one, two, or three minor openings and closings before the vocal folds close completely. EGG has demonstrated that the multiphasic pattern occurs more frequently in male speakers than in female speakers (Chen, Robb, & Gilbert, 2002). Pulse is characterized by a wave that has sharp, short pulses followed by a long closed glottal interval (Childers, 1991). Also, as one would expect, there are fewer cycles per second in pulse than in modal register.

Figure 6.2 Sample Lx waves

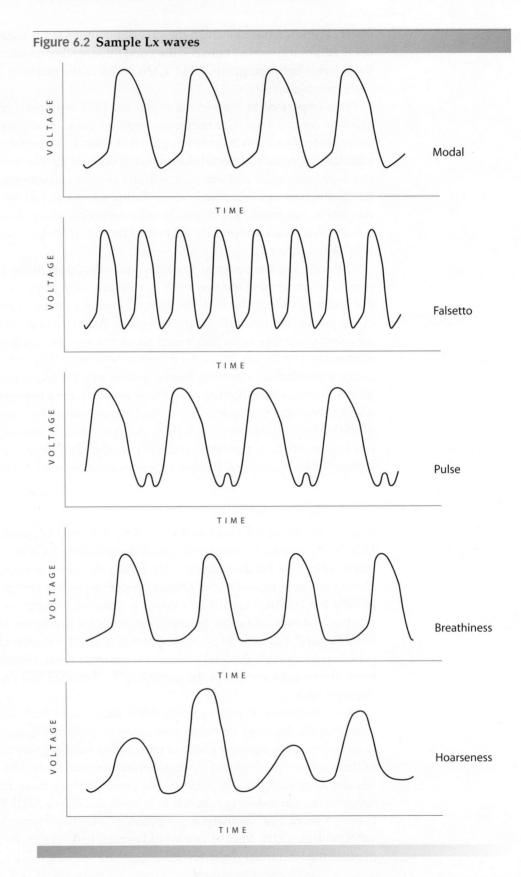

In falsetto, the number of Lx cycles is greatly increased. The waveform looks more nearly sinusoidal (almost like a pure tone), reflecting the extreme longitudinal tension and possible incomplete closure of the folds during vibration (Childers, 1991; Salomão & Sundberg, 2009). Because of incomplete closure, the waveform does not show the less steep gradual opening and the steeper closing pattern typical of modal register. This shape typically indicates that the closed phase is absent, with the motion of the vocal folds remaining periodic but alternating between a more open glottis and a less open glottis (Nair, 1999).

EGG Slope Quotients

Other ways of utilizing the EGG waveform have been developed that are quantitative in nature and do not rely on visual inspection and subjective interpretation. These measures are based on the duty cycle and the various proportions of time that each phase takes to complete. EGG slope quotients are indications of vocal fold behavior during vocal fold contact (Fisher, Scherer, Guo, & Owen, 1996). EGG slope quotients have been obtained from normal voices and have also been applied to various disorders. In this kind of analysis, phases of the duty cycle are measured in terms of their durations, and quotients are obtained by dividing certain durations into other durations (Table 6.1). Many of the EGG quotients have been validated using high-speed digital imaging (e.g., Bhandari, Izdebski, Huang, & Yan, 2011).

The **closed quotient (CQ)** (also called **contact quotient**) compares the duration of the closed phase to the time of the entire vibratory cycle. Because it reflects the proportion of time that the vocal folds are in contact with each other, it is related to the degree of medial compression being exerted. CQs in modal register typically range from around 0.25 to 0.65 (e.g., Nair, 1999; Salomão & Sundberg, 2009). A higher CQ indicates a longer duration of closure, and a lower CQ reflects shorter closure duration. For example, a CQ of 0.67 indicates a longer closed phase than one of 0.52. A louder voice shows a higher CQ than a softer one, and a pressed or tense voice

Table 6.1 EGG Quotients Derived from the Duty Cycle

Quotient	Measure
Closed quotient/contact quotient (CQ)	Duration of closed phase divided by time of entire vibratory cycle
Open quotient (OQ)	Duration of opening of glottis in relation to entire cycle
Contact index (CI)	Ratio of difference in time between closing and opening phases divided by duration of closed phase
Closed-to-open ratio (C/O ratio)	Relative durations of closed and open phases of duty cycle
Speed quotient (SQ)	Ratio of opening-phase duration to closing-phase duration

generates a higher CQ than a soft or breathy voice. Thus, this measure may provide an objective measure of vocal hyperfunction or hypofunction (Orlikoff, 1991).

CQ has been used to evaluate the use of falsetto register in male speakers and singers. Salomão and Sundberg (2009) reported CQ values for males in falsetto register from 0.13 to 0.43. They noted that, on average, CQ in falsetto was about half of the modal value. Herbst and Ternström (2006) obtained higher CQs, between 0.35 and 0.60, for males singing in falsetto register.

The **open quotient (OQ)** reflects the duration of the opening of the glottis in relation to the entire cycle (Bhandari et al., 2011; Echternach et al., 2010; Roubeau, Henrich, & Castellengo, 2009). The OQ has been used to investigate changes in vocal fold vibratory patterns as male speakers change registers from modal to falsetto. Echternach et al. (2010) reported that in more than half of the speakers in their study modal register was associated with a lower OQ, and OQ increased continuously from modal register, through the transition between registers, and into falsetto. The transition between registers has been reported to be accompanied by a large increase in the OQ, even if the transition is not perceptually audible (Bhandari et al., 2012).

The **contact index (CI)** is based on the ratio of the difference in time between the closing and opening phases divided by the duration of the closed phase. The CI measure is sensitive to the mucosal wave of the vocal fold cover, so it can provide information about the way in which the vocal folds are vibrating in a particular register. A similar measure is the **closed-to-open ratio (C/O ratio)**, which gives information about the relative durations of the closed and open phases of the duty cycle. From this information about how long the glottis is closed compared to how long it is open, the degree of hyper- or hypofunction of a person's voice can be determined. A longer closed phase results in a higher C/O ratio, whereas a lower C/O ratio indicates a shorter closed phase.

The **speed quotient (SQ)** is defined as the ratio of opening-phase duration to closing-phase duration, where the closing phase is the interval between the lowest and highest amplitude values on the Lx waveform and the opening phase is the interval between the highest and lowest amplitude values. An SQ of 1.0 indicates equal opening and closing phases; an SQ greater than 1.0 reflects a longer opening phase and shorter closing phase; and an SQ less than 1.0 occurs when the closing phase is longer than the opening phase (Chen, Robb, & Gilbert, 2002). Modal register is typically characterized by SQ greater than 1.0. Examples of EGG quotients are shown in Figure 6.3.

EGG technology is also used to calculate acoustic information, including F_0, jitter, shimmer, and HNR. Because EGG measures vocal fold contact, it is not subject to the same types of problems seen in acoustic programs and provides a more robust indication of the amount of noise in a voice.

Endoscopy and Videostroboscopy

Endoscopic procedures use either a flexible or rigid endoscope that is inserted into the patient's pharynx to illuminate the larynx. The procedure may be done either via the patient's nose or mouth. When done via the nose, a very thin, flexible tube

Figure 6.3 EGG slope quotients

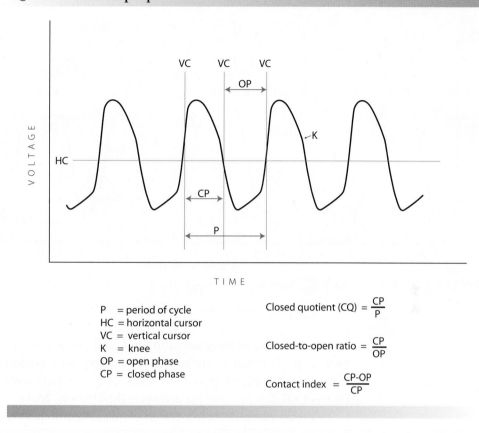

P   = period of cycle
HC = horizontal cursor
VC = vertical cursor
K   = knee
OP = open phase
CP = closed phase

Closed quotient (CQ) $= \dfrac{CP}{P}$

Closed-to-open ratio $= \dfrac{CP}{OP}$

Contact index $= \dfrac{CP-OP}{CP}$

is inserted through the nostril into the pharynx. When done via the oral cavity, a rigid scope is used. Either way, the image is typically projected onto a video monitor, using a magnifying scope and video camera. Laryngeal endoscopy has many advantages. First, the patient is awake, so the risks inherent in general anesthesia are avoided. Second, the procedure allows detailed examination of the structure and function of the larynx. Use of the rigid scope does not permit examination of phonatory function during connected speech as the patient is restricted to phonation of the /i/ vowel. However, the procedure yields a high quality image of the larynx. Vocal fold changes at different pitch levels are also well visualized.

Endoscopy may be used in conjunction with videostroboscopy. Stroboscopy works by shining a light source onto a moving object and periodically interrupting the light source. The observer views only the phase of movement exposed by the light, and any movement that occurs between the flashes of light is not seen (Case, 2002). This generates what is essentially an optical illusion, allowing an observer to view moving objects as though they are stationary or in slow motion (Manfredi, Bocchi, Cantarella, & Peretti, 2011). In laryngeal stroboscopy, the light source is directed through the endoscope to illuminate the larynx. The instrument has two modes based on the timing of the interruptions to the light source. In walking mode (also called running, or traveling, mode) the rate of strobe light illumination is timed to be approximately 2 Hz different from the patient's F_0 (Poburka, 1999).

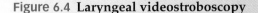

Figure 6.4 Laryngeal videostroboscopy

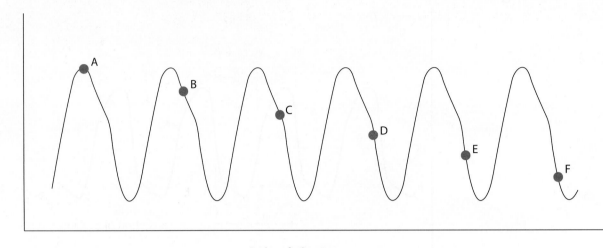

Cycles of vibration

The vocal folds are therefore illuminated at consecutive points over many vibratory cycles (Figure 6.4). The resulting apparent slow motion view of the vocal folds is made up of snapshots of a sequence of cycles, with each snapshot having been taken at a different stage in each cycle (Mathieson, 2001).

Viewers perceive an integrated image rather than a series of disjointed movements because according to Talbot's law, the human eye can only perceive a maximum of five images per second (Kaszuba & Garrett, 2007). Stimuli that are presented faster appear as a single ongoing image because the viewer automatically fills in the missing pieces (Kaszuba & Garrett, 2007). This is similar to what happens when a fan is set into motion. As the fan begins to spin, one sees the blades rotating individually. However, as the fan speeds up, the viewer is no longer able to perceive the blades separately but perceives instead what looks like one blade spinning extremely rapidly. Similarly, when the strobe light illuminates the larynx at a much faster rate than five images per second, the perception of continuous motion of vocal fold vibration is generated. In stopped or locked mode, the light is exactly timed to the individual's F_0, so flashes occur at the same point in each successive cycle. In this mode, the vocal folds appear to be stationary as long as the vibration is regular and periodic (Deliyski, 2007; Hapner & Johns, 2007; Poburka, 1999; Walker & Messing, 2006). Many aspects of vocal fold structure and function can be evaluated via laryngostroboscopy. See Table 6.2.

These parameters may be condensed into a smaller number that is more convenient for examiners to evaluate. Kelley, Colton, Jasper, Paseman, and Brewer (2011) analyzed stroboscopic evaluations from patients with benign lesions of the vocal folds, vocal fold paralysis, functional disorders, and postoperative vocal pathologies. They reported that 11 stroboscopic parameters could be represented by two factors (vocal fold vibration and vocal fold edge), and these factors could be accurately estimated by rating only the amplitude, vibratory behavior, and

Table 6.2 **Laryngeal Parameters Visualized with Laryngostroboscopy**

Parameter	Description
Vocal fold edge	Smoothness of the medial margins of the vocal folds
Glottic closure	Degree and pattern of closing during a cycle of vibration
Extent of opening	Degree of glottal opening when the vocal folds are maximally abducted
Phase closure	Equivalence of open and closed phases
Presence/extent of mucosal wave	Inferior to superior and lateral spread of the margins of the folds
Nonvibrating portion	Lack of vibration of any portion of the vocal fold(s)
Amplitude of vibration	Extent of lateral excursion of the vocal folds
Phase symmetry	Degree to which both folds reach midline and maximum abduction at the same time
Periodicity/regularity	Degree of similarity of successive cycles of vibration
Supraglottic activity	Degree of medial compression or anterior–posterior compression of the false vocal folds
Vertical approximation	Degree to which both folds are on the same vertical plane

edge of the vocal folds. These two factors also differentiated between the four categories of vocal fold pathology and related to the severity of the dysphonia as rated by clinicians.

A disadvantage of stroboscopy is that irregular vocal fold vibration cannot be visualized accurately because the technology relies on periodic vocal fold vibration. Furthermore, interpretation of stroboscopic images is subjective, and rating scales are not standardized (Krausert et al., 2011). Videostroboscopy cannot visualize the inferior margins of the vocal folds, but when used simultaneously with EGG, the onset of vocal fold separation along the inferior surface of the vocal folds can be detected (Krausert et al., 2011).

High-Speed Digital Imaging

Recently, high-speed digital imaging (HSDI) has become a viable option for visualizing the structure and function of the larynx. High-speed equipment can record with sampling rates of 2000 to 5000 frames per second (fps), allowing each individual cycle of vocal fold vibration to be recorded and analyzed (Krausert et al., 2011; Mortensen & Woo, 2008). This overcomes the problem of videostroboscopy, which has a maximum recording rate of 30 fps and cannot capture individual cycles of

Table 6.3 Parameters of Vocal Fold Vibration Examined via High-Speed Digital Imaging

Parameter	Description
Kinematic oscillatory breaks	Complete cessation of vocal fold movement during continuous voicing tasks
Micromotion events	Severe deviation from the cyclic pattern resulting in near, but not complete, cessation of phonatory motion always resulting in abrupt, minute, aperiodic abductory motions of a section of the vocal fold edge compared to the entire mass of the folds
Motion irregularities	Segments consisting of nonrepetitive vibratory cycles
Glottal configuration	No closure, incomplete closure, spindle-shaped closure, posterior gap, anterior gap, complete closure, complete closure with false vocal fold contact, level of vocal folds, length of vocal folds, vocal fold edge, cover characteristics

SOURCE: Information from Patel et al. (2011).

vibration (Patel, Dailey, & Bless, 2008). HSDI also overcomes another limitation of videostroboscopy because it does not depend on a periodic or nearly periodic vibratory pattern for accurate measurement (Deliyski & Hillman, 2010).

The instrumentation allows the recorded glottal cycles to be slowed down and analyzed. Because HSDI is independent of the individual's F_0, it allows for detailed evaluation of vocal fold vibratory patterns in patients who demonstrate voice breaks, diplophonia (perception of a double pitch), and severe dysphonia and is therefore more effective in diagnosing pathological vocal fold vibration (Krausert et al., 2011; Mortensen & Woo, 2008; Patel, Dailey, et al., 2008). High-speed imaging is useful for capturing aspects of vibration such as differences between the left and right vocal folds in terms of phase (i.e., open and closed phases), amplitude, and overall left–right symmetry, as well as glottal closure types and presence and extent of the mucosal wave (e.g., Inwald, Döllinger, Schuster, Eysholdt, & Bohr, 2011; Mehta, Deliyski, Quatieri, & Hillman, 2011). Table 6.3 identifies and defines parameters of vocal fold vibration captured by HSDI. However, HSDI is not widely available, and even when it is, this technology should be viewed as a supplement to stroboscopy and not as a replacement (Patel, Dailey, et al., 2008).

Patel, Dailey, and Bless (2008) compared HSDI and videostroboscopic images of subjects with a variety of voice impairments. The majority of subjects had moderate to severe dysphonia reflected in highly aperiodic vocal fold vibration. Because stroboscopy depends on a relatively periodic signal, vibratory features could not be identified in 62 percent of the dysphonic speakers using stroboscopy alone. However, for speakers with mild voice problems the authors noted that stroboscopy has many advantages compared to HSDI: It is less costly; color images are possible; it has superior spatial resolution; is able to record longer voice samples with both rigid and flexible endoscopes; data reduction and playback are less cumbersome and data storage is more practical for everyday clinical use; and with the recent introduction of distal chip technology, superior images can be obtained using flexible nasoendoscopy. The advantages of HSDI are that this instrumentation allows observers to make judgments of vibratory patterns regardless of the severity of the voice disorder, which is important for patients with moderate or severe hoarseness and patients with neuromuscular conditions.

Videokymography

Videokymography (VKG) is a technique of visualizing the movement characteristics of the vocal folds using a modified video camera and endoscope. The camera can be used at standard rates or at a high-speed rate of almost 8000 images per second (e.g., Manfredi, Bocchi, et al., 2011). One single horizontal line is selected from the entire video image of the vocal folds prior to examination and marked on the screen (Manfredi, Bocchi, Bianchi, Migali, & Cantarella, 2006; Verdonck-de Leeuw, Festen, & Mahieu, 2001). The VKG essentially "zooms in" on this line. During vibration, the movement at the specified location is shown as a series of vertical images over time (Figure 6.5). When used at the high speed, very fine details of the medial and lateral movements of the vocal folds during vibration are captured (Tigges, Wittenberg, Mergell, & Eysholdt, 1999). Unlike videostroboscopy, which

Figure 6.5 Videokymography

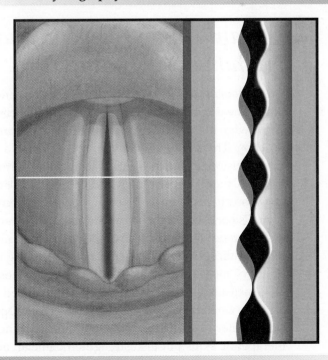

provides a reconstructed moving image of the vocal folds, VKG provides the actual motion. Thus, even highly aperiodic vocal fold vibration can be accurately imaged (Baken & Orlikoff, 2000).

Švec, Šram, and Schutte (2007) used VKG to analyze the vibratory patterns in normal and vocally disordered speakers. They described 10 aspects of vibration that were apparent from the analysis. Aspects included partial or complete absence of vocal fold vibration; interference with vibration of surroundings (e.g., false vocal folds or fluids); cycle variability; closure duration (e.g., absent, short, long); left–right asymmetry (e.g., amplitude differences, frequency differences, phase differences); decreased sharpness of lateral peaks (reflects vertical phase difference); reduced or absent mucosal wave; opening versus closing duration; medial peaks (increased sharpness); and cycle aberrations of any type. The authors noted that some of these features can be derived from stroboscopy. However, VKG also reveals details of vocal fold patterns that cannot be assessed through stroboscopy, such as slight variations in mucosal waves, opening versus closing duration, and cycle aberrations. This kind of information can supplement that obtained via traditional videostroboscopy.

The digital version of VKG (digital kymography [DKM]) is extracted from high-speed videoendoscopy (Manfredi, Bocchi, et al., 2011). DKM can measure multiple "slices" of the vocal folds during vibration rather than just one slice. This allows evaluation of features of vocal fold vibration at different points along the glottis and can therefore assess vibration in an anterior–posterior direction (Krausert et al., 2011). It has been shown that kymographic images correspond to acoustic and perceptual voice quality problems (e.g., Verdonck-de Leeuw et al., 2001).

Advantages of Acoustic and Visual Analysis of Phonatory Function

An understanding of the phonatory system and the acoustic and visual methods of measuring laryngeal structure and function allows clinicians to apply this knowledge in the diagnosis and treatment of numerous problems related to vocal function. There are many advantages to using acoustic and visual information in the provision of clinical services to speakers with voice disorders (Table 6.4).

Analyzing a speaker's vocal output to estimate the condition of his or her vocal mechanism is particularly attractive because information about an individual's condition may be carried in vocal parameters such as F_0, intensity, jitter, and shimmer (Doherty & Shipp, 1988). These measures offer a starting point for rehabilitation and provide a means of assessing the patient's progress. With more objective measures of voice quality, such as those provided by acoustic analysis, EGG measures, videoendoscopy, and high-speed digital imaging, evaluation of the problem can be more precise so that the most appropriate treatment for the patient can be determined. Measures of vocal function not only supplement the clinician's therapeutic skills but also strengthen clinician accountability. Increasingly, third-party payers such as insurance companies and HMOs will only pay for benefits if

Table 6.4 Clinical Advantages of Acoustic and Visual Measures of Phonatory Function

Provide a starting point for rehabilitation and a means of assessing the patient's progress
Strengthen clinician accountability
Can be used as feedback during therapy, as well as serve as outcomes measures to determine the effectiveness of intervention strategies
Can help to detect early changes in speech and voice that cannot be perceived by ear
Can be used to screen speakers for the potential presence of voice disorders
Help to validate a clinician's perceptual judgments of disordered voice and speech by providing norms that can serve as a basis of comparison between vocally healthy and vocally disordered speakers

it can be shown that the treatment is effective. Instrumental measures are invaluable in providing objective documentation of the patient's progress. In addition, information from acoustic and visual analyses can be used as feedback during therapy, as well as serve as outcomes measures to determine the effectiveness of intervention strategies. Instrumental analysis can help to detect early changes in speech and voice that cannot be perceived by ear (Silbergleit, Johnson, & Jacobsen, 1997). Such measures can also be helpful in screening speakers for the potential presence of voice disorders. For example, Jotz, Cervantes, Abrahão, Settanni, and de Angelis (2002) screened a large number of young boys with no reported voice disorders and reported that a high proportion of these boys exhibited some degree of dysphonia. Noise-to-harmonics ratio (NHR) was significantly higher in these speakers, and subsequent flexible laryngoscopy for the boys who failed the screening demonstrated that many of them had either vocal nodules or cysts. Finally, acoustic and visual measures are vital to validate a clinician's perceptual judgments of disordered voice and speech by providing norms that can serve as a basis of comparison between vocally healthy and vocally disordered speakers. Several well-controlled studies demonstrate the link between acoustic measures and the status of a speaker's vocal health. Werth, Voigt, Döllinger, Eysholdt, and Lohscheller (2010) conducted an extensive acoustic evaluation of recorded voices from speakers with a variety of voice disorders and from vocally healthy speakers. They reported that for both males and females, the median values of jitter, shimmer, and normalized noise energy (NNE) were consistently increased for the pathological voices, and HNR was decreased. Carding et al. (2004) examined jitter, shimmer, and NHR in individuals with voice pathologies before and after treatment, in individuals with voice pathologies with no intervention, and in individuals with healthy voices. Intervention resulted in improvements in all three measures. Jitter discriminated between speakers who had received treatment and those with a normal voice. Both groups of subjects with abnormal voices demonstrated significantly higher mean shimmer scores than healthy voices. Individuals with dysphonia who had not undergone voice therapy obtained a lower mean NHR than in the other two groups.

Laryngeal Aging

The voice changes dramatically over the lifespan, from the high-pitched crying of the infant to the thin, quavery voice often associated with the very old. These changes occur as the structures of the respiratory and laryngeal systems develop, mature, and decline, in conjunction with changes in neuromotor control of respiration and phonation. Other factors, such as an individual's overall health, the type and amount of voice use, smoking, consumption of alcohol, presence of gastric reflux, and the individual's psychological state, can also profoundly influence the voice over the course of time.

Acoustic Changes over the Lifespan

Newborns and infants, with their tiny vocal folds, have an average F_0 ranging from 400 to 600 Hz (e.g., Hirschberg, 1999; Michelsson & Michelsson, 1999; Robb et al., 2007). In the childhood years, the larynx and vocal folds start to increase in size. The vocal folds lengthen, and differentiation of the layers of the lamina propria begins. The primary acoustic manifestation of these changes is a drop in F_0 from the infant level to around 230 to 250 Hz by the preteen years. Refer to Table 5.6.

Puberty is a time of enormous growth and change, affecting many bodily systems, including the larynx. Growth is regulated by the male and female sex hormones, which can be classified as androgens (male) or estrogens (female). These classes of hormones are present in both males and females, although in different proportions. Greater levels of androgens (testosterone) are found in males, and greater levels of estrogen are present in females. While laryngeal growth occurs in both sexes, it is particularly pronounced in males due to the release of androgens (Gugatschka et al., 2010; Puts, Hodges, Cardenas, & Gaulin, 2007; Raj, Gupta, Chowdhury, & Chadha, 2010). Growth of the laryngeal cartilages contributes to the overall enlargement of the larynx, with male larynges increasing two to three times more than their female counterparts in both anteroposterior dimensions and weight (Kahane, 1982). The vocal folds also grow in length, with a reported average increase of 11.57 mm in males and 4.16 mm in females (Kahane, 1982). This translates into an increase of 63 percent for males and 34 percent for females (Kahane, 1982). In general, the male's F_0 decreases steadily throughout this period. For males, the decrease in F_0 corresponds to a pitch drop of around one octave, while the F_0 decrease for females corresponds to a pitch drop of around 2.5 semitones.

All laryngeal structures (cartilages, joints, soft tissues, muscles) start to show evidence of degenerative changes by the third or fourth decade of life. These structural changes can result in changes in the function of the vocal mechanism, including less precise control of frequency and amplitude. The term **presbylaryngis** is sometimes used to characterize the aging of the laryngeal mechanism. **Presbyphonia** refers to the vocal changes resulting from the aging process. Presbyphonic changes have been found to be relatively common in groups of healthy elderly individuals and can adversely impact the person's quality of life (e.g., Golub, Chen, Otto, Hapner, & Johns, 2006; Turley & Cohen, 2009). Commonly reported vocal effects include bowing of the vocal folds resulting from atrophy of the thyroarytenoid muscle, incomplete glottal closure during phonation, and resulting breathiness and hoarseness (Tanner, Sauder, Thibeault, Dromey, & Smith, 2010). Both genetic and environmental factors probably influence the aging process (Tanner et al., 2010).

One acoustic effect that is often reported in elderly speakers is a change in F_0 (Table 6.5 and refer to Table 5.6). Some researchers have reported an increase in F_0 in elderly men (Harnsberger, Shrivastav, Brown, Rothman, & Hollien, 2008; Linville, 2004; Xue & Deliyski, 2001), while female F_0 tends to decrease with age by around 10 to 35 Hz (Brown et al., 1991; Ferrand, 2002; Higgins & Saxman, 1991; Linville & Fisher, 1985; Teles-Magalhaes et al., 2000). F_0s in older women range from approximately 160 to 186 Hz, compared to the range in young women of approximately 191 to 224 Hz. The lowering may be accounted for, in part, by postmenopausal edema, which increases vocal fold mass, decreases the rate of vibration, and changes the contour and shape of the vocal folds (e.g., Biever & Bless, 1989; Pontes, Brasolotto, & Behlau, 2005; Reubold, Harrington, & Kleber, 2010).

Physiological health is an extremely important variable in aging of the voice. Many researchers have shown that elderly individuals in good health tend to have younger-sounding voices than younger individuals in poor health. Orlikoff (1990) highlighted this important point by comparing jitter values between young healthy men, older healthy men, and older men with hypertension (high blood pressure). While the values for all three groups fell within normal limits, the elderly subjects with hypertension fell much closer to the upper limits, while the young subjects' values fell closer to the lower limits. The elderly healthy subjects' values fell in between the lower and upper limits. Prakup (2011) examined jitter in elderly singers and nonsingers. Singers reportedly demonstrated less jitter than nonsingers. Further, naïve listeners perceived male and female singers as being significantly younger than nonsingers, and perceived age was positively correlated with degree of jitter in the voice. HNR measures have also demonstrated acoustically that laryngeal function changes with aging. Ferrand (2002) compared three age groups of normally speaking women: young adults, middle-aged adults, and elderly adults. The young and middle-aged women obtained similar HNRs, but the elderly women's HNRs were significantly lower than the other two groups. Other studies have corroborated that elderly speakers' voices demonstrate greater vocal fold instability and increased noise levels (Gotham-Rowan & Laures-Gore, 2006; Harnsberger, Brown, Shrivastav, & Rothman, 2010).

EGG quotient data have demonstrated less complete vocal fold closure in elderly men than in younger men (Higgins & Saxman, 1991). This is consistent with physiological evidence of laryngeal degeneration in aging men, including degeneration of the vocal ligament and mucosa, ossification of the laryngeal cartilages, and bowing of the vocal folds due to muscle atrophy. By contrast, the elderly women in Higgins and Saxman's (1991) study did not show a lack of complete glottal closure. This too is consistent with laryngeal physiology. It has been well established that laryngeal degeneration in women starts later and is less extensive than that of men. Using EGG, Ma and Love (2010) examined F_0 and contact quotient in younger and older women and men. Consistent with other acoustic data, older women obtained a lower average F_0 than younger women; older men obtained a slightly higher average F_0 than younger men. Older males exhibited a significantly smaller contact quotient than younger males, reflecting less complete

Table 6.5 Selected F_0 Values (in Hz) for Young, Middle-Aged, and Older Adults Reported in the Literature

Ma & Love (2010)			
	Young men	**Middle-aged men**	**Older men**
/a/	120.95		123.50
Phrase	108.03		110.00
Reading	114.26		114.63

	Young women	**Middle-aged women**	**Older women**
/a/	224.05		186.05
Phrase	191.41		160.15
Reading	196.97		171.39

D'haeseleer et al. (2011)			
	Young women	**Middle-aged women**	**Older women**
/a/	202.00	190.00	
Speech	200.00	184.00	

Schneider & Bigenzahn (2003)			
	Young women	**Middle-aged women**	**Older women**
Speech	217.00		

Ferrand (2002)			
	Young women	**Middle-aged women**	**Older women**
/a/	209.68	204.49	175.23

Xue & Deliyski (2001)			
	Young women	**Middle-aged women**	**Older women**
/a/	243.97		187.70

	Young men	**Middle-aged men**	**Older men**
	145.22		127.62

vocal fold contact during vibration. However, older women showed a greater contact quotient (i.e., increased vocal fold contact) than younger women. The decrease in vocal fold contact in older men likely results from atrophy of the vocal folds due to aging. The increased glottal contact for older women may be due to the presence of increased edema.

Laryngeal stroboscopy has also been used to evaluate vocal function in elderly speakers and has indicated vocal fold bowing and incomplete closure in many individuals, as well as the presence of acid reflux, muscle tension dysphonia, vocal fold masses, edema, and vocal fold paresis (Gregory, Chandran, Lurie, & Sataloff, 2011; Pontes et al., 2005; Takano et al., 2010). Taken together, these findings from acoustic, EGG, and endoscopic measures demonstrate the importance of accounting for the variable of age when assessing and treating vocal pathology. Otherwise, the effects of normal aging on laryngeal behaviors could be mistaken for those of laryngeal pathology.

Neurological Disorders

Patients with neurological disorders that affect phonation are very commonly treated in hospitals, clinics, private practices, nursing homes, preschools, and elementary and secondary schools. A wealth of acoustic and visual information has been obtained from individuals with a wide variety of neurological disorders including amyotrophic lateral sclerosis, Parkinson's disease, unilateral vocal fold paralysis, spasmodic dysphonia, and paradoxical vocal fold motion.

Amyotrophic Lateral Sclerosis

Amyotrophic lateral sclerosis (ALS) is a progressive neurological disease in which all the motor functions of the body deteriorate. The degeneration is due to damage to the motor nerves that supply the voluntary muscles of the body, including those involved in speech production. Speakers with ALS demonstrate a variety of acoustic changes including increased levels of jitter, smaller maximum phonational frequency ranges, abnormal F_0 levels, and reduced ranges of frequency during connected speech (Silbergleit et al., 1997; Strand, Buder, Yorkston, & Olson Ramig, 1994). Some of these changes may be detected acoustically even when the speakers perceptually sound normal. Acoustic analysis may therefore provide a means by which early oral–facial and laryngeal signs of the disease can be detected. Knowing that neuromuscular weakness is present despite the normal-sounding voice, clinicians can offer intervention at early stages of the disease in order to maintain the patient's vocal function for as long as possible. Acoustic analysis has also indicated that the vocal characteristics of patients with ALS are not uniform but vary greatly from individual to individual. While changes in F_0 seem to be present consistently in patients with ALS, some speakers have lower-than-normal F_0 levels, while others demonstrate higher-than-normal F_0 levels. In addition, some but not all individuals with ALS exhibit a reduced range of F_0 during connected speech. This type of information is critical in planning effective therapy tailored to each individual's particular voice and speech deficits.

Parkinson's Disease

The underlying pathophysiology in Parkinson's disease (PD) is the reduction in the neurotransmitter **dopamine**. The depletion of dopamine results in the characteristic signs and symptoms of PD, including muscle rigidity, **bradykinesia** (difficulty and/or slowness in initiating movements), and tremor. Patients with PD often suffer from voice difficulties, including hoarseness, reduced loudness, and reductions in pitch range. In many cases, the voice difficulties are the first sign of PD (Logemann, Fisher, Boshes, & Blonsky, 1978). Acoustic characteristics that have been reported for individuals with PD include higher F_0, higher levels of jitter, lower intensity levels during connected speech, decreased frequency variability, and decreased dynamic range (Gamboa et al., 1997; Midi et al., 2008). The higher F_0 and decreased frequency variability may indicate increased laryngeal tension (Goberman & Blomgren, 2008; Harel, Cannizzaro, & Snyder, 2004). These acoustic data support the perceptual impressions of restricted pitch and loudness ranges, which are the common complaint of speakers with PD. Furthermore, these measures have the added advantage of quantifying the precise degree of loss of frequency and intensity ranges compared to normal.

Acoustic manifestations of loss of laryngeal control may be present years before the individual demonstrates clinical signs of the disease. Harel et al. (2004) analyzed F_0 variability in conversational speech in one speaker with PD and one healthy speaker. Speech samples were collected from more than five years before the speaker with PD was diagnosed, as well as several years following diagnosis and treatment with anti-Parkinson medications. The authors reported a decrease in F_0 variability starting several years prior to diagnosis and extending until the start of medical treatment. Once the speaker began taking the medication, the F_0 variability in conversational speech normalized. The authors suggested that acoustic analysis may be helpful to track the progression of the disease as well as the patient's response to treatment.

Acoustic measures have been used to evaluate the effectiveness of pharmacological and surgical treatments for PD. The most commonly used drug for PD is levodopa (L-dopa). L-dopa is converted into dopamine in the brain by means of "converter" cells, thus replacing the dopamine that is lacking. This reduces the primary problems of rigidity and tremor. However, acoustic measures of voice in patients with early-stage PD taking L-dopa show increased levels of jitter, shimmer, and NHR, indicating reductions in vocal stability despite the medication (Midi et al., 2008).

Surgical treatments for PD include **fetal cell transplantation (FCT)** and **deep brain stimulation (DBS)**. In FCT, suitable fetal cells are transplanted into the appropriate site in the patient's brain. The aim of this procedure is to replenish the missing dopamine and thus alleviate the symptoms. Baker, Ramig, Johnson, and Freed (1997) reported that, although FCT surgery was effective in improving overall motor performance of the patients studied, acoustic analysis failed to demonstrate improvements in the patients' phonation capacities. DBS involves insertion of implant wires into a specific brain area and implantation of a pulse generator in the patient's chest. When activated by the patient, the device transmits electrical impulses to the brain, which has the effect of reducing the rigidity and blocking the tremors (Benabid, 2003; Trépanier, Kumar, Lozano, Lang, & Saint-Cyr, 2000). However, acoustic analysis has demonstrated mixed results in terms of patients' voices. Some researchers have reported no improvements in voice (e.g., Valálik, Smehák, Bognár, & Csókay, 2011; Xie et al., 2010); others have reported reduced jitter and increased vocal stability (Mate, Cobeta, Jimenez-Jimenez, & Figueiras, 2011).

EGG has been used to compare different types of treatment for patients with PD. Reduction in vocal intensity is a common complaint of speakers with PD. Ramig and Dromey (1996) compared two treatments designed to increase vocal loudness. One treatment, the respiratory treatment (RT), was designed to increase the activity of the respiratory musculature to generate increased volumes and sub-glottal air pressure for speech. The other treatment, known as the Lee Silverman Voice Treatment (LSVT), targeted increased vocal intensity through improved vocal fold adduction. EGG analysis demonstrated that the patients who received LSVT increased their vocal fold adduction and corresponding loudness levels, whereas the group that received only RT showed no improvements in vocal fold adduction and loudness. This objective finding allowed the authors to suggest that treatment approaches that focus solely on respiration to increase loudness may be counterproductive in patients with PD.

The effectiveness of FCT in patients with PD has also been examined by means of EGG measures. Baker et al. (1997) obtained acoustic and EGG recordings for three consecutive days before surgery and some months postsurgery. The patients' limb movements did show notable improvements after surgery. However, the EGG measures did not differ much between before and after surgery. This was consistent with perceptual measures that indicated that listener ratings of speech presurgery were not remarkably different from ratings after FCT surgery.

Unilateral Vocal Fold Paresis/Paralysis

Paresis refers to a slight or partial paralysis, resulting in partial loss of muscle strength and movement. The intrinsic laryngeal muscles may be paretic if either the recurrent laryngeal nerve or superior laryngeal nerve is damaged. Although the vocal folds are able to move, their ability to adduct, abduct, or regulate their tension is reduced, particularly when the individual performs repetitive phona-tory tasks (Heman-Ackah & Batory, 2003; Rubin et al., 2005). The condition may be unilateral or bilateral. The degree of loss of mobility usually depends on the severity of the injury and can range from mild to severe. Diagnosing vocal fold paresis can be challenging because regular laryngoscopy may only show subtle vocal fold irregularities. Mortensen and Woo (2008) used high-speed digital im-aging in conjunction with kymography to confirm a diagnosis of unilateral vocal fold paresis. While endoscopic examination of the speaker's larynx was normal, HSDI and kymography showed that each vocal fold had separate and distinct vibratory patterns and each vibrated at slightly different frequencies. Because this pattern is often associated with paresis, the authors referred the individual for further testing. CT scanning of the chest and neck uncovered a mass on the patient's thymus gland (thymoma), which was affecting the nerve and causing the paresis. Following the removal of the thymoma, the speaker's vocal function normalized.

Unilateral vocal fold paralysis (UVFP) results from damage to the vagus nerve and its laryngeal branches (recurrent laryngeal nerve and superior laryngeal nerve). Paralysis of one vocal fold in the paramedian position results in breathiness and weak intensity levels. Individuals with UVFP have been reported to demonstrate increased levels of jitter, shimmer, and NHR (e.g., Inwald, Döllinger, Schuster, Eysholdt, & Bohr, 2011; Zhang, Jiang, Biazzo, & Jorgensen, 2005).

Many patients undergo surgical procedures to correct the glottal insufficiency, such as vocal fold injection, vocal fold **medialization thyroplasty**, and/or **arytenoid adduction**. Injection of a substance such as collagen or fat into the affected vocal fold increases its bulk and thereby facilitates more complete glottal closure during vibration. Medialization thyroplasty involves placing a synthetic implant behind the paralyzed vocal fold in order to push it closer to the midline and enhance glottal closure. Arytenoid adduction surgically rotates the arytenoid cartilage on the affected side to move the paralyzed vocal fold to a more medial position. Acoustic measures are widely used to evaluate the effects of these treatments, and outcomes reported by many researchers support the effectiveness of these surgical procedures. Outcomes include increased vocal stability and decreased noise in the voice, as indicated by decreases in F_0SD, jitter, shimmer, and NHR (Choi, Chung, Lim, & Kim, 2008; Hartl, Hans, Crevier-Buchman, Vaissière, & Brasnu, 2009; Little, Costello, & Harries, 2011).

EGG measures have also been used to analyze patterns of vocal fold vibration in speakers with UVFP. Choi et al. (2008) reported increases in patients' closed quotient following surgery, reflecting a decrease in the width of the glottal gap during vocal fold vibration. Zagólski and Carlson (2002) and Zagólski (2009) compared phases of vocal fold opening and closing between women with UVFP and healthy speakers. They reported that most of the women with UVFP showed a delay in achieving maximum vocal fold contact resulting in a prolonged closing phase, as well as a shorter opening phase and prolonged open phase. In some patients the vocal folds regained some motion after a period of time, and in these speakers the various phases of vibration showed more normal patterns.

Videostroboscopy is widely used to assess glottic closure before and after treatment of UVFP. In addition to visual inspection of vibratory parameters, researchers have reported several methods of analyzing open and closed quotients of the vibratory cycle during phonation by counting individual frames of stroboscopy recordings. Frame-by-frame analysis of vocal fold opening, open, closing, and closed phases can provide information regarding problems in vocal fold closure (glottic insufficiency). One such method involves calculating the proportion of frames in which the glottis is closed in relation to the total number of frames per glottic cycle. Vocally normal speakers have been shown to have 50 percent closed duration, whereas speakers with glottic insufficiency were shown to have closure durations of less than 40 percent (Carroll, Wu, McRay, & Gherson, 2011). Another way in which glottal closure can be evaluated with stroboscopy is by counting the number of pixels in specific video frames and dividing this number by the square of the average length of the right and left vocal folds. Kimura, Nito, Imagawa, Tayama, and Chan (2008) used this method in combination with perceptual and aerodynamic measures to evaluate patients' voices before and after vocal fold medialization surgery and/or vocal fold injection laryngoplasty. The authors reported that both techniques were successful in increasing relative glottal area, demonstrating more complete vocal fold closure following treatment.

Bielamowicz, Kapoor, Schwartz, and Stager (2004) reported a similar technique. These researchers measured glottal gap ratio by selecting one image of the vocal folds during the most closed portion of the glottal cycle and one from the most open phase of the glottal cycle. They obtained the ratio by dividing the average glottal area during the closed phase (in pixels) by the average glottal area during the open phase (in pixels). A smaller glottal gap yields a ratio close to 1 and vice versa. Individuals with vocal fold paralysis demonstrated a significantly larger glottal gap than individuals with healthy vocal folds.

Videokymography (VKG) has been used to examine fine details of vocal fold vibratory patterns in patients with UVFP. Kimura et al. (2010) used kymography plus acoustic analysis to compare patients' voices before and after arytenoid adduction surgery. Prior to surgery, jitter and shimmer measures were increased. VKG showed that the paralyzed vocal fold did not reach the midline, resulting in incomplete glottal closure for all participants. VKG also revealed different vibration frequencies in the left and right vocal folds. After surgery, VKG showed marked improvements in phonation, including reductions in the size of the glottal gap, improved glottal closure, and identical or nearly identical frequencies in the left and right vocal folds for all patients.

Spasmodic Dysphonia

Spasmodic dysphonia (SD) is a neurological voice disorder in which the individual suffers spasms of the vocal folds. Depending on which intrinsic laryngeal muscles are involved, the spasms may cause the vocal folds to either adduct (adductor spasmodic dysphonia [ADSD]) or abduct (abductor spasmodic dysphonia [ABSD]) inappropriately during phonation. In ADSD, the **laryngospasms** cause the vocal folds to adduct so tightly that they are very difficult to set into vibration. The voice quality of individuals with this disorder is called *strained-strangled* because of the severely strained and tense quality. **Botox injection** has become the gold standard for treatment and is used to alleviate the laryngospasms. The toxin is injected into the affected muscle, which in the case of ADSD is usually the thyroarytenoid muscle. The toxin temporarily weakens or even paralyzes the muscle. Therefore, during vibration, the vocal folds are unable to close with too much medial compression, allowing for much easier phonation. Often, though, the patient's voice after Botox injection is breathy and weak, especially for the first week or two. However, the effects of the injection are not permanent, and the patient's voice starts to lose the breathy quality and become more strained as time goes on. The person is typically reinjected every 3 to 6 months, depending on how long the effects last.

Outcomes measures using acoustic analysis and EGG have demonstrated very good results with Botox injection. Silverman, Garvan, Shrivastav, and Sapienza (2010) acoustically evaluated the effects of Botox injection prior to the injection; at 3, 7, and 12 weeks postinjection; and immediately prior to reinjection. For their outcomes measure, the authors divided the speakers' acoustic output into type 1 signals (nearly periodic), type 2 signals (contain subharmonics), and type 3 signals (aperiodic). Type 1 signals were designated as desirable; types 2 and 3 were considered undesirable. They reported that following injection, all participants demonstrated increased percentages of type 1 signals and decreased occurrence of type 2 and 3 signals during sustained phonation and connected speech.

Another type of surgery that has recently been used to treat ADSD is thyroplasty type II. This procedure lateralizes the vocal folds by means of titanium bridges, thus preventing them from adducting too tightly. This surgical method is advantageous because unlike Botox injection, it is permanent and does not cause side effects of breathiness. Sanuki, Yumoto, Minoda, and Kodama (2010) reported on the results of type II thyroplasty in patients with ADSD. Jitter, shimmer, FOSD, and HNR improved significantly and were within near normal ranges following surgery.

EGG quantifies vocal fold contact area and can therefore provide helpful information in voice disorders in which hyper- or hypofunction is the major problem. This is particularly useful in ADSD because the laryngospasms typically obscure the vocal folds during direct viewing with videostroboscopy or endoscopy. Fisher, Scherer, Swank, Giddens, and Patten (1999) used EGG to quantify patterns of vocal fold contact following Botox injection for SD in five patients. They reported that the greater the degree of vocal hyperadduction prior to injection, the greater was the likelihood of a strong hypofunctional response during the early postinjection period. They also noted that the EGG allowed visualization of adductory differences between individuals and within individuals over time. They suggested that longitudinal application of EGG measures may be helpful in identifying factors that can predict the response to Botox of an individual patient or subgroups of patients.

Paradoxical Vocal Fold Motion

Paradoxical vocal fold motion (PVFM) is a respiratory/laryngeal disorder characterized primarily by inappropriate spasms of the vocal folds during the inhalation phase of breathing. The major symptoms of PVFM are **stridor** and **dyspnea**. Stridor refers to a wheezing sound during breathing; dyspnea is the person's subjective sensation of difficulty and/or discomfort during breathing. Vocal symptoms are also common, particularly during an attack, and can include hoarseness, strain, breathiness, and aphonia (complete lack of voicing). Because of the respiratory component, this disorder is often misdiagnosed as asthma, and it is common for individuals to be treated incorrectly with asthma medications, and even intubation and/or tracheotomy. It is therefore crucial to distinguish between asthma and PVFM in order to provide the most appropriate treatment.

The diagnosis is most certain when the person's vocal folds are shown on endoscopy to close as he or she inspires (Patel, Jorgensen, Kuhn, & Merati, 2004). In addition to inappropriate vocal fold adduction, videostroboscopy has demonstrated false vocal fold adduction, anterior–posterior constriction of the supraglottic larynx, decreased amplitude of vibration, and decreased mucosal wave (Yelken, Gultekin, Guven, Eyibilen, & Aladag, 2010). Many secondary laryngeal abnormalities have also been found on stroboscopy, including inflammation, nodules, and laryngomalacia (excessively flaccid cartilages) (e.g., Patel et al., 2004). These stroboscopic signs are present in many speakers with PVFM, even when they are asymptomatic (Treole, Trudeau, & Forrest, 1999).

There have been several reports of higher-than-normal jitter and shimmer values and lower-than-normal HNR values in speakers with PVFM (e.g., Murray & Lawler, 1998; Vertigan, Theodoros, Winkworth, & Gibson, 2008; Yelken et al., 2010). These acoustic findings reflect the subtle laryngeal abnormalities demonstrated by videostroboscopy even during times when the individual is not undergoing overt respiratory symptoms.

Benign Mucosal Lesions, Muscle Tension Dysphonia, and/or GERD

Lifestyle, personality, and occupational factors have long been thought to play a causative or maintaining role in many benign conditions of the vocal folds, including nodules, polyps, contact ulcers, muscle tension dysphonia (MTD), and hoarseness related to gastroesophageal reflux disease (GERD). Nodules are benign growths that develop on the epithelium of the vocal folds as a consequence of vocal hyperfunction and resulting inflammation of the folds. Polyps are benign growths on the vocal fold mucosa that may result from laryngeal hyperfunction as well as from other causes, such as allergies. An ulcer is a lesion on a mucous surface caused by superficial loss of tissue. Contact ulcers of the vocal folds occur when the mucosa covering the vocal processes collides repeatedly with a hard surface. This causes the mucosa to break down, creating the ulcer. Muscle tension dysphonia (MTD) describes dysphonia that results from hypercontraction of the intrinsic and extrinsic laryngeal muscles as well as muscles in other areas such as the face, jaw, tongue, neck, and shoulders (Lee & Son, 2005; Mathieson et al., 2009; Nguyen & Kenny, 2008; Van Houtte, Van Lierde, & Claeys, 2010). The tension is noticeable in the patient's neck, jaw, shoulders, and throat, and the individual often reports pain in these areas, as well as excessive vocal effort and vocal fatigue. Often, the patient's larynx is elevated in the neck due to increased tension of the extrinsic laryngeal muscles (Van Houtte et al., 2010). Gastroesophageal reflux (GER) refers to the movement of stomach contents into the esophagus. GER is a normal physiologic process occurring mostly after meals. However, sometimes excess reflux, or increased occurrences of reflux, can cause gastroesophageal reflux disease (GERD). GERD refers to a broad array of diseases associated with injury to the esophagus or adjacent organs from the highly acidic gastric contents (called refluxate) into the esophagus or above into the pharynx and oral cavity (Sataloff et al., 2006). Reflux that enters the pharyngeal area and comes into contact with the posterior larynx is called **laryngopharyngeal reflux (LPR)**. This kind of acid injury to the larynx results in edema, which can affect the mass and tension of the vocal folds and interfere with vocal fold vibration (Selby, Gilbert, & Lerman, 2003).

Acoustic measures have been used extensively in the evaluation, treatment, and outcomes measurement of benign mucosal lesions, muscle tension dysphonia, and/or GERD/LPR. For example, Oguz et al. (2007) reported that jitter values were elevated in speakers with LPR compared to those without LPR, likely resulting from tissue irritation and inflammation caused by the acid reflux. Antireflux medications have been reported to be effective in improving the symptoms of reflux, decreasing ratings of hoarseness and roughness and improving levels of jitter, shimmer, and HNR (e.g., Selby et al., 2003; Vashani et al., 2010).

Jitter, shimmer, HNR, and the voice range profile have been used as outcomes measures following behavioral and surgical treatments for a variety of laryngeal disorders. For example, Uloza, Saferis, and Uloziene (2005) examined speakers with a variety of disorders including nodules and polyps before and after surgery to remove the growths. In the 2-week period following surgery, acoustic analysis demonstrated significant decreases in jitter, shimmer, and NNE. Speyer, Wieneke, van Wijck-Warnaar, and Dejonckere (2003) used the voice range profile to compare the effects of behavioral voice therapy in a group of dysphonic speakers. Measurements were taken before and after the voice therapy, as well as three months after the cessation of therapy. The authors reported an increase of the VRP in the low-frequency range following therapy, and these changes were still evident 3 months after completion of therapy.

Acoustic measures can also be a valuable source of visual feedback for individuals with voice disorders. Mora et al. (2010) used an acoustic program to treat adult males with hypofunctional voices. The program included a collection of games with voice-controlled animated graphics that represented pitch and amplitude extracted in real time. The games focused on voicing, timing, and pitch and amplitude control. Average F_0, jitter, shimmer, and NHR normalized after 3 months of therapy. The authors noted that using visual feedback shortened the duration of therapy compared to speakers who underwent similar therapy but without the use of acoustic feedback.

EGG has been used to measure patterns of glottal closure and acoustic parameters in patients with a wide variety of benign vocal fold lesions such as nodules and polyps. Lim, Choi, Kim, and Choi (2006) used EGG to examine changes in F_0, jitter, shimmer, HNR, and closed quotient in patients before and after surgery for Reinke's edema (RE). RE is a condition of polypoid degeneration in which the vocal folds become very swollen and edematous, typically as a result of heavy smoking. The authors reported that the greater was the degree of edema, the lower the F_0, the higher the F_0SD, the higher the jitter and shimmer values, and the higher the closed quotient. After surgery the F_0 was increased to almost normal values for both males and females, shimmer and HNR values improved, and the closed quotient improved.

Endoscopy, with or without stroboscopy, is helpful in demonstrating the mechanics of vocal fold vibration before and after treatment for vocal pathologies. Lan et al. (2010) performed laryngeal surgery for 20 patients with vocal fold polyps. Surgery was performed under topical anesthesia. Because the patients were awake, they were able to phonate, and the vocal folds and vocal fold vibration could be assessed by stroboscopic and auditory evaluation during the procedure. Patients were reassessed several months after the surgery. Follow-up videostroboscopy showed improvement in the degree of glottic closure, vocal fold regularity, phase symmetry, and mucosal wave. Speyer, Wieneke, and Dejonckere (2004) evaluated speakers with a diverse array of voice problems before and after therapy. Laryngostroboscopy demonstrated overall improvement on vibratory parameters, with greater effects for speakers with greater degrees of vocal abnormality before treatment.

Endoscopy has also been useful in establishing the laryngeal signs and symptoms of GERD and/or LPR. These findings include edema and redness of the arytenoids, excessive amounts of tissue in the interarytenoid region, and inflammation of the vocal folds (Belafsky, Postma, & Koufman, 2001; 2002). The presence of these signs is often a cue for the individual to be prescribed anti reflux medications or surgery, and many studies have shown a notable decrease or complete resolution of symptoms following treatment (e.g., Suskind, Zeringue, Kluka, Udall, & Liu, 2001; Tashjian, Tirabassi, Moriarty, & Salva, 2002).

Another clinical use of endoscopy is as a treatment technique to provide visual feedback to individuals with voice disorders. Rattenbury, Carding, and Finn (2004) used transnasal flexible laryngoscopy (TFL) as a form of treatment for individuals with muscle tension dysphonia. They separated their patients into two groups. One group received traditional voice therapy; the other group received TFL-assisted voice therapy. Participants in the TFL group received feedback from their own endoscopic evaluations in addition to traditional voice therapy. Acoustic measures (jitter and shimmer) were used as outcomes. The jitter and shimmer measures showed a significant reduction after treatment in both groups. However, the TFL-assisted group took less time to complete the therapeutic regimen than the traditional therapy group. The authors suggested that using flexible endoscopy as a treatment tool is more efficient than traditional therapy and can be helpful in maintaining the speaker's motivation during the therapy process. More efficient use of time can also have positive financial considerations for the patient.

While much important information is provided by acoustic and EGG measures, the information regarding vocal fold vibration is indirect, and it is not possible to interpret the actual movement patterns of the vocal folds (Patel, Liu, Galatsanos, & Bless, 2011). Further, disorders such as adductor spasmodic dysphonia and muscle tension dysphonia are difficult to distinguish by these means, because these disorders are both characterized by extremely aperiodic voice signals (Patel et al., 2011). Even with endoscopy, it is difficult to differentiate ADSD and MTD because both demonstrate glottal and supraglottic constrictions and excessive involvement of intrinsic and extrinsic muscles (Patel et al., 2011). It is critical to distinguish between these two disorders, however, because clinical management approaches are completely different. ADSD is typically treated with Botox injection, while MTD usually responds well to behavioral voice therapy. In an attempt to distinguish between ADSD and MTD, Patel et al. (2011) used HSDI to compare vibration patterns between individuals with ADSD and MTD (Table 6.3). They also evaluated vocal hyperfunction (lateral or anterior–posterior compression of the glottis). The authors reported that the physiological features of motion irregularities, micromotion, and hyperfunction were different between groups. Irregularity of vocal fold motion was the only significant predictor of ADSD.

Laryngeal Cancer

Individuals who have cancer of the larynx undergo various medical and/or surgical procedures to treat the condition. Depending on the site and the extent of the cancer, the patient may need radiation therapy, chemotherapy, a combination of the two, or surgical removal of parts of or the entire larynx. Cure rates for the cancer are high, particularly if the disease is caught early. Often, however, the person is left with a dysphonic voice. In the case of complete removal of the larynx (**total laryngectomy [TL]**), the individual is not able to produce voice in the normal way. In this case, several approaches for alternative voicing sources are available. These include use of an artificial larynx (AL), esophageal speech (ES), and/or tracheo-esophageal speech (TES). These forms of voice production fall in the general category of alaryngeal speech. The AL electronically generates a sound. The individual holds the device to his or her neck and the tone is transmitted through the tissue into the vocal tract, where it is articulated. Esophageal speech (ES) refers to voice that is produced by taking air into the esophagus and then releasing it through the pharynx. As the air is released, it vibrates the ring of muscle that forms a sphincter between the lower portion of the pharynx and upper portion of the esophagus. This sphincter, called the pharyngoesophageal segment (PE segment), forms the **neoglottis**. Vibration of the neoglottis produces sound. Tracheoesophageal speech is a variant of ES. This form of voicing relies on a surgical connection (puncture) that is made between the back wall of the trachea and the front wall of the esophagus. A one-way prosthesis is inserted into the puncture, which allows air from the trachea to be channeled to the esophagus and released through the PE segment. As with ES, the PE segment is vibrated to produce voice. The prosthesis prevents contents from the esophagus from entering the trachea.

Vocal frequency and intensity characteristics have been used as a yardstick for successful voice restoration in alaryngeal speakers. ES and TES are typically much lower in F_0 and amplitude than normally produced speech. Reported F_0 values for individuals with total laryngectomies average 77.29 Hz for male esophageal speakers and 97.59 Hz for male tracheoesophageal speakers, compared to 120.30 Hz for normal laryngeal male speakers (Arias, Ramon, Campos, & Cervantes, 2000).

Historically, speech–language pathologists have characterized proficient esophageal speech as having a higher F_0 and higher amplitude level than poor esophageal speech. Slavin and Ferrand (1995) tested this assumption by acoustically analyzing the speech of esophageal speakers who were all judged perceptually as being highly proficient speakers. The average frequency for the entire group of speakers was 69 Hz, considerably lower than the normal values for adult speakers presented in Table 6.5. However, Slavin and Ferrand (1995) found that these individuals clustered into four groups, with each group characterized by a different frequency and amplitude profile. For example, individuals in one group had higher than average mean F_0 and greater frequency variability than the group mean. Speakers in a different group had lower mean F_0 and less frequency variability. A third group of speakers obtained an F_0 around 69 Hz, but these individuals had relatively high amplitude levels (around 70 dB SPL). Understanding that different patterns of frequency and amplitude characterize individual esophageal speakers can allow clinicians to be more flexible in choosing rehabilitation strategies geared to the individual's specific anatomical characteristics and communication needs.

Estimates of noise in the voice signal have also been used to characterize alaryngeal voice qualities. Extremely high jitter levels and extremely low HNR levels have been reported in the voices of alaryngeal speakers (Arias et al., 2000). Van As-Brooks, Koopmans-van Beinum, Pols, and Hilgers (2006) developed a signal typing system for TES voices based on visual inspection of the harmonic structure of vowels shown in narrowband spectrograms. Signals were classified as Type I if the signal was stable and harmonic; Type II if the signal was stable and at least one harmonic at the F_0 was evident; Type III if the signal was unstable or partly harmonic; and Type IV if the signal was barely harmonic in its structure or if there was a complete absence of harmonics. Comparison of acoustic and perceptual judgments showed that Type I and II signals were perceived as more normal than the other signal types.

EGG has been used to explore the acoustic characteristics of alaryngeal speech. Recall that EGG does not rely on identifying a periodic signal for analysis. EGG is therefore not as susceptible to the effects of aperiodicity in the voice and provides a more robust acoustic indication of vocal irregularities. Kazi and colleagues (Kazi et al., 2008; Kazi et al., 2008a; Kazi et al., 2008b; Kazi et al., 2009) have reported on a series of studies using EGG to examine speaking characteristics of alaryngeal speakers as well as to investigate the effects of different types of treatments on early and advanced laryngeal cancer. In one study the authors analyzed isolated vowels and connected speech in groups of male and female TES speakers. Both groups demonstrated significantly lower F_0 values than laryngeal speakers, and measures of jitter, shimmer, and NNE were poorer. Average F_0 for the laryngeal male speakers was 122.3 Hz, compared to 105.2 Hz for male TES speakers; average F_0 for laryngeal female speakers was 226.4 Hz, compared to female TES speakers of 112.4 Hz. In another study, Kazi and colleagues analyzed F_0, jitter, shimmer, and NNE before radiotherapy for early laryngeal cancer, and at various times following the completion of treatment. A year following completion, the perturbation and noise measures improved and were closer to normal limits. Kazi et al. (2008a) recorded voice in patients with advanced laryngeal cancer; half of the group had undergone chemoradiotherapy and half had TL with TES speech. The researchers used EGG to analyze F_0, jitter, shimmer, and NNE before treatment and during long-term follow-up (up to 12 months). The group receiving chemotherapy obtained significantly better values than the TE speakers across all measured parameters. The average F_0 was higher than that in TE speakers (around 124 Hz, compared to 88 Hz), and jitter values were lower for the group that received chemoradiation. The authors noted that chemoradiation can preserve not only laryngeal structure but also vocal function. In a similar study, Singh et al. (2008) used EGG to compare F_0, jitter, shimmer, and NNE in three groups of speakers. One group had undergone **vertical partial laryngectomy (VPL)** that preserved a certain portion of the larynx, one group used TES, and one group was normal laryngeal speakers. Not surprisingly, F_0 was significantly lower in the TE speakers than the normal speakers, and jitter, shimmer, and NNE measures were significantly lower (i.e., better) in the normal speakers. However, the acoustic measures of both laryngeal cancer groups were very similar to each other, leading the authors to conclude that VPL is not necessarily a better treatment option in terms of vocal function.

While acoustic and EGG measures provide useful information regarding vocal output, vocal vibratory patterns can only be inferred from the output. Videostroboscopy can directly visualize the larynx or the neoglottis in alaryngeal speakers. However, as noted above, stroboscopy requires a stable periodic signal for reliable and valid voice analysis. High-speed digital imaging and kymographic analysis of vocal fold or neoglottal vibration in alaryngeal speakers lend themselves more readily to analysis of aperiodic voices because these techniques do not rely on a periodic signal. HSDI and kymography have been useful in characterizing movements of the neoglottis or of true and false vocal fold vibration following different types of partial laryngectomy procedures (e.g., Dedivitis, Sertorio, & Pfuetzenreiter, 2009; Mehta, Deliyski, Zeitels, Quatieri, & Hillman, 2010; Saito et al., 2010). Detailed examination of the vibratory source can help to determine the best intervention strategies and can also be used as an outcomes measure following treatment.

Hearing Impairment

Auditory feedback is important in the control of F_0, voice intensity, and voice quality (Hocevar-Boltezar, Vatovec, Gros, & Zargi, 2005). Individuals with hearing impairment have been shown to present with disturbances in vocal function, including atypical variations in F_0 and intensity, abnormal intonational contours, and abnormalities in vocal quality. Hearing-impaired speakers often demonstrate dysphonia characterized by hoarseness, strained phonation, and higher pitch and intensity levels (Baudonck, D'haeseleer, Dhooge, & Van Lierde, 2010). One common finding in hearing-impaired speakers is a higher-than-normal F_0. Increased F_0 may result from laryngeal constriction and tension due to the speaker's reliance on tactile rather than auditory feedback (Lenden & Flipsen, 2007). Factors such as laryngeal elevation, increased phonatory effort, and difficulty controlling vocal fold tension can also contribute to the high F_0 (Dehqan & Scherer, 2011; Poissant, Peters, & Robb, 2006). Another common finding is problems in pitch and loudness control, as well as aberrant stress patterns (e.g., Campisi, Low, Papsin, Mount, Harrison, 2006; Holler et al., 2010; Lenden & Flipsen, 2007). In addition, vocal stability has been reported to be decreased in children with profound hearing loss, as shown by higher-than-normal levels of jitter and shimmer and lower-than-normal values for HNR (Dehqan & Scherer, 2011; Garcia, Rovira, & Sanvicens, 2010). Intervention for hearing-impaired speakers can be more effective when visual feedback is provided in order to compensate for the loss of auditory feedback. For example, Chernobelsky (2002) used EGG to treat deaf adolescent boys who spoke with abnormally high F_0 (average 436 Hz). The author had the boys cough and then extend the voiced vocalization into vowels. Using the EGG, all four boys were able to lower their F_0 to an average of 184 Hz after 8 to 10 sessions, and the decreased F_0 was maintained after 12 months.

Cochlear implantation (CI) is often extremely beneficial in increasing the amount of auditory feedback available to the speaker in terms of timing, intensity, and frequency of sound (Holler et al., 2010). Many studies have investigated the effects of CI on acoustic measures of voice. Hocevar-Boltezar et al. (2005) tested children before CI and 6, 12, and 24 months after CI. Jitter, shimmer, and NHR values improved significantly. Further, the children implanted prior to age 4 years demonstrated improved control of pitch and loudness more quickly and to a greater extent than those implanted after age 4 years. Lenden and Flipsen (2007) evaluated the prosodic and vocal characteristics of two groups of hearing-impaired children over a 12- to 21-month period of time. One group used hearing aids; the other group used cochlear implants. Reportedly, the hearing aid users showed difficulties with pitch control, while the CI users did not. Overall, the CI users did not demonstrate problems with loudness or voice quality, although resonance quality and use of stress did continue to be an issue. The authors noted that the prosody and voice characteristics of children who use CI are less problematic than for children who use hearing aids. This suggests that the auditory information provided by CI improves vocal motor function and voice quality. CI has been shown to be effective in improving control of F_0 and F_0 variability as well as vocal stability (e.g., Evans & Deliyski, 2007; Hassan et al., 2011; Poissant, Peters, & Robb, 2006; Ubrig et al., 2011).

Despite the advantages of CI, problems with pitch and loudness control often persist (Cousineau, Demany, Meyer, & Pressnitzer, 2010). Peng, Tomblin, Spencer, and Hurtig (2007) examined the ability of children and young adults with cochlear implants to imitate appropriate intonation patterns in a yes–no question that requires a rising pitch level at the end of the utterance. They reported that the speakers were perceptually judged as not consistently using the appropriate patterns. This was borne out by the acoustic analysis, which indicated that the children did not show mastery of the F_0, intensity, and duration characteristics required for rising intonation patterns even though the participants had been using the device for several years. Acoustic measures can provide a rational basis for targeted speech therapy to modify these aspects of vocal function following cochlear implantation.

Transsexual Voice

As currently used, the term *transsexual* refers to individuals whose gender identity is fundamentally in conflict with their biological sex and who unambiguously identify with the non-natal gender (Denny, 2004). The individual feels strong discomfort with his or her biological identity and the corresponding roles, expectations, and attitudes that society expects in accordance with traditional male and female genders. It is not uncommon for the person to live for years in accordance with the societal rules for the natal gender (Thornton, 2008). Many such individuals have served in the military or have worked in law enforcement, construction, or some other stereotypically masculine field. Eventually, a transsexual person may seek help and may decide to undergo surgical procedures for changing gender identity.

Most individuals who complete sex reassignment surgery are male-to-female (MTF) transsexuals. Often, the surgery is extremely successful in terms of visual appearance, with the help of appropriate hormone treatment, breast augmentation, electrolysis, and facial plastic surgery. However, the so-called "trans woman" is often left with a voice that is perceived as masculine, at odds with her new appearance. The person's pitch levels, intonational patterns, voice quality, and overall communicative characteristics often remain in the masculine domain.

The goal of voice treatment is to emphasize and highlight the markers of female speech. Markers include a higher pitch, greater intonational range and pitch variability, increased vocal expression, rising intonation on statements, breathier voice quality, feminine patterns of phrasing, and nonverbal visual markers such as increased eye contact, increased hand/arm gestures, and increased use of touch (Parker, 2008).

F_0 is the most salient cue to gender identification for trans speakers as well as for biological men and women (Gelfer & Mikos, 2005). Therefore, raising an individual's pitch has typically been targeted as the most important goal of treatment. Research has established a cutoff F_0 of around 150 to 173 Hz, below which speakers are perceived as male and above which speakers are perceived as female (e.g., Brown, Perry, Cheesman, & Pring, 2000; Gelfer & Schofield, 2000; Wolfe, Ratusnik, Smith, & Northrop, 1990). The range between approximately 145 to 165 Hz forms a gender-ambiguous F_0 zone in which the speaker's gender is not identifiable (Adler, Hirsch, & Mordaunt, 2006; Thornton, 2008). This zone forms the initial target for pitch-raising exercises.

Pitch range and variability are aspects of intonation that are strong markers of gender identity. Female speakers typically use a wider range of F_0s and a more varied pattern of pitch inflections, while male speakers tend to use a more restricted F_0 range and fewer inflectional patterns (Ferrand & Bloom, 1996). Studies have demonstrated that trans speakers' voices identified as female are characterized by more pitch inflections both upward and downward, less extensive downward shifts, a greater proportion of upward shifts, and fewer level intonation patterns (e.g., Gelfer & Schofield, 2000; Wolfe et al., 1990). Women's intonational patterns differ from men's not only in range but in phrase endings. Women tend to use more rising inflections at the end of utterances, often giving their speech a somewhat tentative sound. In fact, a speaker who uses a lower pitch but a more feminine intonational pattern and style tends to sound more feminine than one who uses a higher pitch but fewer feminine patterns.

Holmberg, Oates, Dacakis, and Grant (2010) analyzed voice range profiles (VRPs) of MTF trans speakers and compared the acoustic information to perceptual ratings of their voices as male or female. They reported that the more low-frequency energy in the speaker's voice, the less likely she was to be perceived as female. While F_0 and rated gender were strongly correlated, two of the participants with the highest female ratings had relatively low F_0 values (150 and 135 Hz), below the frequency usually considered as the limit for a female-sounding voice. In contrast, two other participants with higher F_0 levels (both 165 Hz) received low ratings. MTF maximum SPL (85 dB) was very close to the maximum SPL for men (86 dB) and higher than the maximum SPL for women (80 dB). MTF minimum SPL (67 dB) was higher than those for both men (65 dB) and women (64 dB). Based on this information, the authors suggested that lowering SPL may contribute to a more successful female voice.

Palmer, Dietsch, and Searl (2011) used endoscopy and stroboscopy to examine laryngeal aspects of voice in MTF speakers when they were using their feminine voice. They reported that rather than complete glottal closure during phonation, as expected for a male larynx, glottal closure was incomplete in most of the speakers. This resulted in a more extended open phase during vibration. In addition, most of the speakers showed vocal hyperfunction. Because female speakers typically show a slight degree of posterior opening during vibration, which gives the female voice a slight degree of breathiness, the authors suggested that incomplete closure may work well for a trans speaker to create a more female-sounding voice. In order to facilitate this laryngeal position, visual feedback using laryngeal imaging procedures may be beneficial.

Summary

Techniques to visualize laryngeal structure and function include electroglottography, endoscopy, videostroboscopy, high-speed digital imaging, and videokymography.

Advantages of acoustic and visual methods of voice analysis include more precise evaluation of the problem, providing a starting point for rehabilitation, providing a means of assessing the individual's progress, increased clinician accountability, feedback during therapy, outcomes measures, a means to detect early changes in speech and voice, and a way to validate a clinician's perceptual judgments of disordered voice and speech by providing norms that can serve as a basis of comparison between vocally healthy and vocally disordered speakers.

Vocal changes over the lifespan have been well documented by acoustic, EGG, and endoscopic measures; F_0 levels decrease dramatically for boys during puberty, remain stable until the later years of adulthood, and then may increase in males and decrease in females.

Speakers with amyotrophic lateral sclerosis demonstrate a variety of acoustic changes, including increased levels of jitter, smaller maximum phonational frequency ranges, abnormal F_0 levels, and reduced ranges of frequency during connected speech.

Acoustic characteristics that have been reported for individuals with Parkinson's disease include higher F_0, higher jitter, lower intensity, decreased phonational range, and decreased dynamic range.

Diagnosis of vocal fold paresis may be facilitated by the use of high-speed digital imaging in conjunction with kymography.

Acoustic, EGG, videostroboscopic, and high-speed digital imaging techniques have demonstrated that vocal fold injection, vocal fold medialization thyroplasty, and arytenoid adduction are effective methods of increasing glottal closure in patients with unilateral vocal fold paralysis.

Outcomes measures using acoustic analysis and EGG have demonstrated very good results with Botox injection for patients with adductor spasmodic dysphonia.

Acoustic measures have been used extensively in the evaluation, treatment, and outcomes measurement of benign mucosal lesions, muscle tension dysphonia, and GERD/LPR; transnasal flexible laryngoscopy has been shown to be effective as a form of treatment for individuals with muscle tension dysphonia.

High-speed digital imaging has been used to compare vibration patterns between adductor spasmodic dysphonia and muscle tension dysphonia.

Frequency and intensity characteristics have been used as a yardstick for successful voice restoration in alaryngeal speakers.

Use of EGG, high-speed digital imaging, and kymography have demonstrated specific vibratory patterns of the neoglottis following partial and total laryngectomies and voice restoration methods.

Acoustic and visual analysis methods are particularly effective in conditions in which pitch plays a dominant role, including hearing impairment and transsexual voice.

REVIEW EXERCISES

1. Explain the relationship between EGG shape, EGG slope quotients, and vocal fold vibration.

2. Identify advantages and disadvantages of endoscopy, videostroboscopy, high-speed digital imaging, and videokymography.

3. Identify three clinical situations in which the measurement of acoustic and visual vocal factors might be useful, and explain why.

4. Discuss the rationale for the development of separate average F_0 and F_0 variability norms for men, women, and children.

5. Explain how acoustic and visual measures can be used to supplement perceptual evaluations in patients with disorders that affect vocal function.

6. Discuss the electroglottographic measures of contact quotient and closed-to-open ratio in relation to vocal disorders involving hyper- or hypoadduction.

7. Identify advantages and disadvantages of high-speed digital imaging and kymography for individuals with highly aperiodic voices.

8. Choose a vocal disorder and compare the types of information that can be obtained about vocal function with acoustic, electroglottographic, and endoscopic measures.

INTEGRATIVE CASE STUDIES

① Jaime

Background Information

Jaime is a speech–language pathologist in an elementary school, which is part of a large school district. An important part of her job is to screen all entering kindergartners in the school district for any speech or language problems. She downloaded the free acoustic program Praat and is eager to implement a new screening protocol that she developed for identifying possible voice disorders in the children.

Acoustic Measures

Jaime's protocol includes several F_0 and intensity variables, including average F_0, SFF, and average intensity. For average F_0, the child is asked to hold the vowel /a/ for 5 seconds; SFF is taken from a picture-description task.

Average intensity is also taken from these activities. During these activities, Jaime also listens carefully to the children's voices and rates them perceptually.

After screening 150 children (87 girls and 63 boys), Jaime is able to obtain means for these different acoustic measures. Jaime did not think it was necessary to separate the data for the girls and boys, and she obtained all her information from the averages for all the children. The average F_0 for /a/ for all the children was approximately 248 Hz; SFF yielded an average of 242 Hz. Average intensity was 59 dB. Based on these normative values that she derived, Jaime was able to identify several children whose means fell outside these ranges. For example, Peter obtained an F_0 of 224 Hz for /a/, 215 Hz for his

SFF, and an average intensity of 77 dB. This was consistent perceptually with his low-pitched and somewhat loud voice. Emma's values were 258 Hz for /a/, 254 Hz for SFF, and 56 dB for average intensity. Jaime was surprised about the F_0 measures because, perceptually, Emma's voice sounded extremely low pitched for her age. Emma was also hoarse and complained that her throat was sore. Both of these children were referred to an ENT for laryngeal examination.

Clinical Questions

a. What are the possible advantages and disadvantages of using acoustic measures in conjunction with traditional perceptual methods of screening?

b. What may be the advantages and/or disadvantages of Jaime's using her own normative data to make comparisons rather than using values from reported literature?

c. Should the values of the two children who failed the screening have been compared to the single-group averages that Jaime derived from the screenings? Why or why not?

d. What could account for the lack of consistency between the perceptual and acoustic results in Emma's case?

② Mrs. Salerno

Background Information

Mrs. Salerno, age 37 years, scheduled an appointment at your busy speech clinic regarding concerns about her voice. She reported recently starting a new job as a telemarketing agent for a large electric company. Her 8-hour workday consists of making phone calls to potential clients to persuade them to switch electric companies. Mrs. Salerno noted that her voice has become increasingly "strained" over the past year. She commented that her voice "seems to fade out," and at times she has difficulty producing any sound. Mrs. Salerno reported that her voice difficulties are becoming progressively worse, and it is becoming more difficult to speak. She is concerned that her vocal difficulties are interfering with her job responsibilities, as well as with her social life. Mrs. Salerno reported that she has seen numerous doctors, but none has been able to shed light on her problem. You conduct a thorough speech examination. Upon review of the results, and in collaboration with other medical professionals, it is determined that Mrs. Salerno presents with adductor spasmodic dysphonia.

Clinical Observations

Your first impression of Mrs. Salerno is that she is a sociable, outgoing woman who exhibits some degree of difficulty when speaking. Her vocal quality can be described as "harsh," as well as "strained/strangled," with a "whisper-like" quality to it at times. In addition, her voice has frequent breaks, which occasionally cause her to become unintelligible. You also noted that the client has a slight eye twitch whenever she exhibits difficulty with producing speech.

Acoustic/Visual Measures

Mrs. Salerno underwent flexible laryngoscopy. It was noted that her vocal folds vibrated normally when she sustained the vowel /i/, when she whispered, and when she sang "Happy Birthday." However, spasms of the true and false vocal folds were observed during connected speech. Acoustic analysis of isolated vowels demonstrated jitter and shimmer values of 2.6 percent and 1.3 dB, respectively; HNR was –2.7 dB. Spectrographic analysis revealed a high level of type 2 and 3 signals compared to type 1 signals. The average closed quotient obtained via EGG was 0.82.

Clinical Questions

a. Based on the above information, would you recommend Botox injections to alleviate Mrs. Salerno's voice symptoms? Why or why not?

b. What changes would you expect to see in the client's acoustic and visual data immediately after Botox injection?

c. Would you expect to see other changes in the data toward the middle and end of the treatment cycle? Why or why not?

d. Mrs. Salerno's job is very important to her, and her vocal difficulties cause her to worry. Can stress worsen her already strained/strangled voice? Explain.

e. What other health care professionals might you want to consult in order to provide the client with a comprehensive treatment plan?

③ Mr. Lopez

Background Information

Mr. Juan Lopez, a 70-year-old retired pilot for the U.S. Air Force, was recently diagnosed with amyotrophic lateral sclerosis during a visit to his medical institution, due to concerns about noticeable facial weakness and difficulty swallowing. The speech–language pathologist at the medical institution reported that the patient demonstrated dysarthria characterized by hoarseness, weak voice, and hypernasality. Mr. Lopez was referred to your office as an outpatient for services concerning preservation of verbal communication as well as options for augmentative communication devices in the future.

Clinical Observations

During the intake interview, you noted Mr. Lopez's hoarse vocal quality, hypernasality, and imprecise articulatory movements. Also evident was vocal weakness characterized by low volume. The client's wife asserted that her husband demonstrates evident vocal tiredness during conversation, and his hoarse vocal quality appears to be worsening. During the interview, Mr. Lopez needed to pause at non-junctural points in an utterance in order to replenish his breath supply.

Acoustic Observations

Using acoustic instrumentation, you obtained Mr. Lopez's speaking fundamental frequency.

Average SFF during conversation was 168 Hz, well above the average for a healthy male of Mr. Lopez's age. Jitter, shimmer, and HNR values during sustained vowel /a/ were 2.5 percent, 2.3 dB, and 1.4 dB, respectively. Maximal phonational frequency range was 0.76 octaves. Average intensity during connected speech was 46.8 dB.

Clinical Questions

a. In addition to the acoustic measures mentioned above, what other instrumental measures might be helpful in evaluating the client's vocal function? Provide a rationale for each additional measure.

b. What are possible causes for the increased noise evident in Mr. Lopez's vocal output?

c. Would it be beneficial to construct a voice range profile for Mr. Lopez? Why or why not?

d. Given your knowledge of the relationship between frequency and amplitude capabilities of the human phonatory system, how would a voice range profile differ for Mr. Lopez compared to a healthy speaker of his age and sex?

7

The Respiratory System

STUDENT LEARNING OBJECTIVES

After reading this chapter you will

○ Identify the major structures of the respiratory system.

○ Understand how the lungs move due to pleural linkage.

○ Discuss lung volumes and capacities and their relationship to speech breathing.

○ Describe the differences between life breathing and speech breathing.

○ Understand the air pressure and flows involved in respiration.

○ Know how speech breathing patterns develop and change over the lifespan.

The primary purpose of respiration is ventilation. Ventilation is the process of moving air into and out of the airways and lungs in order to exchange oxygen (O_2) entering the lungs and carbon dioxide (CO_2) leaving the lungs. Adequate respiratory function is also essential for voice production. The ability to speak depends on a steady outflow of air that is vibrated by the vocal folds to produce sound. The sound is then further modified by the articulators to generate the specific phonemes of whatever language is being spoken. Without this outflow of air, there would be no speech. The subject of air—how it flows into and out of the lungs; how breathing patterns change when breathing for speech, rather than for purely vegetative, life-sustaining purposes; the pressures and flows of air in different locations of the body during breathing and speaking—will be addressed in this chapter. The chapter begins with a description of the pulmonary airways. This provides a framework for further exploration of the mechanics of respiration in relation to normal and disordered speech production. Keep in mind that many structures of the respiratory system, including the larynx, the oral cavity, and nasal cavities, are involved not only in breathing but in phonation and articulation, as well as swallowing. This multipurpose organization of structures and systems is extremely efficient and is made possible by an extraordinary degree of control and coordination by the nervous system. The respiratory system is divided into the pulmonary apparatus and the chest wall.

Pulmonary Apparatus

The pulmonary apparatus includes the lungs and airways and is the means whereby air containing oxygen (O_2) is conducted to the lungs and transported to all the cells of the body and carbon dioxide (CO_2) is transported from the body back to the lungs and exhaled. The pulmonary apparatus is made up of the trachea, bronchi, bronchioles, alveoli, and lungs. The trachea, bronchi, and bronchioles are often referred to as the bronchial tree.

Bronchial Tree

The **bronchial tree** consists of a branching system of hollow tubes that conduct air to and from the lungs. Similar to a tree, the bronchial system begins with a larger tube (the trunk of the tree, in the analogy), which then divides into smaller and smaller tubes (the branches and twigs) (Figure 7.1).

Directly beneath the larynx lies the trachea, corresponding to the trunk of the tree in the analogy. The trachea is a hollow tube, about 10 to 16 cm long in adults and approximately 2.0 to 2.5 cm in diameter. The trachea is made up of 16 to 20 rings of cartilage, which are closed in the front and open in the back. Between the cartilages and forming the back wall of the trachea is smooth muscle, and overlying the cartilages and muscle is a mucous membrane. The combination of cartilage and smooth muscle allows both great flexibility and support for the trachea. The support prevents the trachea from collapsing when negative pressures generated during inhalation occur within it. On the inside surface, the trachea is lined with a layer of ciliated pseudostratified columnar epithelium. The epithelium contains mucous-producing cells and millions of tiny hairlike projections called **cilia**. The cilia continuously move in a wavelike motion. As they slowly move downward, they pick up particles of dust, pollution, bacteria, and viruses. As they quickly move upward, this material, held together in a sticky blanket of mucus, is forcefully expelled into the throat and swallowed or coughed out. Thus, the cilia act as a filtering system to clean the air going into the lungs. See Figure 7.2.

The trachea splits into two branches called primary or **mainstem bronchi** (singular: bronchus). Each mainstem bronchus is slightly less than half the diameter of the trachea. The right bronchus enters the right lung, and the left bronchus enters the left lung. Each primary bronchus divides into secondary bronchi, which supply the lobes of the lung. Each secondary bronchus, in turn, subdivides into tertiary (segmental) bronchi, which go into the small segments of the lungs. The structure of the bronchi is very similar to that of the trachea, being composed of rings of cartilage, as well as membrane and smooth muscle. The segmental bronchi continue to branch into smaller and smaller tubes. Eventually, the bronchi divide into tiny bronchioles, which at this point lose their cartilage and are composed of only smooth muscle and membrane. The bronchioles further branch into terminal bronchioles and then respiratory bronchioles. In total, the bronchial tree contains 20 to 28 subdivisions (Hixon & Hoit, 2005; Seikel, King, & Drumright, 1997; Zemlin, 1998). With each successive subdivision, the branches become smaller and narrower but increase in number. Consequently, the total surface area of the smaller branches is larger than that of the next larger branch (Seikel et al., 1997). This provides an enormous amount of surface area for respiration.

The respiratory bronchioles open into **alveolar ducts** (Figure 7.3). Each alveolar duct leads to an alveolus, which is a microscopic, thin-walled, air-filled structure. There are millions of alveoli in the lungs, with an average of 480 million, and larger lungs having up to 900 million (Ochs et al., 2004). Each alveolus is surrounded by a dense network of tiny blood capillaries. Within each alveolus is a substance called **surfactant**. Surfactant keeps the alveoli inflated by lowering the surface tension of their walls, thus preventing them from being pulled inward during inspiration. The alveoli and the capillaries are extremely thin walled, allowing for the easy exchange of gases between them.

Figure 7.1 **Bronchial tree**

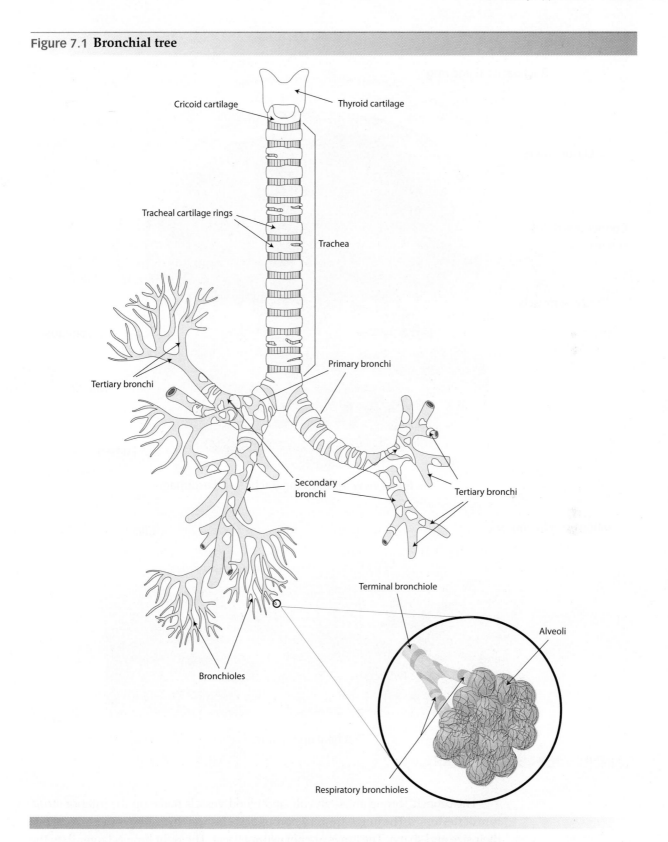

Cricoid cartilage

Thyroid cartilage

Tracheal cartilage rings

Trachea

Tertiary bronchi

Primary bronchi

Secondary bronchi

Tertiary bronchi

Terminal bronchiole

Alveoli

Bronchioles

Respiratory bronchioles

Figure 7.2 **Trachea**

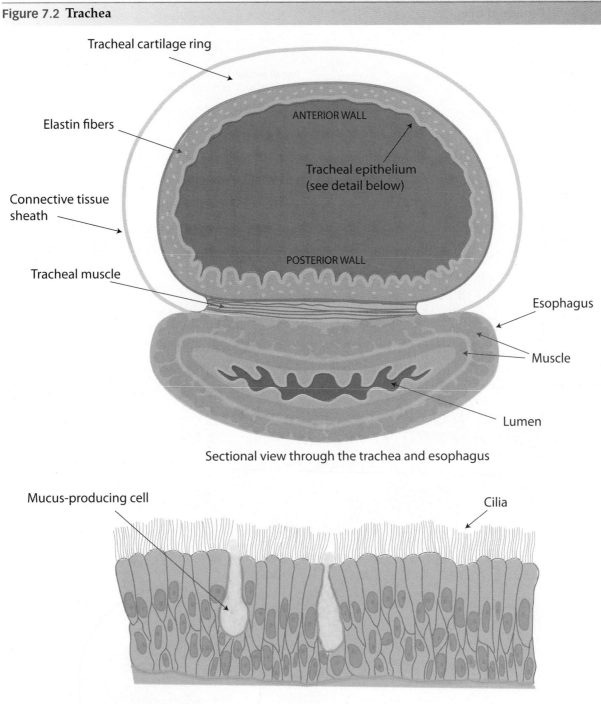

Tracheal cartilage ring

Elastin fibers

Connective tissue sheath

Tracheal muscle

ANTERIOR WALL

Tracheal epithelium (see detail below)

POSTERIOR WALL

Esophagus

Muscle

Lumen

Sectional view through the trachea and esophagus

Mucus-producing cell

Cilia

Tracheal epithelium

The bronchi, bronchioles, alveoli, and blood vessels make up the interior structure of the lungs. The lungs are very porous and elastic, which allows them to change their size and shape. The lungs are not symmetrical. The right lung is larger than the left and is composed of three lobes, which are separated by grooves. The left lung is smaller than the right, to make space for the heart on the left side. The left lung is

Figure 7.3 Alveoli

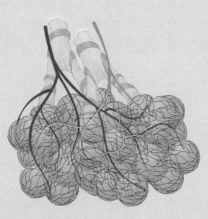

The bronchioles terminate in clusters of tiny balloon-like alveoli that inflate and deflate during breathing.

The alveoli are covered by a network of capillaries.

The exchange of inhaled oxygen and waste carbon dioxide takes place across the extremely thin walls of these pulmonary capillaries and alveoli.

Inhaled O_2 passes through the thin alveolar and pulmonary capillary walls and attaches to the hemoglobin of the red blood cells.

CO_2 (produced as waste by cells) is carried by the red blood cells and passes through the capillary and alveolar walls and is exhaled.

O_2

CO_2

therefore composed of only two lobes (Figure 7.4). The lungs in the newborn infant are a pinkish color, while the effects of environmental pollution and other toxins such as cigarette smoke contribute to a grayish or blackish color in adults.

Chest Wall

The pulmonary apparatus is enclosed within the chest wall. The chest wall is made up of the rib cage, abdominal wall, abdominal contents, and diaphragm. The rib cage and diaphragm make up the thoracic cavity, which houses the lungs (Figure 7.5).

The thoracic cavity is bounded by the sternum (breastbone) and rib cage on the front and sides, the spinal column and vertebrae at the back, and the diaphragm muscle at the bottom. The rib cage is composed of 12 ribs on either side,

Figure 7.4 Lungs

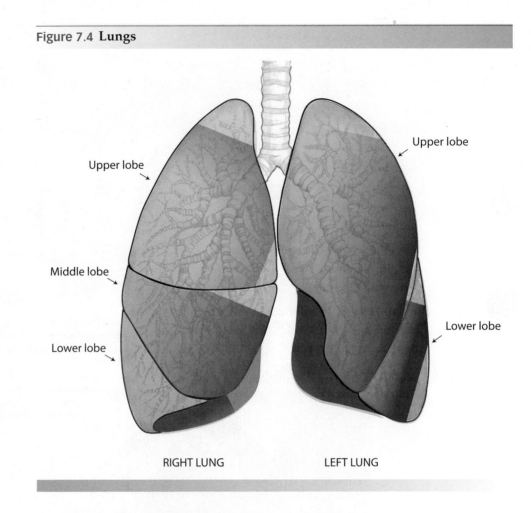

which are attached by means of cartilage to the sternum. The pectoral girdle also forms part of the rib cage. This structure includes the two collar bones (clavicles) in front and two shoulder blades (scapulae) at the back. Many muscles attach to the rib cage and to the pectoral girdle. The lungs are thus well protected and are maintained in an airtight fashion. In a healthy, uninjured individual, the only way that air can get into and out of the lungs is through the bronchial tree.

The abdominal wall forms the boundaries of the abdominal cavity and is divided into the posterior, lateral, and anterior walls. The abdominal wall is composed primarily of muscles and sheets of tendons that wrap around the front, back, and sides. The shape of the abdominal wall depends on the person's age, muscle mass, muscle tone, weight, and posture. The abdominal contents include all organs within the abdominal cavity, such as the stomach, intestines, lower esophagus, colon, appendix, liver, kidneys, pancreas, and spleen.

The diaphragm muscle forms the roof of the abdominal cavity and the floor of the thoracic cavity. This is a large, dome-shaped muscle that stretches from one side of the rib cage to the other. It attaches along the lower margins of the rib cage, the sternum, and the vertebral column (Seikel et al., 1997). The center portion of the diaphragm is composed of a flat sheet of tendon called the **central tendon**

Figure 7.5 Thoracic cavity

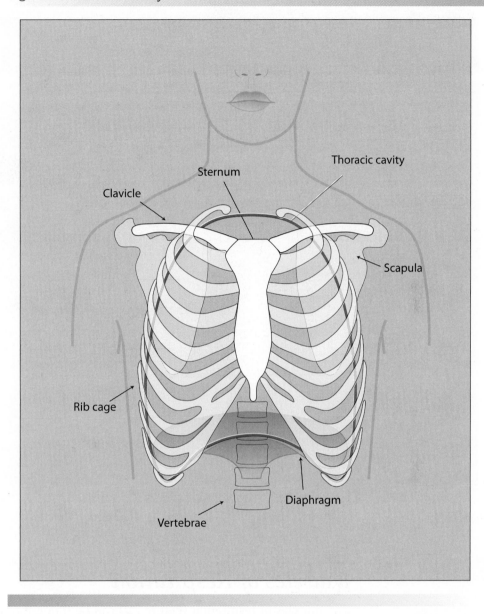

(Figure 7.6). The diaphragm is extremely sensitive to the shifting around of the abdominal contents, which plays an important role in breathing, particularly for speech. In its relaxed state, the diaphragm is shaped like an inverted bowl, in which position the middle portion extends somewhat upward. When it contracts, the diaphragm flattens out, with the middle portion lowering. When the diaphragm contracts, the volume of the thoracic cavity is increased in a vertical direction. In addition, because the diaphragm is attached to the lower rib cage, contraction raises the lower rib cage, and the thoracic cavity is thereby increased circumferentially as well (Hixon & Hoit, 2005).

Figure 7.6 Diaphragm

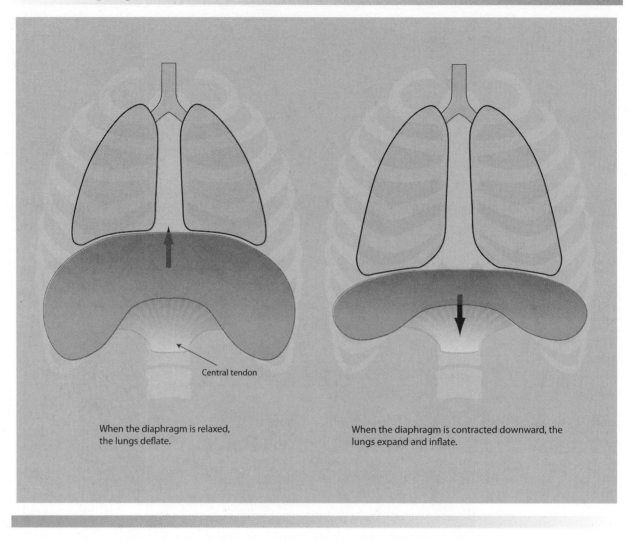

Central tendon

When the diaphragm is relaxed, the lungs deflate.

When the diaphragm is contracted downward, the lungs expand and inflate.

Muscles of Respiration

The muscles of respiration (Figure 7.7) can be thought of as either participating fully in the respiratory process or as helping in the process as the need arises. Many muscles can potentially be recruited for respiration depending on the kind and level of activity. For instance, just breathing quietly while reading a book requires less oxygen than does running, and fewer muscles are therefore involved in quiet breathing than in breathing while running. Muscle activity also changes for vegetative (life-sustaining) breathing and breathing for speech.

The diaphragm plays a crucial role in respiration by increasing and decreasing the volume of the thoracic cavity. Another very important set of muscles for respiration is the external intercostals. There are 11 pairs of external intercostal muscles that run between the ribs. Each pair originates on the lower surface of the rib, and the fibers course downward and forward at an oblique angle, inserting into the upper

Figure 7.7 Muscles of respiration

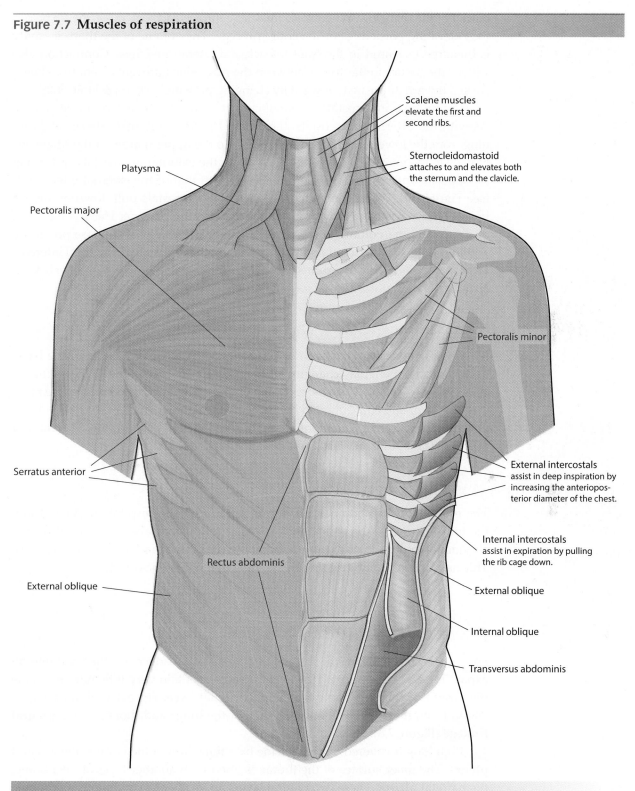

Scalene muscles elevate the first and second ribs.

Sternocleidomastoid attaches to and elevates both the sternum and the clavicle.

Platysma

Pectoralis major

Pectoralis minor

Serratus anterior

External intercostals assist in deep inspiration by increasing the anterioposterior diameter of the chest.

Internal intercostals assist in expiration by pulling the rib cage down.

Rectus abdominis

External oblique

External oblique

Internal oblique

Transversus abdominis

border of the rib below. When these muscles contract, each one raises the rib below, thus elevating portions of or the entire rib cage. The volume of the thoracic cavity is therefore increased in the front-to-back and lateral directions. Contraction also stiffens the tissues in the spaces between the ribs, which prevents them from being sucked inward or pushed outward by changing pressures (Hixon & Hoit, 2005).

The internal intercostals are similar in structure to the external intercostals. As with the external intercostals, there are 11 pairs of internal intercostals, running from the lower margin of the rib above to the upper margin of the rib below. However, the internal intercostals are deep to the external intercostals and run at an opposite angle (downward and backward) to that of the external intercostals (see Figure 7.7). When contracted, the internal intercostals pull down on the rib immediately above and lower portions of or the entire rib cage. This has the effect of decreasing the volume of the thoracic cavity. Because of their close proximity and the fact that they run in opposite directions, the external and internal intercostals together form a strong protective barrier for the lungs and heart, as well as an airtight cavity that is essential for respiration.

Accessory Muscles of Respiration

Many other muscles that attach to the rib cage, as well as muscles of the back, neck, and abdomen, play changing roles in respiration, according to the ventilatory needs of one's body. The more deeply an individual needs to breathe, the more muscles he or she will call on to help elevate the rib cage and enlarge the volume of the thoracic cavity. Therefore, many of these muscles are known as **accessory muscles of respiration**. They are listed in Table 7.1.

Muscles of the Abdomen

The muscles of the abdomen play an important part in respiration. As a group, the four muscles of the abdomen work as a unit to compress the contents of the abdominal cavity, which exerts upward pressure on the diaphragm (see Table 7.1). This has the effect of decreasing the volume of the thoracic cavity.

Pleural Linkage

For respiration to occur, the lungs must increase and decrease their volume by expanding and contracting. However, the lungs contain very little muscle, so the only way that they can move is by some external force. The external force is generated through the structure and linkage of the lungs and thorax, called **pleural linkage** (Figure 7.8).

Each lung is covered on the outside by a thin sheet of membrane, the **visceral pleura**. The inner surface of the thorax is lined with another layer of membrane, the **parietal pleura**. These two pleural layers are really one continuous membrane folded back on itself rather than two separate membranes. Between these two pleurae (singular: pleura) is a very small potential space, the **pleural space**, which contains **pleural fluid**. The pressure inside this space (**intrapleural pressure** [P_{pl}])

Table 7.1 Accessory Muscles of the Neck, Thorax, and Abdomen and Their Functions in Respiration

Muscle	Function
Neck	
Scalenes	Elevate ribs 1 and 2
Sternocleidomastoid	Elevate rib cage
Thorax	
Costal levators	Elevate rib cage
Pectoralis major	Elevate rib cage
Pectoralis minor	Depress ribs 3 to 5
Serratus anterior	Elevate ribs 1 to 9
Serratus posterior inferior	Depress ribs 9 to 12
Serratus posterior superior	Elevate rib cage
Subclavius	Elevate rib cage
Subcostals	Lower rib cage
Transverse thoracic	Depress rib cage
Abdomen	
External oblique	Compress abdomen
Internal oblique	Compress abdomen
Rectus abdominis	Compress abdomen
Transverse abdominis	Compress abdomen

is negative. The difference between the pressure inside the lungs (alveolar pressure [P_{alv}]) and the intrapleural pressure is called **transpulmonary pressure**. Under normal conditions, the transpulmonary pressure is always positive; intrapleural pressure is always negative; and alveolar pressure changes from slightly positive to slightly negative as a person breathes (West, 2005) (Table 7.2).

Table 7.2 Lung Pressures

Pressure	Location	Positive/Negative
Intrapleural pressure (P_{pl})	Between visceral and parietal pleurae	Negative
Alveolar pressure (P_{alv})	Within the lungs	Changes from positive to negative
Transpulmonary pressure	Difference between P_{pl} and P_{alv}	Positive

Figure 7.8 Pleural linkage

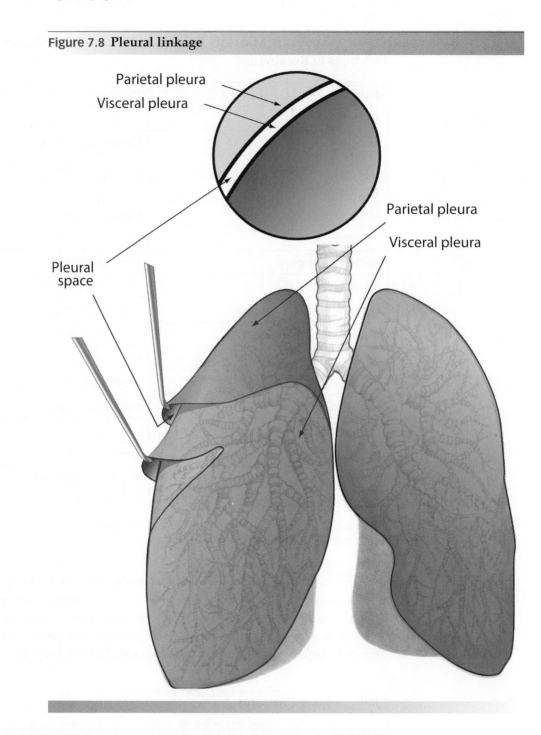

Parietal pleura
Visceral pleura
Parietal pleura
Visceral pleura
Pleural space

The pleural space is negative in pressure due to the opposing recoil forces of the lung and chest wall (Lai-Fook, 2004). That is, the elastic recoil of the lungs pulls the visceral layer inward, while the elastic tendency of the thorax pulls the parietal layer outward. The space between the pleurae is therefore permanently slightly expanded, which lowers the intrapleural pressure. When two structures are close together and the pressure between them is negative, the two tend to be sucked closer together. Because the pressure in the pleural space is negative, the lungs and thorax are permanently pulled close together and, in effect, function as one unit. Whatever the thorax does, or however the thorax moves, the lungs are drawn along as well. When the thorax expands due to muscular activity, the lungs expand as well. When the thorax decreases in volume, so do the lungs. Keep in mind that there are no structural attachments such as ligaments or tendons between the thorax and lungs, only the negative pressure in the pleural space keeps them connected. Without pleural linkage, the thorax would be in a more expanded state and the lungs would be in a more deflated state.

The pleurae not only play a crucial role in linking the lungs to the thoracic cavity but also provide a smooth, friction-free surface for the lungs and thorax to move against each other. If there was no fluid between the surfaces of the lungs and thorax, each cycle of respiration would bring the two directly into contact, creating friction and pain. The pleurae also serve as protection for the lungs. Each lung is encased in its own airtight visceral pleura. If one pleura is penetrated, such as by a knife or gunshot wound, the lung will collapse, a condition known as **pneumothorax**. However, the other lung will remain intact and airtight, and the individual's survival is not necessarily compromised.

Moving Air Into and Out of the Lungs

Air is moved into and out of the lungs by increasing and decreasing the air pressure inside the lungs. When P_{alv} is negative, air from the atmosphere is forced to enter the respiratory system, because air always moves from an area of higher pressure to an area of lower pressure. This is inhalation, or inspiration. When P_{alv} is positive, air from inside the lungs is forced out of the respiratory system to the atmosphere. This is the process of exhalation, or expiration.

Inhalation

To bring air into the lungs, the P_{alv} must become negative so that air will be forced to flow into the respiratory system. To decrease P_{alv}, the volume of the thoracic cavity and lungs must be enlarged. This is done by contracting the diaphragm, which flattens out and increases the vertical dimension of the thorax. Simultaneous contraction of the external intercostal muscles pulls the entire rib cage upward and slightly outward, increasing the back-to-front and side-to-side dimensions of the thorax. Due to the pleural linkage as well as to a drop in P_{pl}, the lungs expand to fill the increased space. As soon as the lungs begin to expand, the P_{alv} falls below P_{atmos}. As the P_{alv} decreases, air from the atmosphere flows into the respiratory system through either the mouth or nose. The air travels throughout the bronchial tree, eventually reaching the alveoli in the lungs. There the fresh oxygen diffuses into the blood capillaries surrounding the alveoli and is carried by the circulatory system to every cell in the body.

Exhalation

For air to exit the respiratory system, the P_{alv} must be higher than P_{atmos}, so the volume of the lungs must decrease. To achieve this, the diaphragm relaxes back to its dome-shaped position, decreasing the vertical dimension of the thorax. The external intercostal muscles relax, allowing the rib cage to return to its original position, and decreasing the back-to-front dimensions of the thorax. Correspondingly, the lungs also decrease in volume. As lung volume decreases, P_{alv} increases to about +2 cm H_2O relative to P_{atmos}. Air carrying carbon dioxide is brought to the alveoli via the circulatory system, diffuses into the alveoli, and flows out of the lungs and respiratory system. At the end of each inhalation and each exhalation the P_{alv} equals the P_{atmos}, and for a brief instant air does not move either into or out of the system. The cycle of breathing in and out then begins again.

Rate of Breathing

Respiration begins at the instant of birth and continues until the instant of death. Respiration occurs when we are awake and asleep, when we breathe vegetatively for life, and when we modify our breathing for speech. Rate of breathing is measured in breaths per minute (BPM). Table 7.3 shows how the rate of breathing changes from infancy to adulthood and how it also depends on level of activity.

Differences in the rate of breathing between children and adults occur because the structures and functions involved in respiration mature from infancy through childhood and adolescence. Numerous anatomical and physiological changes occur during the first year of life, including the following: The alveoli increase in number and size; the alveolar ducts increase in number; The alveolar surface area increases; lung size and weight increase; the thoracic cavity enlarges and changes in shape; the angle of the ribs changes with upright posture; rib cage muscle bulk increases; and pleural pressure becomes more negative (Boliek, Hixon, Watson, & Morgan, 1996). Maturation of the nervous system also contributes to the development of more mature breathing patterns with increasing age.

Table 7.3 **Rates of Breathing in Breaths per Minute (BPM) According to Age, Gender (male: M; female: F; not specified: NS), and Activity**

Age	Gender	Activity	BPM
Infants	NS	Awake	40–70
	NS	Asleep	24–116
5 years	NS		25
7 years	M + F		19
10 years	M		16
	F		18
15 years	NS		20
Adults	NS	Quiet breathing	12–18
Adults	M	Heavy activity	21
Adults	F	Heavy activity	30

SOURCE: Information from Seikel et al. (1997); Zemlin (1998); Hoit, Hixon, Watson, & Morgan (1990).

Lung Volumes and Capacities

Respiration deals with volumes and pressures of air and airflows. A system of classifying certain volumes of air in relation to respiration was established in 1950. These volume classifications are useful because they allow both laboratory and clinical measurements to be made in various populations of individuals. Volumes can be compared in children and adults, or between normally developing children and children with cerebral palsy, or between young adults and elderly adults, and so on. Using these volumes also allows comparisons of how breathing changes in different positions and with different tasks, including speech.

Respiratory volumes and capacities are measured using a method called spirometry. A **spirometer** is a device that measures the amount of air an individual inhales or exhales and the rate at which the air is moved into or out of his or her lungs. Spirometers record either volume (the amount of air exhaled or inhaled within a certain time) or flow (how fast the air flows in or out). Spirometers are widely used and are available in portable and/or computer-based versions. Lung volumes and capacities are measured in relation to resting expiratory level.

Resting Expiratory Level

Resting expiratory level (REL) refers to a state of equilibrium in the respiratory system. In this state, the natural tendency of the lungs to collapse is balanced by the natural tendency of the thorax to expand. If the lungs and thorax could be separated, the lungs would deflate instantly and the thorax would expand. The opposing forces of the lungs and thorax keep the lungs always slightly expanded and the thorax always slightly compressed in relation to each other. When P_{alv} equals P_{atmos}, these two opposing forces are in equilibrium, so air does not go into or out of the system. This state of affairs occurs very frequently; in fact, every time one completes a breath in or a breath out, the P_{alv} and P_{atmos} are in equilibrium for a brief instant before the next inhalation or exhalation begins again. The end point of a normal quiet exhalation is the resting expiratory level, which, because it occurs at the end of every exhalation, is also called the **end-expiratory level (EEL)**. At this level, there is still more air in the lungs that could be exhaled by using the expiratory muscles to pull down on the rib cage, compress the abdominal contents, and decrease lung volume even further.

Lung volumes and capacities are measured in relation to REL. Lung volumes are single, nonoverlapping values; lung capacities include two or more lung volumes. Volumes and capacities are expressed in liters (l) or milliliters (ml). Lung volumes and capacities are listed in Table 7.4.

Lung Volumes

Lung volumes refer to the amount of air in the lungs at a given time and how much of that air is used for various purposes, including speech (Solomon & Charron, 1998). Lung volumes include tidal volume (TV), inspiratory reserve volume (IRV), expiratory reserve volume (ERV), and residual volume (RV). Figure 7.9 shows graphically the relationships among various lung volumes and capacities.

Table 7.4 Lung Volumes and Capacities

Lung Volumes (single volumes, no overlap)	
Tidal volume (TV)	Volume of air inhaled and exhaled during a cycle of respiration
Inspiratory reserve volume (IRV)	Volume of air that can be inhaled above tidal volume
Expiratory reserve volume (ERV)	Volume of air that can be exhaled below tidal volume
Residual volume (RV)	Volume of air remaining in the lungs after a maximum expiration and that cannot be voluntarily expelled
Lung Capacities (including two or more volumes)	
Vital capacity (VC)	Volume of air that can be exhaled after a maximum inhalation (IRV + TV + ERV)
Functional residual capacity (FRC)	Volume of air remaining in the lungs and airways at the end-expiratory level (ERV + RV)
Total lung capacity (TLC)	Total amount of air the lungs can hold (TV + IRV + ERV + RV)
Inspiratory capacity (IC)	Maximum volume of air that can be inspired from end-expiratory level (TV + IRV)

Tidal volume

Tidal volume (TV) refers to the volume of air inhaled and exhaled during a cycle of respiration. Tidal volume varies, depending on age, build, and degree of physical activity. Values for adult males during quiet breathing range from around 600 to 750 ml (0.6–0.75 l). A mild degree of physical exertion increases TV to approximately 1670 ml. Further increasing physical activity increases TV to about 2030 ml (Zemlin, 1998). In general, females inhale and exhale less air during each cycle of breathing than do males, about 450 ml for quiet breathing (Seikel et al., 1997). Children, with their smaller lungs, have a lower TV than adults, ranging from approximately 200 ml at age 7 to just under 400 ml at age 13. The gender difference in TV seen in adult males and females becomes more evident in children as they develop. Table 7.5 shows that at ages 7 and 10, boys and girls have similar values for TV. By age 13 boys have a larger TV, and by age 16 boys and girls have attained essentially adult values of 560 ml for boys and 410 ml for girls.

Inspiratory reserve volume

Inspiratory reserve volume (IRV) refers to the amount of air that can be inhaled above TV. If one breathes in normally, considerably more air can still be inhaled

Figure 7.9 Lung volumes and capacities

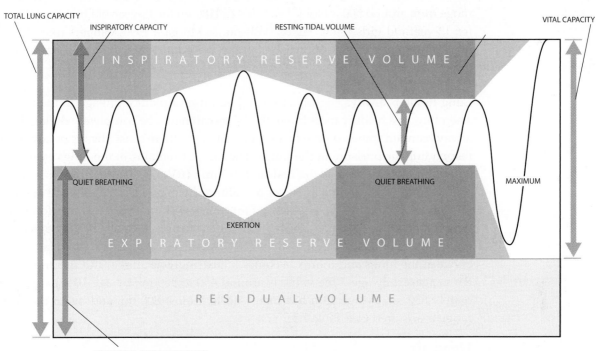

instead of breathing it out right away. This additional amount of air is the IRV. The value for adults ranges from about 1500 to 2500 ml. The IRV can be used by speakers to obtain more air for a particularly long or particularly loud utterance.

Expiratory reserve volume

Expiratory reserve volume (ERV) is the amount of air that can be exhaled below TV. Following a normal tidal exhalation, it is possible to continue exhaling for a while.

Table 7.5 Lung Volumes and Capacities (ml) for Boys (B) and Girls (G) at Ages 7, 10, 13, and 16

	7		10		13		16	
	B	G	B	G	B	G	B	G
TLC	2120	2090	3140	2980	4330	3740	6200	4980
VC	1670	1580	2510	2340	3550	2990	5080	3780
IC	1140	1090	1740	1550	2370	2050	3260	2430
FRC	980	970	1400	1430	1970	1690	2940	2560
ERV	530	480	770	780	1180	940	1810	1350
RV	450	490	630	640	790	760	1120	1210
TV	200	190	260	280	390	350	560	410

SOURCE: Information from Hoit, Hixon, Watson, & Morgan (1990).

Some muscle movement around the abdominal area may be felt as ERV is accessed. Values for this volume in adults range from 1000 to 2000 ml. Values for children range from around 500 ml for 7-year-olds to 1180 ml for 13-year-old boys and 940 ml for 13-year-old girls (Hoit, Hixon, Watson, & Morgan, 1990). Singers might use a large portion of ERV to sustain a long phrase without replenishing the air.

Residual volume

Lung tissue is always slightly stretched because of pleural linkage to the thorax. Therefore, in a healthy individual, the lungs can never be completely deflated and always contain some volume of air. Consequently, there must always be some corresponding air pressure in the lungs. The air that remains in the lungs even after a maximum exhalation is the **residual volume (RV)**. This amount of air, around 1000 to 1500 ml in adults, can never be voluntarily expired. Newborns do not have the same amount of RV as adults. Infant lungs are much larger in relation to the thorax than are adult lungs. Thus, infant lungs are not expanded to the degree that adult lungs are, resulting in a smaller RV. As the child matures, the relationship between the lungs and thorax becomes increasingly adultlike, and the amount of RV increases. By age 7 the value is around 450 to 500 ml, by age 10 it is approximately 630 ml, by age 13 it has increased to almost 800 ml, and by 16 the adult range is acquired (see Table 7.5).

Dead air

A small amount of volume of air in the lungs and airways is known as **dead air**. This is about 150 ml worth of air that is inhaled but is not involved in O_2–CO_2 exchange (Klocke, 2006). This air, at any time, is in the upper respiratory passage and in the bronchial tree. It is the very last to be inhaled and is therefore the first to be exhaled during the next cycle of respiration (Zemlin, 1998). Correspondingly, the last 150 ml of air that is expired from the alveoli during exhalation remains in the dead air spaces and is the first to reenter the alveoli (even though it still has CO_2 in it).

Lung Capacities

Lung capacities combine various lung volumes, and include vital capacity (VC), functional residual capacity (FRC), inspiratory capacity (IC), and total lung capacity (TLC). One of the most important of these, in terms of speech production, is vital capacity.

Vital capacity

Vital capacity (VC) is the combination of tidal volume, inspiratory reserve volume, and expiratory reserve volume (TV + IRV + ERV). Worded slightly differently, VC is the maximum amount of air that a person can exhale after having inhaled as deeply as possible. Vital capacity represents the total amount of air available for all purposes, including speech. It does not include residual volume, which is not under voluntary control. Like the other lung volumes, VC depends on the age and size of the individual. For example, 5-year-old girls and boys have a VC of about 1000 ml and 1250 ml, respectively (Zemlin, 1998). By age 7, VC is around 1500 to

1600 ml, and it increases to about 2000 ml by age 9. By 13 years of age, the amount has increased by approximately 1000 ml for boys and 500 ml for girls. By age 17 years, boys have a VC of around 4500 ml, while the value for girls is about 3750 ml. The average value of 5000 ml is typically used for VC in adults. Vital capacity has been shown to decrease slightly with advancing age, which some researchers have linked to a decrease in voice production capabilities in older adults.

Functional residual capacity

Functional residual capacity (FRC) is the amount of air remaining in the lungs and airways at the end-expiratory level. Thus, FRC combines the expiratory reserve volume and the residual volume (ERV + RV). FRC averages approximately 2500 to 3500 ml in young adults. In 7-year-olds, FRC is a little under 1000 ml, and it increases to the 1400 ml range at age 10 and to around 1700 to 2000 ml by 13 years. By age 16, adult levels are reached.

Inspiratory capacity

Inspiratory capacity (IC) is the amount of air that can be inhaled from end-expiratory level and is the combination of TV plus IRV (TV + IRV). Consistent with age-related increases in tidal volume and inspiratory reserve volume, IC increases from around 1100 ml in 7-year-old children to approximately 2500 to 3500 ml at age 16.

Total lung capacity

Total lung capacity (TLC) refers to the total amount of air that the lungs are capable of holding, including tidal volume, inspiratory reserve volume, expiratory reserve volume, and residual volume (TV + IRV + ERV + RV). Like the other volumes and capacities, TLC is developmental, increasing with age and influenced by gender. Values for 7-year-old boys and girls are in the 2000 ml range; 10-year-olds have a TLC ranging from the high-2000s to low-3000s ml. By age 13, a gender difference emerges, with boys averaging around the mid-4000 ml range and girls around the 3700 ml range. By age 16, the difference is more pronounced, with males demonstrating values in the 6000 ml range and female values in the 5000 ml area.

As can be seen in Table 7.5, lung volumes and capacities increase from infancy through puberty, and adult values are apparent by age 16. Lung volumes and capacities seem to stay stable until the later adult years, when they start to decrease with advancing age. Hoit and Hixon (1987) provided averages for some lung volumes and capacities for three age groups of adults: young adults (25-year-olds), middle-aged adults (50-year-olds), and elderly adults (75-year-olds). Table 7.6 shows that both vital capacity and expiratory reserve volume decrease somewhat with increasing age. This decrease may be implicated in some kinds of speech problems. Table 7.7 provides a comparison of lung volumes and capacities in children and adults at various ages.

Lung volumes and capacities are often expressed as percentages of VC. REL is around 38 to 40 percent VC in the upright position. This means that one can inhale

Table 7.6 Group Means of Three Age Groups of Subjects (25, 50, and 75 years) for Some Lung Volumes and Capacities, in ml

	25	50	75
TLC	6740	7050	6630
VC	5350	5090	4470
FRC	3120	3460	3440
ERV	1730	1500	1280

SOURCE: Information from Hoit & Hixon (1987).

60 to 62 percent more air above REL (IRV) in order to fill the lungs to their maximum capacity. Conversely, at REL the lungs still hold 38 to 40 percent of air that could be exhaled down to 0 percent VC. Below 38 to 40 percent VC, the individual is drawing on ERV to exhale. Figure 7.10 is a schematic representation of some lung volumes expressed as percentages of VC.

Table 7.7 Selected Respiratory Measurements (in l) at Different Ages for Males and Females

Measure	Age	Male Mean	Female Mean
TLC	7	2.12	2.07
	10	3.14	2.98
	13	4.33	3.74
	16	6.20	4.98
	25	6.74	5.03
	50	7.05	5.31
	75	6.63	4.86
VC	7	1.67	1.58
	10	2.51	2.34
	13	3.55	2.99
	16	5.08	3.78
	25	5.35	3.93
	50	5.09	3.60
	75	4.47	2.94
IC	7	1.14	1.09
	10	1.74	1.55
	13	2.37	2.05
	16	3.26	2.43
	25	3.62	2.61
	50	3.59	2.38
	75	3.19	2.27

Table 7.7 (*Continued*)

Measure	Age	Male Mean	Female Mean
FRC	7	0.98	0.97
	10	1.40	1.43
	13	1.97	1.69
	16	2.94	2.56
	25	3.12	2.42
	50	3.46	2.93
	75	3.44	2.59
ERV	7	0.53	0.48
	10	0.77	0.78
	13	1.18	0.94
	16	1.81	1.35
	25	1.73	1.32
	50	1.50	1.22
	75	1.28	0.67
RV	7	0.45	0.49
	10	0.63	0.64
	13	0.79	0.76
	16	1.12	1.21
	25	1.39	1.10
	50	1.97	1.71
	75	2.16	1.92
RTV	7	0.20	0.19
	10	0.26	0.28
	13	0.39	0.35
	16	0.56	0.41
	25	0.56	0.46
	50	0.71	0.55
	75	0.53	0.54

Key to the abbreviations: Total lung capacity-TLC, vital capacity-VC, inspiratory capacity-IC, functional residual capacity-FRC, expiratory reserve volume-ERV, residual volume-RV, resting tidal volume-RTV.

SOURCES: Information from Melcon et al. (1989); Hoit & Hixon (1987); Hoit et al. (1990).

Differences between Breathing for Life and Breathing for Speech

Although it sounds like a simple enough process, breathing is actually an amazingly complex function that is integrated with other body functions, including metabolism, regulation of body temperature, fluid and acid–base balance, and

Figure 7.10 Schematic of lung volume as a percentage of vital capacity

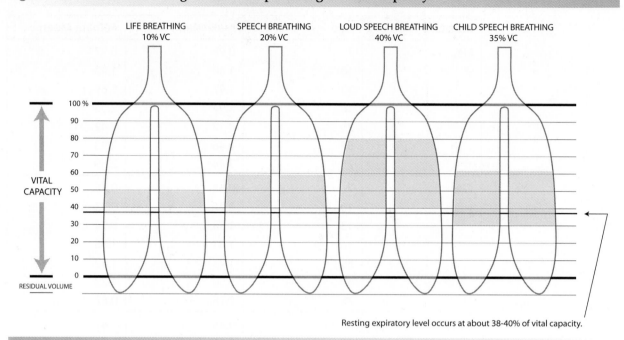

LIFE BREATHING
10% VC

SPEECH BREATHING
20% VC

LOUD SPEECH BREATHING
40% VC

CHILD SPEECH BREATHING
35% VC

VITAL CAPACITY

RESIDUAL VOLUME

Resting expiratory level occurs at about 38-40% of vital capacity.

others (Boliek et al., 1996). Furthermore, breathing for vegetative purposes (often called life breathing or quiet breathing) and breathing to generate a power supply for speech involve different motor strategies. Breathing for life is usually (although not always) an unconscious, automatic process; the rate and extent of breathing are determined by the needs of one's body at a particular moment in time. An individual takes in greater amounts of air when performing vigorous exercise than when sitting quietly and reading a book, for example. These different levels of air intake are determined reflexively, depending on the O_2 and CO_2 levels in the blood.

Breathing for speech complicates the process because the need for appropriate ventilation is integrated with linguistic considerations. These include the need to take breaths at linguistically appropriate places in order not to interrupt the flow of speech, the need to take an appropriate amount of air for the utterance to be produced, and the need to generate an adequate length of exhalation to be able to say more than a few syllables in one breath. The respiratory system is also involved in the prosodic aspects of speech, such as variations in F_0 and intensity, syllable and word stress, and emphasis (Metz & Schiavetti, 1995). Human speech represents fine control and precise neural integration of the activity of seventy to eighty muscles from respiratory, laryngeal, pharyngeal, palatal, and facial muscle groups (Davis, Zhang, Winkworth, & Bandler, 1996). For speech breathing, the automatic nerve signals to the many different muscles involved in respiration and speech production must be replaced by voluntary nerve signals to the same muscles (Smith & Denny, 1990).

Based on ventilatory, linguistic, and prosodic demands, five major changes occur when switching from breathing for life to breathing for speech: the location of air intake, the ratio of time for inhalation versus exhalation, the volume of air inhaled per cycle, the muscle activity for exhalation, and chest wall shape. See Table 7.8.

Table 7.8 **Five Changes That Occur When Switching from Life Breathing to Speech Breathing**

Change	Life	Speech
Location of air intake	Nose	Mouth
Ratio of time for inhalation versus exhalation	Inhale: 40% Exhale: 60%	Inhale: 10% Exhale: 90%
Volume of air	500 ml 10% VC	Variable, depending on length and loudness of utterance, 20 to 25% VC
Muscle activity for exhalation	Passive: Muscles of thorax and diaphragm relax	Active: Thoracic and abdominal muscles contract to control recoil of rib cage and diaphragm
Chest wall position	Abdomen displaced outward relative to rib cage	Abdomen displaced inward relative to rib cage

Location of Air Intake

Both inhalation and exhalation in life breathing typically occur through the nose, unless the individual has some kind of blockage due to a cold, enlarged adenoids, or deviated septum. Breathing through the nose is healthy because inhaled air is warmed, moistened, and filtered as it passes through the nasal cavities. Inhaling through the nose reportedly increases the temperature and relative humidity (RH) of the air from 22 degrees C and 30 to 40 percent RH up to 31 to 32 degrees C and 95 to 99 percent RH at the level of the pharynx (Bien, Okla, van As-Brooks, & Ackerstaff, 2010; Zuur et al., 2009). Inhaling and exhaling for speech occurs through the oral cavity. This is a much more efficient location for speech breathing because it allows for a quicker inhalation and production of oral sounds on the exhalation.

Ratio of Time for Inhalation Versus Exhalation

In life breathing, the proportion of the respiratory cycle taken for inhalation is nearly the same as for exhalation, with inhalation consuming about 40 percent of the cycle and exhalation taking up about 60 percent of the cycle. The ratio of inhalation time to exhalation time changes dramatically for speech breathing. Inhalation time shortens to about 10 percent of the total cycle, whereas exhalation time extends to about 90 percent of the cycle. Exhalation for speech can last up to 20 to 25 s, instead of the approximately 2-second duration in life breathing. This ratio is efficient for speech, which is produced on the expiratory phase of respiration. Speech would be very choppy if one had to pause every few seconds for an air refill and if each inhalation took 2 seconds. By shortening the inhalatory phase and lengthening the exhalation phase, one can generate a smooth and uninterrupted stream of speech. This pattern of quick inspirations and more extended exhalations holds true even for infants and very young children.

Volume of Air Inhaled and Exhaled per Cycle

Tidal volume for life breathing is approximately 500 ml on average, depending on age and gender. 500 ml is 10 percent of the average vital capacity of around 5000 ml. Inhalation for life breathing begins at REL (38–40 percent of VC) and goes up by 10 to 12 percent, to 50 percent of VC. The individual then exhales back down to REL. The volume inhaled for speech is variable, depending on the length and loudness of the upcoming utterance. Volumes for normal conversation typically occur in the midrange of VC (40–60 percent) and are around twice as much as those involved in life breathing (Porter, Hogue, & Tobey, 1995; Solomon & Charron, 1998). At 60 percent of VC, the corresponding alveolar pressure is approximately 10 cm H_2O, which is sufficient for most normal conversational utterances. The midvolume range of VC is highly efficient because it requires very little respiratory muscle activity (Huber, 2008). For longer and louder utterances, speakers inhale to higher lung volumes and continue the exhalation into lower volumes (Huber, 2008). Thus, speakers use around 20 to 25 percent of vital capacity per utterance, compared to 10 percent for quiet breathing. Percentage of VC increases for loud speech to around 40 percent of VC. Inhalation for loud speech is initiated at higher percentages of vital capacity (up to approximately 80 percent). Children use a higher percentage of VC for speech, generally beginning speech at around 65 percent VC and ending at about 30 percent. Children also exhale below REL for speech purposes much more than adults (Stathopoulos, 1997). Classically trained singers use considerably larger volumes during singing, sometimes even using the full vital capacity (Watson & Hixon, 1985; Watson, Hixon, Stathopoulos, & Sullivan, 1990).

Muscle Activity for Exhalation

For both life and speech breathing, inspiration is an active muscular process requiring contraction of the diaphragm and external intercostal muscles to increase the volume of the thoracic cavity and lungs. For life breathing, exhalation is a passive process, relying solely on elastic recoil forces. By contrast, muscle activity plays a crucial role in controlling exhalation for speech. To understand the difference between exhaling for life compared to speech, we need to examine the process of exhalation in more detail.

During exhalation, the thoracic cavity and lungs must decrease in volume in order for the P_{alv} to increase and cause the outflow of air from the lungs. The decrease in volume is achieved by three forces that cause the thorax and lungs to return to their original positions. First, gravity acts to pull downward on the raised rib cage. Second, the external intercostal muscles relax, allowing the rib cage to return to its original position. The diaphragm also relaxes and resumes its dome shape, thus decreasing the vertical dimension of the thorax. Third, elasticity of the respiratory tissues and lungs returns the tissues that have been extended back to their original positions. Together, these restoring forces are called **recoil forces**. The more the thoracic cavity and lungs are expanded during inspiration, the greater the recoil forces that are generated.

The air pressures generated by the passive recoil forces are referred to as **relaxation pressures**. Relaxation pressures are graphed on a relaxation pressure curve, with VC on the vertical axis and P_{alv} on the horizontal axis (Figure 7.11). The 0 point represents resting expiratory level, the state of equilibrium during which

Figure 7.11 Relaxation pressures

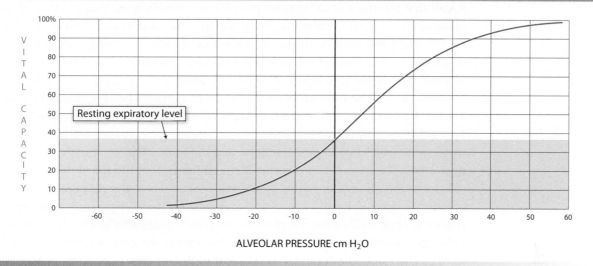

ALVEOLAR PRESSURE cm H₂O

$P_{alv} = P_{atmos}$ (38–40 percent VC). Numbers to the right of 0 represent positive pressures; numbers to the left of 0 represent negative pressures.

After an inspiration, recoil forces begin to return the structures to the rest position, generating a positive P_{alv}. As shown in Figure 7.11, at 100 percent VC, P_{alv} is around 60 cm H₂O. As lung volume decreases, the positive P_{alv} decreases as well. Below REL, the P_{alv} becomes negative, and the system begins to recoil in the inspiratory direction. At lung volumes above 38 percent VC, the inspiratory process requires muscular force, and expiratory forces are passive. At lung volumes below 38 percent VC, the expiratory process requires muscular force, and the inspiratory process is passive (Zemlin, 1998).

For speech, one inhales up to approximately 60 percent VC, yielding a P_{alv} of about 10 cm H₂O (Figure 7.11). For speech purposes, rather than allowing passive recoil forces to operate, the rate of recoil must be controlled in order to prolong the exhalation. When speaking at pressures above REL, the muscles of inspiration continue to contract. The continuing contraction in the inspiratory direction generates a counteracting checking force that prevents the thoracic cavity and lungs from deflating too quickly. To access the expiratory reserve volume and continue speaking below REL, the abdominal muscles are recruited. Contraction of the abdominal muscles forces the abdominal wall to press inwards on the abdominal contents. The abdominal contents are therefore pushed headward against the diaphragm. The continuing upward pressure on the diaphragm further decreases the volume of the thorax and lungs so air continues to be exhaled. The internal intercostal muscles may also contract to depress the rib cage. Speaking at lung volumes below REL thus requires considerable muscular effort in order to prevent the rib cage from recoiling outward in an inspiratory direction. The degree of muscle activity for speech exhalation varies, depending on factors such as the intensity of the utterance, emphasis on specific parts of the utterance, and linguistic stress on particular words and syllables.

Chest Wall Shape

Recall that the chest wall includes the rib cage, diaphragm, abdominal wall, and abdominal contents. When breathing for life, the abdominal wall is displaced slightly outward relative to the rib cage. For speech breathing, the abdomen is displaced further inward relative to the rib cage, causing the abdominal contents to push the diaphragm upward (Bailey & Hoit, 2002; Kalliakosta, Mandros, & Tzelepis, 2007). The upward pressure on the diaphragm has the effect of expanding the lower rib cage. The muscle fibers of the diaphragm are stretched by the upward displacement of the abdominal contents; this enables the muscle fibers to generate quick, strong contractions that are necessary for speech (Kalliakosta et al., 2007; Solomon & Charron, 1998). In addition, keeping the abdomen inward relative to the rib cage provides a platform against which the rib cage can move to control the varying lung volumes and air pressures necessary in connected speech (Bailey & Hoit, 2002). Movement of the rib cage is more efficient in changing lung volumes than movement of the abdomen because of the greater surface area of the lung (about three-quarters) that is adjacent to the rib cage (Connaghan, Moore, & Higashakawa, 2004; Kalliakosta et al., 2007). Therefore, the rib cage wall needs to move only one-quarter of the distance that the abdominal wall does to achieve the same change in alveolar pressure (Kalliakosta et al., 2007).

Speech Breathing for Isolated Vowels and Connected Speech

Although the basic process of speech breathing is the same, there are some differences in the control of respiration for isolated utterances such as vowel prolongations and connected speech. Sustaining a vowel requires a steady outflow of air, despite changes in lung volumes and pressures. It has been shown that for this type of utterance, lung volume decreases at a constant rate, while P_{alv} increases abruptly at the beginning of the utterance, maintains a steady level throughout the utterance, and then decreases abruptly at the end of the utterance. The volumes of the rib cage wall and abdominal wall decrease throughout the utterance (Hixon & Hoit, 2005). The inspiratory and expiratory muscles are active during the entire utterance, with different muscles contracting and/or relaxing at different times throughout the utterance in order to maintain the steady outflow of air required to sustain the vowel prolongation.

Connected speech is more variable than a sustained vowel in terms of pitch and loudness changes, rate of speech, duration of the utterance, and linguistic stress. Despite these variations, a steady outflow of air and relatively constant P_{alv} are still required. Speakers tend to position the chest wall at the beginning of the breath group for the utterance, usually between the end of the inspiratory phase and the beginning of the expiratory phase (Hixon & Hoit, 2005). During this transition, the abdominal wall is pulled inward and the rib cage wall is held outward to facilitate optimal positioning for speech. During connected speech, the rib cage wall and abdominal wall volume decrease at relatively constant rates, with a faster rate of decrease for the rib cage wall (Hixon & Hoit, 2005). As the utterance continues, the rib cage wall and particularly the abdominal wall continue to exert muscle force in order to maintain the positive P_{alv} and expiratory outflow. When small and quick changes in P_{alv} are needed in order to stress specific syllables or words, the contracted abdominal wall provides a stable basis and the muscles of the rib cage wall contract to effect these changes (Hixon & Hoit, 2005). Thus, for speech breathing, the abdominal muscles are continuously activated to facilitate movement of the diaphragm for quick inspiration and movement of the rib cage for rapid adjustments during expiration (Hixon & Hoit, 2005).

Breathing Patterns for Speech

Measurements of pressure, flow, volume, and chest wall shape have been used to establish patterns of breathing for speech. As discussed above, during speech the abdomen is smaller and the rib cage is larger than in their respective relaxation positions. This positioning is efficient for speech, because when the abdominal wall moves inward, it pushes the diaphragm upward and expands the lower rib cage. This allows the diaphragm to make quick, strong contractions, which facilitates the quick inspirations and the constantly changing pressures needed for speech (Hixon, Goldman, & Mead, 1973). During speech, the rib cage and abdomen move continuously to generate the necessary changes in lung volume. Most lung movement is accomplished through rib cage adjustments because a greater portion of the surface of the lung is adjacent to the rib cage than to the diaphragm. Therefore, the rib cage is more efficient than the abdominal wall at moving air from the lungs (Solomon & Charron, 1998). Research using kinematic analysis has shown that just before a person starts to speak, he or she automatically positions the chest wall in such a way as to quickly and efficiently generate the necessary pressures (Baken & Cavallo, 1981). These chest wall movements (known as **prephonatory chest wall movements**) are influenced by the speaking task, such as the length of the upcoming utterance. Prephonatory chest wall movements also depend on the person's lung volume when speech is initiated. At typical lung volumes, the respiratory structures can passively generate P_{alv} of around 5 to 8 cm H_2O, which is more than enough for normal speech. Therefore, the chest wall might not need much setting up for speech. At lower lung volumes that do not produce enough P_{alv} for speech, the chest wall may need to quickly make muscular adjustments immediately before beginning to speak (McFarland & Smith, 1992). Milstein and Watson (2004) examined the percentage of VC for target phrases used by adult men and women at typical, high, and low lung volumes. For the low lung volumes, speakers initiated the phrase at an average of 19 percent VC and terminated at an average of 14 percent. For the typical condition, participants initiated speech at an average of 51 percent VC and terminated the phrase at an average of 45 percent. In the high-volume task, individuals began the phrase at an average of around 89 percent VC and ended around 80 percent. As the lung volume increased, speakers' intensity levels increased as well. Voice quality changes were also apparent between conditions, and listeners were able to use the quality cues to identify speech produced at lower and higher levels of lung volumes.

Analysis of movement patterns (kinematic analysis) has also provided information about the lung volumes used for speech. Recall that speech is produced in the midrange of VC (Manifold & Murdoch, 1993; Mitchell, Hoit, & Watson, 1996). However, lung volumes differ both between individuals and within individuals producing different utterances. The amount of air breathed in is strongly influenced by the loudness of the intended utterance. When speaking very loudly, one inhales a greater volume of air in a shorter amount of time in order to preserve speech fluency while meeting the normal bodily demands of gas exchange (Russell, Cerny, & Stathopoulos, 1998). On the other hand, during very soft speech, individuals typically begin utterances at a much lower lung volume.

Kinematic analysis has also shown that lung volumes, pressures, and flows are influenced by linguistic considerations, such as clause boundaries and the number of clauses in a sentence (Winkworth, Davis, Adams, & Ellis, 1995). People tend to time their inspirations with naturally occurring breaks in the linguistic message, which enhances the overall fluency of speech. Pauses for breath that do not occur at grammatical junctures disrupt the flow of speech and result in the perception of disfluent speech. It has been reported that individuals who stutter often pause at linguistically inappropriate places in a sentence, which contributes to the perception of stuttering (Eisen & Ferrand, 1995).

Another speech breathing pattern relates to the complexity of the speaking activity. More complex speaking tasks seem to result in a smaller number of syllables per breath group, slower speaking rate, and greater average volume of air expended per syllable (Mitchell et al., 1996). The type of phoneme being said also influences respiration. Voiceless stops and fricatives require a high flow of air through the system, while voiced stops and fricatives need a lower flow (Russell & Stathopoulos, 1988). Differences also exist in respiratory function between regular conversational speech and whispering. During whispering, individuals tend to terminate breath groups at lower lung volumes, use fewer syllables per breath group, and expend more air per syllable. Also, P_{trach} is lower when a person whispers than during normal conversational speech (Stathopoulos, Hoit, Hixon, Watson, & Solomon, 1991). Table 7.9 lists typical patterns of speech breathing.

Table 7.9 **Patterns of Speech Breathing Related to Chest Wall Shape, Volume, and Linguistic Influences**

Chest Wall Shape
Abdomen smaller, rib cage larger than during relaxation
Volume
Midrange of VC Approximately twice the volume of quiet tidal breathing
Linguistic influences
Inspirations timed with naturally occurring breaks in the linguistic message Complexity of speaking task Intended loudness Type of phoneme Whispering

Changes in Speech Breathing Over the Lifespan

Like other neuromotor skills, efficient speech breathing is a process that develops over time, in conjunction with anatomical and physiological changes in the young child's respiratory system. Speech breathing progresses through periods of emergence, refinement, and adaptation (Boliek, Hixon, Watson, & Jones, 2009). The emergence period extends from birth to age 3 years. During this period, there are striking differences in respiratory biomechanics between infants and adults. Infants produce changes in lung volume by displacing the diaphragm rather than the rib cage because the rib cage is unable to produce sufficient inspiratory forces (Reilly & Moore, 2009). Infants also show a different relationship between the lungs and thorax whereby the passive forces that collapse the lungs are around three times stronger than the passive forces that expand the rib cage (Papastamelos, Panitch, England, & Allen, 1995). In adults the FRC and EEL both occur, as the opposing recoil forces of the lungs and thorax are in equilibrium. Because of the stronger passive lung recoil in the infant, babies must use inspiratory muscle activity during expiration in order to maintain their EEL at a much higher volume than their FRC (Kosch & Stark, 1984). Despite these differences, infants and young children initiate vocalizations in the midrange of predicted VC and at the beginning of the exhalation, similar to older children and adults (Boliek et al., 1996; Boliek, Hixon, Watson, & Morgan, 1997; Boliek et al., 2009; Hoit et al., 1990). As the baby develops, anatomical and physiological changes result in large changes in the biomechanical features of the chest wall (Reilly & Moore, 2009). These include increases in the size of the lungs with associated increases in lung volumes (Table 7.8); increases in the diameter and relative stiffness of the airways with an overall decrease in airway resistance; and ossification of the ribs, spinal column, and sternum, resulting in increased chest wall stiffness and compliance of the respiratory system (Boliek et al., 2009; Reilly & Moore, 2009).

Refinement is defined as the time during which speech in the young child has emerged but continues to progress toward the adult model (Boliek et al., 2009). Refinement of speech breathing is a long developmental process that continues well into the adolescent years. During the adaptation period, the child's efficiency in breathing for speech continues to become increasingly adultlike as he or she continues to grow physically and, at the same time, becomes more linguistically adept. Lung width, lung length, and total capacity continue to increase until 14 to 16 years of age (Stathopoulos & Sapienza, 1997).

Features of Speech Breathing in Children

Because of their smaller airways, young children generate higher pressures for speech than older children, and older children often use higher pressures than adults (Stathopoulos, 1986). 4- to 6-year-old children have been shown to terminate their breath groups below EEL, often near the lowest portions of the range (Boliek et al., 2009; Stathopoulos & Sapienza, 1997). Young children tend to inhale more deeply and begin speaking at larger lung volumes than do older children and adults (Solomon & Charron, 1998). This may be in order to take advantage of higher passive recoil forces at relatively high lung volumes. The larger lung volumes are reflected in the percentages of VC children use for speech purposes

Table 7.10 **Mean Percentage of Rib Cage Contribution (% RC) to Volume Change in Resting Tidal Breathing at Different Ages**

Age	Male	Female
4	52.85	52.85
5	61.35	61.35
6	51.07	51.07
7	69.36	60.50
10	64.64	59.51
13	75.51	63.39
16	71.23	80.44
25	80.95	69.71
50	80.59	79.38
75	85.02	89.39

SOURCES: Information from Boliek et al. (2009); Hoit & Hixon (1987); Hoit, Hixon, Watson, & Morgan (1990); Melcon et al. (1989).

compared to adults. Solomon and Charron (1998) found that infants use 25 percent and toddlers 13 percent of their predicted VC for a variety of vocalizations. Hoit, Hixon, Watson, and Morgan (1990) reported that 7-year-old children used approximately 18 percent VC for reading and conversational speech compared to older children, who used 12 to 18 percent VC. The percentage of rib cage contribution to changes in lung volume increases as the child develops. Table 7.10 shows the percentage of rib cage contribution increasing from around 50 percent at age 4 years to 70 to 80 percent at age 16 years.

Features of Speech Breathing in Older Adults

Changes occur in older adults' respiratory patterns for speech, resulting from changes in anatomy and physiology over the span of years. Changes include a more convex thoracic shape, increased ossification and calcification of the costal cartilages, decreased strength of the respiratory muscles, loss of alveolar surface tension and pulmonary capillary blood volume, and decreased overall lung size (Huber & Spruill, 2008; Sperry & Klich, 1992). These changes result in decreased chest wall compliance; diminished elastic recoil pressures in the midlung volume range; reductions in VC, IRV, and ERV; and increases in RV (e.g., Hoit & Hixon, 1987; Huber, 2008; Huber & Spruill, 2008; Sperry & Klich, 1992). Sperry and Klich (1992) compared younger and older women's speech breathing. The groups were found to differ in lung volumes and also in speech breathing patterns. For example, the younger group had an average VC of 3356 ml, and the older group had an average VC of 2456 ml. The older adults did not start to phonate immediately after inhaling and wasted two to three times more air than did the younger speakers. To overcome the changes in respiratory efficiency, older individuals have been shown to initiate speech at higher lung volumes (i.e., inhale more deeply), with correspondingly higher recoil pressures. In comparison to younger adults, older adults have been reported to demonstrate larger rib cage and lung volume initiations and excursions, larger volumes of air expended per speech breath and per syllable, and fewer syllables per breath (Hoit & Hixon, 1987; Huber & Spruill, 2008; Melcon, Hoit, & Hixon, 1989). One reason for initiating speech at higher lung volumes may be that inspiratory muscle force is better preserved than expiratory muscle function. Thus, it may be easier for older speakers to achieve higher lung volumes to begin speech than to use expiratory muscle effort to go to lower lung volumes (Huber & Spruill, 2008). Huber and Spruill (2008) noted that older adults also moved the abdomen for speech breathing more than younger adults, possibly as a compensation for the reduced elastic recoil of the lungs and thorax. However, despite the changes in respiratory function with aging, healthy older adults are typically well able to generate and maintain adequate respiratory support for speech.

Summary

The respiratory system consists of the pulmonary system (lungs and airways) and the chest wall system (rib cage, abdomen, and diaphragm).

Inhalation and exhalation occur when P_{alv} decreases and increases, forcing air into and out of the system.

Lung volumes and capacities refer to different amounts of air in the lungs at a given time; these amounts change over the lifespan.

Five important changes occur with breathing for speech rather than for life: location of air intake, ratio of inhalatory to exhalatory time, volume of air per cycle, muscle activity for exhalation, and chest wall position.

Breathing patterns for speech are influenced by linguistic considerations, including speaking task complexity, clause boundaries, and loudness of the intended utterance.

Speech breathing changes over the lifespan due to changes in the structure and function of the respiratory system.

REVIEW EXERCISES

1. Draw a diagram of the pulmonary system and describe each of the components.

2. Explain how the lungs are able to expand and contract even though they contain very little muscle.

3. Define the four lung volumes and four lung capacities.

4. Describe how the respiratory system changes over the lifespan in terms of rate of breathing, lung volumes and capacities, and speech breathing.

5. Identify and describe the five differences between breathing for life and breathing for speech.

6. Explain the concept of resting expiratory level and discuss its role in the measurement of lung volumes and capacities.

CHAPTER

CLINICAL APPLICATION

Evaluation and Treatment of Respiratory Disorders

STUDENT LEARNING OBJECTIVES

After reading this chapter you will

○ Define spirometric measures and understand the basis of pulmonary function testing.

○ Appreciate the role of respiratory kinematic analysis in measuring lung function.

○ Identify measures of air pressures and flows in respiration.

○ Identify dyspnea and stridor as the primary symptoms of airway obstruction.

○ Describe four principles important in the clinical management of speech breathing disorders.

○ Identify respiratory parameters that are affected in individuals with neurological disorders such as Parkinson's disease, cerebellar disease, cervical spinal cord injury, and cerebral palsy.

○ Understand how speech breathing is affected in patients who are mechanically ventilated.

○ Appreciate the role of respiratory function in individuals with voice disorders.

○ Compare and contrast respiratory characteristics in individuals with asthma and those with paradoxical vocal fold motion.

In order to understand the role of respiration and respiratory breakdowns that can affect speech production, it is important to become familiar with measurement of respiratory variables. This chapter focuses on the measurement of lung volumes, pressures, and flows during nonspeech and speech activities. Pulmonary function testing is described. Attention then turns to the major symptoms of respiratory dysfunction and to clinical management of speech breathing in individuals with neurological disorders, voice disorders, asthma, and hearing impairment, as well as those who are mechanically ventilated.

Measurement of Respiratory Variables

Respiratory function is measured in terms of lung volumes, air pressures and flows, and chest wall positioning and movement, Lung volume, pressures and flows, and chest wall positioning are closely related to each other. The positioning of the chest wall (and, due to pleural linkage, of the lungs) results in a particular volume of air in the lungs. The volume of air within the lungs directly influences the pressure in the lungs, and the volume change over time causes air to flow into and out of the respiratory system.

Because of the relationships among these respiratory parameters, it is possible to measure one parameter directly and then to make inferences about other parameters. For example, researchers and clinicians often measure chest wall shape and use this information to estimate lung volume changes. This kind of information is extremely useful in characterizing aspects of breathing in normal and disordered speech.

Lung volumes can be measured directly with a spirometer or estimated from rib cage and abdominal movement. Direct measurement of lung volumes and flows using a spirometer is called pulmonary function testing.

Pulmonary Function Testing

Pulmonary function testing (PFT) is a term that covers a variety of tests designed to assess the amount of air an individual is able to inhale and exhale, as well as how efficiently the person moves air into and out of the lungs. Spirometry is the most common method of PFT (Gildea & McCarthy, 2010; McCarthy & Dweik, 2010). Common spirometric measures are defined in Table 8.1.

Norms have been developed for selected spirometric measures based on age, gender, body height and size, and race. An individual's obtained values are compared against the norms in terms of percentage of predicted value. For example, a person who obtained 75 percent of the predicted value would be considered as showing a mild level of respiratory dysfunction. See Table 8.2. The most widely used parameter to measure the mechanical properties of the lungs is the forced expiratory volume in 1 second (FEV_1) (Gildea & McCarthy, 2010). This measure reflects the functioning of the large- and the medium-sized airways and occurs at about 75 to 85 percent of the forced vital capacity (FVC) in healthy individuals. The FEV_1 is typically reduced in airway disorders.

Spirometry is also used to generate a graph called a **flow-volume loop (FVL)**. This graph shows velocity of airflow on the y-axis and air volume on the x-axis. To generate the FVL, the individual is instructed to inhale as deeply as possible and then exhale as much as possible into the spirometer, followed immediately by a maximum inhalation from the spirometer (Bass, 1973). Expiratory airflow is shown as positive going on the graph, and inspiratory airflow is indicated by a negative-going trace. A normal FVL has a characteristic shape in which the expiratory portion (called a *limb*) rises rapidly to the peak flow rate and is then followed by a sharp decrease as the individual exhales toward residual volume. The inspiratory limb is a more symmetrical curve. The FVL is a very useful index of respiratory function because different airway diseases show characteristically different flow volume relationships than normal. Figure 8.1 shows FVLs for common respiratory diseases such as asthma. The primary symptom of asthma is difficulty on exhalation due to inflammation and swelling of the bronchial airways. The graph shows a corresponding flattening of the expiratory limb. An individual with respiratory muscle weakness that hinders his or her air intake might show inspiratory and expiratory limbs that are markedly smaller than normal.

Table 8.1 **Spirometric Measures and Definitions**

Measure	Definition
FVC	Amount of air that can be exhaled forcefully after a maximum inhalation
FEV_1	Amount of air that can be exhaled forcefully in one breath in 1 second
FEF	Amount of air that can be exhaled measured in an interval of time
FEF25%	Amount of air forcibly expelled in the first 25% of the total FVC
FEF50%	Amount of air forcibly expelled in the first 50% of the total FVC
FEF 25%–75%	Air flow during the middle half of the total FVC
PEFR	Maximum flow rate during FVC maneuver
MVV	Maximum amount of air that can be inhaled and exhaled in 12–15 seconds
SVC	Amount of air that can be slowly exhaled after a maximum exhalation
TLC	Total amount of air capable of being held in the lungs
FRC	Amount of air remaining in the lungs at the end of a normal exhalation
ERV	Amount of air able to be exhaled following a normal exhalation
FEV_1%	Ratio of FEV_1 to FVC, indicating what percentage of the total FVC was exhaled during the first second of forced exhalation
FEF_{50}/FIF_{50}	Ratio between FEF at 50% of exhaled vital capacity and FIF at 50% of inhaled vital capacity

NOTE: FVC–forced vital capacity; FEV–forced expiratory volume; FEF–forced expiratory flow; PEFR–peak expiratory flow rate; MVV–maximum voluntary ventilation; SVC–slow vital capacity; TLC–total lung capacity; FRC–functional residual capacity; ERV–expiratory reserve volume; FIF–forced inspiratory flow; VC–vital capacity.

Table 8.2 **Severity of Reductions in FVC and FEV_1 in Relation to Percentage of Predicted Value**

Severity	Percentage of Predicted Value
Mild	70–79%
Moderate	60–69%
Moderately severe	50–59%
Severe	35–49%
Very severe	Less than 35%

SOURCE: Information from McCarthy & Dwei (2010).

Figure 8.1 **Flow-volume loops**

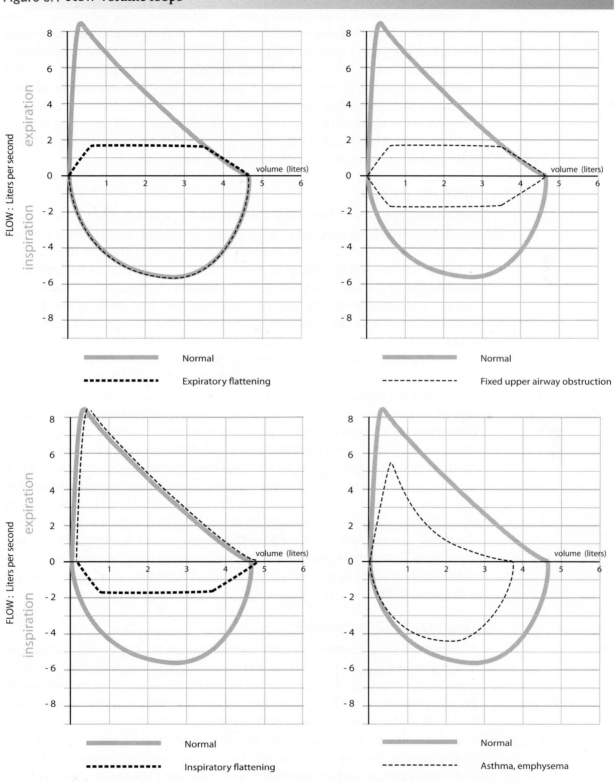

Respiratory Kinematic Analysis

Spirometers are useful in determining static volumes and flows but cannot be used to measure lung volumes during speaking. In speaking situations, **respiratory kinematic analysis** is used, in which lung volumes are estimated from rib cage (RC) and abdominal movement. The RC and abdomen displace volume as they expand and contract during inhalation and exhalation. The movements of these structures therefore reflect the changing volumes of the thorax and abdomen. Measures can be obtained of tidal volume, minute ventilation, and other lung volumes and capacities. Movements of the rib cage and abdomen can be measured with either a plethysmograph or with linearized magnetometers.

Plethysmography

Plethysmographs are of two major varieties: body plethysmographs and respiratory inductance plethysmographs. A body plethysmograph involves the individual being enclosed in a small, airtight chamber. With the person's nostrils clipped shut, he or she is instructed to breathe or pant against a mouthpiece. As the individual breathes, the air pressure and volume in the chamber (and against the mouthpiece) change in accordance with the movements of the chest wall. Because the chamber is airtight, an accurate measure of the individual's lung volume can be calculated (Gold, 2005).

A respiratory inductance plethysmograph (RIP) consists of two elastic bands, each of which covers a coil of wire. One elastic band fits around the chest and one around the abdomen (Figure 8.2). As the person's chest and abdominal walls expand and contract, the changes in his or her cross-sectional areas are measured. These changes are sent to an amplifier and recorder, or computer. This method allows the degree of movement of the RC and abdomen to be assessed independently, and the movements can also be combined to calculate lung volume. RIP is less cumbersome than body plethysmography, as it allows breathing parameters to be assessed without a nose clip. A portable version is commercially available in which the rib cage and abdominal sensors are built into a fitted elastic garment. The person wears this garment while performing exercises or other activities (Witt et al., 2006). This permits individuals to perform normal activities outside the clinic and laboratory while their respiratory function is monitored (Grossman, Wilhelm & Brutsche, 2010).

Linearized magnetometer

A **linearized magnetometer** is composed of two coils of wire. An electric current is passed through one coil and generates an electromagnetic field, which in turn induces an electric current in the other coil. The strength of the voltage induced by the electromagnetic field depends on the distance separating the coils. If one coil is placed on a person's back and the other directly opposite, on a point along his or her thorax or abdomen, the changes in the diameters of the rib cage or abdomen can be calculated in relation to the changing strength of the current. Respiratory measures generated with linearized magnetometers typically include lung volume, RC excursions, and abdominal excursions (e.g., Mendes, Brown, Sapienza, & Rothman, 2006). Excursions are calculated by measuring the

Figure 8.2 **Respiratory inductance plethysmography**

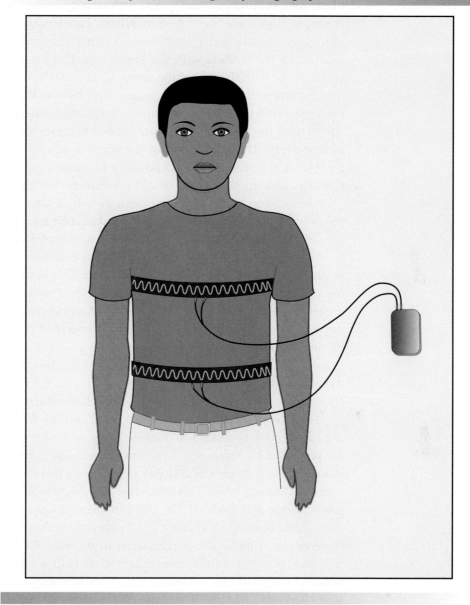

volume of the lungs, RC, or abdomen at the beginning and end of an utterance. The volume of air expended equals the initiation value at the beginning of the utterance minus the termination value at the end of the utterance.

Air Pressures

The pressures necessary for speech include pressure inside the lungs (P_{alv}), pressure below the vocal folds (subglottal pressure [P_s] or tracheal pressure [P_{trach}]), and pressure inside the mouth (oral pressure [P_{oral}]). Air pressures can be measured with a **manometer**, of which there are several types. An air-gauge manometer has dials that are calibrated to show pressure changes in terms of cm H_2O. A person blows into an attached mouthpiece, generating pressure, which displaces the dials. A simple manometer described by Hixon, Hawley, and Wilson (1982) makes use of a glass of water, a drinking straw, a paper clip, and masking tape. The straw is attached to the glass with the paper clip. The masking tape is marked off in centimeters, with the top of the water level equal to 0 cm. The individual blows into the straw until a bubble is created and rises to the surface of the water. The principle underlying this procedure is that however deeply the end of the straw is submerged, the amount of pressure needed to create the bubble is at least as much as that depth. Thus, if the end of the straw is located at 3 cm, the person would have to exert at least 3 cm H_2O pressure to create a bubble. If the end of the straw is located at 8 cm, the person would need to exert at least 8 cm H_2O, and so on.

Manometers measure static pressures, which are useful for determining how much pressure a person can generate and sustain for a period of time. For example, an individual's maximum inspiratory and expiratory pressures can be determined by having him or her suck as hard as possible and blow as hard as possible at the resting tidal EEL (Hixon & Hoit, 2005). This kind of measure can be helpful for evaluating how much pressure an individual with a neurological problem or a cleft palate can build up (Decker, 1990). Another measure is to have the person develop a target pressure and hold it for a specified period of time. For example, he or she may be instructed to generate a pressure of 5 cm H_2O and maintain it for 5 seconds. However, manometers do not provide a permanent record of the obtained values, and they are also not useful for measuring the dynamically changing pressures that occur during speech breathing.

For pressures within the oral and nasal cavities that change very rapidly during speech, it is necessary to convert pressure changes into electrical signals that are processed by computer. A pressure transducer is fitted into a tube that can be placed in the speaker's oral cavity or mounted in a mask placed over the mouth and face (Decker, 1990). This procedure allows pressure variations to be stored for later viewing and analysis. The pressure needed for conversational speech is low, around 5 to 10 cm H_2O. This is a small proportion of the total pressure that a person can generate. Most 5-year-old children can generate 35 to 50 cm H_2O when blowing as hard as possible. Adults can generate 60 cm H_2O or more. Although the pressures needed for normal conversational speech are low, they have to be sustained for different amounts of time. Therefore, the muscles of the chest wall must produce carefully graded forces over the span of the utterance (Solomon & Charron, 1998). Pressures for conversational speech also vary instant by instant, depending on the emphasis on a syllable or word, the changes in vocal amplitude, and the specific phoneme. For louder speech, both children and adults generate greater tracheal pressures to increase intensity (Stathopoulos & Sapienza, 1993). To increase vocal intensity by 8 to 9 dB, a person would have to double P_{trach} (Titze, 1994).

Tracheal and alveolar pressures are not usually measured directly because the procedure involves inserting a needle into the trachea, which is a highly invasive procedure. Fortunately, P_{trach} is easy to measure indirectly by measuring P_{oral}. A small tube connected to a pressure transducer is placed inside the speaker's mouth just past the lips, and the pressure inside his or her mouth during the closure portion of a stop consonant is measured (Smitheran & Hixon, 1981). The strongest oral pressures generated during the closed portion of a voiceless stop consonant (e.g., /p/) are almost identical to P_{alv} and P_{trach}. Why should this be? For the /p/ sound, an individual closes his or her lips, raises the velum to close the velopharyngeal passage and prevent air escaping into the nose, and opens the vocal folds. Because the person is still exhaling, the pressures throughout the system (i.e., P_{alv}, P_{trach}, and P_{oral}) are essentially the same at this moment. So, if P_{oral} is measured at this instant, it can be said with some confidence that P_{oral} is equal to P_{trach} and to P_{alv}. Using this indirect method, pressures have been compared in normally speaking children and adults and between individuals with and without speech disorders.

Airflow

Airflow (volume velocity) is a measure of a volume of air moving in a certain direction at a particular location per unit of time. Airflow is measured in milliliters per second (ml/s), liters per minute (l/min), or milliliters per syllable (ml/syll). A **pneumotachometer** is a device that calculates airflow. The person breathes into a mouthpiece, and the flow of air is converted into a pressure differential across a mesh that has a fixed resistance. The advantage of using a pneumotachometer is that both oral and nasal airflows can be measured during speech tasks. Airflow through the speech production system is strongly related to the structures above the trachea that open and close to valve the airway (Solomon & Charron, 1998). These structures include the larynx and the articulators. Air flows into and out of the lungs due to muscular and recoil forces. The outward flow of air through the system is modified by the various resistances to the flow created as the larynx and other articulators open and close. If the larynx allows too much air to flow through the glottis during vocalization, the voice will be heard as breathy. If too little air is permitted through the glottis because the vocal folds are closed too tightly, the voice may be perceived as tense and strained. Resonance of the voice is also affected by airflow and the resistance to flow. If the soft palate does not offer enough resistance to the airflow, too much air flows into the nasal cavities, resulting in hypernasality and nasal emission. On the other hand, if some kind of blockage, such as enlarged adenoids, causes too much resistance to the flow of air through the nose, the person sounds hyponasal.

Flow rates in milliliters per syllable (ml/syll) have been calculated for children and adults. The amount of flow per syll appears to depend on age. Boliek, Hixon, Watson, and Morgan (1997) reported that toddlers used about 100 ml/syll; Hoit, Banzett, Brown, and Loring (1990) reported that children aged 7 to 16 years used approximately 35 to 60 ml/syll. Table 8.3 provides flow rate information based on data reported in the literature and provided by Baken (1996).

Table 8.3 **Average Flow Rates (in ml/s) for 7-year-old Boys and Girls, Adult Men, and Adult Women for Sustained /a/**

Boys	Girls	Men	Women
95.9	71.6	112.4	93.7

SOURCE: Information from Baken (1996).

In addition to ml/syll, flow has also been calculated in terms of the maximum, or peak flow, during specific phonemes. A speech sound such as a fricative that is produced with high pressure and flow might show a pressure of 7 cm H$_2$O and a flow of around 500 ml/s (Raphael, Borden, & Harris, 2007). Peak airflow during the release of stop sounds is also high, approximately 600 ml/s for children and 900 ml/s for adults (Stathopoulos & Weismer, 1985; Subtelny, Worth, & Sakuda, 1966; Trullinger & Emanuel, 1983). The lower peak flows shown by children may be due to a combination of physical and physiological factors, such as children's smaller vocal tracts, greater vocal tract resistances, and lower elastic recoil of the lungs (Solomon & Charron, 1998).

Individuals who exhibit greater-than-normal airflows during speech may valve the airstream inefficiently, allowing too much air to escape. This is often seen in people with neurological diseases. However, it is important to keep in mind that abnormalities of airflow during speech cannot be attributed only to the respiratory system because the larynx and other articulators contribute to airflow measures (Solomon & Charron, 1998).

Respiratory Function and Speech Production

Respiratory and/or laryngeal disorders that obstruct the airway can interfere with ventilation and pose a life-threatening risk to the individual. Adequate respiratory function is also essential for speech production. Difficulty with inhaling and/or exhaling air, with obtaining an adequate amount of air, or with maintaining appropriate breath support can adversely affect speech production. Neurological disorders can interfere with speech breathing; disorders such as asthma and paradoxical vocal fold motion can negatively affect respiratory and laryngeal function. Breathing for speech may also be affected in individuals who are mechanically ventilated (i.e., who have life support for breathing), in people with voice disorders, and in hearing-impaired individuals.

Classification of Respiratory Problems

Respiratory problems are classified as obstructive, restrictive, or central (Table 8.4). Obstructive problems are those in which narrowing or blockage of the airways occur due to factors such as a foreign body within the airways, inflammation of the airways, spasms of the smooth airway muscle, or other obstructions to airflow (Mehanna & Jankovic, 2010). Typically exhalation is affected in obstructive problems. Examples of obstructive diseases are asthma, bronchitis, emphysema, and chronic obstructive pulmonary disease (COPD).

Restrictive lung diseases are those that restrict lung expansion and are characterized by reduced lung volume. Restrictive difficulties occur due to factors such as loss of lung elasticity, diseases of the pleura and/or chest wall, or neuromuscular dysfunction (Kanaparthi, Lessnau, & Sharma, 2012; Mehanna & Jankovic, 2010). Causes include lung diseases such as fibrosis or connective tissue diseases, neuromuscular diseases, and diseases of the pleura. People with restrictive problems typically have more difficulty on inhalation because of the reduced ability to expand the thorax and lungs.

Table 8.4 **Types of Respiratory Problems**

Symptoms	Causes
Obstructive	
Coughing	Asthma
Wheezing	Bronchitis
Shortness of breath	Emphysema
Chest tightness	COPD
Restrictive	
Difficulty expanding lungs	Intrinsic pulmonary fibrosis
Reduced lung volume	Sarcoidosis
Chest pain	Pneumonia
Dry cough	Neuromuscular diseases
Wheezing	Asbestosis
Shortness of breath after exercise	Radiation fibrosis
Coughing up blood	
Recurrent respiratory tract infections	
Central	
Hypoventilation	Drugs
	Stroke
	Amyotrophic lateral sclerosis
	Brain tumor
	Muscular dystrophy
	Obesity

Central problems in respiration are caused by neurological dysfunction in the respiratory brain centers in the brain stem (Mehanna & Jankovic, 2010). For example, inadequate ventilation (**hypoventilation**) may occur from a stroke that damages the brain stem. Hypoventilation may also be a side effect of certain drugs that depress nervous system function. Hypoventilation results in reduced oxygen and increased concentrations of carbon dioxide in the bloodstream, and it can be fatal.

Symptoms of Respiratory Disorders

The two primary symptoms of airway difficulty are dyspnea and stridor. **Dyspnea** is defined as subjectively perceived discomfort in breathing that can vary from mild to extreme (American Thoracic Society, 1999; Hoit, Lansing, & Perona, 2007;

Lansing, Im, Thwing, Legezda, & Banzett, 2005). The sensation arises from interactions between sensory receptors in the lungs, airways, thorax, and blood vessels, multiple brain areas, and physical and psychological patient characteristics (De Peuter et al., 2004). The individual may perceive the sensation as shortness of breath, or as the need to work hard to breathe, or as chest tightness, or as any combination of these. Shortness of breath is usually due to high levels of CO_2 in the blood (Gracely, 2001; Hixon & Hoit, 2005; Liotti et al., 2001). The feeling of having to work hard arises when the person needs to use high levels of respiratory muscle activity to breathe, usually due to fatigue, pulmonary diseases such as asthma, or neurological diseases that affect the respiratory muscles (Hixon & Hoit, 2005; Lansing et al., 2005). The sensation of chest tightness results when the airways are constricted, typically due to asthma. Dyspnea may occur during speech, particularly in individuals with respiratory difficulties arising from chronic obstructive pulmonary disease, lung cancer, and cervical spinal cord injury (Hoit et al., 2007). Speech-related dyspnea may also occur in healthy individuals during times of high stress or emotion.

Stridor refers to an audible sound that occurs during inspiration and/or expiration. The sound, which may be high or low pitched, results from turbulent air flow as the air passes through a narrowed or obstructed segment in the airway (Benson, Baredes, Schwartz, & Kumar, 2006; Sakakura et al., 2008). Inspiratory stridor is the most common type of stridor (Holinger, 1998) and typically is caused by an obstruction at laryngeal, nasal, or pharyngeal locations (Benson et al., 2006). The obstruction results from the collapse of soft tissues due to negative pressures generated in the airway during inspiration. Expiratory stridor most commonly is caused by an obstruction within the trachea and bronchi and is not typically related to changing pressures within the airway. Stridor can result from acute infections such as epiglottitis, a foreign body in the airway, laryngeal conditions (e.g., laryngomalacia, subglottic stenosis, tumors), neurological problems, pulmonary difficulties, cardiovascular problems, and gastroesophageal reflux disease (GERD) (e.g., Giannoni et al., 1998; Leung & Cho, 1999; Murphy & Ren, 2009; Nielson et al., 1990; Sakakura et al., 2008; Zoumalan et al., 2007).

Principles of Clinical Management of Speech Breathing Disorders

Four principles are important in the clinical management of speech breathing problems. First, although the amount of air needed to produce speech is only around 20 percent of VC, this amount of air must be managed efficiently for speaking purposes. Some clinical researchers have suggested that if a patient can generate a steady stream of P_s of 5 cm H_2O for 5 s or longer, the respiratory system may be sufficient to support speech (Netsell & Hixon, 1992). However, although some individuals with respiratory difficulties may be able to perform this static kind of task, they may not be able to coordinate the more dynamic and complex respiratory maneuvers that are required for speech breathing. Thus, in a clinical situation, it is critical to measure the patient's respiratory function in both nonspeech (static) and speech (dynamic) tasks. Second, treatment needs to be tailored to the patient's specific respiratory difficulty. For example, patients with too much muscular tone may need treatments that will help them relax their muscles. Patients with posture problems may benefit from braces or girdles for abdominal support. Patients with cerebellar problems often need treatment to improve their balance and sense of position. Patients with too little muscular tone require exercises that increase the strength of the muscles used for inhalation and exhalation. Third, the sequence of clinical activities should focus first on pressure variables, then on volume variables, and finally on chest wall shape (Hixon & Hoit, 2005). Pressure is the primary focus because alveolar, subglottal, and oral pressures are crucial for voice and speech production; volume is the next priority because the amount of available lung volume affects the quantity of speech and chest wall shape is the final factor in maximizing the patient's ability to develop the quick inspirations and extended expirations necessary for fluent speech production (Hixon & Hoit, 2005). Finally, because breathing for speech differs from nonspeech breathing, exercises should be practiced in speech contexts rather than in nonspeech contexts (Hixon & Hoit, 2005).

Neurological Disorders

Neurological disorders can adversely impact speech breathing for several reasons. The difficulty may be with the respiratory muscles themselves or with the nervous supply to the respiratory muscles. The muscles may be spastic (excessive tone) or flaccid (too little tone). Generalized weakness can hinder the individual from sitting or standing properly, thus interfering with breath support for speech. Postural problems are particularly evident in neurological disorders such as Parkinson's disease, cerebellar problems, spinal cord injury, and cerebral palsy.

Parkinson's disease

Parkinson's disease (PD) is a progressive neurological disease characterized by a rigidity of muscles that restricts the range of movement of the affected structures. PD is typically associated with speech that is monotonous, distorted in terms of articulation, breathy, low in intensity, and weak. The weakness and low vocal intensity are important factors in communication because they decrease the clarity and intelligibility of the person's speech (Ramig, 1992). The breathy, weak voice is probably due in part to decreased respiratory support (Ramig, Countryman, Thompson, & Horii, 1995). Many patients with PD have restrictive respiratory problems. Because of the muscular rigidity and reduced range of rib cage movement, patients with severe PD are not able to inhale fully, and they show reductions in VC, FEV_1, and FVC (De Letter et al., 2007; De Pandis et al., 2002). Even when patients are taking anti-Parkinson's medications such as levodopa, these respiratory differences persist (e.g., De Letter et al., 2007). Dyspnea is often present when the patient exerts himself or herself, and the dyspnea can become progressively more severe as the disease progresses (Mehanna & Jankovic, 2010; Vercueil, Linard, Wuyam, Pollak, & Benchetrit, 1999). Another feature of speech breathing in individuals with PD is reduced movement of the rib cage and greater displacement of the abdomen (Huber, Stathopoulos, Ramig, & Lancaster, 2000; Solomon & Hixon, 1993).

Examination of speech breathing patterns using linearized magnetometers in conjunction with acoustic and linguistic data indicated that speakers with PD produced shorter breath groups and fewer syllables per second. Many individuals with PD initiated speech at lower lung volumes, and considerably more of these speakers than healthy individuals finished breath groups below REL (Bunton, 2005). Bunton (2005) suggested that increasing abdominal activity below REL is advantageous in the case of PD because use of the abdominal musculature compensates for the rigidity of the chest wall and allows the speaker to maintain and control adequate respiratory support for speech.

The decline in cognitive and linguistic capacity that is often seen in patients with PD may also contribute to the differences in speech breathing behavior. Huber and Darling (2011) used respiratory inductance plethysmography (RIP) to determine lung volume usage during both structured reading and extemporaneous speaking in individuals with PD compared to those without. They reported several findings. First, during longer utterances, speakers with PD terminated speech at lower lung volumes; by contrast, control speakers inhaled to higher lung volumes to achieve the necessary breath duration. Second, individuals with PD took longer to inhale before an utterance in extemporaneous speech but not in reading. The authors speculated that this may have allowed the speakers more time to formulate their thoughts. Third, persons with PD used more of their VC per syllable compared to healthy speakers, probably due to difficulties controlling the flow of air through the larynx.

Many individuals with PD can probably generate adequate P_{trach} for speech. However, even when tracheal/subglottal pressures are adequate, many speakers cannot build up as much P_{oral} as individuals without the disease. This suggests that an individual with PD probably loses pressure through the lips or through the velopharynx (Solomon & Hixon, 1993). Speakers with PD may be able to produce enough respiratory driving pressures for speech but may have difficulty with controlling the airstream using the articulators. The lower-than-normal P_{oral} seen in some speakers with PD may contribute to their lack of intelligibility because of inadequate pressure buildup in the oral cavity necessary for sounds such as stops and fricatives.

Because the respiratory system has been reported to be one of the first speech-production subsystems affected in PD, strategies to improve breathing function are often targeted in treatment programs. These strategies should be based on the patient's breathing physiology. For example, teaching patients to speak in short phrases may be more successful than trying to increase lung volume because the rigidity of the chest wall limits achievement of higher volumes. One main complaint in PD is reduced vocal intensity. Increasing intensity is often targeted in treatment and is accomplished by increasing P_{trach}, as well as by increasing the strength of vocal fold closure. Strategies include increasing respiratory effort through tasks such as breathing in and out as much and as forcefully as possible; sustaining voiceless sounds, such as /s/ and /f/, for as long as possible; taking deep breaths frequently; speaking at the beginning of the exhalation without wasting breath; and sustaining vowels for as long as possible (Ramig et al., 1995). Silverman et al. (2006) described a program of expiratory muscle strength training using a pressure-threshold device. The aim is for the individual to generate enough expiratory pressure to open a spring-loaded valve and to sustain this pressure throughout the exhalation. The rationale proposed by the authors is that strength training can help the individual increase P_{alv}. Increasing P_{alv} can facilitate production of longer utterances, increased loudness levels, and improved voice quality (Baker, Davenport, & Sapienza, 2005; Silverman et al., 2006).

Cerebellar disease

The cerebellum is important in the coordination of voluntary movement, as it regulates the speed, direction, force, and amplitude of movement. If the cerebellum is injured due to disease or trauma, the smooth coordination of muscle groups is lost, and movements tend to be jerky and uncoordinated. The person looks like he or she is intoxicated, with an unsteady, lurching gait. If the speech-production system is affected, the person's voice may fluctuate unpredictably in pitch and loudness, and the individual loses the ability to make the fine adjustments to F_0 and intensity that are necessary for stress and emphasis. Speech therefore becomes slow, and syllables tend to be produced with excess and equal stress, giving an almost robotic sound to the speech. This type of speech is called *scanning* speech. In some individuals, an underlying respiratory disorder may contribute to the speech problems since the respiratory system is involved in the regulation of loudness, pitch, and stress.

Research has shown that some speakers with cerebellar disease have total lung capacities within normal limits but have reduced vital capacities (Murdoch, Chenery, Stokes, & Hardcastle, 1991). The reduction in VC is probably the result of the breakdown in the coordinated action of the components of the chest wall, such as abrupt changes in the motions of the rib cage and abdomen and motion jerks. Some patients in a study by Murdoch et al. (1991) even breathed in during exhalation for speech, a pattern the authors termed "inspiratory gasps." The gasps seemed to be caused by momentary breakdowns in the control of the outgoing airflow for speech. The authors also reported that the majority of the patients with cerebellar problems initiated utterances below normal lung levels. Many began their utterances at a lung volume just barely higher than their resting tidal end-expiratory levels, and two speakers actually initiated utterances below REL.

Understanding the underlying respiratory patterns of individuals with cerebellar disease could be very important in tailoring intervention strategies. For example, a patient who begins his or her utterances at an abnormally low lung volume could be taught to begin each utterance at a higher lung volume.

Cervical spinal cord injury

Individuals who have suffered cervical spinal cord injury (CSCI) often have respiratory problems. Injury to the part of the spinal cord that supplies nerve impulses to the muscles of respiration can result in weakness or paralysis. If the diaphragm is affected, the person may not be able to breathe at all and will need mechanical ventilation. Even when the diaphragm is not affected and the individual is able to breathe by him- or herself, speech may be affected if the person has difficulty generating adequate pressures and flows. This could result in reduced loudness, imprecise consonant production (because of the problem in generating the P_{oral} necessary for stops and fricatives), abnormally short breath groups, and slow inspirations (Hoit, Banzett, et al., 1990).

Many individuals with CSCI report dyspnea, particularly during speaking (e.g., Grandas et al., 2005). This occurs because it is more difficult to balance ventilatory and linguistic demands when the respiratory system is compromised.

While resting tidal volume and breathing rate may be normal, patients with CSCI demonstrate reduced inspiratory and expiratory muscle strength as well as reductions in VC, TLC, FRC, and ERV (Stepp et al., 2008; Tamplin et al., 2011). Patients with quadriplegia resulting from CSCI have been reported to use accessory respiratory muscles (sternocleidomastoid and trapezius) to increase vocal intensity (Tamplin et al., 2011). Hoit, Banzett, et al. (1990) reported that most patients with CSCI in their study began and ended their exhalations for speech at larger lung volumes than normal. Also, the injured individuals had larger abdominal volumes, whereas healthy speakers kept the abdomen at smaller volumes during speech breathing. Most of the speakers with spinal cord injuries produced fewer-than-normal syllables per breath. However, similar to that of healthy individuals, average flow per syllable ranged from about 35 to 80 ml. Hoit, Banzett, et al. (1990) noted that some of the patients compensated for their muscular impairment by taking in larger amounts of air. This increased the resulting recoil pressure so that they would not have to rely on the muscles of exhalation to speak. The downside of this compensatory strategy was that the number of syllables produced per breath was reduced. Despite this minor disadvantage, this kind of strategy could be very useful as a clinical tool. Individuals with CSCI can be taught to take in larger amounts of air to help them increase loudness and project their voices better.

Massery (1991) provided an excellent example of the importance of clinical management of speech breathing in patients with CSCI problems. He described a child of not quite 4 years of age with a CSCI. During the initial evaluation, the child could produce only two syllables per breath. Treatment focused on chest wall development, such as body positioning, muscle strengthening, and coordination exercises. After 2 months, the child was able to produce eight syllables per breath and spoke in full sentences.

Cerebral palsy

Many children and adults with cerebral palsy (CP) face problems with respiratory function that affect their speech production to lesser or greater degrees. Different forms of CP may affect respiratory function in different ways. *Spastic* CP is a condition in which the affected structures are hypertonic and weak. With involvement of the chest wall muscles, the person's inhalations tend to be shallow, and expirations are forced and uncontrolled (Massery, 1991). *Athetoid* CP is characterized by the presence of involuntary movements that interfere with normal voluntary movements. This condition is more likely to result in irregular and uncontrolled breathing, with involuntary bursts of air during inhalation and/or exhalation. These sudden movements are probably due to abnormal involuntary movements of the chest wall (Solomon & Charron, 1998). With *ataxic* CP, the person lacks coordination, resulting in irregular rate, rhythm, and depth of tidal breathing.

All the parameters of respiratory function (pressure, flow, volume, and chest wall shape) may be affected in individuals with CP. Pressures and volumes may be lower than normal, with difficulty in accessing IRV and/or ERV. Thus, children with CP are not able to pull air into or force air out of the lungs voluntarily as well or as much as able-bodied children (Solomon & Charron, 1998). The compromised respiratory muscles can result in a person with CP needing to use a much larger proportion of the already-reduced VC for speech. In addition, speakers with CP may valve the airstream inefficiently at any location of the vocal tract, including the larynx, velopharynx, or other articulators. This wastes air, so airflows are typically abnormally high during speech.

The shape of the chest wall is an extremely important variable in treating children with CP. Recall that the most efficient position of the chest wall for speech is one in which the abdomen is smaller and the rib cage larger than during relaxation. Deformities of the chest wall are common in children with CP (Davis, 1987). This is likely due to hypertonic and/or weak muscles, as well as to postural problems. Children with spastic CP spend a lot of time in a flexed position. This causes breathing that worsens with development, along with deterioration in vocal quality and loudness (Workinger & Kent, 1991). The child's attempts to compensate for the abnormal tone might also contribute to the increasing difficulty in breathing for speech. Children with athetoid CP become more posturally stable as they mature, and their speech may become more intelligible.

Strengthening the muscles of the chest wall may improve a child's ability to generate greater P_{trach} and a correspondingly louder voice (Solomon & Charron, 1998). Strengthening the respiratory muscles can also help increase VC and improve endurance for breathing. The child may then be able to produce more syllables in one breath and to talk for longer periods of time. This was demonstrated by Cerny, Panzarella, and Stathopoulos (1997), who used a muscle-conditioning protocol in which children with low muscle tone wore a face mask that provided resistance against the outgoing breath stream. They wore the mask for 15 minutes each day, 5 days a week, for 6 weeks. Even though speech itself was never targeted during training, the children showed increases in P_{trach} and vocal loudness during both normal and loud speech, demonstrating the efficiency of working on the underlying respiratory difficulty.

Other respiratory exercises are designed to improve speech breathing coordination. A child can be taught to inspire quickly and deeply and to exhale in a slow and controlled manner while speaking. The deep inhalation results in increased lung volume and greater pressures available for speech. To control the expiration, the child must use his or her inspiratory muscles to counteract the passive recoil forces at high volumes (Netsell & Hixon, 1992). Other techniques are used to focus only on inspiration or on expiration (e.g., sniffing and blowing exercises) or on switching voluntarily between the two (Solomon & Charron, 1998).

Improving postural support can be very helpful in treating respiratory function. An individually adjusted seating system can change the positioning of the individual's body in ways that improve his or her posture. This in turn can increase VC so the person can exhale for longer amounts of time. Boliek (1997) described the respiratory function of a preschooler with spastic CP and accompanying respiratory problems. When unsupported, the child began phonation below REL, with a breathy and strained vocal quality. With appropriate support, the child began speaking at higher lung volumes and ended utterances at or above REL.

Another way of improving posture and respiration for speech is by using abdominal trussing. Corsets, braces, wraps, and belts can be used to push

Table 8.5 Respiratory Findings Reported for Individuals with Neurological Disorders

Parkinson's disease
Reduced VC, FVC, FEV$_1$
Dyspnea
Reduced rib cage movement
Increased abdominal displacement
Finish breath groups below REL
Cerebellar disease
Normal TLC
Reduced VC
Inspiratory gasps
Initiate utterances close to or below REL
Cervical spinal cord injury
Dyspnea
Normal resting TV
Reduced VC, TLC, FRC, and ERV
Larger abdominal volumes
Larger lung volumes to begin and end exhalations for speech
Cerebral palsy
Reduced pressures and volumes
Difficulty accessing IRV and/or ERV
Need to use greater proportion of VC for speech
Difficulties with posture and chest wall positioning

SOURCES: Information from Bunton (2005); Davis (1987); De Letter et al. (2007); De Pandis et al. (2002); Grandas et al. (2005); Huber et al. (2000); Mehanna & Jankovic (2010); Murdoch et al. (1991); Solomon & Charron (1998); Solomon & Hixon (1993); and Vercueil et al. (1999).

the individual's abdomen inward, lift the rib cage, and force the diaphragm upward. This makes exhalation more efficient, so lung volume, maximum inspiratory and expiratory pressures, maximum flow, and maximum phonation time all increase; and speakers can pause at more linguistically appropriate places (Watson, 1997).

Table 8.5 lists the most commonly reported respiratory findings in individuals with neurological disorders.

Mechanical Ventilation

Understanding respiratory patterns in speech production is important in the treatment of individuals who are dependent on a mechanical respirator to breathe. The person is attached to a ventilator by a tube called a *cannula* that fits tightly into a *stoma* (hole) in his or her neck that leads to the trachea. The ventilator has an inspiratory phase, during which air is pumped into the person's respiratory system. In this phase, P_{trach} increases because of the increase in the density of the air within the trachea. Exhalation occurs as the individual's thorax and lungs recoil, forcing the pumped air out of the system. P_{trach} decreases during exhalation. In some cases, if the patient's ventilatory function is greatly compromised, no air is allowed to flow into the upper airway but is directed fully into the trachea. However, some individuals are able to speak using the air from the ventilator. In this case, a small portion of the air that is pumped into the trachea is allowed to flow upward through the larynx and vocal tract so that it can be used to power speech.

Although some people who are mechanically ventilated are able to speak, they often have difficulties doing so. Several problems exist. First, the individual may be unable to control the timing of ventilator cycles. Second, the tracheal pressures generated by the ventilator are abnormally high and change rapidly. Third, these individuals must balance the aeromechanical requirements of speech production with the body's air exchange needs (Hoit, Shea, & Banzett, 1994). Differences in speech breathing behavior have been found between normal speech and ventilator-dependent speech (Table 8.6). Hoit et al. (1994) reported that the tidal volumes of most ventilator-dependent individuals were as much as three times larger than those of healthy persons. Recall that normal TV for quiet breathing is around 500 ml. The participants in the Hoit et al. (1994) study had TVs ranging from 700 to 1470 ml. Hoit et al. (1994) also found differences in P_{trach}, which for these ventilator-dependent patients ranged from 13.9 to 26 cm H_2O, compared to 5 to 10 cm H_2O in normal speech. In addition, rather than producing speech on an exhalation, the ventilator-dependent patients began to speak as P_{trach} rose during inspiration and stopped as P_{trach} fell during expiration. These patients usually began speaking 0.3 to 0.7 s after the onset of inspiration and stopped speaking around 0.7 to 1.1 s after the inspiratory flow ceased. The time at which the individual stopped speaking was usually influenced by the linguistic structure of the utterance. However, sometimes these patients stopped speaking when P_{trach} dropped below about 2 cm H_2O. For the most part, individuals did not take advantage of the full speaking time available to them. Average speaking duration ranged from 59 to 81 percent of the patient's potential speaking time. Therefore,

Table 8.6 **Respiratory Findings Reported for Mechanically Ventilated Individuals**

Excessively high TV
Higher-than-normal P_{trach}
Speech produced on inspiration

SOURCE: Information from Hoit et al., 1994.

speakers produced a smaller-than-normal number of syllables per breath. Based on these findings, Hoit, Banzett, et al. (1990) suggested that a promising strategy for maximizing speech duration is to encourage the patient to continue speaking as far into the expiratory portion of the cycle as possible, until voicing begins to fade with the falling P_{trach}. However, although this strategy can increase speaking time, it might also result in frequent linguistically inappropriate breaks in the speaker's discourse. Hoit, Banzett, et al. (1990) suggested that these breaks may actually be beneficial because they signal the listener that the speaker plans to continue talking.

Patients who require mechanical ventilation are often good candidates for placement of a speaking valve, such as a Passy-Muir valve. This is a one-way valve that fits into the stoma in the patient's neck. When the patient wants to speak, the valve can be closed using positive pressure generated in the trachea. The air is therefore prevented from exiting the trachea and consequently is exhaled through the larynx. This allows the patient to use the larynx to generate voice.

Voice Disorders

Many voice disorders such as nodules and polyps and vocal fatigue are associated with respiratory dysfunction (Table 8.7).

A substantial amount of research has established that individuals with vocal nodules demonstrate different speech breathing behaviors than healthy speakers. Sapienza and Stathopoulos (1994) examined respiratory and laryngeal function in children and women with bilateral nodules. They reported that individuals with nodules produced larger lung volume excursions, characterized by both higher lung volume initiation and lower lung volume termination. They suggested that the high volumes may be a compensation for the greater flow of air through the glottis caused by incomplete approximation of the vocal folds. Iwarsson and Sundberg (1999) noted that compared to the individuals without nodules, their subjects with nodules initiated a shouting task at lower lung volumes, spent a higher percentage of their vital capacity per second in all tasks, inhaled more frequently but to a lesser lung volume, and demonstrated fewer syllables per breath group. It appeared that the patients did not take advantage of the higher recoil pressures generated by inspiring to higher lung volumes. Schaeffer, Cavallo, Wall, and Diakow (2002) compared speech breathing patterns in speakers with and

Table 8.7 **Respiratory Findings Reported for Individuals with Voice Disorders**

Higher- or lower-than-normal lung volume initiations for speech
Speech initiated at volumes below REL
Higher percentage of VC per second in speaking tasks
Lower lung terminations for speech
Decreased lung volumes at higher intensities
Higher-than-normal P_{trach}

SOURCES: Information from Iwarsson & Sundberg, 1999; Lowell et al., 2008; Sapienza & Stathopoulos, 1994; and Schaeffer et al., 2002.

without vocal fold lesions. They reported that not only did the dysphonic speakers end speech at significantly lower lung volumes (i.e., below REL), but a large proportion of these speakers consistently began speech below REL. Speech breathing for the dysphonic group occurred at very different ranges in VC than it did for the nondysphonic individuals. Further, the group with vocal pathologies was less efficient in managing speech breathing, as talking at volumes below REL places greater demands on the muscles of the respiratory system.

The increased strain on the respiratory muscles that occurs when speaking at low lung volumes can have the additional effect of stiffening the vocal folds during phonation (Milstein, Qi, & Hillman, 2000). Excessive use of laryngeal muscle force during phonation (hyperfunctional voice production) is often associated with higher P_{trach}, indicating increased respiratory effort. Respiratory patterns reported in conjunction with hyperfunctional voice disorders include shallow breathing, poor coordination of expiration and phonation, and clavicular breathing. Some patients with hyperfunctional voice disorders complain of a loss of breath and respiratory fatigue during voice production (Sapienza & Stathopoulos, 1995). The fatigue may be due, at least in part, to the greater muscular force needed for speech at lower lung volumes. This was illustrated in a study by Lowell, Barkmeier-Kraemer, Hoit, and Story (2008). These researchers used linearized magnetometers to measure lung volume changes in teachers with and without voice disorders. Teachers with voice disorders started and ended their breath groups at smaller lung volumes, particularly during a simulated teaching condition. When asked to speak at louder intensities, the teachers with voice disorders decreased their lung volume initiations and terminations. This is opposite of what most speakers do to increase loudness, and it requires greater expiratory muscular pressure, especially at the end of breath groups. The greater muscular forces used may contribute to the symptoms of effort, work, and fatigue reported by the teachers with voice disorders.

Therapeutic intervention aimed at decreasing the use of lung volumes below REL has been reported as beneficial in individuals with dysphonia. Schaeffer (2007) measured respiratory and phonatory function in speakers with moderate to severe dysphonia before and after therapy. Therapy focused on facilitating the coordination of respiration and phonation. Speakers were taught to pause and release their breath at appropriate intervals in order to replenish their air supply more efficiently and to maintain voicing until the end of the breath group. Following the course of therapy, RIP and EGG measures showed that the participants used similar lung volumes to those reported for healthy speakers. Furthermore, after therapy the participants' voices were rated as having improved in voice quality.

Asthma

Asthma is a chronic disorder in which the large and small airways become narrower than normal. Bronchial narrowing results from inflammation and swelling of the mucosal lining of the airways, as well as from contraction of the bronchial smooth muscles (Dorinsky, Edwards, Yancey, & Rickard, 2001; Ihre, Zetterson, Ihre, & Hammarberg, 2004). The airway obstruction may be reversible or partially reversible either spontaneously or with treatment. See Figure 8.3.

Figure 8.3 Normal versus asthmatic airway

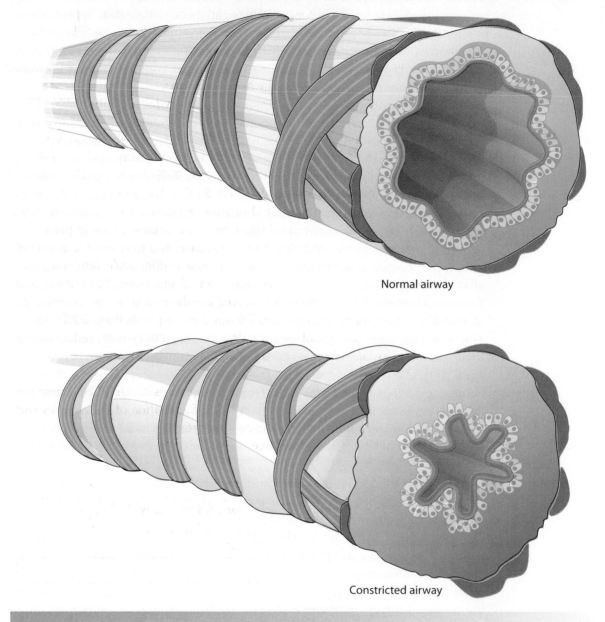

Normal airway

Constricted airway

While asthma is a chronic disease, it is also characterized by acute flare-ups ("attacks"). Symptoms in the chronic or steady state include nighttime coughing, dyspnea with exertion but not at rest, chronic throat clearing and cough, and chest tightness. Acute attacks are characterized by dyspnea, labored breathing, wheezing on expiration, and chest tightness (Saunders, 2005). An attack may be so severe that the individual needs to be hospitalized.

There are many triggers for asthma attacks, including pet hair and dander, dust, allergies, changes in the weather, viral infections, exercise, mold, pollen, chemicals, smoke, uncontrolled GERD, and stress. Exercise is a common trigger. Speaking and singing have also been reported as triggers for asthma (e.g., Cohn, Sataloff, & Branton, 2001).

Asthma is diagnosed by means of pulmonary function tests. Typically, the variables measured are VC, TLC, RV, and peak expiratory flow rates (PEF). PEF is the maximum flow rate generated at any time during a forceful exhalation (Eid, Yandell, Howell, Eddy, & Sheikh, 2000). PEF measures the rate of flow of air from the large airways (i.e., bronchi and trachea). Other measures of airflow include FEV_1 (forced expiratory volume in 1 s), FVC (forced vital capacity), FEV_1/FVC ratio (FEV_1 divided by FVC), and $FEF_{25-75\%}$ (forced expiratory flow between 25% and 75% of VC) (e.g., Eid et al., 2000; Jenkins et al., 2003). FEV_1 has been reported to reflect the function of the large- and medium-sized airways, while $FEF_{25-75\%}$ is a measure of the smaller airways (Drewek et al., 2009; Stelmach, Grzelewski, Bobrowska-Korzeniowska, Stelmach, & Kuna, 2007). FEV_1 in particular is used internationally to establish a probable diagnosis of asthma, to predict continuation of asthma from childhood to adulthood, to predict relapse following termination of treatment, to grade the severity of the disease, and to assess the effects of treatment (e.g., Appleton, Adams, Wilson, Taylor, & Ruffin, 2005; Tantisira et al., 2006). FEV_1 and FEV_1/FVC ratio are typically lower than predicted in asthma, and the more severe the disease, the more reduced are the expiratory measures (e.g., Birnbaum et al., 2009; Firoozi, Lemière, Beauchesne, Forget, & Blais, 2007). Flow-volume loops in asthma typically show a flattened expiratory limb, reflecting the obstructive nature of the disease. Oxygen levels are consistently reduced, particularly during acute attacks. See Table 8.8.

The primary treatment for asthma is inhaled corticosteroids (ICS). These are designed to reduce or eliminate the underlying inflammation of the airways and decrease the excessive mucous production associated with the disease. ICS use has been shown to be extremely effective in controlling asthma symptoms (Balter,

Table 8.8 Respiratory Findings Reported for Individuals with Asthma

Flattened expiratory limb on a flow-volume loop
Reductions in FEV_1
Reductions in FEV_1/FVC ratio
Cough
Dyspnea
Chronic throat clearing
Chest tightness
Labored breathing
Wheezing/stridor on expiration
Reduced oxygen levels

SOURCES: Information from Birnbaum et al. (2009); Firoozi et al. (2007); and Saunders (2005).

Adams, & Chapman, 2001; Roland, Bhalla, & Earis, 2004). There are also medications available that combine a corticosteroid with a bronchodilator that reduces smooth muscle constriction of the airways. These medications act to improve lung function, reduce asthma symptoms and acute attacks, and decrease the rate of emergency room visits and hospital admissions. The efficacy of asthma medications has been demonstrated by improvements in FEV_1 and $FEF_{25-75\%}$ (Stelmach et al., 2007). FEV_1 and $FEF_{25-75\%}$ have been widely used to compare the efficacy of specific drugs (e.g., Dorinsky et al., 2001; Patel, Van Natta, Tonascia, Wise, & Strunk, 2008).

A large percentage of children with asthma reportedly also have speech and voice disorders (Keating, Turrell, & Ozanne, 2001). Children with asthma and other airway disorders commonly use mouth breathing. This is less healthy than nose breathing, as the air inhaled through the oral cavity is not warmed, moistened, and filtered in the same way as the air inhaled through the nasal cavities. It has been shown that oral breathing dehydrates the mucosal layers of the airways and the vocal folds and contributes to increased vocal effort (Sivasankar & Fisher, 2002). Asthma can also cause dyspnea and clavicular/thoracic breathing rather than the more efficient abdominal breathing for speech. Lack of breath support can in turn result in inadequate vocal volume and dysphonia. Further, the labored breathing and wheezing that are characteristic of asthma can inflame the vocal folds and further contribute to poor vocal quality. Another concern is that while the use of inhaled corticosteroids is very effective in controlling asthma symptoms for many individuals (Balter et al., 2001; Roland et al., 2004), laryngeal side effects such as hoarseness have been reported in a sizable number of ICS users (e.g., Kim, Moon, Chung, & Lee, 2011; Roland et al., 2004; Stanton, Sellars, MacKenzie, McConnachie, & Bucknall, 2009; Williamson, Matusiewicz, Brown, Greening, & Crompton, 1995).

Paradoxical Vocal Fold Motion

Paradoxical vocal fold motion (PVFM) is a disorder in which the coordination between the respiratory and laryngeal systems is disrupted by inappropriate spasmodic vocal fold adduction during the inhalation phase of breathing (Holmes et al., 2009). The major symptoms of PVFM are stridor, dyspnea, and chronic cough. The stridor is typically heard when the patient inhales. In asthma the stridor usually occurs on the exhalation. However, it is not uncommon for the exhalation phase to be affected as well because once the laryngospasm has begun during inspiration, the hyperadduction may carry over for a brief interval into the exhalation phase (Andrianopoulos, Gallivan, & Gallivan, 2000). In addition, many individuals with PVFM also have asthma (e.g., Doshi & Weinberger, 2006; Gurevich-Uvena et al., 2010; Koufman & Block, 2008; Morris, 2006; Newman, Mason, & Schmaling, 1995; Parsons et al., 2010). Other features are also common in both PVFM and asthma, including GERD, postnasal drip, and allergies (Gurevich-Uvena et al, 2010; Parsons et al., 2010). The overlap in signs and symptoms and the presence of stridor and dyspnea make the diagnosis of PVFM very challenging, and symptoms are often misdiagnosed as asthma or reactive airway disease. It is not uncommon for patients with PVFM to undergo aggressive asthma treatment, which is usually not effective (Morris, 2006). In some cases, individuals have undergone invasive interventions such as intubation or even tracheostomy (Newman et al., 1995).

Pulmonary function testing is an integral component of diagnosing PVFM. One of the distinguishing characteristics of PVFM is that spirometric values are normal when the individual is asymptomatic. Even when an individual with PVFM is experiencing severe respiratory symptoms, blood oxygen levels are typically normal (Hicks, Brugman, & Katial, 2008; Noyes & Kemp, 2007) or may be mildly abnormal (oxygen and carbon dioxide may be slightly reduced during an acute attack). Individuals with PVFM may show a reduced VC and abnormal inspiratory volumes (Murry, Cukier-Blaj, Kelleher, & Malki, 2011). Some individuals with PVFM show a reduction in the ratio of FEV_1/FVC compared to individuals without PVFM (Morris, Deal, & Bean, 1999). However, patients who are symptomatic may demonstrate reductions in both the FEV_1 and FVC, resulting in a normal FEV_1/FVC ratio (Morris & Christopher, 2010). The FEF_{50}/FIF_{50} is another spirometric measure that can help in the diagnosis of PVFM. This variable compares the middle portion of the expiratory airflow to the middle portion of the inspiratory airflow. The normal ratio is less than or equal to 1, whereas it is often greater than 1 in patients with PVFM (Hicks et al., 2008; Morris & Christopher, 2010). In other words, individuals with PVFM often show greater flow on expiration than on inspiration. See Table 8.9.

Flow-volume curves tend to be different in persons with PVFM than in those with asthma. Individuals with PVFM often demonstrate flattening or blunting of the inspiratory limb of the loop, reflecting a reduction in the amount of inhaled air which may be present even when the individual is asymptomatic (e.g., Buddiga, 2010; Christopher & Morris, 2010). In some cases, the expiratory portion of the flow-volume loop may also be flattened (Chiang, Goh, Tang, & Chay, 2008). This may occur in cases where the paradoxical vocal fold movement continues into the exhalation phase of respiration and hinders the outflow of air. It can also occur in individuals with coexisting PVFM and asthma. People with asthma but without PVFM show blunting only of the expiratory limb. This is consistent with the obstructive nature of the disease due to bronchial narrowing and inflammation. See Figure 8.1.

Treatment for PVFM is aimed at relieving the patient's airway obstruction and can be divided into that for an acute attack and/or long-term therapy. Clinical management can include behavioral voice therapy, pharmacological therapy, respiratory procedures, or any combination of these. Speech therapy focusing on breathing management has become the primary intervention of

---

Table 8.9 **Respiratory Findings Reported for Individuals with PVFM**

Stridor on inhalation
Normal to mildly abnormal blood oxygen levels during attack
Reduction in FEV_1/FVC ratio
FEF_{50}/FIF_{50} greater than 1
Flattened inspiratory limb on flow-volume curve

SOURCES: Information from Buddiga (2010); Hicks et al. (2008); Morris et al. (1999); Morris & Christopher (2010); and Noyes & Kemp (2007).

choice for chronic PVFM (Morris, 2006). Speech therapy has been shown to be very helpful for individuals to manage the symptoms of the disorder (e.g., Jines & Drummond, 2006). Because speech–language pathologists are trained in laryngeal anatomy and physiology, they are well equipped to teach a patient how to control his or her laryngeal function for respiration. Speech therapy typically encompasses patient education, respiratory retraining, raising awareness and relaxation, and vocal hygiene, including reduction of coughing and throat clearing.

Respiratory retraining techniques are designed to teach a patient to respond to the feeling of throat constriction with a more relaxed breathing pattern (Blager, 2006). An individual practices using abdominal rather than thoracic muscles to inhale and exhale. This involves expanding the abdominal wall on inhalation and contracting the abdominal muscles when exhaling (e.g., Altman et al., 2002; Morris, 2006). The patient simultaneously maintains his or her shoulders, neck, and jaw in a relaxed position. This respiratory pattern helps to remove the focus from the larynx. Respiratory retraining has been reported as very effective in the long-term management of people with PVFM (e.g., Murry, Tabaee, Owezarzak, & Aviv, 2006).

Summary

Lung volumes can be measured directly with a spirometer or estimated from rib cage and abdominal movement.

Pulmonary function testing refers to a variety of tests designed to assess the amount of air an individual is able to inhale and exhale, as well as how efficiently the person moves air into and out of the lungs.

Respiratory kinematic analysis is used to estimate lung volumes from movements of the rib cage and abdomen, using plethysmography or linearized magnetometers.

Air pressures can be measured with manometers or pressure sensors placed within the oral cavity.

Airflow through the respiratory system is measured via pneumotachometry.

Obstructive lung diseases are marked by difficulty in exhalation due to narrowing or blockage of the airways.

Restrictive lung diseases are those that restrict lung expansion and are characterized by reduced lung volume.

Central problems in respiration are caused by neurological dysfunction in the respiratory brain centers in the brain stem.

Dyspnea refers to subjectively perceived discomfort in breathing, which may be perceived as shortness of breath, the need to work hard to breathe, and/or chest tightness.

Stridor is defined as an audible sound that occurs during inspiration and/or expiration, resulting from turbulent air flow as the air passes through a narrowed or obstructed segment in the airway.

Four important principles in the clinical management of speech breathing problems are measuring the patient's respiratory function in both static and dynamic tasks; tailoring treatment to the patient's specific respiratory difficulty; sequencing clinical activities in terms of pressure variables, volume variables, and chest wall shape; and practicing exercises in speech contexts rather than in nonspeech contexts.

Patients with Parkinson's disease often show reduced movement of the rib cage and greater displacement of the abdomen during speech breathing, which is opposite the normal pattern.

Patients with cervical spinal cord injury may not be able to breathe on their own and may need mechanical ventilation; if such a person can breathe, he or she may have difficulty generating adequate pressures and flows for speech.

Many children and adults with cerebral palsy face problems with respiratory function affecting pressure, flow, volume, and shape.

Patients with cerebellar disease sometimes show a reduced vital capacity, resulting from the breakdown in the coordination of chest wall activity.

Speakers with voice problems such as nodules tend to end speech at significantly lower lung volumes than healthy speakers, and they may even begin speech below REL.

FEV_1 and FEV_1/FVC ratio are typically lower than predicted in individuals with asthma, and the more severe the disease, the more reduced are the expiratory measures.

Pulmonary function testing can reveal different patterns on a flow-volume loop for individuals with asthma and those with paradoxical vocal fold motion.

REVIEW EXERCISES

1. Describe the use of spirometric measures in pulmonary function testing.

2. Identify the ways in which air pressures and airflows for speech are measured and describe advantages and disadvantages of each measure.

3. Do you agree or disagree with the suggestion that, if a patient can sustain a steady stream of subglottal air pressure of 5 cm H_2O for 5 s, the respiratory system may be sufficient to support speech? Provide a detailed rationale for your answer.

4. How does the muscle rigidity that is a hallmark of Parkinson's disease affect respiration and speech production?

5. Make a table of similarities and differences in respiratory function in patients with cerebellar disease and in those with cervical spinal cord injury.

6. Compare respiratory function in spastic, athetoid, and ataxic cerebral palsy.

7. Identify two problems in respiratory and speech function in individuals who are mechanically ventilated.

8. Explain how speaking at low lung volumes can affect voice production.

9. Compare and contrast the respiratory characteristics of individuals with asthma, those with paradoxical vocal fold motion, and those who suffer from both conditions.

INTEGRATIVE CASE STUDIES

① Mr. Stevens

Background

Mr. Stevens is a 78-year-old man who was diagnosed with Parkinson's disease 5 years ago. He was referred by his neurologist to your outpatient rehabilitation center for a speech evaluation and possible treatment. Family members, including Mrs. Stevens and their three adult children, have complained about having difficulty understanding him. Mrs. Stevens reports that his voice is extremely soft, that he sounds "breathless," and that he "mumbles." The children all live out of state and communicate mostly with their parents through phone calls, since their parents do not own a computer. Of late, Mrs. Stevens is finding it more and more difficult to get her husband to talk to the children on the phone. She's hoping that speech therapy will improve his ability to communicate.

Clinical Observations

Upon meeting Mr. Stevens, you are struck by his stooped posture, and you note that his head hangs forward, both when standing and sitting. As his wife indicated, his speech intelligibility is reduced due to low intensity, lack of normal prosody, and slurred speech.

Respiratory Measures

Using a portable spirometer, you obtain Mr. Stevens vital capacity both in his typical stooped posture and with postural support that helps to improve the alignment between his head and chest. In addition, you have Mr. Stevens sustain the /a/ vowel for as long as possible in order to determine his maximum phonation time. This activity is also done under the two conditions of his stooped and improved posture. Spirometric measurements under the stooped postural condition indicate a VC of 2800 ml, compared to the norm of 4470 ml for his age group. When provided with postural support, his VC improved to 3500 ml. Maximum phonation time also improved from 3.5 seconds with extremely breathy voice to 9 seconds with a stronger voice quality.

Clinical Questions

a. How can the diagnostic information provided above be used to set treatment goals for this patient?

b. What other respiratory measurements might be helpful in the diagnosis and treatment of this patient?

c. What kinds of respiratory exercises may be implemented to improve Mr. Stevens's speech breathing?

d. How could treatment focusing on respiration improve the client's vocal intensity levels?

② Bella

Background

Bella, age 15, is the star player on her junior varsity soccer team. She has had mild asthma since she was 5 years old and uses a rescue inhaler when necessary. Recently, she has started to complain that when on the field, she experiences a sensation of breathing difficulty, and this causes her to become very anxious. During her last game, she had to be escorted off the field as she "couldn't get her breath," even with the inhaler. Her doctor has referred her to your clinic for a thorough evaluation.

Clinical Observations

Upon your initial meeting with Bella, you note that she is friendly and self-assured. Although she is accompanied by her mother, she seems to be comfortable handling most of the communication herself. She relates that she becomes very shaken and anxious when she has "breathing spasms." She also comments that these spasms "feel different" from the mild asthma attacks that she has experienced since she was a little girl. You suspect from this description that Bella might have paradoxical vocal fold motion in addition to the existing asthma.

Respiratory Measures

Using a spirometer, you measure Bella's VC, FVC, FEV_1, and FEF_{50}/FIF_{50}.

❸ Mike

Background

Mike is a 17-year-old male with spastic cerebral palsy (CP) and is wheelchair bound. He has come to a clinic that specializes in CP for his annual speech evaluation. Mike is accompanied by his parents, who express concern regarding his breathing during speech. They report that Mike "talks really softly and can't seem to get any louder." In addition, they note that Mike's voice sounds like it has become tense and strained. Due to parental concerns, a full respiratory assessment has been included as part of the evaluation.

Clinical Observations

Mike has an unsupported rigid posture while seated in his wheelchair. His trunk deviates to the right side, and his head is hyperextended 120 degrees in an upward manner. The wheelchair appears to lack the support necessary to keep his trunk centered and his head at a 90-degree angle. The clinician notes that Mike's vocal quality is pressed, and his loudness is reduced. The client's inhalations are shallow, and respiratory movements are noted primarily in the thoracic area. Exhalations are forced and uncontrolled.

Clinical Questions

a. What spirometric values would you expect to see for Bella?

b. Do you think that spirometric values could be used to distinguish the asthma from the paradoxical vocal fold motion characteristics? Why or why not?

c. What additional measures might be helpful to make a more definitive diagnosis of paradoxical vocal fold motion?

d. What are some measures that asthma and PVFM have in common?

Respiratory Measures

Pulmonary function testing is conducted, and findings are compared to normative values specific to 17-year-old Caucasian males, 5'9" in height. The following measures are obtained:

VC	3286 ml
TV	289 ml
IRV	679 ml
ERV	566 ml

Clinical Questions

a. How might wheelchair positioning/support play a role in maximizing Mike's respiratory functioning?

b. What other respiratory measures would be helpful in assessing Mike's breathing support for speech?

c. Based on the clinical observations of shallow breathing, what would you expect a flow-volume loop to look like for Mike?

d. Based on clinical observations of thoracic breathing and reductions in Mike's spirometric measures, what are some therapeutic techniques that might help improve his breath support for speech?

CHAPTER

9

The Auditory System

STUDENT LEARNING OBJECTIVES

After reading this chapter you will

○ Identify the structures and functions of the outer, middle, and inner ears.

○ Understand the relationship of the basilar membrane in the cochlea and the traveling wave.

○ Compare conductive and sensorineural loss in terms of degree and configuration.

○ Understand the impact of hearing loss on speech perception.

○ Explain the acoustic patterns in the perception of vowels and consonants, such as formants, formant transitions, categorical perception, and redundancy.

The ear acts as a transducer—a device that converts energy from one form to another. For example, a microphone transduces sound waves into electrical energy, and a loudspeaker converts electrical energy into acoustic pressure waves. The ear converts acoustic pressure waves to mechanical energy in the middle ear, and it converts mechanical to electrical energy in the inner ear. The ear in some ways can also be likened to a spectrographic analyzer because the auditory system detects changes in the frequency and intensity of sound waves over time. To understand the transformations of the acoustic signal that take place in the ear, it is important to gain an understanding of the structures involved, including the outer, middle, and inner ears. Problems with auditory function in any part or parts of the ear result in different types of hearing loss and can interfere with speech perception. The processes involved in assigning meaning to the sounds that a listener hears are considered.

Outer Ear

Two parts make up the outer ear, the pinna (or auricle) and the external auditory meatus, or ear canal. The pinna is the external "flap" on the side of the head, often referred to as "the ear." Most of the pinna is made of flexible elastic cartilage, with the exception of the inferior, or bottom, part, known as the lobule (or lobe). The pinna is attached to the side of the cranium by ligaments. Although the pinna does contain some muscles, they are vestigial in humans (Dickson & Maue-Dickson, 1982). The main function of the pinna is to help channel sound waves into the ear canal. This is particularly true for high-frequency sounds and for localization in the vertical plane and in front–back distinctions (Hofman & van Opstal, 2003). The pinna also protects the entrance to the external auditory meatus and, because

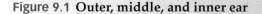

Figure 9.1 Outer, middle, and inner ear

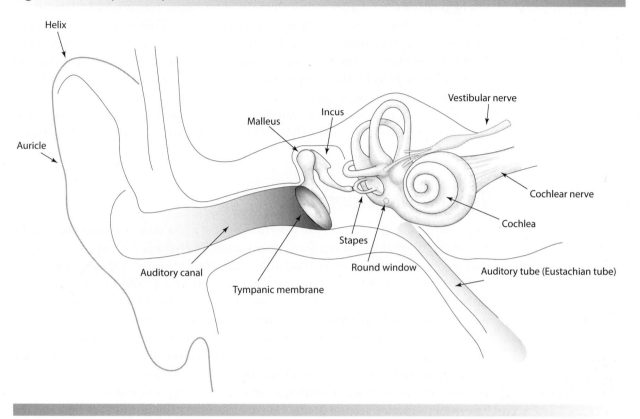

humans have two pinnae, one on each side of the head, they help in the localization of sound. However, compared to animals, the pinna in humans does not play a particularly important role in sound detection.

The external auditory meatus leads from the pinna to the eardrum, or tympanic membrane (TM) (see Figure 9.1). In adults, the meatus is an S-shaped tube about 2.5 to 3.5 cm long and about 6 mm in diameter (Kent, 1997b). The canal terminates at its medial end at the tympanic membrane. The lateral one-third to one-half of the canal is cartilaginous, and the medial one-half to two-thirds is bone. The entire canal is lined with a layer of epidermis. The cartilaginous part of the canal contains glands that secrete oil and a waxy substance known as cerumen. These serve to lubricate the ear canal and to hinder the entry of insects. The lateral part of the canal also contains cilia. The cilia move in a wavelike fashion, which helps to propel the cerumen, together with small particles of dust or other substances, toward the outside.

The ear canal has several functions. First, by virtue of its length and shape, and the presence of cerumen and cilia, it protects the more delicate middle and inner ears. Second, the ear canal plays an important part in terms of sound detection, because it is a quarter-wave resonator, open at the pinna end and closed at the tympanic membrane. As with any quarter-wave resonator, the lowest resonant frequency (RF) of the canal is calculated by multiplying the length of the tube by 4 and dividing this number into the speed of sound. Based on a length of 2.5 cm, the

RF of the ear canal is 3400 Hz: 2.5 cm $\times$ 4 = 10 cm; 34,000/10 = 3400 Hz. Due to this high-frequency resonance, the external auditory meatus resonates and boosts the amplitude of high-frequency sounds entering the ear. This is helpful for sounds such as /s, z, ʃ, ð/, which have much of their acoustic energy in frequencies above 2000 Hz. Together the pinna and ear canal create a broad resonance, resulting in approximately 10 to 15 dB of amplification of the spectrum between 2500 and 5000 Hz at the tympanic membrane, relative to the sound source (Greenberg, 1996). This increase in high-frequency amplitude enables humans to detect sounds that would not otherwise be audible if the TM were located at the surface of the head.

Tympanic Membrane

The tympanic membrane is the interface between the outer ear and the middle ear. In the normal ear, it is a semi transparent, oval-shaped sheet of membrane that is concave on its external (lateral) surface. This gives the TM a conical shape, with the point of the cone facing the middle ear space. The tip of the cone is called the umbo. The membrane is held in position by a ligament and is composed of external, middle, and internal layers. The external (lateral) layer is contiguous with the epidermis of the ear canal. The internal (medial) layer is mucous membrane and is continuous with the mucous membrane that lines the cavity of the middle ear. Between these two is a fibrous layer that contains radial and circular fibers, both providing support to the tympanic membrane structure. The small, superior section of the TM contains fewer fibers and is designated the pars flaccida; the remaining section is known as the pars tensa. A part of one of the bones of the middle ear, the malleus, is embedded in the TM, contributing to its conical shape.

The primary function of the tympanic membrane is to vibrate when acoustic pressure waves impinge on it. Because part of the malleus is embedded within the TM, the vibration of the TM is transmitted to the malleus and to the other two bones in the middle ear, the incus and the stapes. The TM is extremely sensitive to tiny variations in pressure and responds to an extraordinary range of pressures across a wide range of frequencies. Thus, the TM is involved in the process of transducing pressure waves to mechanical vibration.

Middle Ear

Lying directly behind (medial to) the TM is the middle ear. The middle ear is a tiny space, about 6 mm wide and about 4 mm deep (Kent, 1997b), with a volume of about 2 ml. The space is divided into two sections—the tympanic cavity, or tympanum, and the epitympanic recess, or attic. As its name implies, the attic lies superior to the tympanic cavity. In the normal ear, the middle ear is an air-filled cavity, ventilated and drained by the Eustachian tube. It contains three small bones, the malleus, incus, and stapes, collectively referred to as the ossicles; ligaments that hold the ossicles in place; and two muscles.

Eustachian Tube

The Eustachian tube (sometimes called the auditory tube) is about 35 mm in length. The frontmost two-thirds of the tube lies within a canal made of cartilage, and the posterior one-third lies within a bony canal. The tube runs from the nasopharynx to the middle ear. The pharyngeal opening of the tube is a slit approximately 8 mm high and 1 mm wide. This end of the tube is normally closed, except when one swallows or yawns, when it opens through the action of the tensor veli palatini and the levator veli palatini muscles. The opening to the bony section is normally open. The inside of the tube is lined with epithelium.

The Eustachian tube is extremely important for middle ear function as it serves to keep the middle ear space ventilated and drained through two functions. First, the tube acts to equalize the air pressure between the otherwise closed middle ear and the external atmosphere because air from the atmosphere enters the middle ear when the tube opens. If anything prevents the tube from opening, the equalization of air pressures becomes difficult or impossible. The result is a negative pressure condition in the middle ear cavity (relative to the atmosphere), which presents as a "blocked" sensation in the ear. If this condition is not resolved, fluid from the middle ear space may begin to accumulate, which can result in a middle ear infection.

The second function of the Eustachian tube is to help clear mucus from the middle ear by draining the mucus to the pharynx, where it is swallowed. If mucus is not cleared, it can lead to otitis media, a middle ear infection. Young children are particularly susceptible to middle ear infections because their Eustachian tubes run nearly horizontally, so fluids do not drain as easily as they do in adults.

Ossicles

The three ossicles are the smallest bones in the human body. They are connected to each other, to the TM on one side, and to a part of the inner ear called the oval window on the other (most medial) side. The malleus, or hammer, has two major parts—the head and the handle, or manubrium. The manubrium is embedded in the TM, while the head extends into the epitympanic recess. The tip of the manubrium coincides with the umbo. The incus, or anvil, is connected to the malleus, and the stapes, or stirrup, is attached to the incus and to the oval window. The malleus measures about 8 mm in length. The incus is also about 8 mm in length. It has a rounded body from which two processes extend. The stapes has a body, with an anterior and posterior crus (leg) converging on it from either side. The oval-shaped footplate of the stapes fits into the oval window of the inner ear and is held in place by the annular ligament. This ossicular chain, as it is sometimes called, is supported by ligaments and forms the mechanical vibrating element of the auditory system.

Muscles of the Middle Ear

The two muscles of the middle ear are the tensor tympani and the stapedius. The tensor tympani muscle is about 20 mm in length and runs parallel to the Eustachian tube. The tensor tympani originates at the tendon of the tensor veli palatini muscle, passes through a bony canal in the temporal bone of the cranium, emerges into the tympanic cavity, and connects with the manubrium of the malleus. A contraction of the tensor tympani pulls the malleus inward (medially).

The stapedius muscle is much shorter than the tensor tympani, about 6 mm, and runs from the posterior wall of the tympanic cavity to the head of the stapes. A contraction of the stapedius pulls the stapes posteriorly (Zemlin, 1998). The stapedius muscle is involved in a reflex known as the acoustic, or stapedial, reflex. This reflex occurs when the stapedius muscle contracts strongly in response to intense sound of 80 dB HL (hearing level) or more, stiffening the ossicular chain and the tympanic membrane. The reflex occurs bilaterally, meaning that a loud sound introduced to either ear will elicit the reflex in both ears. The contraction of the stapedius has the effect of reducing the pressure applied to the oval window, which in turn reduces the sound intensity by around 10 dB, notably in the low frequencies. The reflex does not occur instantaneously but takes some fractions of a second to act. Therefore, sounds that occur very suddenly can be transmitted to the inner ear before the reflex has had time to occur. Also, as with any other muscle, the stapedius eventually fatigues. Consequently, in a noisy environment, the reflex becomes less effective at damping loud sounds. The middle ear muscles are also activated before and during vocalization, effectively reducing the level of one's own voice at the cochlea. These muscles also contract in response to non auditory stimuli, such as tactile stimulation of the face.

3 Functions of the Middle Ear

The middle ear performs several crucial functions in hearing. First, it increases the amount of acoustic energy that gets transmitted into the inner ear by overcoming the impedance mismatch between the middle and inner ears. Impedance is a measure of the difficulty of signal transmission through a medium, such as a gas or liquid; its inverse is admittance, which is a measure of how easily signals are transmitted through a medium. Different mediums can offer more or less opposition to sound waves. Liquids have a higher impedance to sound waves than does air. When sound waves traveling through air come to a fluid, the difference in impedance acts as a barrier, and most of the sound energy is therefore reflected rather than being transmitted. The middle ear is filled with air, whereas the inner ear is filled with fluid. The boundary between these two areas is the oval window, located in the medial wall of the middle ear space and in which the stapes footplate is seated. When sound waves propagating through the air in the middle ear come into contact with the fluid in the inner ear, almost all of the incident energy is reflected, and very little is transmitted to the fluid. To overcome this impedance mismatch, it is necessary to increase the amplitude of the pressure changes at the oval window. The middle ear achieves this pressure amplification in three ways. The first and most effective way in which pressure amplification is achieved relies on the difference in the surface area of the TM compared to the oval window. The area of the TM is about 0.85 cm², although only about 0.55 cm² is active in vibration. The area of the oval window is about 0.03 cm² (Raphael et al., 2007). The difference in surface area results in a gain of about 17:1 (Seikel, King, & Drumright, 1997; Zemlin, 1998). Because pressure is equal to force over a surface area, a given force exerts greater pressure over a smaller area than over a larger one. Therefore, the pressure changes causing vibration of the much larger TM become more intense when they are transmitted by the ossicles to the smaller oval window, yielding an increase of approximately 25 dB (see Figures 9.2 and 9.3). The second way in which the middle ear increases pressure at the oval window is through the lever action of the ossicles. Leverage increases the force at the stapes footplate by a factor of about 1.3, or approximately 2 dB, in comparison to the force at the malleus. The third factor,

Figure 9.2 Pressure amplification through leverage

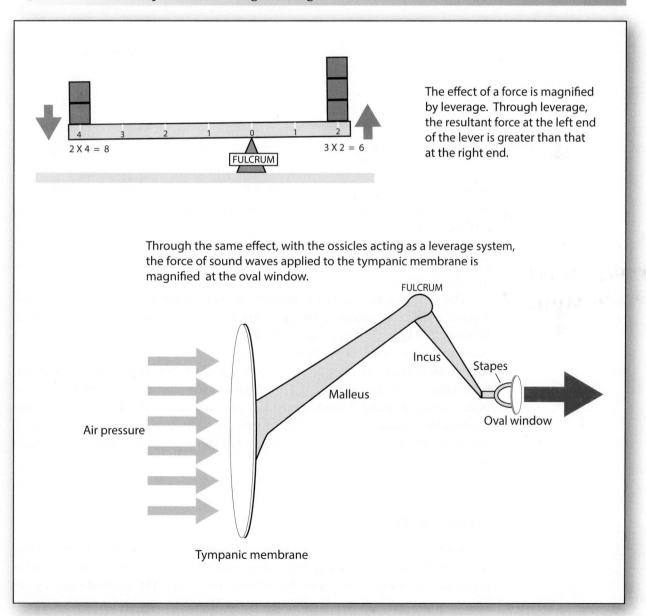

The effect of a force is magnified by leverage. Through leverage, the resultant force at the left end of the lever is greater than that at the right end.

$2 \times 4 = 8$

FULCRUM

$3 \times 2 = 6$

Through the same effect, with the ossicles acting as a leverage system, the force of sound waves applied to the tympanic membrane is magnified at the oval window.

FULCRUM

Incus

Stapes

Malleus

Oval window

Air pressure

Tympanic membrane

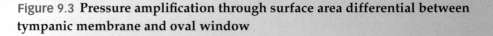

Figure 9.3 Pressure amplification through surface area differential between tympanic membrane and oval window

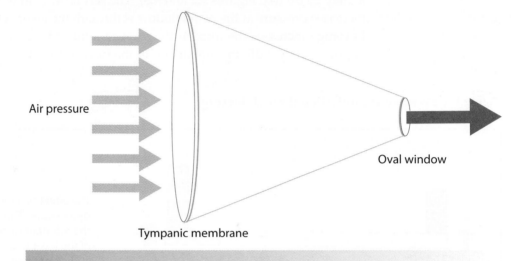

The energy of the air pressure that moves the tympanic membrane is concentrated on the much smaller oval window, creating an amplification effect.

Air pressure

Oval window

Tympanic membrane

often referred to as the "buckling effect," involves the conical shape of the TM, which results in greater movement of the membrane along the curved portion. All together, these effects increase the pressure at the oval window by about 30 dB. This is still not enough to pass along all the acoustic energy arriving at the TM. Only about half the sound energy arriving at the TM is actually transmitted into the inner ear.

The second function of the middle ear is to attenuate loud sounds by the acoustic reflex, brought about by the contraction of the stapedius muscle. The third function is to keep the air pressure inside the middle ear cavity and in the ear canal equal by means of the Eustachian tube. For the TM to vibrate properly, the pressure in the middle ear must be equal to that in the canal. Higher pressure within the middle ear pushes out on the TM, causing discomfort and interfering with the transmission of sound. Lower middle ear pressure causes the TM to be retracted, which also causes discomfort and interferes with sound transmission. These changing air pressure conditions can be felt during airline travel as the plane ascends and descends.

Inner Ear

The inner ear lies deep within the temporal bone and is composed of the cochlea, the semicircular canals, and a connecting vestibule between them. The cochlea is involved with hearing, whereas the semicircular canals and vestibule are important for balance. The following discussion focuses on the cochlea, with its extraordinary ability to function as a frequency and intensity analyzer.

Cochlea

The cochlea is housed in the petrous portion of the temporal bone, just medial to the tympanic cavity. It is a snail-shaped, bony, spiral canal (Figure 9.4) that makes two- and three-quarter turns around a bony core, known as the modiolus. Projecting from the modiolus, like the turns of a screw, is a bony shelf, the osseous spiral lamina, through which the nerve fibers contacting the hair cells are able to pass. The cochlear turns decrease in size from the base to the apex. The apex is that point of the canal farthest from the middle ear. If the cochlea were straightened out, it would measure around 5 cm (Pickles, 1988). Inside the bony canal is a membranous canal that takes the same snail shape. Between the bony canal and the membranous canal is fluid, the perilymph (*peri* = around). Within the membranous canal is a different kind of fluid, the endolymph (*endo* = within). The membranous canal is attached to the osseous spiral lamina and also to the outer wall of the bony canal (by the spiral ligament), forming three separate chambers, or scalae. The membranous canal is often referred to as the cochlear duct, or simply the cochlear partition. The base of this duct is the basilar membrane (BM). The roof of the duct is formed by the vestibular, or Reissner's, membrane. The space above the vestibular membrane is known as the scala vestibuli, and the space below the BM is the scala tympani. Between these two is the cochlear duct, or scala media. The scala vestibuli terminates at the oval window, which is covered by the footplate of the stapes. Another opening between the middle and inner ears, the round window, is the terminus of the scala tympani. This opening is covered with membrane. The cochlear duct does not completely fill the bony canal, extending almost, but not quite, to the apex of the canal. Where the cochlear duct ends, the scala vestibuli and scala tympani meet each other. This point of communication is the helicotrema.

Lying within the cochlear duct, sitting on the basilar membrane and running along its entire length, is the organ of Corti. This structure consists of several types of supporting cells and the sensory cells for hearing. The sensory cells are called the inner and outer hair cells, named for the tiny hairlike projections (**stereocilia**) that extend from their tops. The tips of the stereocilia of the outer hair cells are embedded in the tectorial membrane, a gelatinous structure that forms the roof of the organ of Corti.

There are about 3500 inner hair cells arranged in a single row along the length of the basilar membrane, and there are about 12,000 outer hair cells in three to five rows along the BM length. The shape of the inner hair cells resembles a flask, while the outer hair cells have a test-tube appearance. The two types of hair cells differ not only in their number and shape but also in their function. The outer hair cells are capable of movement, and their movement amplifies the signal and enhances the tuning of the basilar membrane. This in turn improves both auditory sensitivity and frequency selectivity, or ability to resolve the frequency components of a complex sound. When the inner hair cells are activated, they release neurotransmitter to excite the auditory nerve fibers contacting the base of the cell. When the BM vibrates, the stereocilia on the hair cells are sheared (bent) by the tectorial membrane; this shearing action stimulates the auditory nerve to fire. The hair cells thus serve as transducers, transforming fluid vibrations into electrical energy (Rosen & Howell, 1991).

Figure 9.4 Cochlea

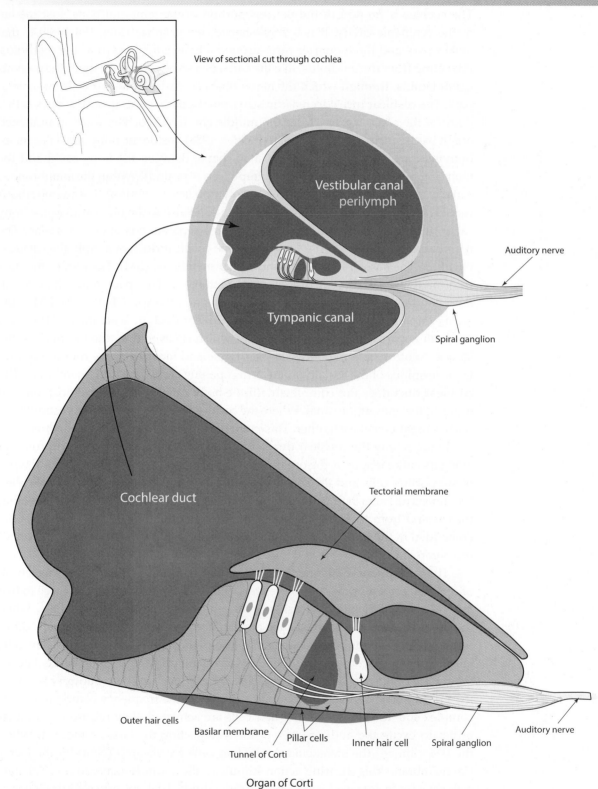

View of sectional cut through cochlea

Vestibular canal perilymph

Tympanic canal

Auditory nerve

Spiral ganglion

Cochlear duct

Tectorial membrane

Outer hair cells

Basilar membrane

Pillar cells

Tunnel of Corti

Inner hair cell

Spiral ganglion

Auditory nerve

Organ of Corti

Basilar Membrane

The basilar membrane, because of its structure, plays a crucial role in the cochlea's ability to perform a frequency and intensity analysis of all incoming sounds. The BM is not equally wide along its entire length (Figure 9.5). At its base, closest to the middle ear, the BM is only about 0.04 mm wide, increasing in width to around 0.36 mm at its apex, farthest from the middle ear (Buser & Imbert, 1992). This is in contrast with the bony cochlea itself, which decreases in width from base to apex. Not only does the width of the BM increase from base to apex, but so too does its stiffness. The membrane is stiffest at its narrow basal end and is about 100 times more

Figure 9.5 Schematic representation of the unrolled basilar membrane, showing its differential frequency response

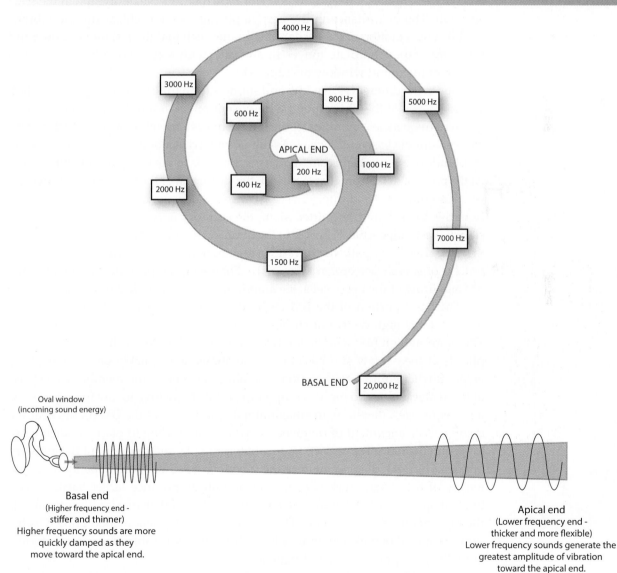

compliant at its wider apical end, making it more responsive to high frequencies at the base and lower frequencies at the apex. These different levels of width and stiffness of the BM are the factors that create the cochlea's capacity to perform a frequency analysis of sounds (Figure 9.5).

Cochlear Function

Events in the cochlea are set into motion through the footplate of the stapes, which sits in the oval window. When the tympanic membrane is set into vibration by increases and decreases in air pressure pushing and pulling at its surface, the vibration is transferred to the ossicles by the manubrium of the malleus, which is firmly attached to the TM. The movement of the malleus in turn sets the other ossicles, including the footplate of the stapes, into vibration. As the footplate moves inward and outward in the oval window, the vibration disturbs the perilymph in the scala vestibuli. The disturbance in the perilymph causes the cochlear duct to vibrate, establishing a motion in the basilar membrane, such that the BM moves down and up as the stapes footplate moves in and out (with a corresponding out-and-in motion of the round window membrane).

Due to the differences in width and stiffness from the base to the apex of the BM, different areas of the BM respond with greater or lesser amplitude of vibration to different frequencies. Vibration of the BM produces a traveling wave, which always moves from the base to the apex. As the wave travels along the BM, it increases in amplitude to a peak displacement that corresponds to the frequency of stimulation. At the point of maximum displacement, the stereocilia of the hair cells are activated, which stimulates the auditory nerve to fire at that frequency. The nerve impulses from the cochlea are transmitted along the auditory nerve, a branch of the eighth cranial (vestibulocochlear) nerve, to the brain stem. The impulses then continue up the central auditory pathway to various regions in the cortex of the brain, where the process of speech perception takes place. Following the peak displacement of the BM and firing of the nerve cells, the amplitude of the wave declines rapidly.

The basal portion of the BM responds to pressure waves at all frequencies, but due to its high degree of stiffness, it is most responsive to high frequencies. Therefore, at high frequencies, the wave motion of the BM reaches maximum amplitude at the narrow stiff base of the membrane and quickly becomes damped before traveling much farther along the BM. The apex of the membrane, because of its greater width and higher compliance, is most sensitive to low frequencies. At low frequencies, therefore, the maximum displacement of the BM occurs near the apex. This arrangement of frequency sensitivity according to place is called tonotopic organization. Tonotopic organization is maintained throughout the auditory system. The peak displacement of the traveling wave will also depend on the intensity of the signal. Signals of greater amplitude produce larger basilar membrane displacement. A low-frequency signal of high intensity significantly affects the high-frequency (basal) end. This accounts for the phenomenon known as the upward spread of masking, in which low frequencies are able to mask, or interfere with, the perception of higher frequencies.

The cochlea essentially performs a Fourier analysis of complex sounds into their component frequencies. Raphael et al. (2007) noted that the sound of /i/

would result in many traveling waves moving along the basilar membrane, with at least two areas of maximum displacement: one near the base of the cochlea for the higher formants and one near the apex for the lower formant. For the word /si/, the high-frequency /s/ would displace the membrane maximally even closer to the base of the cochlea. Also, the traveling waves would be aperiodic during /s/ and become periodic during /i/.

Rosen and Howell (1991) compared the BM to a series of filters, with each point on the BM corresponding to a band-pass filter with a different center frequency (F_c). From the base to the apex of the cochlea, the F_c of each band-pass filter becomes lower and therefore resonates most strongly to successively lower frequencies in the sound wave. These filters are theoretically infinite and overlapping, but it is common to consider them as discrete and adjacent. In this view, the range of human hearing is defined by about 25 filter bands, the bandwidths of which are relatively narrow. This gives the cochlea an extraordinary degree of frequency resolution and helps explain why listeners with only a moderate loss in sensitivity often have great difficulty with speech recognition. The loss of the outer hair cell cochlear amplifier increases the auditory filter bandwidth and reduces frequency resolution. Spectral details tend to be smeared, with more interaction between parts of the speech in different frequency ranges. Rosen and Howell (1991) noted that, whereas a normal auditory system keeps "each frequency in its place," listeners with widened auditory filters have frequencies much more mixed up. This is supported by the common subjective report of individuals with hearing loss who describe being able to "hear" but not being able to "understand" the speech of others.

Perception of Speech

Discussion so far has focused on how people hear. The discussion now turns to how one perceives the sounds that are heard—that is, how a listener assigns meaning to an acoustic sound wave that stimulates the auditory system. Speech perception is a very interesting phenomenon because what one consciously perceives are not the acoustic features that make up the phonemes, such as voicing, formants, voice onset time, and so on, but linguistic events, such as phonemes, syllables, phrases, and sentences. Speech perception is a search for meaning, which is based on the ability to discriminate between and identify the acoustic–phonetic features of the speech waveform. In fact, a central question in the study of speech perception is how listeners are able to segment a continuously changing stream of sound into separate units of meaning. This question is deceptively simple, but numerous researchers investigating various aspects of perception, and many theories, are devoted to trying to answer it.

Segmentation Problem

When listening to someone talking, an individual perceives a sequence of separate sounds combined in innumerable different ways to form syllables, words, and phrases. The perceiver, in turn, combines these into meaningful ideas and information. However, at the acoustic level, the sound waves carrying the linguistic information are continuous and are not segmented into identifiable units corresponding to each specific phoneme. The problem is even more complicated because phonemes are extremely variable in their production. Ranges of formant frequencies overlap for vowels produced by different speakers. Phonemes are also influenced, due to coarticulation, by preceding and following sounds. The acoustic waveform for the /k/ phoneme will differ, for example, depending on whether the following vowel is an /i/ or an /u/. Producing sounds at different rates of speech or stressing syllables differently also results in different acoustic waveforms. Rate of speech, patterns of stress and intonation, dialect, and many other factors also contribute to variability in phoneme production. Thus, there is not a one-to-one correspondence between individual phonemes and their acoustic underpinnings.

Somehow a listener transforms continuously changing sound waves into the distinct, separate linguistic units of speech. This variability leads to the question of how listeners perceive individual sounds as constant (e.g., an /i/ always sounds like an /i/), even when the acoustic features that underlie the sounds are constantly changing. Some theorists propose that there are invariant and unchanging properties of phonemes that are always present, despite the variability in production, and that this is what listeners use to recognize phonemes. An opposing point of view is that, because of the dynamic and constantly changing nature of speech, phonemes do not possess invariant properties; rather, listeners use dynamic information in conjunction with contextual clues and their own linguistic knowledge to decode speech. This continues to be a hotly debated question that has not been resolved to date.

Role of Redundancy in Speech Perception

Although speakers have a good idea of the acoustic structure of sounds, experiments with filtered and distorted speech have shown that not only are acoustic cues ambiguous, but many of them can actually be eliminated without any adverse effect on speech perception (Denes & Pinson, 1993). The fact that multiple acoustic cues are embedded within single phonemes, as well as the fact that information from many phonemes converges on a specific sound, probably helps in perception. What is equally important for decoding speech is that most perception occurs in context. Speakers of any language know from experience which sounds go together and which do not. When one hears a speaker start to produce the /n/ sound, for example, as English speakers, we know that the following sound must be a vowel. One would not expect to hear an /nd/ sequence at the beginning of a word, although such a sequence might well be heard at the end of a word (e.g., end). Individuals have similar expectations of other linguistic parameters, such as syntax (word order) and semantics (meaning). Thus, contextual and linguistic information serve to enhance speech perception and the decoding of an acoustic signal into meaningful units. Familiarity with the subject matter can make speech recognizable even when the acoustic cues alone are ambiguous or insufficient because of noise or poor speaker intelligibility (Denes and Pinson, 1993).These multiple sources of cues are often referred to as "redundant." Boothroyd (1978) provided an excellent illustration of these redundancies. In listening to the sentence

"I bought some new shoes," both of the listener's ears are stimulated (physiologic redundancy). The listener also has access to the full acoustic spectrum (acoustic redundancy). There are clues to the final consonant in the consonant itself and in the formant transitions and duration of the preceding vowel (phonetic redundancy). The phoneme /z/ is one of only a few phonemes that can be added to /u/ to make a meaningful English word (lexical redundancy). The word *some* indicates that the last word will be plural (syntactic redundancy), and the listener's knowledge of the world informs him or her that shoes come in pairs (semantic redundancy).

Instrumental Analysis of Vowel and Consonant Perception

Much research has been done since the 1950s to try to understand how the transformation from acoustic to phonemic knowledge occurs. Most of this research has focused on the phonetic level—that is, on the acoustic characteristics that form patterns that individuals are able to perceive as distinct sounds. Two types of instruments have been particularly valuable in expanding knowledge in this area. The first is the spectrograph, which provides detailed information about the acoustic structure of speech sounds. The other is an instrument developed in the 1950s, the **Pattern Playback (PP)**. The PP works in reverse to the spectrograph: Whereas the spectrograph visually displays the acoustic characteristics of individual sounds, the PP converts visual patterns into sounds. The PP has been extremely useful because it allows researchers to synthesize speech and to manipulate various acoustic cues in a systematic way.

Many experiments have been done in which listeners' perceptions of sounds were tested to see how they responded to the manipulations. In these studies, the PP was fed spectrogram-like patterns that it scanned with a light beam and then played back the corresponding auditory sound wave. Artificial speech was generated as the PP played back stylized patterns that were painted on a plastic belt. Different patterns were painted to generate many different sounds. Researchers experimented with formants by manipulating the number of formants, their frequencies, and their durations. Since about 1970, the PP has been replaced by computers, which do essentially the same manipulations but far more quickly and with much-improved sound quality.

Much of the research using the spectrograph and the PP or computerized programs for synthesizing speech has focused on the different classes of speech sounds, such as stops, vowels, and fricatives. These types of sounds have been manipulated in various ways to determine how listeners perceive them and assign them to different classes. The following discussion examines perception of vowels and consonants.

Perception of Vowels and Diphthongs

Vowels are characterized by distinct patterns of vocal tract resonances, the formants, which depend on vocal tract dimensions. Vowels are both longer in duration and more intense than consonants; their frequency components are also generally lower than those of consonants. The vowel with the greatest intensity is /a/, as in the word *thaw*, which is about 25 dB greater than the weakest consonant, /θ/, also as in the word *thaw* (Fletcher, 1953). Vowels form the main portions, or nuclei, of syllables. Research has shown that the formants of a particular vowel are not all equal in terms of how much they contribute to a listener's perception of that vowel. When formants are close in frequency, such as F_1 and F_2 are for back vowels and F_2 and F_3 are for front vowels, the listener integrates the two into one perceptual unit, which is the equivalent of an average of the two closely spaced formants. Thus, front vowels are perceived on the basis of the frequency of F_1 and an average of F_2 and F_3, whereas back vowels are perceived on the basis of the average of F_1 and F_2, as well as F_3 (Strange, 1999). Vowel formant frequencies, however, are variable. Even when a vowel is said by itself, in isolation, formant frequencies differ for the same vowel when it is produced by different speakers. On the other hand, different vowels can overlap considerably in their formant frequencies when produced by the same speaker or by different speakers. Consequently, there is no strict one-to-one correspondence between vowels and their formant frequencies, yet this blurring of the boundaries between vowels is not usually a problem for listeners. Individuals are somehow able to compensate for the differences or similarities in formant frequencies within and between vowels.

Researchers have proposed various theories as to why the lack of consistent formant values for particular vowels is not a problem for listeners. Why should it be possible for an individual to perceive as /i/ a sound with formant values for F_1, F_2, and F_3 of 270, 2290, and 3010 Hz, respectively, but perceive equally clearly as /i/ a sound with F_1 of 345 Hz, F_2 of 2470 Hz, and F_3 of 3325 Hz? One theory suggests that it is not the absolute frequency values that are important in perception but rather the relationships among the formant frequencies. In the preceding example, even though the absolute values are different, each /i/ sound is characterized by a very low F_1 and by a very high F_2 and F_3, which are close together in frequency. Thus, when a young child and an adult male say /i/, the formant values for the two productions are very different because of the differences in vocal tract lengths. Each production, however, is characterized by a similar pattern of formant relationships, and it is the pattern, rather than the absolute formant frequency values, that is the basis of the perception.

A related theory posits that the ratio of F_2 to F_1 is the important factor in vowel recognition. High front vowels such as /i/ have very low F_1 and very high F_2; thus, the ratio of F_2 to F_1 is very large, whereas the F_2/F_1 ratio is much smaller for high back vowels such as /u/, which have F_1 and F_2 closer together. For example, F_1 and F_2 for /i/ are around 270 and 2290 Hz for men, 310 and 2790 Hz for women, and 370 and 3200 Hz for children. Based on these figures, the F_2/F_1 ratios would be 8.48, 9.00, and 8.65 for men, women, and children, respectively. These ratios are similar among the three groups. The ratios for /u/ work out to be 2.90 for men (F_2 = 870 Hz, F_1 = 300 Hz), 2.57 for women (950/370 Hz), and 2.72 for children (1170/430 Hz). As with /i/, the ratios are similar across the three groups, while the ratios for the two different vowels are quite different. Table 9.1 shows the ratios for front, back, and central vowels, based on the average formant frequency data reported in Chapter 2 (Table 2.2). Ratio differences are clearly apparent among the front vowels but are less clear for the back vowels. Furthermore, the ratios for

Table 9.1 F_2/F_1 **Ratios for Men (M), Women (W), and Children (C) for Front, Back, and Central Vowels**

Front Vowels				
	/i/	/ɪ/	/ɛ/	/æ/
M	8.48	5.10	3.47	2.61
W	9.00	5.77	3.82	2.38
C	8.65	5.15	3.78	2.30

Back Vowels				
	/u/	/ʊ/	/ɔ/	/a/
M	2.90	2.32	1.47	1.49
W	2.57	2.47	1.56	1.44
C	2.72	2.52	1.56	1.33

Central Vowels				
		/ə/		/ɚ/
M		1.86		2.76
W		1.84		3.28
C		1.87		3.25

/æ/, a low front vowel, overlap considerably with those for /u/ and /ʊ/, the two high back vowels. This overlap between the F_2/F_1 formant ratios also results in ambiguity.

The picture is even more complicated when it comes to understanding how people perceive vowels in connected speech. When vowels are produced in context, the acoustic contrast among them lessens because of coarticulation. The articulators move around constantly, so the formants are very seldom in a steady state but rather are constantly transitioning. The F_1/F_2 vowel space becomes reduced, resulting in **target undershoot**, in which the formant patterns of different vowels become similar to each other. The amount of undershoot depends on which phonemes precede and follow the particular vowel, as well as on the speaker and the speaking style. Some speakers reach vowel targets even when they talk very quickly, while others show less undershoot when they speak more slowly (Strange, 1999).

Even though the formant frequencies of vowels shift and become reduced in connected speech, listeners generally do not have any problem identifying them.

This suggests that listeners use other cues aside from formant frequencies to make judgments about vowel identity in connected speech. Strange (1999) and her colleagues have manipulated aspects of vowels, including vowel duration, formant transitions, and steady-state portions of vowels. Their research has shown that, even when the vowel nucleus of the syllable has been cut out, vowel perception is highly accurate as long as dynamic spectral information is present, such as the direction and slope of formant transitions and duration information. When duration information was also cut out, the dynamic spectral information was more helpful than the formant frequency in identifying the vowel. Thus, the perception of coarticulated vowels appears to be based on dynamic spectrotemporal patterns within the syllable. In other words, the changing formant patterns yield the most important acoustic information for identifying coarticulated vowels. In addition to acoustic information that is present in the vowel itself, listeners also use information that is external to the vowel, such as the F_0 and formants of preceding vowels and consonants. That is, individuals use information about the size, age, and gender of the speaker available in the person's speech patterns to interpret ambiguous vowels (Strange, 1999).

While the acoustic features of vowels and consonants influence perception, the context of the ongoing speech also plays an important role. The listener's knowledge of the speaker, the social context, the topic, the rules of grammar, and environmental conditions (e.g., quiet, noisy) all contribute to successful speech perception. For example, if two people are having a conversation about their friend Ed, it is unlikely that one of them will perceive the /ɛ/ in Ed as /æ/, as in add, even though the speaker's formant frequencies for /ɛ/ may be close to or even overlap considerably with his or her formant frequencies for /æ/. Both participants' knowledge of the topic and their expectations of hearing Ed's name in the conversation reduce the ambiguity of the similar formants of /ɛ/ and /æ/.

Diphthongs

Diphthongs are perceived on the basis of their formant transitions, which change from the steady state of one vowel and transition to the steady state of the second vowel in the diphthong unit. It has been found that it is not the exact formant frequencies that are important in identifying diphthongs; how fast the formants change is the most salient cue. This suggests that listeners are more sensitive to the acoustic consequences of the tongue moving in the appropriate direction than to the final position that the tongue achieves for the sound.

Consonants

Consonants are produced with much more rapid movements of the articulators than are vowels. There is also a much greater variety of consonant types than vowels, and the acoustic cues that enable perception of consonants tend to be more complex than those of vowels. Several features of consonant perception are described below.

Categorical Perception

The way that many consonants are perceived is different from how vowels are perceived because many consonants are perceived categorically. That is, if a series of consonant sounds was heard by a listener, with the sounds differing in one acoustic aspect by small equal steps, the listener would perceive some of the sounds as the same phoneme until a boundary was reached. On the other side of this boundary, known as the **crossover**, the listener would hear the other sounds as a different phoneme (see Figure 9.6). Thus, if there were 10 sounds in the series, the listener might group all 10 into only two different categories. This has been shown in tests of categorical perception, in which speech sounds are synthesized so as to differ in only one or two acoustic aspects in predetermined steps.

In one early test, Peter Eimas and his colleagues created a series of /ba/s and /pa/s. The researchers expected that the sounds in the series would be perceived as changing gradually from /ba/ to /pa/, with many sounds in the middle of the series sounding ambiguous. Instead, the listeners reported hearing a series of /ba/s that abruptly changed to a series of /pa/s. Furthermore, when the researchers asked the listeners if they could hear the difference between two adjacent /ba/s or /pa/s in the series, they could not do so, even though the two /ba/s or /pa/s were acoustically different. Listeners could only perceive the difference between adjacent stimuli at the crossover point, when the sound changed abruptly from the phoneme /b/ to the phoneme /p/ (Kuhl, 1991). It is characteristic of categorical perception that sounds that are perceived as being in the same category are hard to tell apart, whereas it is easy to differentiate those that are perceived as being from different categories. Simply put, it is easy to recognize the difference between /p/ and /b/, whereas it is not easy to distinguish between two /b/ sounds, even if they are acoustically different. The fact that listeners are not able to distinguish among members of the same phoneme class probably facilitates perception, since irrelevant differences can safely be discounted, while only those differences that contribute to the perception of different speech sound categories are taken into account by the listener.

Figure 9.6 Categorical perception

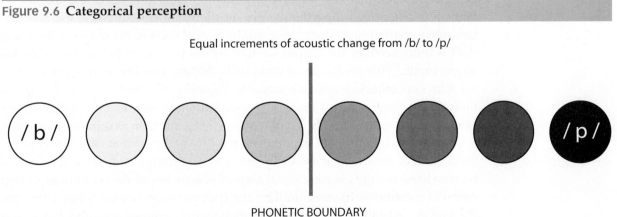

Equal increments of acoustic change from /b/ to /p/

PHONETIC BOUNDARY
(Perception of sound changes abruptly)

Categorical perception has been shown to occur for VOT and for place of articulation for stops and fricatives. Strange (1999) reported on an investigation in which researchers constructed a continuum of 14 stop-vowel syllables, in which the syllables differed only in the direction and extent of the F_2 transition of the stop. The F_2 transition changed in small, evenly spaced steps from a low-onset frequency and rising transition (typical of a labial stop), through intermediate-onset frequencies (typical of an alveolar stop), to a relatively high-onset frequency and falling transition (typical of a velar stop). Most listeners reported hearing all stimuli unambiguously as either "bay," "day," or "gay," showing that place of articulation for stops is perceived categorically. Categorical perception also occurs for other acoustic features, such as duration of transitions that are important in differentiating stops such as /b/ from glides such as /w/.

Multiple Acoustic Cues

In natural (not synthetic) speech, listeners use several different acoustic features to categorize a consonant. For example, a listener may use both VOT and onset of F_1 frequency to decide whether a stop is voiced or voiceless. A low F_1 onset frequency and a shorter VOT are characteristic of voiced stops, whereas a higher F_1 onset frequency and a longer VOT are associated with voiceless stops. However, acoustic cues show what are known as trading relations between them. For example, one study found that F_1 onset frequency traded with VOT cues for voicing. Stimuli with low F_1 onset, typically associated with voiced stops, could be perceived as voiceless stops if the VOTs were lengthened. Stimuli with a higher F_1 onset, typically associated with voiceless stops, were perceived as voiceless even when accompanied by shorter-than-usual VOTs (Strange, 1999). Other acoustic features such as vowel duration, frication noise duration, and F_0 cues to fricative voicing have also been shown to trade off. These multiple acoustic features associated with consonants are somehow fused into the perception of a single phoneme by the listener.

Influence of Coarticulation

Listeners do not just use acoustic information from one specific phoneme to make a decision regarding the identity of that phoneme. Because the articulators move continuously during the production of speech, the shape of the vocal tract is influenced by the shapes for the sounds that occur before and after the target sound. This results in continuously shifting acoustic features that interact with and influence adjacent features. Perceptually, therefore, one integrates information that is spread out over several phonetic segments to make a decision about phoneme identity. This was shown in a study in which the researchers synthesized a continuum of fricative sounds (/ʃ/ and /s/) that varied only in the bandwidth of the fricative noise. The noise varied from a wide band for /ʃ/ to a narrow band for /s/, in nine equal steps. Subjects heard the continuum in two different conditions. In one condition the fricative sounds were followed by the /i/ vowel, and in the other condition they were combined with the /u/ vowel (i.e., /si/–/ʃi/, /su/–/ʃu/). The fricative noises that fell in the midrange of bandwidths were heard as /ʃ/ when they were combined with /i/ and as /s/ when they were combined with /u/. Thus, the subjects' perceptions shifted from /ʃ/ to /s/, depending on the vowel context. Rate of speech also influences a listener's identification of consonants. For example, in continua in which VOT is varied, stimuli with intermediate VOTs are heard as voiceless in fast speech and voiced in slow speech.

Perception of Consonants

Liquids

Similar to diphthongs, the liquids /r/ and /l/ are recognized on the basis of their formant transitions. One factor that distinguishes liquids from diphthongs is that the formant transitions in /r/ and /l/ are much more rapid than those in diphthongs. The F_3 frequency is particularly important for differentiating between the liquids. The F_3 in /r/ sounds is usually much lower in frequency than the F_3 in /l/ sounds.

Glides

The glides /j/ and /w/ are characterized by transitions that are shorter in duration than those of diphthongs. Experiments have shown that, when the transition duration is shorter than about 40 to 60 msec, listeners tend to hear a stop. When the transition is greater than 40 to 60 msec but less than 100 to 150 msec, listeners usually judge the sound to be a glide. When the transition exceeds about 100 msec, listeners hear a vowel-plus-vowel sequence (Denes & Pinson, 1993).

Nasals

Nasals are recognized on the basis of their internal formant structure, as well as on the basis of the formant transitions of the vowels occurring before and after the nasal sound. F_1, F_2, and F_3 of nasals are weak in intensity because of antiresonances occurring within the vocal tract. Nasals also have an extra formant, the nasal formant. These two features help listeners to recognize that a sound is a nasal. In synthetic speech, it has been found that when the upper formants are cut out, the nasal formant by itself is enough to judge a sound as a nasal. Researchers have also reported that when a nasal occurs at the end of a syllable, information in the vowel preceding the nasal is enough to identify the nasal. When the researchers cut out the transitions between the vowel and the nasal, as well as the nasal phoneme itself, listeners could still detect nasality in the vowel.

The formant transitions (particularly F_2) between a nasal and a preceding or following vowel are what signal the place of articulation of the nasal (Raphael, Borden, & Harris, 2007). These transitions contain frequency and durational cues. The formant transitions from /m/ are the lowest in frequency and the shortest in duration; those for /n/ are higher in frequency and a bit longer in duration; and those for /ŋ/ are the highest and the most variable in frequency and the longest in duration.

Stops

Stops are perceived on the basis of numerous acoustic cues that are intertwined with the acoustic cues for the vowels and consonants surrounding the phoneme. Part of recognizing a stop involves perceiving the relationships between the stop and its neighboring sounds. Some acoustic cues signal the manner of the stop, some are clues to its place of articulation, and others provide information about voicing status. Cues to manner include a brief interval of silence or attenuation of sound, a transient burst of noise, and rapid formant transitions between the stop and a preceding or following vowel. Research has shown that just inserting an interval of silence between two phonemes can cause a stop sound to be heard. For example, in the word *slit*, if a silent interval is inserted between the /s/ and the /l/, the word will be heard as *split*, with a /p/ being perceived rather than just silence.

The duration of formant transitions seems to play an important part in identifying manner of articulation. For example, investigators have synthesized the stop-plus-vowel combinations of /be/ and /ge/ on the PP, using very brief formant transitions of less than 40 msec. Even though release bursts were not included, listeners were able to recognize the sounds without any difficulty. When the researchers extended the duration of the transitions to 40 or 50 msec, listeners heard glides, rather than stops, at the start of the syllables /we/ and /je/. When they lengthened the transitions to 150 msec or more, listeners perceived not a consonant and vowel sequence but a sequence of two vowel sounds, /ue/ and /ie/ (Raphael et al., 2007).

Place of articulation of stops is also signaled by several acoustic cues, including the frequency of the burst in relation to a vowel, the F_2 transition between the stop and the adjacent vowel, and VOT. VOT differs according to place of articulation, with bilabial stops showing the shortest VOTs (or negative VOTs) and velar stops having the longest VOTs. The F_2 transition seems to be a particularly strong cue in recognizing different stops, at least in synthetic speech. It has been shown in experiments using synthetic speech that the F_2 transition for /p/ and /b/ begins at a low frequency, around 600 to 800 Hz. The alveolars /t/ and /d/ have their F_2 transitions beginning in the midfrequency region, at approximately 1800 Hz. The starting position for the F_2 transition for /k/ and /g/ depends on whether the stop is produced in combination with a back vowel or a front vowel. When combined with a front vowel such as /i/, the stop is made farther forward in the oral cavity. Conversely, the stop is made more toward the back of the oral cavity when followed by a back vowel such as /u/. The starting frequencies for the F_2 transition for velar stops, therefore, can be either around 1300 Hz, appropriate for a high back vowel, or much higher, at about 3000 Hz, appropriate for a high front vowel. However, these starting frequencies for the F_2 transition, which are known as loci (singular: locus), have not been found to be as important in natural speech as they are in synthetic speech. All the formant shifts (for F_1, as well as F_2 and F_3) are probably important cues for listeners to identify the place of articulation of a stop (Kent & Read, 1992). In fact, in experiments in which the bursts of the stops are cut out, listeners can recognize the stop based only on the formant information.

Stops also differ from each other in terms of their voicing. As with manner and place of articulation, several acoustic cues help to identify the voicing status of a stop. The presence or absence of phonation and the degree of aspiration noise when the stop is released play important roles. VOT is also a major indicator of voicing, with voiceless stops in English being characterized by longer VOTs and voiced stops being associated with much shorter (and sometimes negative) VOTs. The relationship between the F_1 and F_2 transitions from the stop to the following vowel can also signal whether the stop is voiced or voiceless. A delay of F_1 relative to the beginning of the F_2 transition is referred to as F_1 **cutback** (Figure 9.7). Research has shown that listeners usually report hearing voiceless stops when the F_1 cutback is 30 msec or more.

The cues for voicing, however, depend to some degree on the position of the stop in the syllable. At the beginning of a syllable, cues include VOT, F_1 cutback, and the F_0 of the vowel following the stop. Vowels that follow voiceless stops tend to have a higher F_0 than those that follow voiced stops. For stops that occur in the final position in a syllable, vowel duration is an important cue. Vowels are longer before voiced stops and shorter before voiceless stops. The duration of the silent interval in a stop can also help to signal its voicing status. Thus, numerous acoustic cues are generated in the production of a stop. Many of these cues are redundant, which helps to make stops easy to perceive for individuals with normal hearing.

Fricatives

Frication noise provides the major cue as to the manner of articulation of fricatives. The noise is longer in duration than that of stops. Sounds tend to be heard as fricatives when the noise is around 130 msec or greater, whereas sounds with noise durations less than around 75 msec are perceived as stops. The frication noise also signals voicing status, being both longer in duration and greater in amplitude for voiceless fricatives than it is for voiced cognates.

Place of articulation of fricatives is perceived on the basis of the spectrum and intensity of the noise. The sibilant fricatives (/s, z, ʃ, ʒ/) have steep, high-frequency spectral peaks, whereas the nonsibilants (/f, v, ɵ, ð/) have flatter spectra. The location of the spectral peaks can also aid in distinguishing between the alveolar and palatal sibilant fricatives. The alveolars /s/ and /z/ have a prominent peak at around 4000 Hz, and the peak for /ʃ/ and /ʒ/ is lower, at around 2500 Hz. The labiodental and linguadental fricatives have very similar spectra, so it is not as easy to tell them apart. Also, the sibilants have a much more intense spectrum than the nonsibilants. In fact, the /ɵ/ is the sound that has the weakest intensity in English.

Aside from these spectral differences, the formant transitions to and from the fricative also play a role in differentiating between the fricatives, although not to as great an extent as for the stops. F_2 transitions to and from adjacent vowels are probably more important for the weaker fricatives than for the sibilants, because the spectral shapes of the weaker fricatives are similar and do not help to distinguish between them.

Figure 9.7 F_1 **cutback**

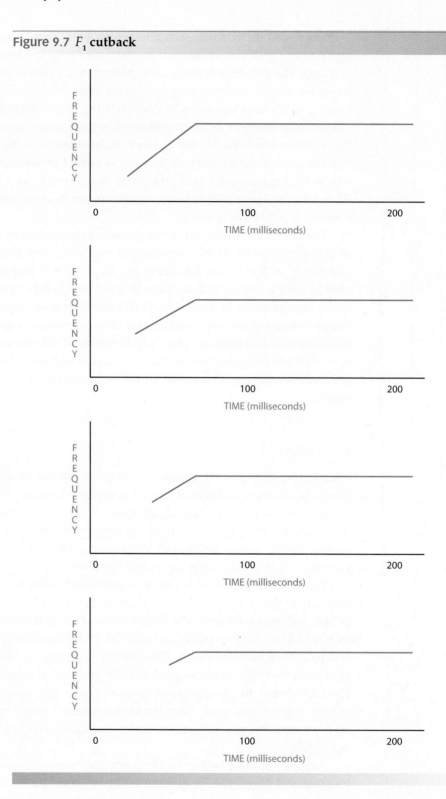

Figure 9.8 Frequency locations and intensity of vowels and consonants

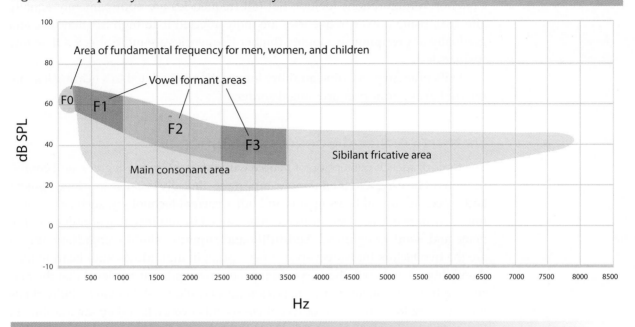

Affricates

Because affricates are produced as a stop plus a fricative, they share acoustic features with both types of sounds. The **rise time** may be particularly important in recognizing affricates versus fricatives. Rise time refers to how long it takes for the amplitude envelope to reach its highest value. The rise time for affricates has been measured at around 33 msec; that for fricatives is longer, about 76 msec (Kent & Read, 1992). The duration of the frication noise is also different, being longer for the fricatives than for the affricates.

Figure 9.8 shows the frequency and intensity regions for vowels and consonants.

Hearing Loss

Hearing loss is typically described in terms of type, degree, and configuration. Hearing loss types include conductive (outer ear and/or middle ear pathology), sensorineural (inner ear or eighth cranial nerve pathology), and mixed (both conductive and sensorineural losses are present in the same ear). The outer hair cell damage occurring in individuals with sensorineural hearing loss compromises the cochlear amplifier, resulting in both a loss of sensitivity and a loss of frequency selectivity or frequency resolution.

The degree of hearing loss refers to the amount of hearing loss and is typically characterized as mild, moderate, moderately severe, severe, or profound. A mild loss reflects a loss of about 25 to 40 dB HL, and a profound loss represents a loss greater than 90 dB HL; the remaining categories fall between those two. Configuration of loss refers to the shape of the loss according to frequency. Common configurations include flat (all frequencies are approximately equally affected), rising (lower frequencies are more affected than high frequencies), and gradually or precipitously sloping (higher frequencies are more affected than low frequencies).

Difficulties in processing auditory information not related to a hearing loss are referred to as auditory processing disorders.

Hearing Loss and Speech Perception

The topic of speech perception of people with different types, degrees, and configurations of hearing loss is extremely important clinically because the development and successful use of hearing aids and other current technology, such as cochlear implants, depends on benefits that can be gained in auditory perception and phoneme and word recognition. **Audibility** and **suprathreshold recognition ability** are the two factors that affect speech perception in individuals with hearing loss. Audibility refers to whether a specific speech cue is present at a level that the person can hear. This level is known as a suprathreshold level. However, individuals with hearing loss often cannot recognize sounds even when they are audible. In this case there is a loss of suprathreshold discriminability and recognition ability, which may be caused by factors such as deficits in identifying frequency and timing cues present in the sound wave. This is likely due to the loss of the cochlear amplifier as a result of outer hair damage, which reduces the frequency resolution of the auditory system. Glasberg and Moore (1986) and Pick, Evans, and Wilson (1977) determined that the auditory filters in impaired ears were wider than in normal ears, contributing to difficulties in complex sound analysis and in speech-recognition performance in noise. When normally hearing listeners are presented with a frequency of 1000 Hz, the nerve fibers respond to a bandwidth of about 100 to 150 Hz around this frequency. This is approximately 10 to 15 percent of the center frequency of 1000 Hz. For listeners with sensorineural hearing loss (SNHL), the filter bandwidth could be as much as three to four times larger than normal, with some people's values approaching 50 percent of the center frequency (Turner, Chi, & Flock, 1999). The resulting frequency resolution is very poor, hindering the individual from making the fine frequency discriminations that are so important in the perception of phonemes.

Both hearing-impaired children and adults have deficits in discriminating between similar acoustic elements, resulting in difficulty in identifying the acoustic–phonetic features of speech. However, the speech recognition performance of adults who acquire hearing loss after years of normal hearing differs substantially from that of children with congenital or pre lingual hearing losses. As an example, an adult who has lost high-frequency hearing and the ability to either detect or recognize the phoneme /s/ is aware that the phoneme is present at the end of the word *cats* based on the redundancies of language. In addition, adults with acquired hearing loss typically maintain excellent speech production skills despite their loss of hearing since audition is not the primary feedback loop for a competent speaker. This is not true of a child during the early years of language development. The inability to hear the crucial /s/ marking grammatical morphemes such as plural, possessive, and tense is likely to impact the child's acquisition of language. The phoneme /s/ acts as a plural marker (cat–cats), as a possessive marker (Jack's hat), as a marker for third-person singular (he walks), and as a copula (it is—it's). Clinically, therefore, enhancing a child's auditory perception of this phoneme is a high priority. Hearing loss reduces the amount of acoustic information available to a child, who cannot integrate the acoustic fragments into a meaningful message (Ross, Brackett, & Maxon, 1991). Unlike normally hearing children who use audition to extract meaning from an utterance, children with hearing impairment must focus on the acoustic–phonetic elements rather than on the global understanding of the message. Therefore, hearing-impaired children who are not identified at an early age and do not receive intervention often do not develop the spoken language level of their normally hearing peers. While digital hearing aids have provided significant advantages in signal processing and improved access to the higher frequencies, full access to spectral information is not available to hearing-impaired children, even with amplification.

As discussed above, the acoustic structure of vowels and consonants provides many different cues to perception. Individuals use multiple cues to identify phonemes. People with normal hearing probably do not need all the cues present in a phoneme to judge its identity because of the redundancy of the situational, linguistic, and acoustic cues. Different acoustic cues usually play more or less of a role in identifying sounds. For instance, young children assign more importance to dynamic information provided by formant transitions and less to more static spectral information, whereas older children and adults seem to be more sensitive to spectral differences between sounds, such as the information contained in the burst of a stop or in the frication noise of a fricative. Some cues that may be of secondary importance to normally hearing listeners may be considerably more salient to people with hearing impairment, as long as they can detect the particular acoustic feature. For example, because the spectral energy of stops and fricatives is greatest in the higher frequencies, spectral cues are often inaudible to a person with a high-frequency hearing loss or to an individual whose hearing aid has a limited high-frequency range. Formant transitions, however, are greatest in intensity in the lower frequencies and may allow the individual to detect the presence of a stop or fricative, despite the lack of available spectral information. In addition, duration cues present in phonetic segments may be accessible to hearing-impaired listeners and may act to signal a particular phonetic cue. For instance, vowels are longer when they precede a voiced consonant than when they precede a voiceless one.

The impaired frequency resolution and resulting lack of ability to detect spectral differences in complex sounds might be expected to interfere with the perception of vowels, which depends to a large degree on the ability to detect subtle differences in formant frequencies. However, many listeners with hearing loss are able to discriminate vowels without any problems, perhaps due to the redundancy of acoustic cues in the signal (Summers & Leek, 1992). On the other hand, many children with high-frequency hearing losses often confuse vowels because of poor frequency resolution and poor audibility. One fairly common vowel confusion is between /i/ and /u/. The F_1 of /i/ and /u/ are fairly close in frequency (270, 310, and 370 Hz for men, women, and children, respectively, for /i/; 300, 370, and 430 Hz for /u/).

Because F_2 for /i/ is relatively high in frequency (between about 2300 and 3200 Hz), it may not be detected by a hearing-impaired child, so he or she does not have access to the salient acoustic information that would help to discriminate this vowel.

While vowel perception does not seem to pose a great problem for most hearing-impaired listeners, consonant perception is more of a challenge. Fricatives in particular are difficult to perceive for many hearing-impaired individuals with high-frequency losses. The cues for fricatives include the duration of the frication noise, the spectrum of the noise, formant transitions, and the amplitude relationship between the fricative and the adjacent vowel in the F_3 region (Hedrick, 1997). The spectral energy of fricatives, particularly the sibilants, is extremely high in frequency, with that of /s/ being above 3500 Hz. Consequently, the spectral information is not accessible to many hearing-impaired individuals, even with amplification. Zeng and Turner (1990) tested the speech recognition performance of normally hearing and hearing-impaired listeners on four fricative vowel syllables (see, fee, thee, and she). When the frication portion was audible to the hearing-impaired listeners, they used it as their primary cue for the fricative, whereas, even when the transition cues were audible, these individuals did not use them for fricative recognition. The normally hearing individuals in this study used transition information to recognize fricatives when the spectral information was experimentally masked and was not audible to them, but the hearing-impaired listeners did not do this. Consequently, it seems that one factor that makes it hard for hearing-impaired people to discriminate fricatives is their lack of ability to use dynamic information from the formant transitions between the fricative and the adjacent vowels.

The most common perceptual errors made by hearing-impaired individuals involve place of consonant articulation, the cues for which are contained primarily in the higher frequencies. Acoustic correlates of stop consonant place of articulation are typically found in the first 20 to 40 msec of a consonant–vowel syllable. Dubno, Dirks, and Schaefer (1987) examined stop consonant (CV) identification ability in hearing-impaired persons using syllable durations ranging from 10 to 100 msec. Normally hearing subjects achieved good identification for CV syllables with 20 to 40 msec durations. Hearing-impaired subjects did much more poorly, even at the longest syllable durations. Hearing-impaired listeners seem to assign less weight to F_2 frequencies than do normally hearing listeners and more weight to other cues that may be more accessible to them, such as F_1 or vowel duration. Another factor that plays a part in speech recognition for people with high-frequency sensorineural hearing loss is the relationship between the amplitudes of the consonant and the adjacent vowels, known as the consonant-to-vowel amplitude ratio (CVR). However, the relationship between CVR and speech recognition is complicated and seems to depend on the specific phonemes involved (Sammeth, Dorman, & Stearns, 1999). Although individuals with hearing loss have difficulty identifying the place of articulation through audition, some information concerning place is available through the visual modality. For example, the linguadental production of /θ/ or the labiodental production of /f/ is readily observable on the face. Consequently, speech recognition performance in the auditory–visual mode is improved over auditory-only performance (Erber, 1975; Grant, Walden, & Seitz, 1998; Walden, Busacco, & Montgomery, 1993).

Summary

The auditory system includes the outer, middle, and inner ears and the auditory nerve pathway.

The middle ear functions to overcome the impedance mismatch between the middle and inner ears, to attenuate loud sounds by means of the acoustic reflex, and to maintain equal air pressures inside and outside the middle ear via the Eustachian tube.

The inner ear transduces the mechanical vibrations of the middle ear to fluid vibrations and to electrical energy using the organ of Corti.

The structure of the basilar membrane facilitates a frequency analysis of all incoming sounds to the cochlea.

Speech perception is a search for meaning, which is based on the ability to discriminate and identify the acoustic–phonetic features of the speech waveform as well as on linguistic and contextual redundancy.

Individuals with hearing impairment do not have access to the multiple acoustic cues used by normally hearing speakers to identify phonemes.

Hearing-impaired listeners are often able to discriminate vowels but have problems in identifying consonants, particularly fricatives.

REVIEW EXERCISES

1. Describe how the structure of the middle ear acts to transmit acoustic pressure waves to the inner ear.

2. Explain the relationship between the organ of Corti and the basilar membrane and discuss the role of the basilar membrane in the frequency analysis of incoming sounds.

3. Explain how categorical perception, multiple acoustic cues, coarticulation, and context influence speech perception.

4. Explain why individuals with high-frequency hearing losses have particular difficulty in perceiving fricatives.

5. Discuss the relationship between phoneme perception and morphological markers in children with hearing impairment.

6. Elaborate on the concept of frequency selectivity and explain its link to normal hearing and to hearing impairment.

10

CLINICAL APPLICATION

Evaluation and Treatment of Disorders Related to Hearing Impairment

STUDENT LEARNING OBJECTIVES

After reading this chapter you will

○ Describe the role of immittance audiometry, otoacoustic emissions, and auditory brain stem testing in the diagnosis of hearing impairment.

○ Describe the components of cochlear implants and different implementation methods used to stimulate the auditory nerve.

○ Appreciate that otitis media is a form of early sensory deprivation and understand its effects on speech perception.

○ Explain the links between speech perception problems and language and reading disability.

○ Understand the relationship between speech perception and articulation problems.

Measurement of Auditory Variables

Problems or pathologies in the peripheral auditory system often result in partial hearing loss or in deafness. It is unusual for a person to have no hearing at all. Typically, even a deaf person has some degree of residual hearing, which can provide information about the timing and intensity patterns of speech. Problems in the central auditory system often result in subtle problems of auditory processing in which the person's hearing sensitivity is normal, but the perception of speech is decreased, particularly when the signal is degraded in some way as by noise or filtering.

As noted in Chapter 9, there are different types of hearing loss, depending on which part of the ear is affected. Together, the outer ear and middle ear are referred to as the conductive mechanism since their function is to conduct sound waves to the inner ear. A **conductive hearing loss** results when something interferes with this transmission. For example, the external auditory meatus might get plugged by cerumen. This would prevent much of the sound energy from reaching the TM. Within the middle ear, several conditions can interfere with or prevent the ossicles from being set into vibration, such as otitis media (ear infection) or otosclerosis, a condition in which the formation of bone around the stapes fixates it in the oval window. The inner ear and auditory (vestibulocochlear) nerve together are referred to as the sensorineural mechanism (*sensori* = hair cells; *neural* = nerve fibers). Conditions that affect these structures result in a **sensorineural hearing loss**. One such condition is intense noise exposure that damages the hair cells in the cochlea, a leading cause of acquired hearing loss in adults. Other major causes of sensorineural hearing loss are aging and genetic factors.

Various diagnostic procedures have been developed to assess middle ear and inner ear function and auditory system integrity. Three instrumental techniques, in particular, have had a large impact on clinical diagnostic practice: immittance audiometry, otoacoustic emissions testing, and auditory brain stem response testing.

Immittance Audiometry

The current method of choice for identifying middle ear problems is based on immittance audiometry. **Immittance** is a measure of how easily a system can be set into vibration by a driving force. The term immittance includes two reciprocal concepts: impedance and admittance. Impedance describes how a system opposes the flow of energy through it and is measured in units called **ohms**. Admittance refers to how easily energy is transmitted through a system and is measured in milliliters (formerly millimhos). The reciprocal nature of admittance and impedance is also expressed in their units of measurement; note that *mho* is *ohm* spelled backward. If a system can be set into vibration easily, its admittance is high and its impedance is low. Conversely, if it takes a lot of force to set the system into vibration, its admittance is low and its impedance is high. Measuring immittance is important in evaluating conductive hearing loss, which is caused by changes in the transmission characteristics of the middle ear vibratory system (Jerger & Stach, 1994). Immittance is measured and displayed on an instrument called an **acoustic-admittance meter**, or more commonly, a **tympanometer**, which is capable of three clinical tests: tympanometry, static-acoustic middle ear admittance, and acoustic reflexes. Performing these tests is quick, easy, and noninvasive, and the procedures have become a mainstay of the standard clinical audiometric evaluation.

Tympanometry

Tympanometry generates a graph called a tympanogram; a tympanogram is a plot of changes in middle ear admittance as air pressure is systematically varied in the external ear canal. The admittance of the middle ear is greatest when the air pressure in the external ear canal and in the middle ear cavity is the same. In this situation the transmission of sound occurs with maximum admittance. If the air pressure in the external ear canal becomes either positive or negative in relation to the air pressure in the middle ear space, the admittance of the system decreases, reducing the transmission of vibration. As soon as the air pressure changes even slightly below or above the level that produces maximum admittance, the energy flow through the system drops quickly and steeply to a minimum value (Jerger & Stach, 1994).

Tympanometric procedure

To obtain a tympanogram, a small device called a probe tip is inserted in the external ear canal. A complete seal is created between the probe tip and the ear canal because the probe tip is made of a flexible plastic that fits snugly in the ear canal, preventing any leakage of air. Four small tubes connect to the probe tip. One tube is connected to a loudspeaker that delivers a tone into the ear canal. This sound is called the probe tone or probe signal. The second tube is connected to a microphone that measures the probe tone in the ear canal. The third tube is connected to an air pressure pump and manometer, and the fourth tube is connected to another receiver used to present stimuli for testing the acoustic reflex (Gelfand, 1997).

During tympanometry, the probe tone signal is presented to the ear as air pressure changes are gradually introduced into the ear canal by means of the air pressure pump and manometer attached to one of the tubes. The air pressure is measured in relation to atmospheric pressure in units of decapascals (daPa) or millimeters of water (mm H_2O). 1 daPa = 1.02 mm H_2O at 20 degrees Celsius (Shanks, Lilly, Margolis, Wiley, & Wilson, 1988). 0 daPa represents atmospheric pressure (P_{atmos}); positive pressure (e.g., +100 daPa) means that the ear canal pressure is greater than P_{atmos}, and negative pressure (e.g., −100 daPa) means that the pressure in the canal is less than P_{atmos}. The tympanogram shows admittance (in ml) on the y-axis and air pressure (typically ranging from −400 daPa on the left to +200 daPa on the right) on the x-axis.

Tympanogram shapes

There are several ways of interpreting tympanograms. In clinical situations, the amplitude, shape, and peak pressure point of the tympanogram are used to provide information about the functioning of the middle ear. A classification system in common clinical use is one reported by Jerger (1970), in which the letters A, B, and C are used to describe tympanograms using a 220 or 226 Hz probe tone frequency.

Figure 10.1 shows that in the normal middle ear, a tympanogram is similar to a bell-shaped curve with a single rather sharp peak. The highest point of the graph, the pressure peak, occurs at around 0 daPa of air pressure (i.e., P_{atmos}) and indicates the greatest admittance of the middle ear at that pressure. The slopes of the curve are quite steep, showing that the admittance decreases quickly as the pressure in the canal becomes either positive or negative. This shape, called type A, is typical of normal middle ear function.

Types B and C are different in shape from type A, reflecting changes in middle ear admittance due to various conditions. A type B tympanogram has a much flatter contour than a type A, usually evincing no peak pressure point (Figure 10.2). This kind of tympanogram can occur with impacted cerumen or in several different middle ear conditions. It is often seen in cases of otitis media, in which the middle ear space is filled with fluid. In this condition the extreme negative pressure condition in the middle ear, coupled with the mass of the fluid, hinders energy flow through the middle ear.

A type C tympanogram has a similar peaked shape to the type A, but instead of the peak being at or close to 0 daPa of air pressure, the peak is in the negative pressure region, to the left of 0 daPa (Figure 10.3). This kind of tympanogram is typical of conditions in which the Eustachian tube does not function normally, so middle ear pressure is not replenished and equalized with P_{atmos}. The lack of equalization causes a decrease of pressure in the middle ear because air is continually

Figure 10.1 Type A tympanogram

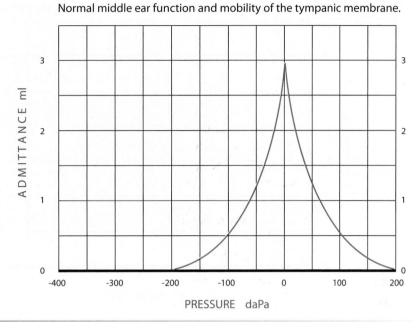

Type A Tympanogram

Normal middle ear function and mobility of the tympanic membrane.

Figure 10.2 Type B tympanogram

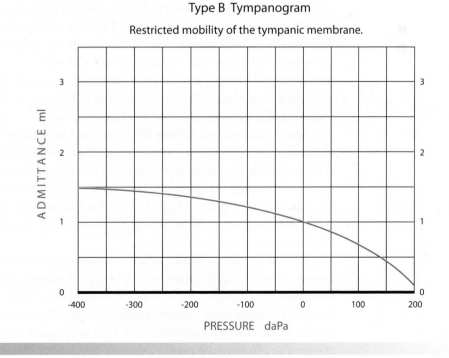

Type B Tympanogram

Restricted mobility of the tympanic membrane.

Figure 10.3 Type C tympanogram

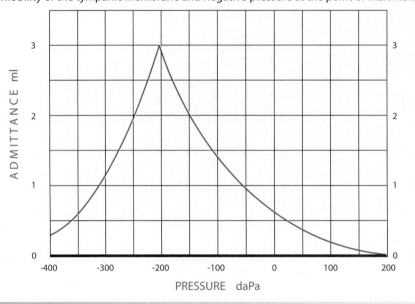

Type C Tympanogram

Normal mobility of the tympanic membrane and negative pressure at the point of maximum mobility.

absorbed by the tissues of the middle ear. During swallowing, the Eustachian tube is opened, which allows the air in the middle ear to be re-equalized with air from the atmosphere. When the tube does not function normally, the pressure cannot be equalized, so the pressure in the ear canal is higher than that in the middle ear. This difference in pressure causes the TM to be pulled inward (medially). To match the lower middle ear pressure and have acoustic energy flow through the system, the pressure in the ear canal must be decreased as well. Once this happens, energy can be transmitted through the system, resulting in a normal tympanogram peak but at a negative pressure, usually below -100 daPa. Thus, a type C tympanogram reflects a condition of negative middle ear pressure.

Any condition that causes the ossicular chain to become stiffer will result in a reduction in energy flow through the middle ear and will attenuate the peak of the tympanogram (Jerger & Stach, 1994). For example, otosclerosis, a disease of the bone surrounding the footplate of the stapes, prevents the ossicles from vibrating. This generates a type A shape but with a lower peak, and it is designated type A_s (where s represents the stiffness of the ossicles or the shallowness of the tympanometric peak) (Figure 10.4).

A break or discontinuity in the ossicular chain results in a much greater than normal peak, in conjunction with the type A shape (Figure 10.5). This happens because, with a break in the chain, the middle ear vibratory system is no longer coupled to the cochlear system, which allows the TM to respond with much greater amplitude to changes in air pressure. This is designated type A_d, with d referring to the greater depth of the peak or to discontinuity in the ossicular chain.

Figure 10.4 Type A$_s$ tympanogram

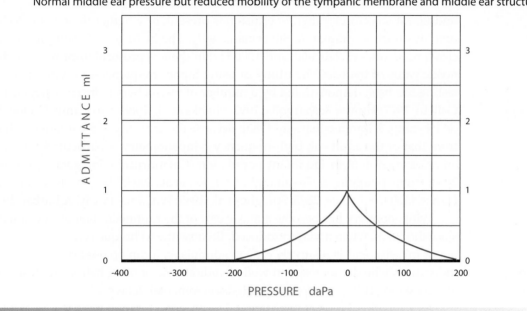

Type A$_s$ Tympanogram

Normal middle ear pressure but reduced mobility of the tympanic membrane and middle ear structure.

Figure 10.5 Type A$_d$ tympanogram

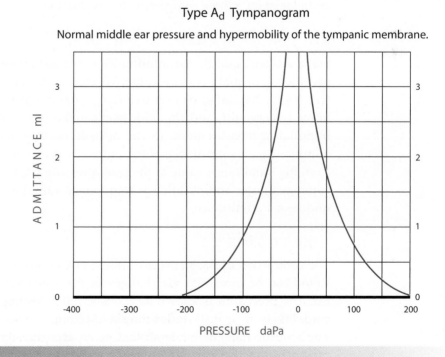

Type A$_d$ Tympanogram

Normal middle ear pressure and hypermobility of the tympanic membrane.

Advantages of tympanometry

Acoustic immittance testing is a sensitive diagnostic tool that provides valuable information about the underlying middle ear condition. From this kind of information, it is possible to determine whether a problem results from stiffening of the middle ear structures, whether effusion is present, or whether there is Eustachian tube dysfunction (Silman & Silverman, 1991). The inclusion of multiple frequencies (probe tones of 220, 660, and 1000 Hz) in the test protocol improves the diagnostic value of the test. The utility of using higher frequencies in tympanometric testing has been demonstrated by a number of researchers (Alberti & Jerger, 1971; Colletti, 1977; Hunter & Margolis, 1992; Shanks et al., 1988; Van Camp, Creten, Van de Heyning, & Vanpeperstraete,1983). Because the anatomy of the infant ear differs from that of the adult ear, high-frequency tympanometry is particularly useful as an assessment tool in the infant population (Calandruccio, Fitzgerald, & Prieve, 2006; Holte, Margolis, & Cavanaugh, 1991; Kei et al., 2003; Margolis, Bass-Ringdahl, Hanks, Holte, & Zapala, 2003; Sprague et al., 1985; Williams, Purdy, & Barber, 1995).

Tympanometry has become a major part of the routine audiological evaluation since the 1970s, when it was introduced. Because the technique is not time-consuming or invasive and is relatively easy to administer, it can be used quite easily with individuals who do not respond well to audiometric or other behavioral tests, such as very young children or people with developmental delays.

As with other kinds of instrumental techniques, tympanometry is an excellent way of documenting changes in a patient's middle ear function resulting from surgical and/or medical treatment for middle ear problems. Tympanometry also serves as a quick and easy screening tool to detect the presence of middle ear pathology in children at all grade levels, including preschool. If a child obtains an abnormal tympanogram, he or she can then be referred to an otolaryngologist or audiologist for a more comprehensive evaluation.

Static-acoustic Middle Ear Admittance

Static-acoustic middle ear admittance is the admittance of the middle ear at a specified ear canal pressure value. When the ear canal pressure is a high positive (i.e., +200 daPa) or negative (i.e., −400 daPa) value, the tympanic membrane is very stiff, and the middle ear makes no contribution to the acoustic immittance measurement. In the measurement of static-acoustic middle ear admittance, the immittance of the outer ear at one of these values is subtracted from the immittance value at the peak pressure point of the tympanogram (the combined outer and middle ear immittance value), yielding the static-acoustic middle ear admittance.

Acoustic Reflex Testing

The contraction of the stapedius muscle in the middle ear in response to a loud sound can be measured via changes in the acoustic immittance of the middle ear. The procedure is known as acoustic reflex testing, and there are two measures involved: acoustic reflex threshold testing and acoustic reflex decay testing. The acoustic reflex is bilateral; that is, an acoustic signal of sufficient intensity presented to either ear will cause the stapedius muscle to contract in both ears.

Consequently, the acoustic reflex can be measured for both ipsilateral (stimulus presented to the ear being measured) and contralateral (stimulus presented to the ear opposite the one being measured) stimulation. The comparison of the values obtained in these two measures can be diagnostically useful. In the acoustic reflex threshold test, the lowest intensity level of the signal (typically pure tone stimuli of 500, 1000, and 2000 Hz) that produces a change in the middle ear admittance is recorded as the acoustic reflex threshold. Across frequencies, listeners with normal hearing have acoustic reflex thresholds between about 85 dB SPL and 100 dB SPL. Normative data for both normal hearing and hearing-impaired listeners have been published (Silman & Gelfand, 1981).

In the acoustic reflex decay test, the acoustic stimulus is presented for 10 seconds at a level 10 dB above the threshold level and the change (decrease) in reflex magnitude is monitored. A decrease of 50 percent is generally considered to be abnormal (Jerger, Harford, Clemis, & Alford, 1974; Olsen, Noffsinger, & Kurdziel, 1975).

Otoacoustic Emissions Testing

Another valuable component of the diagnostic process is the measurement of otoacoustic emissions (OAEs). OAEs are extremely low-intensity sounds (usually < 30 dB SPL) that originate in the cochlea as the outer hair cells process incoming sound. These cochlear sounds are transmitted in the opposite direction. That is, they travel back to the footplate of the stapes, across the ossicular chain to the TM, and into the external ear canal, where they can be measured.

Spontaneous and evoked otoacoustic emissions

OAEs have been categorized into two types, both of which can be attributed to the activity of the outer hair cells. The two major categories are spontaneous and evoked OAEs. Spontaneous otoacoustic emissions (SOAEs) occur without any incoming auditory stimulation in up to 70 percent of people (including infants) with normal hearing (DeVries & Newell Decker, 1992; Norton, 1992; Penner & Zhang, 1997; Prieve, 1992; Talmadge, Long, Murphy, & Tubis, 1993). According to Bright (2002), most SOAEs in adult ears fall between 1000 and 2000 Hz, while those of infants range between 3000 and 4000 Hz. SOAEs also occur more frequently in females than in males and in right ears more than in left. Because SOAEs are not observed in all normal ears, they currently hold little diagnostic value.

Evoked otoacoustic emissions (EOAEs) occur in response to acoustic stimulation to the ear and for virtually everyone with normal hearing. There are several types of EOAEs, depending on the type of stimulus used to evoke them. Transient evoked OAEs (TEOAEs) are elicited using a click or tone burst. Distortion product OAEs (DPOAEs) are elicited using a series of paired pure tones of slightly different frequency and intensity. Because the cochlea is nonlinear, the interaction of these two tones produces distortion products, the most prominent of which is the cubic distortion product (2 f1–f2). The basic procedure used to generate and record OAEs consists of placing a miniature loudspeaker and sensitive microphone in the person's external ear canal by means of a miniature probe which seals the ear canal and reduces external noise. The loudspeaker generates the sound, and the microphone records the emissions.

EOAEs are clinically important because nearly everyone with normal ears demonstrates them, whereas they are absent in people with even mild degrees of sensory hearing loss. For instance, Robinette (1992) measured EOAEs in 105 normally hearing men and 160 normally hearing women between 20 and 80 years. EOAEs were observed in all 265 normal ears but were absent in all ears with sensory hearing loss. Thus, because EOAEs cannot be detected in people with mild or more severe degrees of hearing loss, testing for their presence or absence can be used as an objective, sensitive way of measuring cochlear function. Also, EOAE testing is noninvasive and does not require patients to participate actively in the test. This makes it a particularly effective way of evaluating cochlear function in infants and young children. Furthermore, EOAEs can be tested very quickly, and the technology is not expensive, making this an excellent way of screening infants, babies, and children in clinics and hospital. In fact, OAEs are widely used as the clinical test of choice in neonatal hearing screening programs throughout the United States.

One important point to keep in mind is that for the results to be valid, an individual's middle ear status must also be assessed. This is because a conductive loss would interfere with the acoustic signal in both directions—that is, both traveling through the middle ear to the cochlea and traveling back from the cochlea through the middle ear to the external canal. A child who has otitis media with effusion or another conductive pathology, therefore, cannot be evaluated successfully for EOAEs. However, EOAEs can be used to measure recovery of conductive function after treatment.

To date, the most valuable use of EOAEs is in neonatal screening. Early identification of hearing problems is a crucial factor in rehabilitation because the earlier a problem is detected, the sooner the child can be fitted with appropriate amplification or even cochlear implants. Prior to the creation of the Early Hearing Detection and Intervention (EDHI) grants and subsequent legislation (1999–2000), which provided federal funds for the establishment of infant hearing screening and intervention programs, children born with permanent hearing loss typically would not have been identified and diagnosed until 2½ to 3 years of age. Since the start of these programs, the average age of identification of hearing loss has decreased to 2 to 3 months of age (Harrison, Roush, & Wallace, 2003; White, 2003), making it possible to begin intervention during the critical language period. Studies have shown significantly better spoken language performance in children who were identified and started on an intervention program at an earlier age than those identified and enrolled in programs at later ages (e.g., Kennedy et al., 2006; Moeller, 2000; Yoshinaga-Itano, 2003; Yoshinaga-Itano et al., 1998).

Auditory Brain Stem Response Testing

The auditory brain stem response (ABR) test is a measure of neuroelectric potentials that occur within about 10 msec after auditory stimulation. The procedure involves inserting small foam-tipped earphones in the person's ears to deliver the stimuli, which are typically a series of clicks or tone bursts. Electrical activity generated by the auditory pathway in response to the sounds is recorded by means of surface electrodes attached to the individual's scalp and earlobes. The recording appears as a waveform with a series of five peaks, which represent the activity of the auditory nerve and the brain stem pathway as the stimulus is processed. Waves I and II are assumed to be generated peripherally in the auditory nerve, and waves III, IV, and V are associated with brain stem processing of the stimulus (Ponton, Moore, & Eggermont, 1996). The measures of interest are the latencies (times) and amplitudes of the peaks. For infants and small children, it is preferable to perform the procedure while the child is asleep. In some cases, the child may need to be sedated. Because the ABR is relatively unaffected by the patient's state and does not require his or her cooperation or active participation, this procedure joins EOAE testing as a tool for newborn hearing screening. It is also used to identify auditory system pathology as well as to estimate a person's auditory threshold, to determine hearing loss type and degree, and in intraoperative monitoring.

Evaluation of Speech Perception

Speech perception is an integral part of learning a language and of developing all the numerous bases of language, such as phonology, morphology, syntax, and semantics. Reading and language are also closely related, and speech perception plays an important role in the development of reading skills. Consequently, problems in speech perception can have adverse effects on many different aspects of language and reading. It is extremely important to evaluate the speech perception abilities of hearing-impaired individuals in order to gain a precise understanding of their patterns of perception and, in children, their related production errors. Rehabilitation, in the form of amplification, cochlear implantation, and/or speech–reading training, can then be targeted toward the underlying perceptual errors.

The audiological evaluation of both children and adults typically includes a measure of suprathreshold speech-recognition ability, most commonly with lists of phonetically balanced monosyllabic words presented in quiet. While this test provides a measure of how a listener perceives the various phonemes of English, it provides only a limited picture of how a listener communicates on a day-to-day basis because it eliminates many of the redundancies of communication and is delivered in the artificial environment of a sound room.

For normal hearers, speech recognition can be predicted using one of several methods based on the articulation index (French & Steinberg, 1947) or on another transmission index. The articulation index (AI) divides the speech spectrum into 20 contiguous bands, each of which makes an equal contribution to intelligibility (5%). The signal-to-noise ratio in each band contributes to the total score, which can range from 0 to 1.0. The actual speech-recognition score will depend on the test materials used. As an example, an AI score of .5 will result in a score of 75 percent for monosyllabic words but 97 percent for sentences, reflecting the role of context in speech perception. The AI has been used with hearing-impaired listeners, but other factors related to the hearing loss must be taken into consideration.

One way of evaluating how hearing-impaired individuals perceive consonants and vowels is by phonetically transcribing the phonemes that they recognize in terms of the traditional classification system or other phonetic classification systems. For example, phonetic transcription may indicate that an individual consistently misses the /s/ sound in the final position of words, suggesting difficulty in perceiving this phoneme. From these types of analysis, it is possible to understand the kinds of errors in perception made by the listener, but it is not possible to determine the actual acoustic and perceptual bases for the errors (Ochs, Humes, Ohde, & Grantham, 1989). By using synthetic speech or by digitally manipulating acoustic features of natural speech, it is possible to determine precisely which acoustic features are important for individuals with hearing loss.

Cochlear Implants

Cochlear implants have become popular in the United States and other countries as a means of enhancing hearing in individuals with profound hearing loss. A cochlear implant is an electronic device designed to directly stimulate the auditory nerve by bypassing a person's damaged cochlea. There are currently three cochlear implant manufacturers in the United States: Advanced Bionics Corporation, Cochlear Corporation, and Med-El Corporation. Regardless of manufacturer, part of the device is surgically implanted in the cochlea, and part is worn externally. The external parts of the device include a microphone, speech processor, transmitter, and battery, while the internal parts include a receiver/stimulator and the electrode array. The microphone converts the acoustic signal to an electrical signal, which is sent to the speech processor. The speech processor codes the signal and sends it to the transmitter, which in turn delivers it to the implanted receiver/stimulator. The receiver/stimulator then sends the electrical signals to the electrodes, which stimulate the auditory nerve fibers. The electrodes are arranged throughout the cochlea, taking advantage of its tonotopic organization.

How the signal is represented is extremely important in recreating it in such a way that the implant user can gain the most benefit. For example, the range of frequencies represented is an important factor. Speech frequencies can have a wide range, from the F_0 of an adult male's voice, around 100 Hz, to the extremely high-frequency energy present in the sibilant fricatives. An implant therefore must be able to detect and transmit a wide range of frequencies, arranged in frequency bandwidths. Another consideration is that the signal processor must be able to resolve small frequency differences between sounds. For example, to identify a vowel sound, an implant must be able to resolve the formant frequencies of the vowel (Dorman, 2000), which sometimes differ by only a few hundred hertz.

Information about manner of articulation and voicing is contained in the spectrum of sounds. Spectral shapes are different for stops, fricatives, glides, liquids, and nasals. Recall that a stop has a short duration of aperiodic sound (the burst), whereas fricatives are characterized by longer-duration aperiodic noise. This kind of spectral information can be coded by one electrode. However, information signaling formant frequencies for vowels and place of articulation for consonants is best coded by multiple electrodes (Dorman, 2000). In addition, because of the dynamic nature of speech, with its rapidly changing frequencies and intensities, an implant must be able to resolve not only the formant frequencies but where the formant frequencies are at a given moment in time. In other words, the implant works to resolve rapid changes in formant frequencies over time (Dorman, 2000).

The cochlear implant works by filtering the speech signal into a series of frequency channels. Information about the signal envelope in each channel is transmitted to the electrodes for stimulation of the nerve fibers. Two implementation methods are in use today: continuous interleaved sampling (CIS) and the spectral-maxima strategy (ACE/SPEAK). The major difference between the strategies involves the method of envelope detection, stimulation rate, filter spacing, and shape of compression function (Loizou, 2006). Because simultaneous stimulation of electrodes can result in distortion of the signal spectrum, the CIS strategy modulates the waveforms so that only one electrode is stimulated at any one time. All three manufacturers are able to employ CIS.

The spectral-maxima strategy, known commonly as the SPEAK (spectral peak)/ACE (advanced combination encoder), or m-of-n strategy, transmits information about the spectral peaks in the signal. The n of the m-of-n strategy is the overall number of frequency bands, while m is the number of channels with the highest energy peaks. This strategy typically divides the acoustic signal into around 20 frequency bands to achieve a satisfactory frequency resolution. The 5 to 12 channels (depending on manufacturer and spectral composition of the signal) with the highest energy are determined, and the electrodes associated with these channels are stimulated. The m channels thus represent the formants in the speech signal. Dorman (2000) pointed out that the m-of-n strategy is an excellent way to transmit speech because only the formants are transmitted, and as the formant frequencies change, so do the electrodes being stimulated. Early experiments using the Pattern Playback with normally hearing listeners showed that speech can be transmitted with very good intelligibility based only on information about the location of the formant peaks. In effect, the change in location of the stimulated electrode mimics the normal frequency change in location along the basilar membrane (Dorman, 2000).

Another method of coding speech information is based on feature extraction. The speech signal processor works by representing acoustic cues such as F_0, F_1, F_2, and other high-frequency peaks of energy in the signal. The signal is sampled every few milliseconds to detect changes in the acoustic energy peaks over time. An example of this is the $F_0F_1F_2$ strategy, which stimulates only two electrodes, based on estimates of the F_1 and F_2 frequencies. The stimulation occurs at a rate that corresponds to the F_0 of the signal when the stimulus is voiced and to a random rate around F_0 when the stimulus is not voiced. Another version, the MPEAK strategy, stimulates four electrodes representing F_1 and F_2 and two high-frequency peaks of energy (for voiced sounds), as well as four electrodes representing F_2 and three high-frequency peaks (for unvoiced sounds). These methods have not been as widely implemented as the other methods due to difficulty extracting formant information, particularly in noisy backgrounds, but interest in these methods continues. For a comprehensive review of the history of cochlear implant processing strategies and the current status of processing, the reader is referred to Loizou (1998, 2006).

A recent development in cochlear implants is a new surgical procedure in which patients with residual low-frequency hearing are implanted with a shorter electrode. The procedure gives these individuals access to both low-frequency information (by way of their auditory-acoustic access) and high-frequency information (by way of the electrical stimulation), thus providing improved word recognition and music appreciation (Gantz & Turner, 2004).

Cochlear implants are becoming increasingly accepted as a viable means of enhancing the speech-recognition abilities of children and adults with severe and profound sensorineural hearing loss, with over 220,000 people worldwide (>71,000 in the United States) receiving implants. Many researchers have examined the resulting phoneme perception in implant users. For example, Meyers, Swirsky, Kirk, and Miyamoto (1998) tested the speech perception of children wearing cochlear implants. They used the Minimal Pairs Test, which assesses vowel height and advancement, consonant voicing, and manner and place of articulation. The authors reported that the children's performance depended on how long the implants had been in place. Just prior to implantation, the children's average scores were at chance level. By approximately 1 year post implantation, the average consonant perception score reached a level of 65 percent. The authors found that, on average, children with hearing losses in the 101 to 110 dB HL range received greater speech perception benefits from a cochlear implant than from their hearing aids. This is extremely valuable information, pointing to the possibility of improved speech perception for many children using cochlear implants. With changes in candidacy criteria and improvements in surgical techniques and processing strategies, it is expected that the speech-recognition performance of adults and children using cochlear implants will continue to increase.

Training for Cochlear Implant Users

Training in speech recognition is essential for a person who has received an implant, and visual feedback is crucial for training, at least in the early stages. Electroglottography and spectrography have been used to visualize the phoneme contrasts being trained. As soon as the cochlear implant user can discriminate the contrast through auditory input alone, the visual feedback is withdrawn. Training should occur at both segmental and suprasegmental levels. One of the first discriminations a new cochlear implant user is able to make is the overall temporal structure of the segments, such as counting the number of sounds heard (Cooper, 1991). Intonation is also an extremely important aspect of rehabilitation, and training involves the user's learning to perceive (and, for children, to produce) different F_0 contours. The suprasegmental aspects of speech, such as intonation, stress, duration, and rhythm, are carried in the low frequencies and are often more audible to people with severe and profound losses. Training should capitalize on these aspects so that improved suprasegmental perception becomes a bridge to increased phoneme and word recognition. Visual feedback from spectrograms, electroglottography, and instrumental tracking of F_0 and intensity contours acts as a powerful clinical tool to facilitate the implant user's suprasegmental and segmental recognition.

All three cochlear implant manufacturers in the United States offer training programs for children and adults. Videos and printed materials are also available to help new users develop auditory skills. Implant recipients are able to augment their passive daily listening experiences with a variety of structured listening programs, many of which can be completed in their homes. Research has shown that auditory training is beneficial in improving speech recognition performance (Qian-Jie, Galvin, Xiaosong, & Nogaki, 2005) and tone quality (Gfeller et al., 2002) in adult cochlear implant patients. While a variety of other factors (age at identification of hearing loss, age at implantation, communication mode, etc.) influence how a child's auditory perception and oral language will develop using a cochlear implant, research findings indicate that daily use, time and training are important components (Connor, Hieber, Arts, & Zwolan, 2000; Fryauf-Bertschy, Tyler, Kelsay, Gantz, & Woodworth, 1997; Kühn-Inacker, Shehata-Dieler, Müller, & Helms, 2004).

Otitis Media and Speech Perception

The most common cause of conductive hearing loss is otitis media (OM). Anyone can get OM, but it is particularly prevalent among young children. This happens in part because of the different shape of the Eustachian tube in children and adults. The adult tube lies at an angle of about 45 degrees to the horizontal, whereas it is almost horizontal in young children (Gelfand, 1997). The horizontal position makes drainage of fluids through the tube less efficient, and thus it is more likely that fluid will accumulate in the middle ear. Tube dysfunction can also be caused by an upper respiratory infection, in which edema and fluid block the tube, and by allergies, enlarged adenoids, or structural problems such as cleft palate. When the tube does not open properly, the middle ear cannot be ventilated. Some of the air in the middle ear gets absorbed into the tissues of the middle ear. Consequently, the air pressure inside the middle ear becomes lower than in the surrounding atmosphere, including in the ear canal. This causes the tympanic membrane to be drawn inward, and the air pressure cannot be equalized because of the blockage of the Eustachian tube. Because the middle ear cannot be drained properly, fluids often build up within the middle ear. This is known as otitis media with effusion (OME).

OME is very prevalent in preschool children and can cause temporary conductive hearing losses of approximately 20 to 40 dB (Groenen, Crul, Maasen, & van Bon, 1996). Many young children have repeated bouts of OM, called recurrent OM. Each episode may be associated with a temporary conductive hearing loss. These recurring periods of hearing loss have been linked to problems in perception, subtle language deficits, and academic difficulties. Even though the hearing loss is temporary, if the child has recurring periods of loss during the interval in which he or she is acquiring speech and language, the youngster may be at risk for language problems later. Children with a history of recurring OME in early childhood have been shown to have subtle differences in speech perception from their peers. For example, some children with early OME show poorer VOT perception, and some show less mature weighting strategies for the perception of synthetic

/s/ and /ʃ/ continua. Groenen et al. (1996) tested the voiced–voiceless distinction using VOT continua varying from /b/ (/bak/) to /p/ (/pak/). Children without OME or language impairment were compared to children with a history of OME only and to children with both OME and language impairment. Children with either early OME or language impairment were not as adept at identifying the sounds. Thus, a history of OME appears to result in poorer phonetic processing, irrespective of language impairment. The authors proposed that recurrent OME may be considered a form of early sensory deprivation. Information that is important to the perception and categorization of speech may therefore be less consistent during the years when the child should be acquiring the sound system of his or her native language.

Subtle disturbances in phonetic perception can affect a child's linguistic abilities. Nittrouer (1996a) used synthetic /s/ and /ʃ/ fricatives to test whether children with early OME used similar weighting strategies as their peers without early OME. Children with early OME showed less mature perceptual weighting strategies than children with no OME. Very young children give more weight to dynamic information (e.g., formant transitions) than they do to more static spectral information. As they develop a larger vocabulary, they learn to make more subtle perceptual distinctions between sounds, based more on static spectral cues and with less reliance on dynamic characteristics. Thus, chronic OM clearly puts children at risk for delays in the development of perceptual weighting strategies and phonemic awareness. In turn, this may lead to difficulties with higher-level language functioning and with reading.

Language and Reading Disability and Speech Perception

Difficulties with the perceptual processing of acoustic cues have been found to be important in some forms of language-learning disorders and in reading disabilities. Much research has focused on whether these difficulties arise from problems in the perception of phonemes at the phonetic-acoustic level or from a higher level, more linguistically based impairment. Much of the research is based on the hypothesis that difficulty perceiving the rapidly changing sound waves of speech results in problems relating the acoustic information contained in the phonemes and syllables to the person's mental representation of phonemes. For reading, this may interfere with the process of transforming written symbols to phonetic units (Watson & Miller, 1993). The distinction between a phonetic processing problem and a higher level linguistic problem is important because treatment strategies would differ, depending on the root cause of the problem.

If a child has a hearing loss and, as a result, his or her receptive and expressive language skills are delayed, then it is expected that the child will also present with reading difficulties. Even a mild hearing loss can have an effect (Wake, Hughes, Poulakis, Collins, & Rickards, 2004). However, evidence suggests that early identification and intervention with hearing-impaired children has the potential to positively influence language and literacy outcomes (Carney & Moeller, 1998).

Often a child with a language and/or reading disorder does not have any obvious problems that are causing it, such as mental or emotional challenges or hearing loss. **Specific language impairment (SLI)** is a disorder in which children show a significant problem with language despite having normal hearing, normal nonverbal intelligence, and no known neurological problems. The cause of SLI is not known, but one theory is that these children have a problem with auditory perception that results in the language difficulties. As noted previously, during connected speech, the acoustic signal changes rapidly and continuously in frequency and intensity, and a child who has difficulty perceiving these quick shifts may have difficulty detecting phoneme changes. The difficulty processing rapid acoustic signals is referred to as a **temporal processing problem**. According to Tallal et al. (1996), children who are language-learning impaired often cannot identify fast elements, such as formant transitions or spectral information, that are embedded in ongoing speech. If a child has difficulty perceiving the phonemes of the language, then the child does not have access to complete language input from the environment. This can interfere with higher-order language functions, such as phonological processing skills, morphology, syntax, and semantics.

Research over the past two decades has explored how children with reading difficulties and language problems are able to detect small acoustic differences between sounds. Many of these tests use synthetic speech stimuli rather than naturally spoken speech. For example, Nittrouer (1999) compared children with language-learning difficulty and those with normal language. The first test examined the children's ability to discriminate between voiced and voiceless sounds (/t/ and /d/). Nittrouer (1999) manipulated the duration of the F_1 transition and the spectrum of a 10 msec release burst. The F_1 transitions varied from 40 msec to no transition (0 msec), in equal steps of 5 msec each. Each synthetic item was paired up with a 10 msec burst from a speaker saying /da/ and /ta/. The stimuli thus varied from most /da/-like to most /ta/-like. The children were presented with one item at a time and had to decide if it was a /da/ or a /ta/. In another task, the children listened to sounds on a continuum of /s/ to /ʃ/. The sounds varied in the center frequency of the synthetic fricative noises, from 2200 to 3800 Hz, in 200 Hz steps. Recall that the /s/ is associated with a very high spectral peak, while the /ʃ/ has a much lower-frequency spectral peak. As with the /da–ta/ task, the children were presented with one sound at a time and had to assign it to an /s/ or /ʃ/ category. Both groups of children in Nittrouer's (1999) study used these acoustic cues similarly in deciding on the identity of the sound. The children with language-learning difficulties, however, performed more like younger typically developing children, thus demonstrating subtle delays in perceptual processing of at least some phonemes. Perceptual processing delays were also reported by Elliott and Hammer (1993), who tested older and younger children in three groups: children with a language-learning problem, children in a regular school placement, and children with moderate intellectual impairment. The test activities involved a place-of-articulation continuum (/ba–da–ga/) and a VOT continuum (/ba–pa/). The place continuum differed in frequency characteristics, with different starting frequencies for F_2 and F_3. The VOT continuum differed in the amount of time between the release burst of the consonant and the onset of vibration for the following vowel. The older children performed better than the younger children on most of the tasks. The younger children with language problems performed more poorly than the younger children in regular school placements on every test measure. Children with language problems required a VOT of 23 msec to differentiate /ba/ from /pa/, whereas the typically developing children required only 17 msec. Performance for the children with intellectual impairment was poorer than for the other two groups. The authors suggested that the lower the level of a young child's speech and language skills, the greater the importance of auditory discrimination of small acoustic differences in increasing receptive vocabulary and language skills. The authors proposed that young typically developing children are primarily dependent on auditory stimulation for language learning. As they mature, other influences such as reading become increasingly important, so older children may rely less on audition, and auditory discrimination becomes less important.

Other research confirms that older children do not seem to rely as much on auditory discrimination as do younger children. Bernstein and Stark (1985) followed up the speech-perception abilities in language-impaired children 4 years after the children had first been tested, using synthetic /ba/ and /da/ syllables. Of the 29 children in the follow-up study who were identified as language impaired at time 1, 23 were still language impaired at time 2. However, the authors found some perceptual development among the language-impaired children, suggesting that these children beyond age 8 years do not have difficulties obtaining perceptual information. The authors suggested that early perceptual deficits do not prevent language development, but language develops more slowly than it does for typically developing children. These kinds of perceptual deficits have been shown to be highly correlated with children's scores on language tests, such as the *Peabody Picture Vocabulary Test–Revised* and the *Token Test for Children* (Stark & Heinz, 1996a). In fact, these kinds of acoustic characteristics can be very accurate in predicting whether children will have language-learning disabilities once they reach school age.

Leonard, McGregor, and Allen (1992) provided a specific link between the perceptual processing difficulties of children with SLI and grammatical function. Morphology is often an area of particular difficulty for these children, including inflections such as the third-person singular -s, as well as function words such as the articles *a* and *the*. Interestingly, the morphological features that seem to pose the most difficulty are consonant segments (e.g., third-person singular -s) and unstressed syllables (e.g., *the*), which are characterized by shorter duration than adjacent morphemes and often lower F_0 and amplitude. Children with SLI, however, use some of the same phonetic forms in other contexts. Leonard et al. (1992) noted that the children used the /d/ in *braid* much more than in *played* and the /s/ in *box* more than in *rocks*. They proposed that the difficulty seems to be not so much in perceiving the sound as in both perceiving it and treating it as a morpheme. The child must not only perceive the /d/ in *played* but also relate *played* to *play* and put -*ed* in the proper place. Because these additional operations are not involved in *braid*, acquisition and use of /d/ will be more advanced in *braid*.

The authors also suggested that the duration of the contrastive portion of the stimulus is important for its perception in children with SLI. When the part of the word to be discriminated is shorter than the remaining portion, children with

SLI have greater difficulty than typically developing children of the same age. However, when the duration of the contrastive feature is longer than the rest of the stimulus, these children perform adequately. Leonard et al. (1992) suggested two possible sources of the children's difficulty. The first is that their perceptual abilities are extremely fragile. Therefore, when they need to make difficult discriminations between sounds, any additional processing that needs to be done suffers. The second possibility is that these children have some kind of generalized processing problem so that, when they need to use extra resources for a particularly difficult task, fewer resources are left for other mental operations.

Language and reading are integrally related. Developmental dyslexia is a disorder in which the person's reading ability is significantly lower than what would be predicted on the basis of age and IQ (McAnally, Hansen, Cornelissen, & Stein, 1997). It has been established that children with **developmental dyslexia** do not show as clear-cut categorical perception of synthetic continua as typically reading children. Many individuals with dyslexia have difficulty perceiving consonant contrasts and may confuse sounds that are phonetically similar more often than typical. People with dyslexia may have deficits in processing the temporal order of acoustic information. Stark and Heinz (1996b) reported that children with language impairment find it difficult to discriminate and identify phonemes and also have problems judging the order in which phonemes are heard. Many of these children, according to Stark and Heinz (1996b), go on to have reading disabilities.

It is clear that many children with language and/or reading impairment have difficulties segmenting, discriminating, and identifying speech sounds (Bishop et al., 1999). The temporal characteristics of auditory stimuli are critical for children with language impairment. Very short or very rapid stimuli present serious challenges to children with language impairment. However, these children seem to have less difficulty in discrimination when the stimuli are lengthened or presented at a slower rate. The question is whether such difficulties have their basis in a more fundamental auditory perceptual deficit that affects the processing of all sounds. It is currently thought that the impairment in discriminating brief or rapid events is not specific to auditory processing but also occurs in other sensory areas. However, the difficulty in rapid processing is thought to have an especially severe impact on language development, which is crucially dependent on the ability to distinguish and identify brief and rapid auditory events (Bishop et al., 1999).

Articulatory Problems and Speech Perception

Researchers and clinicians have long suspected that there may be a link between errors in articulation and perception that do not result from problems such as cleft palate or deafness. However the nature of this link is far from clear. Some children have been found to have similar abilities in articulation and perception. Some children misarticulate specific sounds but can perceive the sounds they misarticulate without a problem. Others misarticulate specific sounds and also have difficulty perceiving these sounds.

Investigators have used synthetic speech sounds to try to clarify this link because synthetic speech sounds can be manipulated more easily to show precisely which acoustic cues in the signal influence children's perception and production of the sounds. Raaymakers and Crul (1988) tested adults and 5- to 6-year-old children on synthetically generated words ending in /s/ and /ts/. One group of children misarticulated the /s–ts/ contrast. Another group exhibited various other misarticulations. The authors generated a continuum using the Dutch words *moes* to *moets* by adding periods of silence between *oe* and /s/. They found that the poorer the child's articulation skill, the more variable the child was in his or her response.

Other authors have found similar variability and lack of precision in perceptual performance of children who have articulation difficulties. Hoffman, Daniloff, Bengoa, and Schuckers (1985) looked at children's abilities to discriminate between the /w/ and /r/ sounds. These sounds are differentiated in part by their formant frequencies, with /r/ having a much lower F_3 than /w/. Research has shown that 3-year-old children with developmentally appropriate articulation skills can identify synthesized /l/, /r/, and /w/ sounds that differ in the onset frequencies of the first three formants. Many of these children cannot yet produce the /l/ and /r/ sounds accurately, instead producing them both as /w/. However, 3-year-old children with delayed articulation show a large number of perceptual errors. The authors tested children 6 years to 6 years and 11 months old who substituted /w/ for /r/ and children who produced the sounds correctly, both on synthesized /r–w/ continua. The children who misarticulated demonstrated less precise discrimination and identification of these phonemes than the controls. Approximately two-thirds of the children who misarticulated failed to categorize /r/ and /w/ stimuli when they had to rely only on formant trajectories. The remaining one-third made a categorization that was less well defined than that of the controls.

Children learn to produce the phoneme contrasts and sequences of their language gradually during their first years by matching their own productions to an acoustic model. A child who fails to produce speech correctly may omit a target phoneme, produce that phoneme inaccurately, or substitute another phoneme for the intended one. Sometimes a child neutralizes the contrast between the two phonemes. For instance, a child who substitutes /w/ or a /w/-like sound for /r/ neutralizes the contrast between /w/ and /r/. The child may or may not be able to perceptually discriminate between his or her own productions of the error sound and the intended sound. If the child can discriminate the sounds even when the contrast between them cannot be perceived by another listener, the child may be using subphonemic cues to mark the contrast. Such cues are not audible to adults, although often they can be detected with acoustic instrumentation. In some cases, a child may maintain a contrast but misarticulate both phonemes. For example, when a child substitutes /w/ for /r/ and /j/ for /l/, both /l/ and /r/ are misarticulated, but the contrast between them is maintained (Broen, Strange, Doyle, & Heller, 1983).

Broen et al. (1983) compared the perception of 3-year-olds with misarticulations and children who had developmental misarticulations of /l/ and /r/ using the synthetically produced words *wake–rake*, *rake–lake*, and *wake–lake*. They reported that, although the majority of children in both groups misarticulated /l/ and/

or /r/, the pattern of errors was different. When the children with developmental errors misarticulated /l/ or /r/, they produced /w/ or a /w/-like distortion, neutralizing that contrast for the adult listener. However, these developmentally appropriate misarticulations were not accompanied by perceptual problems. The articulation-delayed children had a much more varied pattern of misarticulations of the /l/, /r/, and /w/ sounds. Some children actually omitted all these sounds. These children also showed problems in the perception of all three contrasts.

Similar perceptual difficulties have been reported with synthetic /s/–/ʃ/ contrasts. Rvachew and Jamieson (1989) investigated the perception of normally speaking adults, normally speaking 5-year-olds, and articulation-disordered 5-year-olds in the synthetically generated words *seat* and *sheet*. The adults and the normally speaking children identified fricatives differing in spectral characteristics with equal consistency. The articulation-disordered children, however, were much more variable. More than half of them were unable to classify the stimuli in the continuum reliably. Some children responded *seat* to almost all the stimuli, whereas others responded in an apparently random manner.

Thus, it appears that children with a functional articulation disorder can be categorized into at least two subgroups: those with speech-perception difficulties and those with normal speech-perception skills. It is very important, therefore, to determine children's perceptual skills in the clinic before implementing therapy procedures for articulation and phonological problems. Some children may need help in honing their perceptual skills before the production problem is treated, whereas other children with normal perceptual skills may be treated immediately for the articulation problem. Rvachew and Jamieson (1989) emphasized that children with articulation problems show speech-perception difficulties that are not general to all speech sounds but that are specific to the child's misarticulated sounds. Therefore, speech discrimination tests that cover a wide range of phoneme contrasts might not be sensitive enough to detect the child's very specific perception problem.

Summary

Immittance audiometry, otoacoustic emissions, and auditory brain stem response testing have become valuable diagnostic tools in the assessment of middle ear and inner ear function.

Individuals with hearing impairment do not have access to the multiple acoustic cues used by normally hearing speakers to identify phonemes.

Hearing-impaired listeners are often able to discriminate vowels but have problems in identifying consonants, particularly fricatives.

Cochlear implants work by filtering a speech signal into a series of frequency channels; information about the signal envelope in each channel is transmitted to the electrodes for stimulation of the auditory nerve fibers. Training in auditory discrimination using visual feedback is essential for cochlear implant users to receive the greatest benefit from their device.

Otitis media is a form of early sensory deprivation that has been linked to subtle speech-perception and linguistic problems.

Children with language and/or reading disabilities may have a temporal processing problem that hinders them from perceiving the phonemes of their language.

Children with articulation problems may or may not have speech perception difficulties related to their specific misarticulations.

REVIEW EXERCISES

1. Draw Type A, B, and C tympanograms and explain what each indicates about a patient's middle ear function.

2. Describe advantages and disadvantages of otoacoustic emissions and auditory brain stem response testing in diagnosis of hearing disorders.

3. Describe the components of a cochlear implant and explain how the device works to provide auditory stimulation to the user.

4. Why is otitis media considered to be a form of sensory deprivation, and what is its effect on language?

5. Explain the term *temporal processing problem* and describe its impact on children with language and/or reading disability.

6. Describe the relationships between phoneme perception and articulation ability in young children.

INTEGRATIVE CASE STUDY

❶ Mr. Williams

Background Information

Mr. Williams, a 69-year-old man, came to your speech and hearing clinic accompanied by his wife of 43 years. Mrs. Williams reported that her husband does not respond to her conversation at home. She is upset, though, that he seems to have no difficulty conversing with his male friends at home, and she feels that his problem is with her, and not with his hearing. The couple enjoys dining out with friends once or twice per week, and Mr. Williams has lately been having difficulty following conversations in these situations. Mr. Williams admits that he feels frustrated in these situations but denies having any difficulty at home. His wife reports that the TV is always on at an uncomfortably high level.

Auditory Measures

Pure-tone testing revealed normal hearing through 1 kHz dropping to a moderate bilateral high-frequency sensorineural hearing loss. Speech-recognition testing indicated only fair recognition of speech. Otoacoustic emission screening showed no emissions bilaterally. Tympanometry was consistent with normal middle ear function.

Clinical Questions

a. Why might Mr. Williams be having difficulty hearing his wife's voice?

b. Why does Mr. Williams have more difficulty in noisy situations than in quiet ones?

c. What specific vowels and consonants would you expect him to have particular problems hearing? Why?

d. With appropriate amplification, do you think Mr. Williams will be better able to perceive his wife's voice? Why or why not?

e. With appropriate amplification, do you think Mr. Williams will be better able to perceive his friends' voices? Why or why not?

11

The Nervous System

STUDENT LEARNING OBJECTIVES

After reading this chapter you will

○ Understand the structure and function of neurons.

○ Identify the functional components of the central nervous system and their influence on language processing and speech production.

○ Describe the origin and target structures of the cranial nerves that are important in speech and hearing.

○ Appreciate the importance of a steady blood supply to the brain.

○ Understand the structure and function of the upper and lower motor neurons involved in speech production.

○ Explain the importance of feedback and feedforward systems in speech motor control.

The nervous system (NS) serves as the control system of the body and is the most important regulator of movement, as well as higher-order processing skills. This includes all the movements involved in speech production, including the regulation and coordination of the speech subsystems: respiration, phonation, and articulation. A normally functioning NS is crucial for normal speech. Disruptions to the NS at any point or location can have devastating effects on speech motor control, as is seen with neurological disorders such as cerebral palsy, stroke, Parkinson's disease, multiple sclerosis, and traumatic brain injury. Higher-order processing includes cognition and language. Disruption to the NS can also produce cognitive deficits in attention and memory, linguistic disorders such as aphasia, and the cognitive-communication disorders associated with right hemisphere damage and dementia.

Hugely complex in structure and function, the NS can be examined from many different anatomical and physiological viewpoints. In this chapter we will begin by describing the basic structure of the NS in terms of the neurons that constitute the brain and spinal cord. The electrochemical nature of nerve impulses will be explained. Different functional portions of the NS will be highlighted, and their relationship to speech motor control will be emphasized. The nerve pathways (tracts) that are formed by bundles of neurons will then be discussed in terms of their function related to speech production. Components of the classical zone of language will be described with respect to current theories of how language is represented in the brain. The chapter closes by exploring various mechanisms used in motor control of the speech subsystems.

The NS is divided into the central nervous system (CNS) and peripheral nervous system (PNS). The CNS consists of the brain and spinal cord. The PNS is further divided into the somatic system and the autonomic system. The somatic division of the PNS consists of the cranial and spinal nerves that transmit and receive nerve impulses to and from all the muscles and glands of the body. The cranial nerves are particularly important for speech as they innervate the muscles of the head and neck. There are two major types of tissues that make up the brain.

Brain Tissue

The brain is made up of billions of densely packed cells that form the nervous tissue of the body. The tissue of the nervous system is specialized to react to stimuli and to conduct impulses to and from areas within and outside of the brain. The brain is a small structure, weighing approximately 1400 g in the mature adult, although individual brains range anywhere from 1100 to 1700 g (Nolte, 2002). Two major types of tissue make up the brain: glial cells and neurons.

Glial Cells

Glial cells are a type of connective tissue and perform a variety of functions, including metabolic support, secretion of cerebrospinal fluid, response to injury, and insulation. These cells are located throughout the NS and make up an extensive support system that is crucial for its proper operation. Glial cells bring nutrients from the blood vessels to each neuron and remove the waste products of metabolism. Different types of glial cells are located in different areas of the NS. The most common glial cells are **astrocytes** (Figure 11.1), which are located throughout the

Figure 11.1 Astrocytes

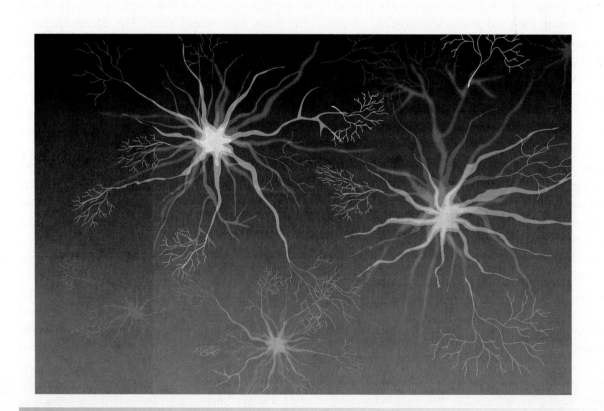

system of nerve cells in the brain. These cells have numerous projections that connect to blood capillaries and thereby assist in transporting substances from the blood to the nerve cells.

Oligodendrocytes in the CNS and **Schwann cells** in the PNS form layers of insulation, called myelin, that wrap around the nerve cells. Other cells called **microglia** help to keep the CNS clean by engulfing and destroying harmful organisms. Unlike nerve cells, glial cells are able to divide and reproduce throughout their lives. Therefore, if nerve tissue dies, the space previously occupied by the neurons tends to be filled by connective tissue. When this occurs, the site can become a focal point of epileptic seizures.

Neurons

Neurons are highly specialized structures that receive, process, and transmit information to, from, and within the NS. There are about 100 billion neurons in the CNS. All neurons have essentially the same structure, although some have modifications depending on their specific function. The basic structure consists of a **soma** (cell body), dendrites, and an axon, all bounded by a cell membrane (Figure 11.2).

The soma is formed by a nucleus surrounded by a mass of cytoplasm. Within the cytoplasm are organelles, which are specialized microstructures involved in various cell functions. For example, **Nissl bodies** synthesize proteins that keep the neuron healthy, while **mitochondria** are involved in cell respiration and the production of energy (Clayman, 1995). Other organelles called **Golgi apparatus** secrete and transport proteins and sugars. It is within the soma that the major metabolic activity of the neuron takes place. Branching off the cell body are numerous short projections called dendrites, which serve to transmit nerve impulses toward the cell body. Dendrites often have small spikes, which increase the surface area available for connections with other nerve cells. Also extending from the cell body is an **axon**, which is a projection that transmits nerve impulses away from the cell body. Axons originate from a small bump at the cell body called the axon hillock. Axons extend longer distances than dendrites and vary in length from less than 1 mm to more than 1 m (Hutchins, Naftel, & Ard, 2002; Webster, 1999). Most axons in the CNS are wrapped in myelin. Much like the insulation around a wire, the myelin sheath insulates and protects the axon. The diameter of the nerve and the thickness of its myelin sheath determine the speed of nerve conduction. The myelin sheath is not continuous along the axon but is interrupted by breaks known as **nodes of Ranvier**. These nodes are involved in speeding up the rate of nerve transmission, as the nerve impulse jumps from one node to the next.

At its endpoint the axon divides into numerous **terminal branches** (also called *telodendria*), which in turn end in small swellings or bumps, the **terminal buttons**. The number of buttons per axon varies, from a few to many thousands. Within the terminal buttons are tiny containers called vesicles, which contain different types of neurotransmitters. Neurotransmitters are chemical substances that act to stimulate or inhibit the impulse. This endpoint is the site of communication with other nerve cells. Between nerve cells is a tiny gap or cleft, called a **synapse**. A synapse may occur between the axon of one nerve and the dendrites, cell body, or axon of another nerve or nerves, of a muscle fiber, or of a glandular cell. A synapse between an axon and another axon is called an axo axonal synapse. A synapse

Figure 11.2 **Neuron**

Figure 11.2 Neuron

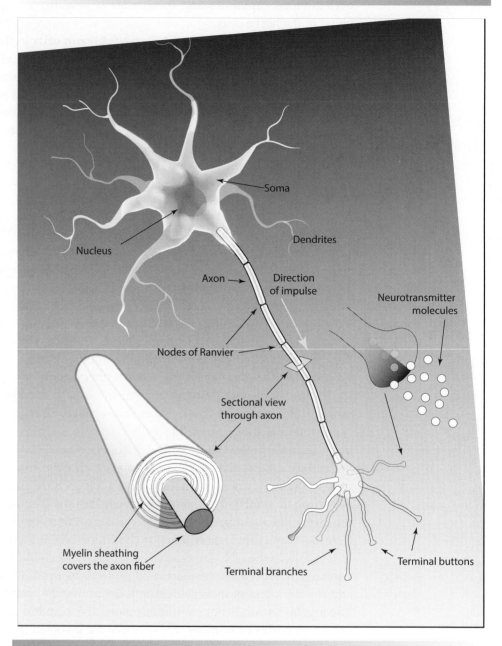

between an axon and a soma is an axo somatic synapse; an axodendritic synapse occurs between an axon and a dendrite. Communication between neurons is accomplished by neurotransmission, the movement of chemicals or electrical signals across a synapse. An axon that synapses with a skeletal muscle fiber is called the **neuromuscular junction** or the *neuromuscular end plate*. A single neuron may synapse with thousands of other neurons and in return may receive axonal input from many other neurons. This results in extraordinarily complex networks of neuronal connections throughout the NS.

Neurons function in groups. That is, axons do not extend to structures as individual projections but are wrapped together in bundles that form nerve pathways or tracts. Pathways are either *sensory* (**afferent**), transmitting information from sensory receptors toward the CNS, or *motor* (**efferent**), transmitting information from the CNS toward muscles and glands. Mixed nerve pathways contain both sensory and motor components.

Types of neurons

Neurons vary in size and shape, as well as in the total number of their receiving and transmitting processes. There are three ways of classifying neurons. One way of classifying neurons is according to their number of processes. Unipolar neurons have a single process, while bipolar neurons have two processes. Most neurons in the human nervous system are multipolar, with multiple dendrites and an axon. Multipolar neurons are further divided into Golgi Type I and Golgi Type II. Golgi Type I, also called projection neurons, have long axons that extend to the PNS and synapse with nerves that innervate muscles or glands. Golgi Type II are local circuit neurons with short axons that synapse on nearby neurons within the CNS. Golgi Type I axons are typically myelinated, while Golgi Type II tend to be unmyelinated (Webster, 1999).

Neurons can also be classified according to their function. Motor or efferent neurons are those that travel away from the NS and cause a response of a muscle or a gland. Sensory or afferent neurons carry information toward the CNS from peripheral structures such as specialized receptors in the skin, sense organs (eye, ear, etc.), and viscera. **Interneurons**, as the name suggests, connect neurons to each other, either locally—that is, within a small area of the CNS—or over longer distances (projection neurons). Most neurons in the human NS are interneurons.

A third way of classifying neurons is based on the type of neurotransmitter contained within its vesicles. For example, neurons containing the neurotransmitter dopamine are referred to as dopaminergic; those containing serotonin are serotonergic, acetylcholine-carrying neurons are cholinergic, and so on. Table 11.1 summarizes these classifications.

Table 11.1 **Ways of Classifying Neurons**

Number of processes	Unipolar
	Bipolar
	Multipolar
	Golgi Type I
	Golgi Type II
Function	Efferent (motor): Toward periphery
	Afferent (sensory): Toward NS
	Interneurons: Within NS
Neurotransmitter	Dopaminergic
	Cholinergic
	Serotonergic

Table 11.2 **Types of Sensory Receptors**

Type of Receptor	Sensory Information	Organ
Teleceptors	Distant environment	Eye, ear
Exteroceptors	Immediate environment	Skin
Proprioceptors	Position of body structures in space	Inner ear, muscles, tendons, joints
Visceroceptors/ interoceptors	Visceral structures	
Mechanoreceptors	Pressure/deformation	Tissue
Thermoreceptors	Changes in temperature	
Nocioreceptors	Tissue damage	
Photoreceptors	Light	Retina
Chemoreceptors	Taste and smell	Tongue, nose
Baroreceptors	Air pressure	Trachea, bronchi

Sensory receptors

In order to make sense of the information from an individual's external and internal environment, the body is richly supplied with different types of receptors. Receptors are specialized nerve cells that respond to changes in the organism or its environment and transmit these responses to the NS. Receptors respond to specific sensory stimuli. For example, receptors in the retina of the eye (rods and cones) respond to light. Receptors of the ear (inner hair cells) respond to sound waves. Receptors in the skin are differentially sensitive to touch, pressure, pain, and temperature. Table 11.2 identifies some different types of receptors.

Neuronal function

Nerves work through a complex progression of electrochemical activities in order to receive, process, and send information to other neurons. To achieve rapid, long distance communication, neurons have evolved special abilities for sending electrical signals along axons. Neurons have unique capabilities for communication within and between cells. The cell body of a neuron communicates with its own terminals via the axon (conduction); communication between neurons is achieved by the process of **neurotransmission**.

Neurotransmission is an electrochemical process. Because of its chemical composition, the inside of a neuron and the extracellular fluid that surrounds it are electrically charged. Conduction begins when an action potential is generated near the cell body portion of the axon. An action potential is an electrical signal that occurs because electrically charged particles, called **ions**, move across the neuronal membrane. An ion carries an electrical charge that is either positive or negative depending on if it is gaining or losing electrons. Whether the charge is positive or negative depends on the concentration of ions. When the neuron is at rest, there is a higher concentration of positive ions (sodium, Na+, and potassium, K+) outside the cell and a higher proportion of negative ions (chlorine, Cl–) within the cell. The sodium concentration within the neuron at rest is around one-tenth of the amount outside the cell (Zemlin, 1998). This imbalance creates a voltage across the cell membrane, called the **resting membrane potential (RMP)**. At rest the interior of the neuron has a voltage of approximately −70 millivolts (mV), while the extracellular space is positively charged. The RMP is maintained by a process called the sodium–potassium pump. During this process, excessive sodium ions inside the cell are pumped out of the neuron as fast as they enter, and K+ ions that may have left the cell are brought back within.

The protein membrane of a neuron acts as a barrier to ions. Neurotransmitters open and close the ion channels as they cross the membrane. The electrical property of the membrane changes when the concentration of ions on the inside of the neuron changes. Normally, the membrane potential of a neuron rests at –70 mV, and the membrane is said to be polarized. The flow of ions in and out of the ion channels during neurotransmission will depolarize the neuron by making the inside of the neuron more positive. The depolarization occurs when channels in the cell membrane that regulate sodium ions open, allowing sodium ions to enter into the intracellular fluid. This causes the electrical charges within and outside the cell to briefly reverse, with the inside becoming positively charged relative to the extracellular fluid and going from −70 mV to around +30 mV, as shown in Figure 11.3.

Figure 11.3 Action potential

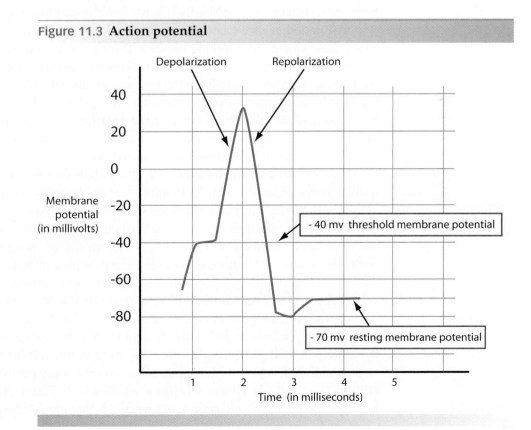

When depolarization reaches a threshold, a large electrical signal is generated. The depolarization affects only a tiny portion of the cell membrane and lasts for a very short time. Then potassium channels in the cell membrane are opened and potassium ions escape into the extracellular fluid. Consequently, the cell membrane once again reverts to the negatively charged state. This reverse process is called **repolarization**. As one portion of the cell membrane reverses its voltage and depolarizes, it causes the adjacent portion of the membrane to depolarize. As each portion of the axon is depolarized, it is followed by the repolarization. The wave of depolarization is called the **action potential (AP)**. When an AP occurs, the neuron is said to have "fired," and a nerve impulse is generated. The signal is then propagated along the axon until it reaches its axon terminals. The AP travels in only one direction, away from the cell body, and it travels in an all-or-none fashion. That is, a neuron either discharges completely or not at all. Once an AP begins, it travels with the same strength along the entire axon. If the threshold is not reached, there will not be an action potential. Not all inputs to the neuron are strong enough to reach the critical threshold necessary for depolarization. Typically, neurons receive electrical input from many other neurons, and these separate inputs are summed together. The addition of separate neural inputs can increase the strength of the stimulation and reach the membrane threshold. There are two types of summation of impulses: temporal and spatial. **Temporal summation** occurs when separate inputs reach the cell membrane with slight time differences. As long as the differences fall within some brief amount of time, they may add together. **Spatial summation** refers to the addition of impulses arriving at slightly different locations on the cell body or dendrites. Impulses arriving close together will combine and increase the strength of the resulting input. Once a nerve has fired, there is a brief period of time (about 0.5 msec) during which it cannot be stimulated, no matter how strong the incoming impulse. During this period, potassium ions flow into the neuron. This is called the **absolute refractory period**. After this brief interval, the neuron undergoes a **relative refractory period**, during which it can be stimulated but only by a stronger-than-usual stimulus. This whole cycle from RMP to AP and back again to RMP takes about 1 msec in most neurons. In other words, most neurons can fire around 1000 times per second (Seikel, Drumright, & Seikel, 2004).

Up to this point the discussion has focused primarily on the generation of an AP, how the cell body of a neuron communicates with its own terminals via the axon in a single nerve. However, in order to transmit information to and from the brain and spinal cord, nerves must communicate with each other. Neurotransmission (communication between neurons) is accomplished by the movement of chemicals or electrical signals across a synapse. A nerve signal travels along one nerve, finally reaching the terminal buttons of the axon. The vesicles within the buttons are stimulated to release their neurotransmitter into the synapse between the activated neuron (the presynaptic neuron) and the next neuron in line (the post synaptic neuron). The neurotransmitter can have one of two actions. It can lower the threshold of the post synaptic neuron and make it easier for it to fire, called an **excitatory postsynaptic potential (EPSP)**; or it can make it more difficult for the post synaptic neuron to fire by raising its threshold, called an **inhibitory post synaptic potential (IPSP)**. The neurotransmitter acts like a key to a lock (Figure 11.4). On the membrane of the post synaptic neuron are receptors that are selectively responsive to

Figure 11.4 Nerve synapse

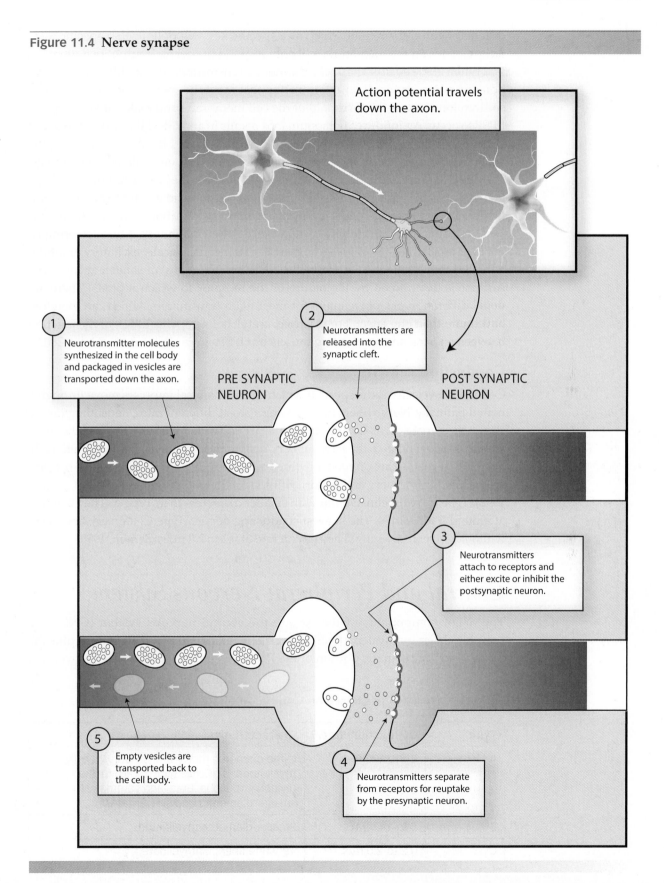

Action potential travels down the axon.

1. Neurotransmitter molecules synthesized in the cell body and packaged in vesicles are transported down the axon.

2. Neurotransmitters are released into the synaptic cleft.

PRE SYNAPTIC NEURON

POST SYNAPTIC NEURON

3. Neurotransmitters attach to receptors and either excite or inhibit the postsynaptic neuron.

5. Empty vesicles are transported back to the cell body.

4. Neurotransmitters separate from receptors for reuptake by the presynaptic neuron.

different neurotransmitters. Much as a specific key will only open a specific lock, receptor sites on the membrane will only respond to specific neurotransmitters.

When the key fits the lock, the neurotransmitter causes either sodium or potassium ion channels to open in the post synaptic membrane. An inflow of sodium ions lowers the threshold of the cell membrane and makes it easier for an EPSP to occur. An inflow of potassium ions results in an IPSP. If the critical threshold at the post synaptic neuron is reached, the nerve fires and the AP travels along the axon. In this manner neural information is transmitted among billions of nerve cells.

There are numerous different neurotransmitters in the NS, including acetylcholine, norepinephrine, serotonin, gamma-amino-butyric acid (GABA), glycerine, glutamic acid, dopamine, adenosine, nitric oxide, and even carbon monoxide (Hutchins et al., 2002). Neurotransmitters can be excitatory or inhibitory, either lowering or raising the cell threshold. However, there is nothing intrinsically excitatory or inhibitory about any neurotransmitter (Nolte, 2002). The effect of a transmitter at any given synapse is determined by the nature of the receptor to which it binds. There are many different types of receptors for most neurotransmitters, which can therefore have more than one effect. For example, acetylcholine causes EPSPs at the junction between an axon and a voluntary muscle but IPSPs in cardiac muscle (Nolte, 2002).

Conduction velocity

Conduction velocity is the speed at which electrochemical impulses move through a neural pathway. Nerve fibers transmit impulses at different rates, depending on the size of the nerve and its degree of myelinization. The larger the nerve, and the more heavily it is myelinated, the faster its conduction rate, and vice versa (see Table 11.3). On this basis nerves are divided into three categories. Type A nerves are large myelinated fibers, both sensory and motor, with conduction rates of up to 120 m/s (Zemlin, 1998). Type B are myelinated but with smaller diameters than Type A. They conduct at around 3 to 14 m/s. The slowest conducting nerves, Type C, are very fine fibers without a myelin covering. They have a rate of 0.2 to 2.0 m/s (Zemlin, 1998).

Central and Peripheral Nervous System

The major components of the NS are the central nervous system (CNS) and peripheral nervous system (PNS). The CNS is comprised of the brain itself plus the spinal cord. The somatic portion of the PNS, which controls voluntary movement

Table 11.3 **Nerve Types Based on Conduction Rates**

Type	Conduction Rate	Characteristics
A	Up to 120 m/s	Large diameter, motor and sensory, heavily myelinated, branches (collaterals) further divided into alpha, beta, and gamma with smaller diameters and slower rates
B	3 to 14 m/s	Smaller diameter, myelinated
C	0.2 to 2.0 m/s	Very fine fibers, unmyelinated

Figure 11.5 Schematic of central and peripheral nervous systems

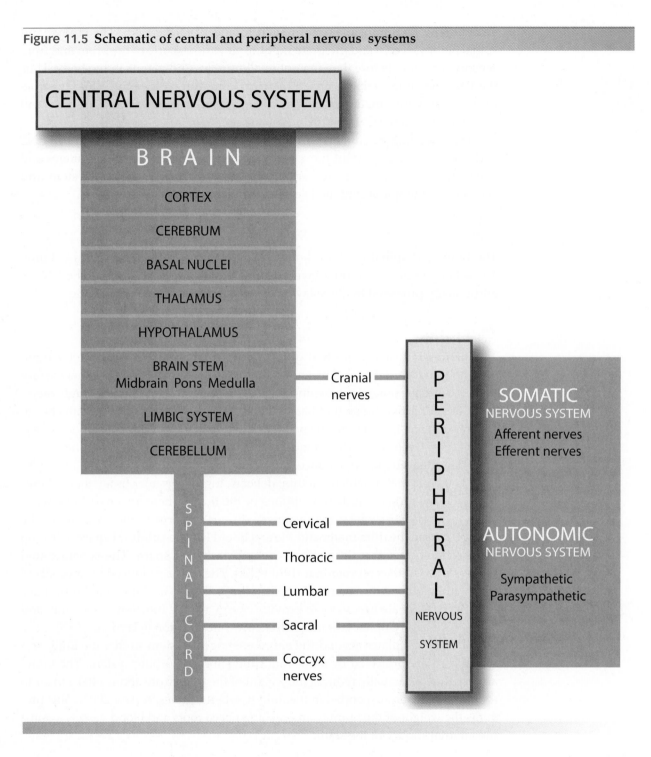

and sensory reception, is made up of 12 pairs of cranial and 31 pairs of spinal nerves (Figure 11.5). The CNS is involved in all aspects of information processing, including interpretation of all incoming sensations; integration of sensory information across modalities; planning, organization, and monitoring of goal-directed behavior, including motor behavior; and memory, language, and abstract functioning in general. The PNS transmits information to and from the CNS. The cranial and spinal nerves receive and integrate input from various parts of the brain and from sensory receptors before they fan out to all muscles and glands in the body. Thus the PNS constitutes what is called the **final common pathway** to all body structures. Sensory information from these structures travels by way of the spinal and cranial nerves to the CNS for further processing.

The following discussion will focus on the primary components of the CNS and PNS that are important for speech and hearing, including the meninges and ventricular system, the cortex and subcortical structures, the brain stem and cerebellum, the spinal cord, and selected cranial nerves.

Central Nervous System

The brain and spinal cord are housed within the skull and the spinal column. These bony structures form a layer of protection for nervous tissue. The CNS is additionally protected by three layers of non nervous tissue, the meninges.

Meninges

The **meninges** form a protective system of tissue and fluid surrounding the brain and the spinal cord. Figure 11.6 shows that immediately deep to the inner surface of the skull is the outermost meningeal layer, the **dura mater**. This is a tough, membranous connective tissue that has two parts, the periosteal layer that attaches to the cranium and the meningeal layer. The dura is well supplied with blood vessels and nerves. Deep to the dura mater is the **arachnoid mater**, so called because it has a delicate web like appearance. This layer has no blood vessels. The innermost layer is the **pia mater**, which is a thin, delicate, highly vascular tissue that adheres closely to the grooves and convolutions of the brain. There are areas in between each of these layers where the meninges do not conform to the contours of the brain. Between the dura mater and the arachnoid lies the **subdural space**; between the arachnoid and the pia mater is the **subarachnoid space**. The subarachnoid space is filled with **cerebrospinal fluid (CSF)**. The CSF is produced by specialized cells within four cavities (ventricles) of the brain. This clear fluid contains proteins and glucose that are necessary to provide energy for cell function in the brain and spinal cord and lymphocytes that help to prevent infection (Clayman, 1995).

The CSF circulates around the entire meningeal system so that the brain and spinal cord are protected by a buoyant fluid shock-absorbing system. The buoyancy of the CSF actually reduces the weight of the brain from about 1400 g in air to around 45 g when suspended in the fluid (Corbett, Haines, & Ard, 2002). This prevents the weight of the brain from crushing nerve roots and blood vessels against the internal surface of the skull.

Ventricles

Four ventricles, or cavities, are located within the brain: two lateral ventricles, one in each hemisphere, the third ventricle, and the fourth ventricle. The two lateral ventricles both connect to the third ventricle by way of the interventricular foramen, and the third and fourth ventricles are connected by the cerebral aqueduct (Figure 11.7).

Figure 11.6 **Meninges**

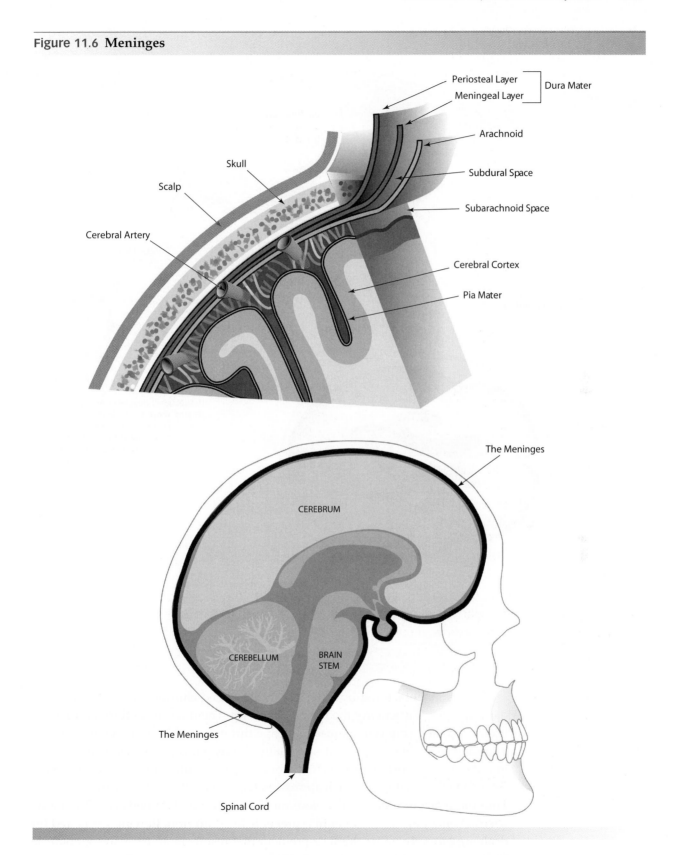

Figure 11.7 Ventricles

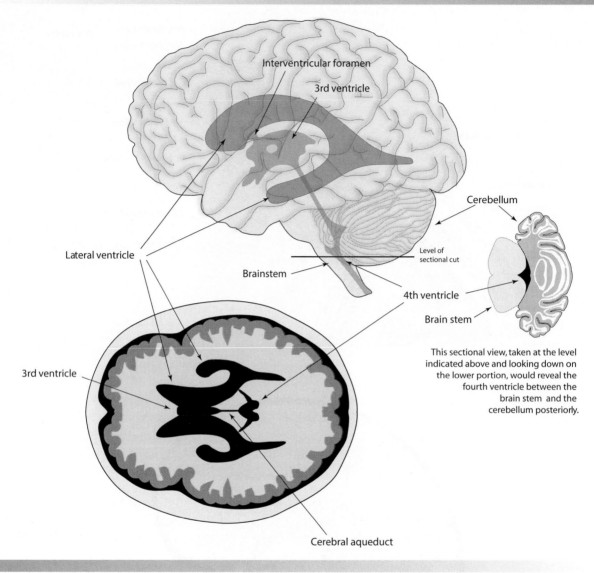

Interventricular foramen

3rd ventricle

Cerebellum

Lateral ventricle

Level of
sectional cut

Brainstem

4th ventricle

Brain stem

3rd ventricle

This sectional view, taken at the level
indicated above and looking down on
the lower portion, would reveal the
fourth ventricle between the
brain stem and the
cerebellum posteriorly.

Cerebral aqueduct

CSF is manufactured by specialized cells called **choroid plexus cells** within the ventricles, particularly the lateral ventricles. The fluid flows through the ventricles and their connecting areas to escape through median and lateral apertures into the subarachnoid space. It eventually drains out of the subarachnoid space into the venous portion of the circulatory system. Adults produce around 450 to 500 ml of CSF per day, of which approximately 330 to 380 ml drains into the veins. Thus the average volume of CSF is about 120 ml in adults (Corbett et al., 2002). Any obstruction within this system that prevents the fluid from flowing freely and/or draining properly or any kind of problem that results in an excessive amount of CSF can cause serious neurological problems.

Functional Brain Anatomy

The brain is divided into two hemispheres, right and left. The hemispheres are connected by means of nerve pathways and each hemisphere is divided into lobes. The outermost layer of the brain is made up of cortex, which is tissue formed by the cell bodies of neurons. The cortex is commonly known as "gray matter." The inner mass of the brain is the cerebrum and is primarily made of nerve axons bundled into pathways and covered with myelin. Because myelin is whitish in color, the inner mass is referred to as "white matter." Deep within the white matter of the brain are circumscribed areas of gray matter, known as the subcortex. These areas include the basal nuclei (also known as the basal ganglia), the thalamus, and the hypothalamus. Located immediately behind the cerebrum is the cerebellum, connected to the cerebrum by nerve pathways. Immediately under the cerebrum is the brain stem, consisting of the midbrain, the pons, and the medulla. The medulla is continuous with the spinal cord. Cranial nerves originate in the brain stem and extend to muscles and glands in the head and neck areas. Spinal nerves originate at different levels of the spinal cord and travel to all the muscles and glands in the rest of the body.

Cortex

The cortex is the outer covering of the brain, and it is extremely convoluted; that is, rather than being a flat, smooth surface, the cortex is irregular and bumpy. There are numerous folds on the cortex where the tissue forms raised surfaces called **gyri** (singular: gyrus), shallow depressions called **sulci** (singular: sulcus), and deeper grooves called fissures. The convolutions serve an important purpose by increasing the surface area of the cortex without increasing the space needed to house it. Certain of the sulci and fissures divide the brain into hemispheres and lobes. As shown in Figure 11.8, the **longitudinal cerebral fissure** divides the brain into two hemispheres. The **central sulcus** roughly separates the brain into anterior and posterior portions. The **lateral fissure** delineates the superior and inferior regions of the brain. The central sulcus and lateral fissure demarcate the brain into four major lobes: frontal, parietal, temporal, and occipital. These lobes are visible on the surface of the brain, but there is another lobe that cannot be seen because it lies deeper within the brain. The deeper lobe, called the insula, is located at the bottom of the lateral fissure but can only be seen when the fissure is opened. Some anatomists also include a sixth lobe, the limbic lobe, which is also not visible on the surface of the brain.

The cortex is composed of three to six layers of nerve cells and varies in thickness from about 1.5 to 4.5 mm (Zemlin, 1998). The nerve cell bodies that make up the cortex vary in their sizes and shapes. The most numerous neurons of the cortex are called pyramidal cells. They range in size from 10 microns (millionths of a mm) in size up to the 70- to 100-micron giant pyramidal cells, called Betz cells. Betz cells are located primarily in the motor cortex. Most of the cortex in the human brain (roughly 95%) is of a type known as **neocortex**. In evolutionary terms, this is the part of the brain that appeared late in human development, and it is greatly expanded compared to other primates. It is the neocortex where higher order and abstract processing occurs. This allows humans to talk, to plan and organize, and to use different types of symbolic functions, including those involved in language and mathematics.

Figure 11.8 Major cortical landmarks and lobes

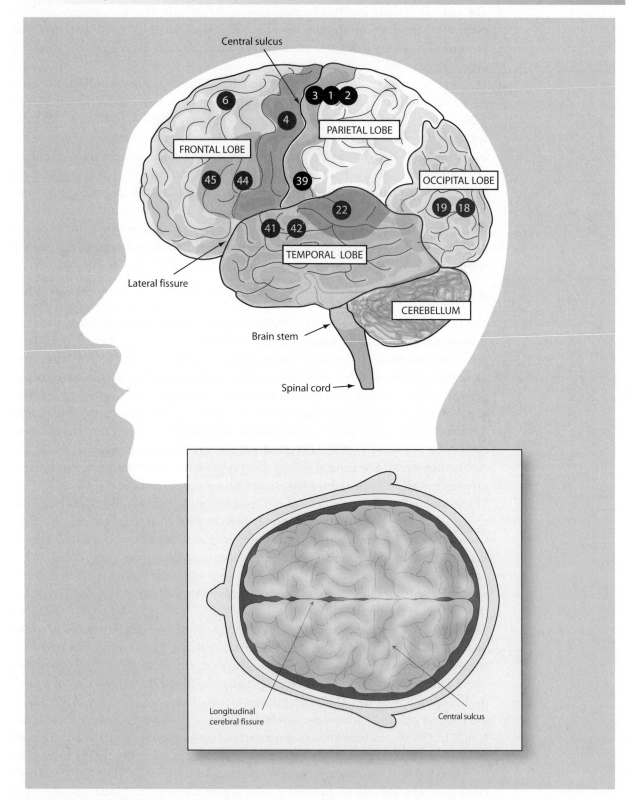

The two hemispheres of the cortex receive input from and provide output to many other regions in the NS, including subcortical structures. Different cortical areas also connect to each other by means of association fibers. Traditionally, the cortex is considered to be made up of primary sensory areas, primary motor areas, association areas, and limbic areas. Different areas of the cerebral cortex are associated with different functions, such as processing of incoming sensory information, planning and sequencing of motor activity, memory storage and retrieval, and emotional functioning.

Lobes of the Brain

The sulci and fissures separate the brain into lobes. Areas within each lobe have been associated with various functions. In 1914, Brodmann divided and numbered areas of the brain based on microscopic analyses of the structure and organization of the cells and tissues that comprise the cortex. Brodmann identified 52 functional areas of human cerebral cortex, and selected areas important for speech and hearing (see Figure 11.8). The numbering system that Brodmann devised is still in use today. Many of the areas that Brodmann identified have been correlated closely to diverse cortical functions using neuropsychological testing and functional brain imaging.

In discussing these areas, several caveats are important to keep in mind. First, these areas are not completely separated, and their boundaries are not precise. Second, the identified areas are not the only brain sites for a particular function. Most human behaviors are extremely complex, involving numerous brain areas that work together synergistically. Third, lobes in the left and right hemisphere are not mirror images of each other in either structure or function. In general, the left hemisphere performs functions that are more linear in nature, while the right hemisphere performs functions that are more holistic in nature. In most people, the left hemisphere is the one that is dominant for language processing, while the right is more involved in the emotional expression of language and intonational patterns of speech. Many years of clinical experience have shown that reasonably predictable deficits are associated with damage at specific cortical sites, so the Brodmann system is useful for diagnostic and clinical purposes (Nolte, 2002). Table 11.4 provides selected Brodmann's areas and numbers important for the understanding and expression of speech and language.

Frontal lobe

The frontal lobe makes up one-third of the cortex (Seikel et al., 2004) and is located anterior to the central sulcus and superior to the lateral sulcus. This is the part of the neocortex that contains areas devoted to language and speech, as well as abstract functions including reasoning, problem solving, personality, and symbolic function. Most motor activity is controlled by the frontal lobe, including primary motor cortex, or M1 (area 4), also known as the motor strip, premotor area (area 6), and supplementary motor area (area 6). Broca's area is located in the lateral portion of the inferior region of area 4 and is numbered areas 44 and 45. The primary motor cortex, M1, is situated on the precentral gyrus, immediately anterior to the central sulcus.

The motor strip is organized so that motor control of different body structures is located within specific portions of the tissue. In other words, rather than the entire motor strip participating in controlling movements of all muscles, specific

Table 11.4 Selected Brodmann's Areas Important for Speech and Hearing

Lobe	Brodmann's Number	Name(s) of Area
Frontal	4	Primary motor area, M1
	6	Premotor area and supplementary motor area
	44, 45	Broca's area (only in dominant hemisphere)
Parietal	3, 1, 2	Primary somatosensory area, S1
	5, 7	Somatosensory association area
	39	Angular gyrus
	40	Supramarginal gyrus
Occipital	17	Primary visual area, V1
	18, 19	Visual association area
Temporal	41	Primary auditory area, A1
	42	Auditory association area
	22	Wernicke's area

portions of the motor strip control specific muscles and structures. In addition, the organization of control occurs in a particular pattern. Starting at the top of the motor strip and progressing inferiorly toward the lateral fissure are portions of cortex responsible for movement of the hip, trunk (thorax and abdomen), arms, hands, neck, and face. Broca's area, numbers 44 and 45, is located at the most inferior portion of the motor strip and is responsible for sequencing and controlling the motor movements required for the production of speech. This organization of motor control according to body part is called **somatotopic organization**. However, the body structures are not represented equally in terms of the amount of cortical tissue devoted to their function. Those structures that require fine levels of motor control for skilled and precise movements have much greater representation on the motor strip than others. The differing amount of neural tissue allocated to motor control of different bodily structures is often represented in a caricature called the **homunculus** (Figure 11.9).

The homunculus shows that the hands and fingers have a much larger area devoted to their control than does the trunk. The structures involved in speech—that is, the larynx, velum, tongue, and lips—have disproportionately large areas dedicated to them, indicating the extremely fine motor control required for speech production. The premotor and supplementary motor areas are also somatotopically organized, although in a less precise fashion than the motor strip. The prefrontal cortex is located anterior to the primary motor and premotor areas and has been associated with intellectual traits such as judgment, foresight, a sense of purpose, a sense of responsibility, and a sense of social propriety (Lynch, 2002).

Figure 11.9 Motor and sensory homunculus

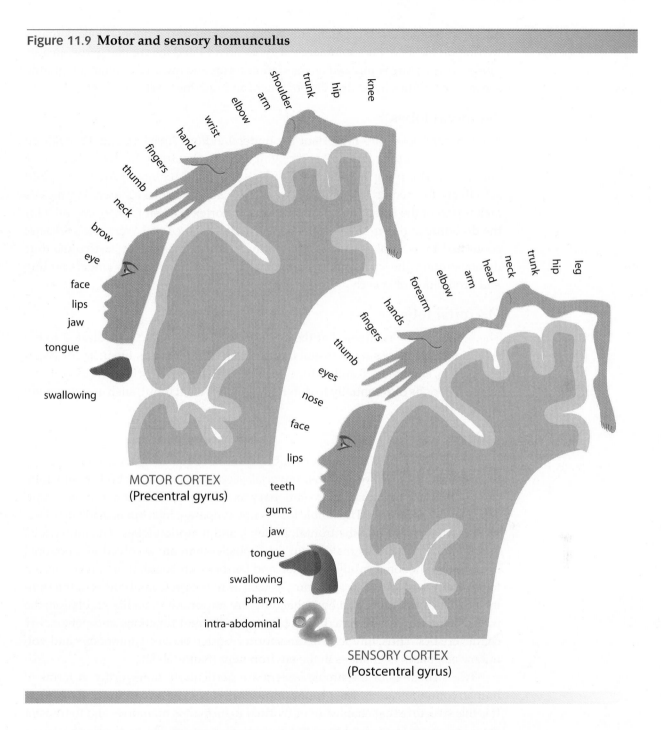

MOTOR CORTEX
(Precentral gyrus)

SENSORY CORTEX
(Postcentral gyrus)

Parietal Lobes

The parietal lobes are located on the postcentral gyrus, immediately posterior to the central sulcus. These lobes deal with bodily sensation including touch, pressure, pain, proprioception, and temperature. The primary somatosensory areas (S1) are 3, 1, and 2 and are represented somatotopically, similar to the motor cortex. These areas receive information from many nerve pathways and react to different types of sensory input (Nolte, 2002). For example, area 3a receives input from muscle receptors (Nolte, 2002). The bottom portion of the parietal lobe contains two important areas: the supramarginal gyrus, area 40, and the angular gyrus, area 39. These two areas are composed of association cortex and are important in integrating sensory modalities including vision, touch, and hearing (Webster, 1999).

Temporal lobes

The temporal lobes are important for understanding. Areas 41 and 42 make up the primary auditory cortex (A1) receiving information from the ear and auditory nerve. Area 41 is mapped tonotopically. That is, specific regions of Area 41 respond selectively to specific frequencies. Area 22 is called Wernicke's area. Wernicke's area is part of the receptive speech association cortex (Webster, 1999), essential for the decoding and comprehension of speech. Broca's area and Wernicke's area are connected by way of an association pathway called the arcuate fasciculus, thus demonstrating the close neuroanatomical relationship between understanding and production of speech.

Occipital lobe

The occipital lobe is situated at the posterior of the brain and is dedicated to the reception and processing of visual information. Area 17 forms the primary visual cortex (V1), and areas 18 and 19 form the visual association cortex. The association cortex responds differentially to different types of visual input, such as movement, color, and shape.

Limbic lobe

The limbic lobe is part of a larger **limbic system**, comprising several brain structures including the hippocampus, amygdala, septal, mammillary bodies, and anterior nuclei of the thalamus. In evolutionary terms the limbic system is more primitive than the neocortex. The limbic lobe is not a separate lobe but is made up of the most medial margins of the frontal, parietal, and temporal lobes. The limbic lobe and the other structures making up the limbic system are involved in emotional and sexual function, feeding behavior, and temperature regulation. It is connected to the brain stem and hypothalamus, as well as to the prefrontal cortex of the frontal lobe. The brain stem and hypothalamus are important in bodily regulation; the prefrontal cortex is associated with higher intellectual functions and personality characteristics. Thus, limbic structures form a bridge between autonomic and voluntary responses to changes in the environment (Nolte, 2002).

Two structures of the limbic system are particularly noteworthy in terms of human communication. The **hippocampus** is involved with learning and memory. It is this structure that enables an individual to form new memories and to transfer these memories from short-term to longer-term memory. This is clearly crucial for communication, in which the person must remember what has been said in order to continue the conversation in an appropriate manner. The **amygdala** is involved in ascribing emotion to events and behaviors. This structure also participates in memory building, in the sense that it facilitates decisions about which facts and events are important enough to be committed to long-term memory. To illustrate, if one meets a friend and chats about this and that, one is not likely to remember for very long the specific details of the conversation. However, if the friend reveals a shocking or exciting piece of news, information that generates emotion, that is much more likely to be remembered.

Cortical Connections

The cortex is the prime information processor of the NS. The pathways of the NS are involved in facilitating the flow of information between different areas. Some pathways deliver information from sensory receptors to the NS and are called afferent or sensory pathways. Others, the efferent or motor pathways, transport impulses from the NS to the muscles and glands of the body. Many nerve fibers interconnect various regions of the NS to each other. There are three main types of interconnecting pathways: commissural, association, and projection.

Commissural fibers

Commissural fibers link two corresponding areas in the right and left hemispheres. The major commissural pathway is the **corpus callosum**, a thick band of white matter that extensively connects the right and left hemispheres. This pathway has a fanlike structure, with fibers radiating between many areas of the two hemispheres, and is the means by which each hemisphere is constantly updated as to the moment-by-moment functioning of the other. Fibers of the corpus callosum are found in the medial parts of the brain and are arranged longitudinally, so that the pathway runs from anterior to posterior regions of the brain. This pathway is sometimes cut in individuals with severe epilepsy. Interestingly, in such cases, the individual can function normally, but literally, the right hemisphere does not know what the left is doing, and vice versa. There are other smaller commissures that link the two hemispheres including the anterior, middle, and posterior commissures, but the corpus callosum is by far the largest and most important.

Association fibers

Association fibers can connect different cortical regions within the same hemisphere or link adjacent areas of cortex. Fibers that connect different cortical regions are longer than those connecting adjacent areas. The pathways formed by the long fibers are called **fasciculi** (singular: fasciculus). Some important pathways include the superior longitudinal fasciculus, which links the four major lobes, and the arcuate fasciculus, which connects parts of the frontal, parietal, and temporal lobes to each other.

Projection fibers

Recall that projection fibers, particularly Golgi Type I fibers, have long axons that extend to relatively distant neural structures and to the spinal cord. Two major bundles of nerve fibers, the **internal capsule** and the **corona radiata**, form the primary links between the cortex and other regions of the CNS. The internal capsule is formed by a large mass of myelinated fibers that runs mainly between the thalamus and the cerebral cortex. The internal capsule forms the main pathway by which most nerve impulses are transmitted to and from the cerebral cortex. The fibers traveling from the cortex to the thalamus are called corticothalamic; those projecting from the thalamus to the cortex are thalamocortical. Some pathways making up the internal capsule also transmit neural information from the cortex to the brain stem (corticonuclear or corticobulbar fibers) and from the cortex to the spinal cord (corticospinal fibers). The corticonuclear and corticospinal motor pathways will be discussed in more detail in a later section.

As the fibers of the internal capsule travel from the basal nuclei, thalamus, brain stem, and spinal cord toward the cerebral cortex, they diverge and flare out in a fan-shaped manner, reaching many areas within the cerebrum and cerebral cortex and joining with other pathways that interconnect different cortical areas. This fan-shaped area is referred to as the corona radiata.

Subcortical Areas of the Brain

As noted above, the cortex is composed of gray matter and is involved in information processing. The main mass of the brain, the cerebrum, is made up of white matter, the mostly myelinated nerve fibers that are involved in the transmission of information. Deep within the cerebrum are several circumscribed areas of gray matter: the basal nuclei, the thalamus, and the hypothalamus. These collections of nerve cell bodies are important in the control and regulation of movement, including movement for speech production (see Figures 11.10–11.12 and Tables 11.5 and 11.6).

Basal Nuclei

The basal nuclei, also called basal ganglia, comprise several areas of gray matter in each hemisphere. These areas are adjacent to each other and include the **caudate nucleus**, the **globus pallidus**, the **putamen**, and the **substantia nigra**. The nuclei are often grouped in different ways; thus, the putamen and globus pallidus together are known as the lenticular nucleus, while the caudate and putamen together form the **striatum**.

The basal nuclei connect with many other structures and pathways, receiving input from the motor and other areas of the cortex and the thalamus, as well as making connections with each other and other nuclei. The pathways to, from, and among the components of the basal nuclei form a series of complex circuits between the cerebral cortex, basal nuclei, and thalamus. One of the major circuits is the motor circuit. Fibers from the primary motor area, premotor area, and supplementary motor area project to the striatum (corticostriatal fibers), which also receives input from somatosensory cortex, substantia nigra, limbic lobe, hippocampus, and amygdala (Ma, 2002; Nolte, 2002). The striatum thus forms the major receiving center of the basal nuclei. Projections from the basal nuclei leave from the globus pallidus and substantia nigra and travel to the thalamus. From the thalamus, nerve fibers project back to the cerebral cortex via the internal capsule and corona radiata, completing the circuit. Because of these interconnections, the basal nuclei are constantly informed about most aspects of cortical function.

One of the primary functions of the basal nuclei is regulating aspects of motor control such as posture, balance, background muscle tone, and coordination of muscle groups. The basal nuclei are also critically important in the indirect control of precise voluntary movements through a neural mechanism called inhibition. Recall

Figure 11.10 Sagittal view of selected brain structures

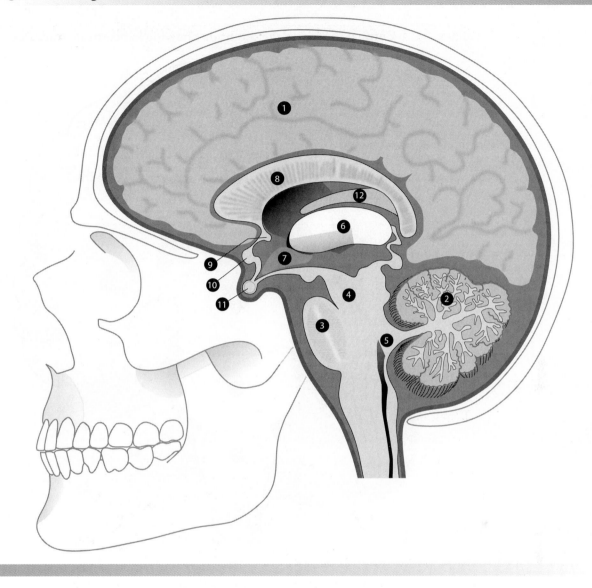

Table 11.5 Selected Brain Structures Seen in a Sagittal Section

1	Cerebrum
2	Cerebellum
3	Pons
4	Midbrain
5	Fourth ventricle
6	Thalamus
7	Hypothalamus
8	Corpus callosum
9	Anterior commissure
10	Optic chiasm
11	Pituitary gland
12	Fornix

Figure 11.11 Coronal section of the cerebrum showing subcortical structures

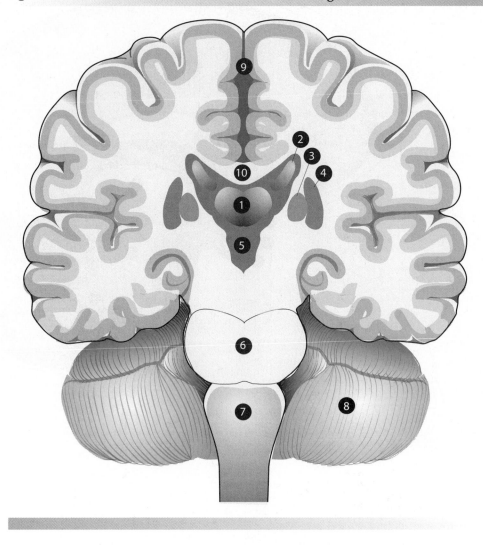

Table 11.6 Selected Brain Structures, Including Basal Nuclei

1	Thalamus
2	Caudate nucleus
3	Globus pallidus
4	Putamen
5	Third ventricle
6	Pons
7	Medulla
8	Cerebellum
9	Central sulcus
10	Corpus callosum

Figure 11.12 Subcortical structures including basal nuclei

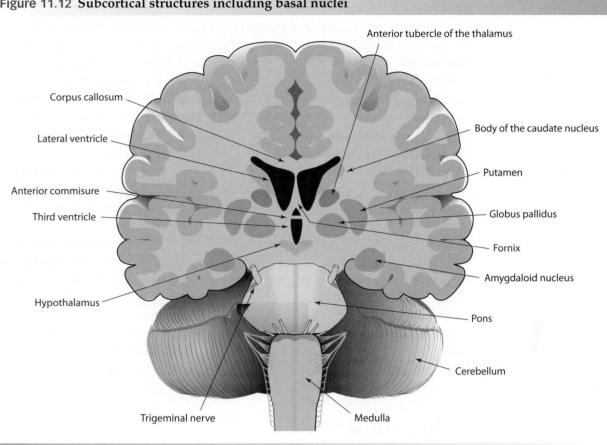

that a post synaptic neuron can undergo an excitatory or an inhibitory post synaptic potential (EPSP or IPSP). With an IPSP, the neuron membrane is hyperpolarized, making it more difficult for an action potential to be triggered. One of the neurotransmitters in the basal nuclei is dopamine, which has an inhibitory effect. Thus, the outflow from the basal nuclei to the thalamus and back to the motor cortex is inhibitory, which serves to refine and smooth the initial neuromuscular output from the cortex. Due to this inhibitory feedback system, damage to the basal nuclei typically results in excessive involuntary movements such as tics and tremors, increased muscle tone and rigidity, and other disruptions of movement control. Parkinson's disease is an example of this kind of disinhibition, in which the patient suffers from rigidity and tremors resulting from destruction or damage to the substantia nigra and/or the pathways between the substantia nigra and striatum (nigrostriatal fibers).

Thalamus

The thalamus comprises a collection of nuclei, some of which are involved with motor function and some with sensory function. Thalamic nuclei that receive and transmit nerve impulses to and from specific cortical areas are known as relay nuclei. Other nuclei, called **association nuclei**, receive and transmit to broader cortical areas.

The thalamus is sometimes called the "gateway to consciousness" because all information traveling to the cerebral cortex, aside from olfaction, passes through the thalamus. The thalamus sorts and interprets neural information and "decides" which signals should be transmitted to the cerebral cortex. The thalamus can be likened to a relay station that collects inputs from many different locations and structures and relays them to many other locations and structures. The nuclei of the thalamus send information to and receive information from the cerebral cortex via the pathways of the internal capsule. The nuclei of the thalamus participate in motor, sensory, and limbic functions. Each nucleus projects to a different part of the cerebral cortex (thalamocortical fibers), and that portion of the cortex reciprocally projects to the originating thalamic nucleus (corticothalamic fibers).

The thalamic nuclei that are most important for speech and hearing are relay nuclei, including the **ventral anterior nuclei (VA)**, **ventral lateral nuclei (VL)**, **medial geniculate body**, and **lateral geniculate body**. The VA and VL nuclei receive input from the basal nuclei and cerebellum and project to the motor areas of the cerebral cortex. These two nuclei are directly involved in motor function. The medial geniculate body processes auditory information and relays it to the auditory cortex in the temporal lobe. The lateral geniculate body processes visual information and transmits it to the visual cortex in the occipital lobe.

Hypothalamus

The hypothalamus is another subcortical gray matter structure, containing nuclei that are involved in sensory and motor control of visceral functions. The hypothalamus, like the thalamus, is also strongly linked to the limbic system. In addition, the hypothalamus regulates hormonal function, body temperature, hunger, sleep–wake cycles, sexual drive, blood pressure, and other functions designed to keep the body's internal environment in a state of equilibrium (homeostasis). The hypothalamus connects with the limbic system, pituitary gland, and brain stem, allowing widespread control of the visceral and emotional behavior that influence how individuals react to the internal and external environments (Hardy, Chronister, & Parent, 2002). However, hypothalamic functioning is not under conscious control.

Brain Stem

The brain stem is a collective term for three separate but tightly linked structures: the midbrain, the pons, and the medulla. The brain stem is crucially important, as it is the site of many reflexes involved in respiration, body temperature, swallowing, and digestion. It is also the site of origin of the cranial nerves. As shown in Figure 11.13, the topmost portion, the midbrain, is located directly underneath the cerebrum. The

Figure 11.13 Brain stem

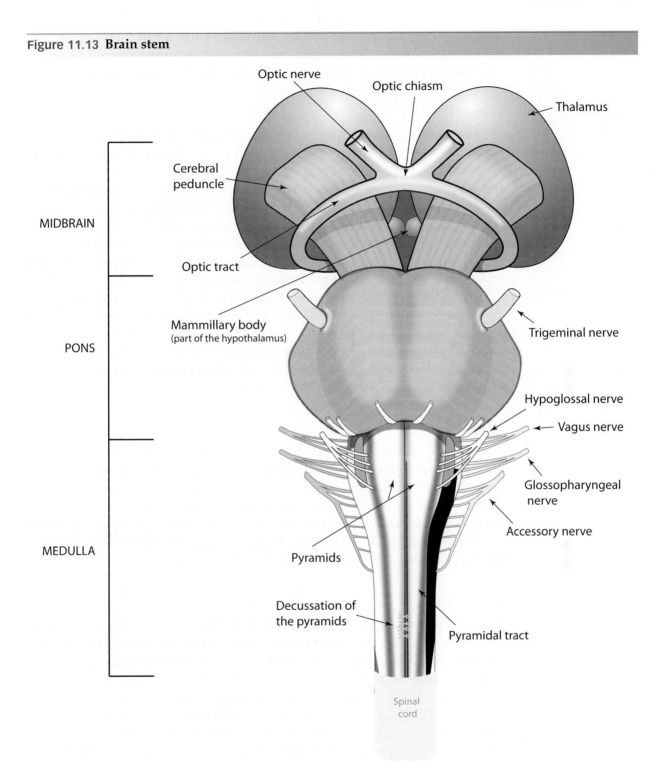

MIDBRAIN

PONS

MEDULLA

Optic nerve

Optic chiasm

Thalamus

Cerebral peduncle

Optic tract

Mammillary body
(part of the hypothalamus)

Trigeminal nerve

Hypoglossal nerve

Vagus nerve

Glossopharyngeal nerve

Accessory nerve

Pyramids

Decussation of the pyramids

Pyramidal tract

Spinal cord

lowermost part, the medulla, connects with the spinal cord. The pons forms a bridge not only between the midbrain and medulla, but also to the cerebellum.

At the core of the brain stem is the **reticular formation**, a loose and diffuse network of nuclei controlling complex patterns of movement involved in breathing, cardiac function, and swallowing. The **reticular activating system** is part of the network, and the nuclei forming this portion of the brain stem control state of alertness and level of consciousness. Damage to the reticular activating system can result in a coma.

Midbrain

The midbrain is a short structure consisting of the two cerebral peduncles and the superior and inferior colliculi (singular: colliculus). The **cerebral peduncles** are continuations of the internal capsule. They are large bundles of nerve pathways including corticospinal, corticonuclear (corticobulbar), and corticopontine fibers traveling via the cerebrum and midbrain to their respective targets. The paired **inferior colliculi** are masses of gray matter that are linked to different parts of the auditory system and that ultimately project to the medial geniculate nucleus of the thalamus. The inferior colliculi also project fibers to the **superior colliculi**, which are involved in visual processing, as well as to the cerebellum and spinal cord. These numerous connections facilitate the integration of information from various areas within the nervous system and play an important role in higher level reflexes such as turning one's eyes to the source of a sound and startle responses to unexpected noises. The cerebral aqueduct, linking the third and fourth ventricles, is located within the midbrain. The midbrain is the point of origin for two cranial nerves: CN III (oculomotor) and IV (trochlear).

Pons

The pons is located inferior to the midbrain and anterior to the cerebellum. *Pons* in Latin means bridge, and this portion of the brain stem includes nerve pathways (superior and middle cerebellar peduncles) that act as a bridge between the cerebellum and the rest of the nervous system. In addition, there are nuclei within the pons that process information arriving from the cerebrum on its way to the cerebellum. Four of the cranial nerves originate at the pontine level: CN V (trigeminal), VI (abducent), VII (facial), and VIII (vestibulocochlear).

Medulla

The medulla is the most inferior portion of the brain stem, continuous with the pons above and the spinal cord below. The medulla is around 2.5 cm long and about 1 cm in diameter (Seikel et al., 2004). It is an important structure, because this is where a large percentage of nerve fibers (80 to 90%) originating at the cerebral cortex cross over (decussate) and continue down the opposite (contralateral) side of the body. Thus, it is the left hemisphere of the brain that controls motor function on the right side of the body, and vice versa. The decussation occurs at a site on the medulla called the pyramids. These are two pyramid-shaped ridges running from the pons to the inferior border of the medulla. Most of the fibers that form the pyramids arise in the motor cortex as corticospinal fibers (Haines & Mihailoff, 2002). Cranial nerve nuclei in the medulla include CN IX (glossopharyngeal), X (vagus), XI (spinal accessory), and XII (hypoglossal). The medulla also connects to the cerebellum by way of the inferior cerebellar peduncles. The medulla mediates many reflexes such as coughing, sneezing, and vomiting.

Cerebellum

The cerebellum is located posterior to the brain stem and inferior to the cerebrum (see Figures 11.10, 11.11, and 11.12). It connects to the brain stem by way of the inferior, middle, and superior **cerebellar peduncles**. The cerebellum is a relatively large structure, accounting for around 10 percent of the weight of the entire CNS. The cerebellum has some interesting similarities to the cerebrum. Like the cerebrum, it is composed of a mass of white matter overlaid by an outer cortex. Also like the cerebrum, deep within the cerebellar white matter are concentrations of subcortical cell bodies. Similar to the cerebral cortex, the cerebellum has two hemispheres that are connected by a thick nerve fiber bundle. In addition, the cerebellum is divided into lobes. However, unlike the cerebral cortex, which exerts contralateral control of movement, the cerebellum works ipsilaterally.

The cerebellar cortex has a different appearance to that of the cerebral cortex. While the cerebral cortex is highly convoluted, the cerebellar cortex is more regular in appearance, with a surface that looks almost like segments of a peeled orange. This characteristic appearance is created by deep straight grooves on the cortex, with smaller indentations within the deeper fissures that result in a series of ridges on the surface called folia (Nolte, 2002). The inner mass of the cerebellum is composed of white matter that is sometimes called "arbor vitae" (tree of life) due to its branching pattern. The nerve pathways that make up this inner mass contain fibers projecting to and from the cerebellar cortex. Deep within the inner mass are four clusters of deep nuclei. These nuclei receive input from and project back to specific portions of the cerebellar cortex, and project as well to the brain stem and thalamus via the cerebellar peduncles.

The parts of the cerebellum can be identified in an anterior–posterior direction as well as a medial–lateral direction. In terms of anterior–posterior, the cerebellum has three lobes: a small anterior lobe, a large posterior lobe, and a very small inferior lobe called the **flocculonodular lobe**. In the medial–lateral direction there are likewise three sections: the midline section called the **vermis** that connects the cerebellar hemispheres and the lateral structures on either side.

The cerebellum receives and sends information from and to many sources. It receives sensory information via the inferior and middle cerebellar peduncles, including proprioceptive and vestibular (balance) information from spinal and vestibular pathways. It also sends motor information from the deep nuclei to the cerebral cortex, traveling via the superior cerebellar peduncles to the thalamus and ending at the motor areas of the cerebral cortex. The cerebellum is richly interconnected with the cortex and spinal cord. Current thinking is that the lateral cerebellum, which receives input from the premotor and association cortical areas, acts to preprogram a movement, whereas the vermis acts to update an evolving movement via its input from the sensorimotor cortical and spinal inputs (Kent, 1997b; Nolte, 2002).

From the above discussion, it is clear that the cerebral cortex, subcortical areas, and cerebellum are linked, allowing for information sharing that is vital to motor function. The cerebellum is involved in balance, posture, background muscle tone, and the coordination of voluntary movements. With its extensive connections to other motor centers as well as its extensive sensory input, it is well suited to its central role in motor control and coordination. The cerebellum coordinates movements in terms of the direction of the movement, the force and speed with which the movement is executed, and the amount of displacement of the structure that is moving. It also ensures that complex movements are carried out with appropriate timing so that smooth synergistic muscular patterns are maintained. As an example, think of the coordination that is involved in a simple task such as picking up a pen from a table. You first have to move your entire arm toward the pen, which also involves the correct degree and displacement of shoulder, upper arm, and forearm movement. As your arm approaches the pen, your fingers must start to close. The force and speed of the arm and finger movements must be precisely regulated: Too much or too little force and speed will result in overshooting or undershooting the target. Similarly, the direction of your arm and fingers must be correct in order to reach the pen. As your fingers close around the pen, their muscular force must be finely graded in order to successfully complete the task. Individuals with cerebellar damage lack this fine coordination, and their movements tend to be jerky due to problems in their timing, force, direction, and speed. Another problem often seen in such an individual is that movements take longer to begin, and the person cannot easily stop the movement or change it once it has been initiated. One way in which the cerebellum performs this precise coordination is by comparing a person's intended movement with the actual neuromuscular command issued by the motor areas of the cerebral cortex and correcting any errors or differences that are detected. The comparison is performed in terms of the status of the muscles (e.g., tension, length, force) involved in the movement, proprioceptive information about the position of relevant structures, and information arriving from the spinal cord, from the basal nuclei, from the vestibular system, and from the cerebral cortex. Thus the cerebellum continuously monitors both sensory and motor information, allowing constant updating of movement patterns and carrying out movements in a smoothly coordinated fashion. The cerebellum, particularly the vermis, also regulates posture as well as patterns of movements such as those involved in walking.

Spinal Cord

The spinal cord is the downward continuation of the brain stem and contains the cell bodies for the 31 pairs of spinal nerves that run to all the muscles of the body, aside from those of the head and neck. The spinal cord is one continuous structure, but it is divided into several sections: cervical (neck), thoracic (chest), lumbar (lower back), sacral (pelvis), and coccygeal (tail bone) (Figure 11.14). Each section serves a specific area of the body, as shown in Table 11.7.

Table 11.7 **Regions of the Spinal Cord and Areas Served by Each Region**

Region	Areas Served
Cervical (C1–C8)	Back of head, neck, shoulders, diaphragm, arms, hands
Thoracic (T1–T12)	Ribs, back, abdomen
Lumbar (L1–L5)	Lower back, thighs, legs
Sacral (S1–S5)	Thighs, buttocks, legs, feet
Coccygeal (Co1)	Thighs, buttocks, legs, feet

Figure 11.14 Spinal cord

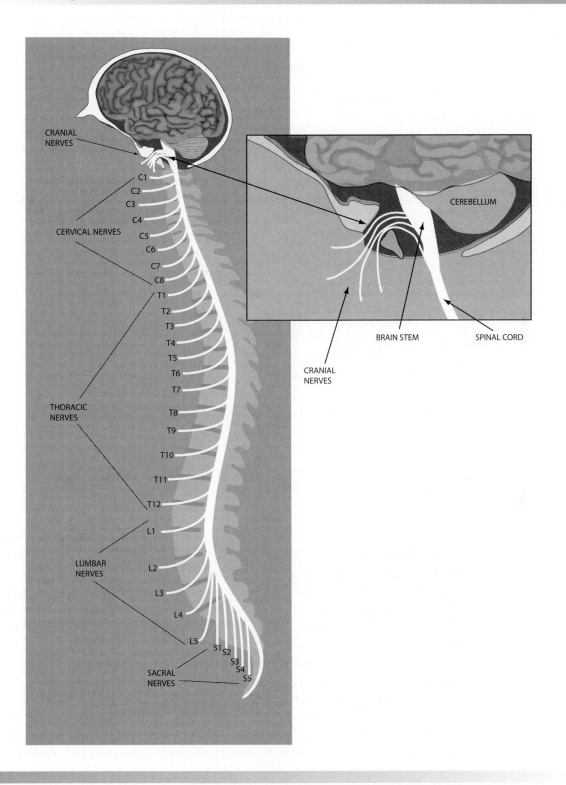

CRANIAL
NERVES

C1
C2
C3
C4
C5
C6
C7
C8

CERVICAL NERVES

T1
T2
T3
T4
T5
T6
T7
T8
T9
T10
T11
T12

THORACIC
NERVES

L1
L2
L3
L4
L5

LUMBAR
NERVES

S1 S2
S3
S4
S5

SACRAL
NERVES

CEREBELLUM

CRANIAL
NERVES

BRAIN STEM

SPINAL CORD

Figure 11.15 Section through the spinal cord

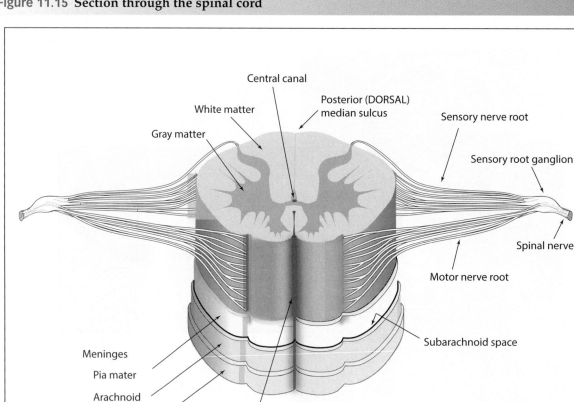

In an adult, the cord is about 42 to 45 cm long and about 1 cm in diameter at its widest point (Nolte, 2002). The spinal cord, like the brain, is enveloped by the meninges, which form a complete protective sheath around the entire CNS (Figure 11.15). Recall that the dura mater is the outermost layer of the meninges. In the spinal column this layer is separated from the vertebrae by the epidural space. The innermost layer, the pia mater, closely follows the spinal cord itself. The subarachnoid space contains cerebrospinal fluid. The spinal cord is also protected by the vertebral column, within which it is situated (Figure 11.16).

Like the brain, the spinal cord is made up of areas of gray and white matter. In the brain the gray matter forms the outer covering and the white matter is located within. This pattern is reversed in the spinal cord, with the white matter on the outside and the gray matter contained within. The shape of the gray matter is often likened to a butterfly with its wings spread. These "wings" actually comprise two sets of horns: The dorsal, or posterior, horns are made up of nerve cell bodies that receive sensory information from all areas of the body, and the ventral, or anterior, horns contain the cell bodies that project fibers to skeletal muscles.

Figure 11.16 Vertebral column and spinal cord

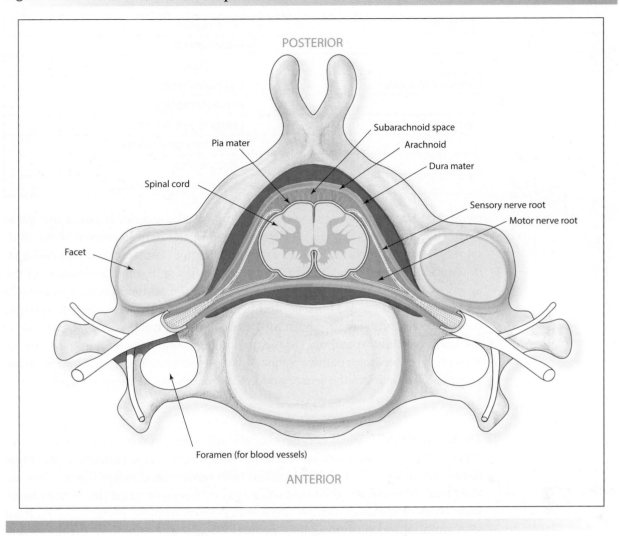

POSTERIOR

Pia mater

Spinal cord

Facet

Subarachnoid space

Arachnoid

Dura mater

Sensory nerve root

Motor nerve root

Foramen (for blood vessels)

ANTERIOR

At some levels of the spinal cord, there are also lateral horns that are involved in visceral functions. The regions where the anterior and posterior horns meet are called the **intermediate zone**. The white matter surrounding the inner core of gray matter is made up of myelinated sensory and motor pathways bundled into large tracts called **funiculi** (singular: funiculus). There are four funiculi: one dorsal, one ventral, and two lateral. All the pathways, both sensory and motor, are situated within the funiculi. Major sensory pathways in the spinal cord include the **spinothalamic tract** and the **spinocerebellar tract**. These pathways transmit information about pain, temperature, touch, and proprioception to the thalamus, cerebral cortex, and cerebellum. The major motor tracts include the **lateral corticospinal tract** (also known as the pyramidal tract), the **anterior corticospinal tract**, the **rubrospinal tract**, and the **lateral vestibulospinal tract**. The lateral corticospinal tract originates primarily in the sensorimotor areas of the cerebral cortex. Most of the descending fibers decussate at the pyramids of the medulla (hence the name

Table 11.8 **Selected Funiculi and Pathways of the Spinal Cord**

Funiculi	One dorsal
	One ventral
	Two lateral
Sensory pathways	Spinothalamic
	Spinocerebellar
Motor pathways	Lateral corticospinal
	Anterior corticospinal
	Rubrospinal
	Lateral vestibulospinal

pyramidal tract) and synapse with the neurons in the anterior horns of the spinal cord. The anterior corticospinal tract is formed by the 10 to 15 percent of descending fibers from the cortical motor areas that do not decussate, but that continue downward on the ipsilateral side to synapse with spinal motor neurons in the anterior horn. The rubrospinal tract originates in the midbrain from a nucleus of cell bodies called the red nucleus, and fibers from each side cross over to synapse contralaterally with anterior horn motor neurons. The cell bodies that give rise to the lateral vestibulospinal tract are located in the vestibular nuclei in the medulla. As with the other motor pathways, fibers synapse with anterior horn motor neurons. Table 11.8 summarizes the sensory and motor pathways of the spinal cord.

Spinal Nerves

Thirty-one pairs of spinal nerves enter and exit the spinal cord by way of spaces called intervertebral foramina located between successive vertebrae. All spinal nerves are mixed—that is, they contain both sensory and motor fibers. They are classified on the basis of their origin (for sensory fibers) or target (for motor fibers). Four types of spinal nerves are identified: general somatic afferents (GSA) from skin surfaces and proprioceptors; general visceral afferents (GVA) from viscera including digestive tract, respiratory system, etc.; general somatic efferents (GSE) to skeletal muscles; and general visceral efferents (GVE) to viscera including glands, smooth muscles, heart, and so on. Refer to Table 11.9.

Each spinal nerve has both a sensory and a motor branch. The sensory branch exits the spinal cord via the posterior horn, and the motor branch enters the cord via the anterior horn. The two branches converge outside the spinal cord to form the spinal nerve (see Figures 11.15 and 11.16).

Table 11.9 **Types of Spinal Nerves, Origins, and Destinations**

Type	Motor/sensory	Origin/destination
GSA	Sensory	Skin, proprioceptors
GVA	Sensory	Digestive tract, respiratory system
GSE	Motor	Skeletal muscles
GVE	Motor	Glands, smooth muscles, heart

The spinal cord functions to institute reflexes. A reflex is an involuntary, stereotyped motor response to a sensory input. Reflexes may be relatively simple and confined to a single cord level (intrasegmental), or complex, involving multiple cord segments (intersegmental) (Haines, Mihailoff, & Yezierski, 2002). A common example of a simple reflex is the knee jerk, or patellar reflex. When the knee tendon is tapped, the front thigh muscle is slightly lengthened. This sensory information travels to the spinal cord via the posterior horn and stimulates the motor portion of the nerve, which in turn causes the involuntary kicking response. Another example is when one puts one's hand too close to a heat source and reflexively pulls it away very rapidly. In this case, the sensory input is the heat. The sensory information travels to the spinal cord and stimulates the motor portion of the nerve to contract the relevant muscles (Figure 11.17). Information is also carried to the thalamus and

Figure 11.17 Spinal reflex

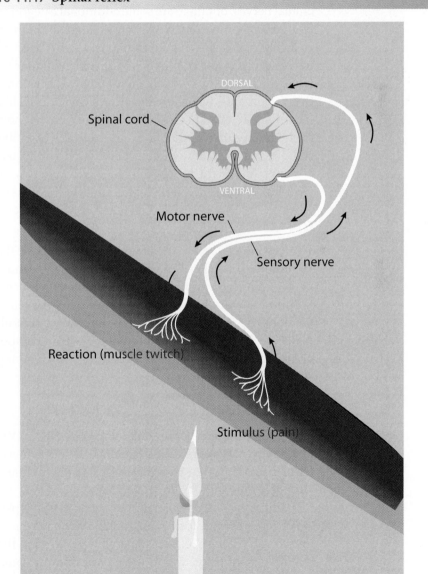

on to the cerebral cortex, so that the individual becomes aware of his or her motor response a split second after it has occurred.

Cranial Nerves

The 12 pairs of cranial nerves transmit information to and from the face and neck regions. The cranial nerves are numbered with roman numerals from I to XII. These nerves are crucial for speech and hearing. Most of the cell bodies of the cranial nerves (III to XII) arise from the brain stem, and the axons project to muscles in the face, head, and ears. The nerves are numbered according to their order of emergence from the brain stem. Thus CN III emerges at the most superior point in the brain stem, and CN XII emerges at the most inferior point (Figure 11.18).

The classification used for spinal nerves (GSA, GVA, GSE, GVE) applies also to cranial nerves, but there are some additional categories in the case of cranial nerves: Special somatic afferent (SSA) nerves transmit information from the "special" senses including hearing, equilibrium, vision, and taste. Special visceral efferent (SVE) nerves carry motor commands to specific voluntary muscles such as those of the face, which develop from an embryological structure called the branchial arch. For this reason, SVE fibers are sometimes called branchial motor fibers. While spinal nerves are all mixed (sensory and motor), cranial nerves can be more specialized, containing primarily GSE fibers or primarily SSA fibers, or they can carry a more complex combination of fibers. Discussion will focus on those cranial nerves that are most important for speech and hearing: CN V (trigeminal), VII (facial), VIII (vestibulocochlear), IX (glossopharyngeal), X (vagus), and XII (hypoglossal).

CN V: Trigeminal

The trigeminal nerve is made up of three branches, the ophthalmic, maxillary, and mandibular branches (Figure 11.19). Both GSA and SVE fibers are found in the nerve. GSA fibers transmit information about touch, pressure, pain, proprioception, and temperature from various areas of the face—the maxillary branch from the upper lip, teeth, and upper jaw; and the mandibular branch from the lower lip and teeth, lower jaw, and oral cavity. The SVE component innervates the muscles of mastication, the tensor veli palatini, the tensor tympani, and some of the extrinsic laryngeal muscles.

CN VII: Facial

CN VII is a complex nerve containing GSA, SVA, GVE, and SVE fibers. The largest component consists of the SVE fibers that supply nerve impulses to the muscles of facial expression, the stapedius muscle in the middle ear, and some of the extrinsic laryngeal muscles (Figure 11.20).

Unlike the other cranial nerves, which receive ipsilateral innervation, the facial nerve receives both ipsilateral and contralateral innervation. Innervation to facial muscles above the eyes is ipsilateral, with axons in the originating motor nuclei in the brain stem projecting to the muscles on the same side. However, projections from the motor neurons to the facial muscles below the eyes are contralateral. This

Figure 11.18 Brain stem origins of the cranial nerves

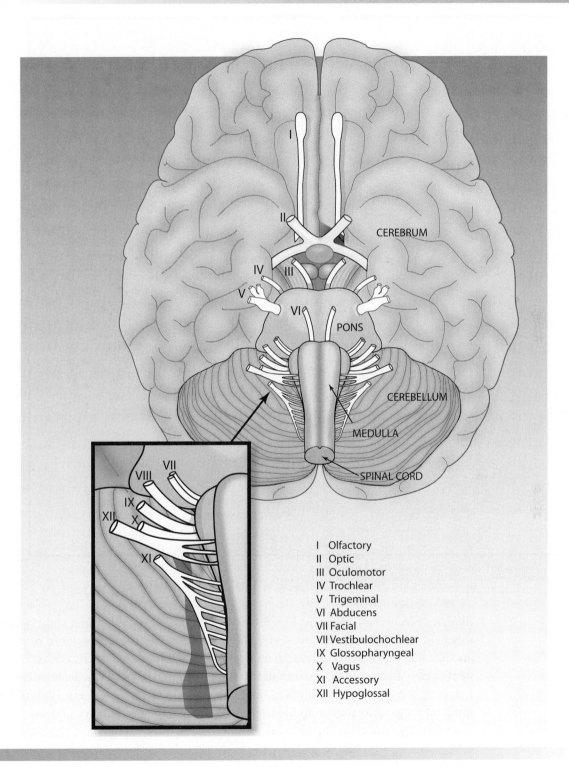

I   Olfactory
II   Optic
III Oculomotor
IV   Trochlear
V   Trigeminal
VI   Abducens
VII Facial
VII Vestibulochochlear
IX   Glossopharyngeal
X   Vagus
XI   Accessory
XII Hypoglossal

Figure 11.19 Trigeminal nerve

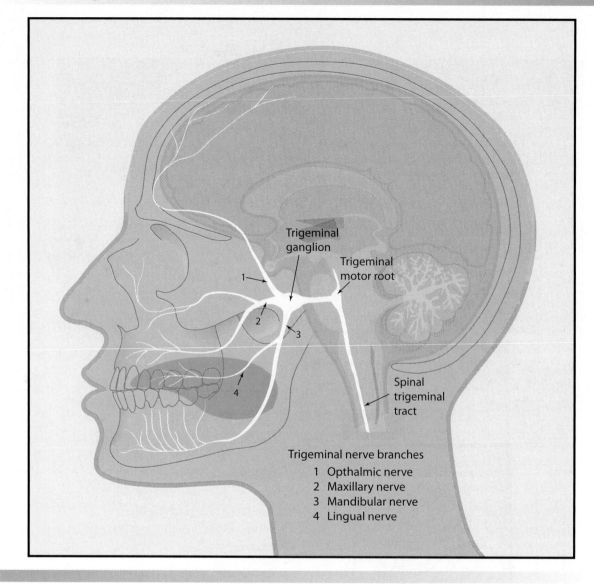

Trigeminal ganglion

Trigeminal motor root

Spinal trigeminal tract

Trigeminal nerve branches
1 Opthalmic nerve
2 Maxillary nerve
3 Mandibular nerve
4 Lingual nerve

difference in nerve supply may be related to the more linked left and right movements of the forehead and eyes, compared to the relative independence of right and left side movements of human mouths and lips (Nolte, 2002). The GSA component of CN VII transmits sensory information from the external ear. Taste information from the anterior two-thirds of the tongue is carried by SVA fibers. GVE fibers transmit motor information to the lacrimal (tear) glands and salivary glands.

CN VIII: Vestibulocochlear

CN VIII has two SSA branches, the vestibular branch and the cochlear branch. The vestibular fibers arise from the semicircular canals, utricle, and saccule in the inner ear and relay information to the CNS about balance and head position. The

Figure 11.20 Facial nerve

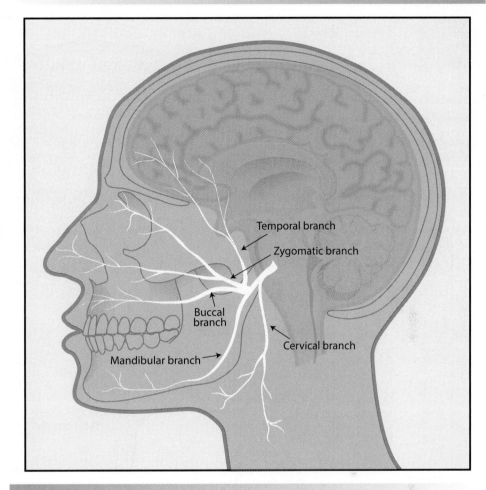

cochlear portion arises from the inner hair cells in the cochlea and transmits auditory information. The nerve also has a small SVE component with motor information from the brain stem to the inner ear (Webster, 1999).

CN IX: Glossopharyngeal

The glossopharyngeal is a complex nerve with GSA, SVA, GVE, SVE, and GVA fibers (Figure 11.21). The GSA fibers are associated with sensation from the external ear. The SVA portion is involved with taste from the posterior one-third of the tongue. The GVE fibers transmit motor information to one of the salivary glands in the oral cavity. The SVE fibers carry neural impulses to some of the pharyngeal muscles. The GVA portion transmits sensory information from the Eustachian tube, posterior one-third of the tongue, and pharynx. In general, the motor fibers are involved in swallowing, and the sensory fibers transmit information about taste, as well as pain, touch, and temperature.

Figure 11.21 Glossopharyngeal nerve

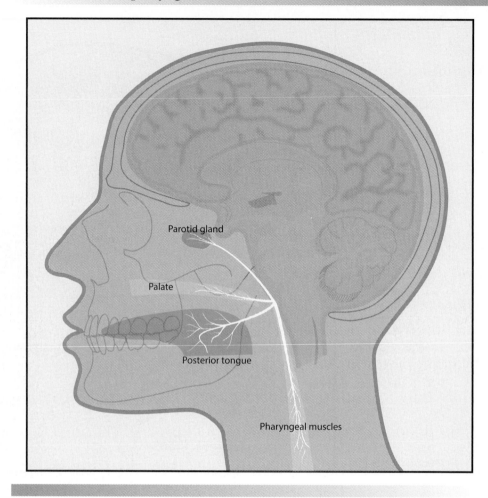

Parotid gland

Palate

Posterior tongue

Pharyngeal muscles

CN X: Vagus

The vagus nerve plays a vital role in heart rate, endocrine function, and digestion, and is also crucial for phonation. The nerve has many branches, which supply visceral organs including the lungs, heart, liver, stomach, pancreas, and others (Figure 11.22). Three branches are integral to speech production: the pharyngeal, superior laryngeal, and recurrent laryngeal nerves.

The pharyngeal, superior laryngeal, and recurrent laryngeal branches are composed of SVE fibers. The pharyngeal nerve innervates the muscles of the soft palate (aside from the tensor veli palatini) and the pharynx. The superior laryngeal and recurrent laryngeal nerves carry neural impulses to the laryngeal muscles. Specifically, the recurrent laryngeal nerve innervates all the intrinsic muscles of the larynx except for the cricothyroid, which is innervated by the superior laryngeal branch. The anatomy of the recurrent laryngeal nerve, unlike other cranial nerves, is not symmetrical on the right and left sides of the body. Before entering the larynx, the recurrent laryngeal nerve descends into the chest and then ascends to enter the larynx. Figure 11.22 shows that on the right side the nerve loops under

Figure 11.22 Vagus nerve

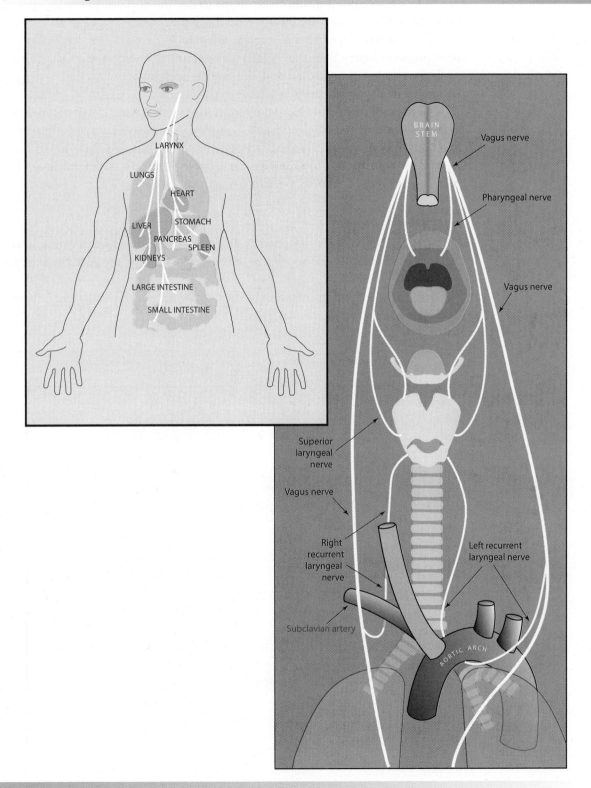

LARYNX

LUNGS

HEART

LIVER   STOMACH

PANCREAS

SPLEEN

KIDNEYS

LARGE INTESTINE

SMALL INTESTINE

BRAIN STEM

Vagus nerve

Pharyngeal nerve

Vagus nerve

Superior laryngeal nerve

Vagus nerve

Right recurrent laryngeal nerve

Left recurrent laryngeal nerve

Subclavian artery

AORTIC ARCH

the subclavian artery of the heart before ascending; on the left side, the nerve descends to a lower point in the chest, loops under the aorta of the heart, and then travels upward to enter the larynx. The difference in the length of the nerve on the right and left sides helps to explain why the left recurrent laryngeal nerve is more prone to injury than the right. This anatomical configuration also accounts for the fact that certain cardiac problems such as congestive heart failure can affect the recurrent laryngeal nerve, resulting in dysphonia.

The vagus also carries GSA fibers from the external ear; SVA fibers from a few taste buds around the epiglottis; and GVE fibers transmitting neural impulses to the heart, smooth muscles in the thorax and abdomen, and various glands. Finally, GVA fibers transmit sensory information from the thoracic and abdominal viscera as well as from the larynx, pharynx, trachea, and esophagus.

CN XII: Hypoglossal

The hypoglossal nerve is composed primarily of GSE fibers innervating intrinsic and extrinsic muscles of the tongue, as well as some of the extrinsic laryngeal muscles (Figure 11.23).

Table 11.10 lists the cranial nerves important for speech and hearing, the types of fibers, and their origins and/or destinations.

Figure 11.23 Hypoglossal nerve

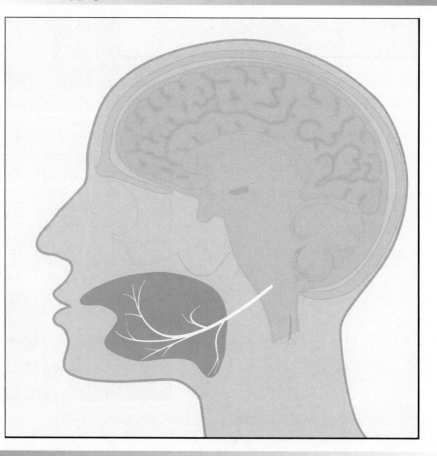

Table 11.10 Selected Cranial Nerves with Types of Fibers and Innervation

CN #	Name	Fibers	Sensory/motor	Innervation
V	Trigeminal	GSA	Sensory	Touch, pressure, pain, proprioception, temperature from facial areas
		SVE	Motor	Muscles of mastication, tensor veli palatini, tensor tympani, extrinsic laryngeal muscles
VII	Facial	SVE	Motor	Muscles of facial expression, stapedius, extrinsic laryngeal muscles
		GSA	Sensory	External ear
		SVA	Sensory	Taste from anterior two-thirds of tongue
		GVE	Motor	Lacrimal and salivary glands
VIII	Vestibulocochlear	SSA	Sensory	Balance, head position, sound
		SVE	Motor	Inner ear
IX	Glossopharyngeal	GSA	Sensory	External ear
		SVA	Sensory	Taste from posterior one-third of tongue
		GVE	Motor	Salivary gland
		SVE	Motor	Pharyngeal muscles
		GVA	Sensory	Eustachian tube, posterior one-third of tongue, pharynx
X	Vagus	SVE	Motor	Soft palate, pharynx, larynx
		GSA	Sensory	External ear
		SVA	Sensory	Taste buds around the epiglottis
		GVE	Motor	Heart, thoracic and abdominal smooth muscles, glands
		GVA	Sensory	Thoracic and abdominal viscera, larynx, pharynx, trachea, esophagus
XII	Hypoglossal	GSE	Motor	Intrinsic and extrinsic muscles of tongue, extrinsic laryngeal muscles

Blood Supply to the Brain

The brain is crucially dependent on a continuous supply of blood for oxygen and glucose to support the metabolic needs of the nervous tissue. Because the brain does not store these energy-producing elements, the blood supply to the brain cannot be interrupted for more than a few minutes. Longer interruptions can cause permanent brain damage and death as the oxygen supply is cut off and nerve cells start to die.

Figure 11.24 Blood supply to the brain

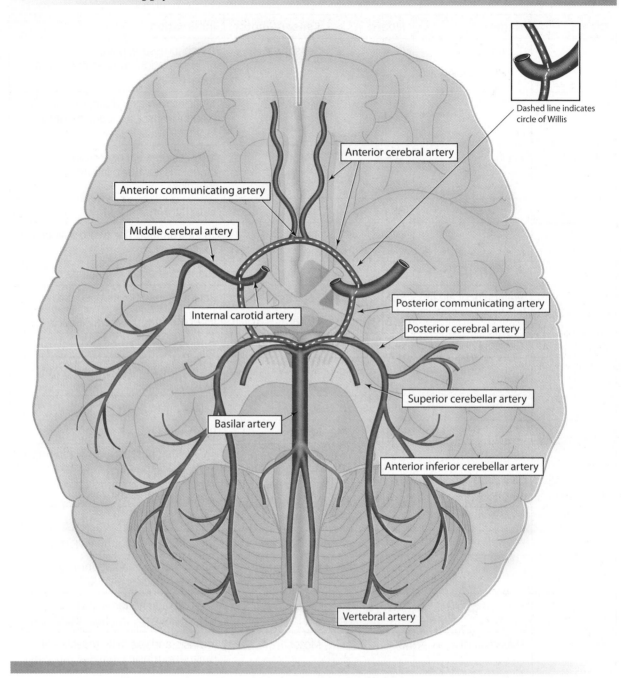

Dashed line indicates circle of Willis

Anterior cerebral artery

Anterior communicating artery

Middle cerebral artery

Internal carotid artery

Posterior communicating artery

Posterior cerebral artery

Superior cerebellar artery

Basilar artery

Anterior inferior cerebellar artery

Vertebral artery

The arteries that supply the brain are patterned in a roughly circular fashion, called the **circle of Willis**. As shown in Figure 11.24, the arteries that form this circle are the internal carotid and the vertebral, as well as branches off these major vessels, such as the anterior and posterior communicating arteries (Figure 11.24).

Once it enters the skull, the internal carotid branches into the anterior and middle cerebral arteries (ACA and MCA) on either side of the brain. The ACA supplies portions of the frontal and parietal lobes, the corpus callosum, the basal nuclei, and part of the internal capsule (Seikel et al., 2004). The MCA provides blood to the temporal lobe, motor strip, and Wernicke's area, among others (Seikel et al., 2004). The two vertebral arteries, one from each side, join to form the basilar artery, which supplies blood to the brain stem. The basilar artery then branches into the posterior cerebral artery (PCA) and the cerebellar arteries. The PCA provides blood to portions of the temporal and occipital lobes, as well as to the upper midbrain and the cerebellum. The cerebellar arteries supply the cerebellum.

The Language Zone

The classical language zone was defined by Dejerine in the early 1900s as a region of the brain that contains the neural substrates that are essential for the conceptualization, production, and perception of language. Located on the lateral surface of the left cerebral hemisphere within the distribution of the middle cerebral artery, it is an area that lies around the lateral fissure and incorporates portions of the frontal, parietal, and temporal lobes. The anterior region of the language zone includes Broca's area in the premotor region of the frontal lobe. Broca's area lies adjacent to the inferior portion of the motor strip and is responsible for the movement of articulatory and phonatory mechanisms. The posterior portion of the language zone includes Wernicke's area, the auditory association cortex located in the posterior portion of the superior temporal gyrus. Two large bundles of nerve fibers lie beneath the cortical surface of the language zone. Broca's area and Wernicke's area are connected by a subcortical white matter pathway called the arcuate fasciculus. The superior longitudinal fasciculus connects the frontal, occipital, and temporal lobes. These two white matter pathways pass through the angular gyrus and the supramarginal gyrus at the posterior border of the lateral fissure where the parietal and temporal lobes meet. Both the angular and supramarginal gyri are association areas that contain numerous neural connections from all over the brain. The supramarginal gyrus seems to be involved in the phonological processing of words and the symbolic integration of symbols for writing. The angular gyrus is apparently involved in visual, auditory, and tactile processing and the integration of symbols for reading. The components of the language zone are shown in Figure 11.25.

The idea of a highly specialized region for language processing has been confirmed using the lesion analysis method. That is, it is widely acknowledged that lesions in the area of the language zone produce predictable patterns of speech and language deficits that characterize the clinical syndromes of aphasia. However, technologies such as computer tomography (CT scans), positron emission tomography (PET), and functional magnetic resonance imaging (fMRI) have challenged the strict localizationist approach to language. Current theory rejects the idea that there is a one-to-one direct correspondence between specific language processes and discrete areas of the brain. Language processing is now believed to arise from multiple and complex neural networks. The language zone is now conceptualized as a major intersection, or a bottleneck, included among several overlapping neural networks that give rise to language. Although many neural connections

Figure 11.25 The language zone

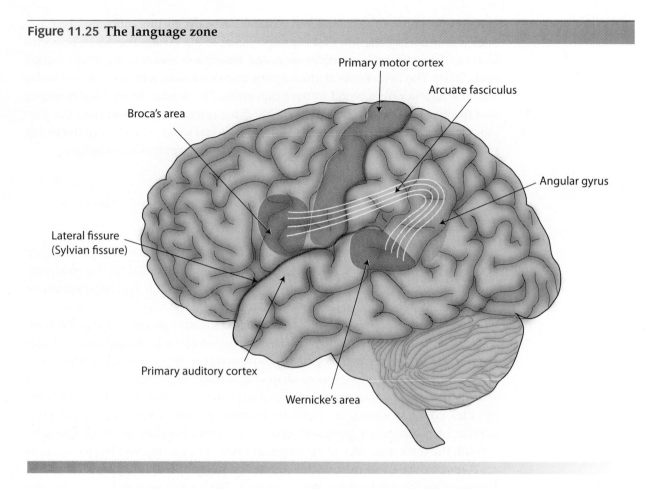

converge in the language zone, evidence based on current technologies suggests that language processing is distributed all over the brain, and includes the subcortex and the right hemisphere. That is, language arises from the connections among the neural networks, not the language zone alone. The idea that language is broadly distributed throughout the brain is termed parallel distributed processing.

Motor Control Systems Involved in Speech Production

Speech production, although seemingly effortless for the most part, requires a huge amount of neural processing to occur. The simplest utterance requires neuromuscular signals from numerous areas of the CNS and PNS to numerous muscles involved in respiration, phonation, and articulation. In addition, background postural muscle tone is an important component of the process. Sensory information from muscles, joints, skin, and tendons plays a crucial part in regulating the motor commands that allow the relevant structures to move in the appropriate sequence, and at the rapid rates involved in speech production.

As an example, take the word *tan*. Just to produce this word, information must be transmitted from the motor areas of the cerebral cortex along nerve pathways involving the basal nuclei, cerebellum, thalamus, and corticospinal and corticonuclear tracts, to the correct spinal and cranial nerves, to the appropriate musculature for each phoneme in the word. Further, the phonemes must be correctly sequenced, so that the utterance emerges as planned and not as *nat* or *ant*. This involves coarticulating the sounds, moving different articulators almost simultaneously while maintaining the separate identity of each phoneme. For the /t/ sound, the tongue tip must be raised, so neural impulses must arrive via CN XII to the superior longitudinal muscles of the tongue. The velum is raised to direct airflow out the oral cavity, so the levator veli palatini is activated via the pharyngeal branch of CN X. /t/ is voiceless, so the posterior cricoarytenoid muscles of the larynx, innervated by the recurrent laryngeal branch of CN X, are contracted to open the vocal folds, while the lateral cricoarytenoid muscles are relaxed. For the vowel, the vocal folds must close, regulated by the nerve impulses arriving via the recurrent laryngeal nerve at the lateral cricoarytenoid and interarytenoid muscles; the tongue body lowers for the vowel, mediated by neuromuscular commands traveling along CN XII to the vertical muscles. The nasal /n/ requires a lowered velum, so the levator veli palatini relaxes, allowing the velum to drop. Once again the tongue tip is raised, and the vocal folds remain closed and vibrating. Consider that all these neuromuscular commands occur within the space of less than a second, and one begins to see the stunning complexity of the system. Consider also that the muscles of respiration are activated via the appropriate spinal nerves, changing from the postures for life breathing to those for speech breathing. Simultaneously, the speaker is either sitting or standing or walking, so the appropriate trunk and limb muscles are being regulated as well. In addition, sensory systems of proprioception from joints and muscles, sound from the auditory system, visual stimuli, and so on are processed alongside the motor information. Now, take one phoneme and multiply all these neuromuscular events for that phoneme by around 20 (we speak at approximately 20 phonemes per second in normal conversational speech), and the importance of the sensorimotor neural control system becomes apparent. Table 11.11 summarizes selected neuromuscular events involved in the production of the word *tan*.

Table 11.11 Selected Neuromuscular Events for the Word *Tan*

Phoneme	Primary Structures	Primary Nerve Pathways
/t/	Tongue tip raised by superior longitudinal muscle	CN XII
	Velum raised by levator veli palatini	Pharyngeal branch of CN X
	Vocal folds opened by posterior cricoarytenoids	Recurrent laryngeal branch of CN X
/æ/	Vocal folds closed by lateral cricoarytenoids and interarytenoids	Recurrent laryngeal branch of CN X
	Tongue body lowered by vertical tongue muscles	CN XII
/n/	Velum lowered by relaxation of levator veli palatini	
	Tongue tip raised by superior longitudinal muscle	CN XII
	Vocal folds remain closed by lateral cricoarytenoids and interarytenoids	Recurrent laryngeal branch of CN X

The following discussion will focus on some of the motor control systems that speakers use for speech production, including the motor cortex, upper and lower motor neurons, and mechanisms of sensory feedback and feedforward.

Motor Cortex

As noted above the motor cortex includes primary, premotor, and supplementary motor areas; each of these areas is equipped with a map, in more or less detail, representing various bodily structures. Far from duplicating each other's functions, however, each motor area regulates movement in different yet complementary ways. The primary motor cortex (M1) in area 4 (see Figure 11.10) controls single muscles or small groups of muscles that work synergistically to perform a complex coordinated movement. This area receives extensive sensory input from the thalamus, from the somatosensory cortex, and from the premotor cortex; it is thus continuously updated about ongoing and anticipated movement. Research has shown that neurons in M1 regulate the amount of force and the direction needed for the desired movement and that these neurons fire in preparation for (i.e., slightly in advance of) an upcoming movement (Mihailoff & Haines, 2002). However, the activity of these neurons can also be modified during a movement, indicating that other sensory and motor information coming from many different nervous system locations is processed while a movement is in progress. It is important to note that the primary motor cortex does not initiate movement, but rather collects and channels information about aspects of movement and then transmits this information to the brain stem and spinal cord to be passed along to the appropriate spinal and cranial nerves for execution.

The premotor and supplementary motor cortices are both located in area 6, anterior to area 4. The premotor area prepares, plans, and organizes information about upcoming movements based partially on sensory information. The sensory input involves balance and visual information that is needed to enable an individual to assess his or her position in space or the position of relevant structures in space, to judge the direction and force of the movement necessary to reach its target, and to make any adjustments to posture that are necessary to keep one's balance while carrying out the movement. This data is transmitted to M1, as well as to the spinal cord and brain stem. Unlike M1, which acts to regulate relatively small groups of muscles, the premotor cortex deals with larger groups of muscles in widely separated parts of the body. The supplementary motor area functions similarly to the premotor cortex. However, while premotor cortex is more involved with movements in response to external environmental stimuli, the supplementary motor cortex plays more of a role in planning complex, internally generated movements (Nolte, 2002). The supplementary motor area has been implicated in such disorders as stuttering, in which there is a breakdown of the complex, coordinated movements necessary for fluent speech.

Upper and Lower Motor Neurons

Two components of the motor control system are the **upper motor neuron (UMN)** and **lower motor neuron (LMN)**. The UMN comprises the nerve cells and their axons arising from various cortical areas and projecting to the brain stem and spinal cord. The LMN includes nerve cell bodies and axons of cranial and spinal nerves that connect with voluntary muscles. Once motor information from cortical areas has been acted upon by the basal nuclei and cerebellum, the final neuromuscular commands are transmitted by the UMN to the LMN and from there to the target structures for movement execution. Spinal and cranial nerves that make up the LMN are often called the final common pathway, since all cortical and subcortical motor information converges onto these nerves.

The two major pathways of the UMN are the corticospinal and corticonuclear (corticobulbar) tracts (Figure 11.26).

The corticospinal tract is a large one, with around 1 million fibers (Nolte, 2002). About one-third of the fibers arise in M1, another one-third in premotor and supplementary motor areas, and the remaining one-third in the somatosensory cortex in the parietal lobe (Figure 11.27). Fibers in this tract synapse directly onto motor nerve cells in the anterior horn of the spinal cord, although along the way branches of these fibers project to other locations including the basal nuclei, thalamus, reticular formation, and sensory nuclei (Nolte, 2002). Most fibers in this tract (around 80 to 90%) decussate in the medullary pyramids and continue contralaterally to their spinal targets, while a small percentage of fibers continue ipsilaterally. The crossed fibers on either side form the lateral corticospinal pathways. The anterior corticospinal pathways are made up of the uncrossed fibers.

The corticonuclear tract is also known as the corticobulbar tract. The term *bulb* refers to the medulla, although this name is now obsolete. The term *corticobulbar* is not anatomically accurate but is still used to refer to all cortical projections that synapse on motor neurons of cranial nerves in the brain stem. The newer term *corticonuclear* was adopted in 1998 by the International Federation of Associations of Anatomists (Mihailoff & Haines, 2002). This term refers specifically to nerve cells and their axons arising from cortical areas and synapsing with motor nuclei of CN V, VII, and XII, as well as the nucleus ambiguus that gives rise to CN X, among other pathways. Only striated muscles that are involved in voluntary movement are supplied by the corticonuclear tract. Whereas fibers in the corticospinal tract arise from several cortical locations, the origin of corticonuclear fibers is more localized to the face and neck portions of the primary motor cortex, as shown in Figure 11.28. The corticonuclear tract innervates the left and right motor nuclei in the brain stem bilaterally, with information from left and right motor cortices traveling ipsilaterally. However, as noted previously, some selected fibers, such as those innervating the lower areas of the face, are contralateral.

Direct and Indirect Systems

The corticospinal and corticonuclear tracts together are referred to as the **pyramidal system**, or **direct system**. This system is involved in controlling fine, skilled voluntary movements, and damage can result in muscles that are weak or spastic. The **indirect system**, or **extrapyramidal system**, refers to nerve pathways from the cortex to the brain stem or spinal cord that do not synapse directly with the motor neurons, but that travel more circuitously via the basal nuclei and cerebellum before synapsing with spinal and brain stem motor nuclei. Damage to the indirect system can result in abnormal involuntary movements such as tics and tremors that interfere with normal voluntary control, as well as postural deficits.

Figure 11.26 Relationship between corona radiata, internal capsule, corticospinal, and corticonuclear pathways

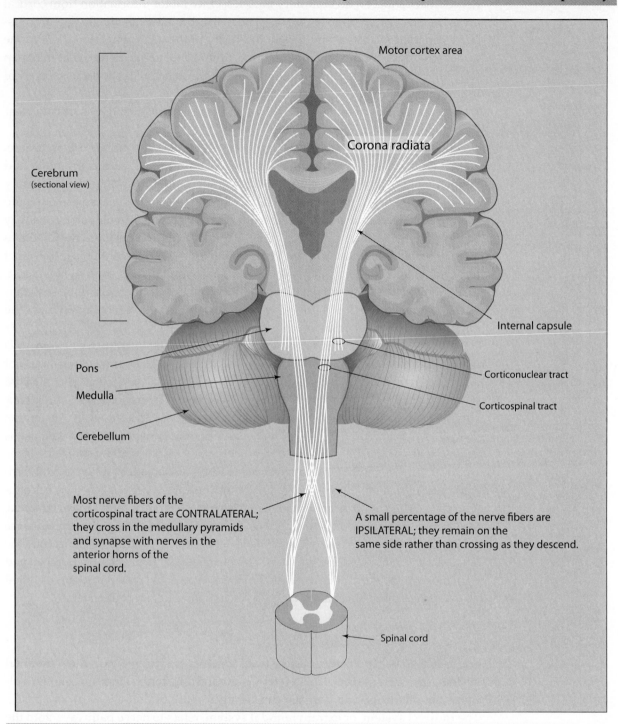

Motor cortex area

Corona radiata

Cerebrum (sectional view)

Internal capsule

Pons

Corticonuclear tract

Medulla

Corticospinal tract

Cerebellum

Most nerve fibers of the corticospinal tract are CONTRALATERAL; they cross in the medullary pyramids and synapse with nerves in the anterior horns of the spinal cord.

A small percentage of the nerve fibers are IPSILATERAL; they remain on the same side rather than crossing as they descend.

Spinal cord

Figure 11.27 Schematic of corticospinal pathway

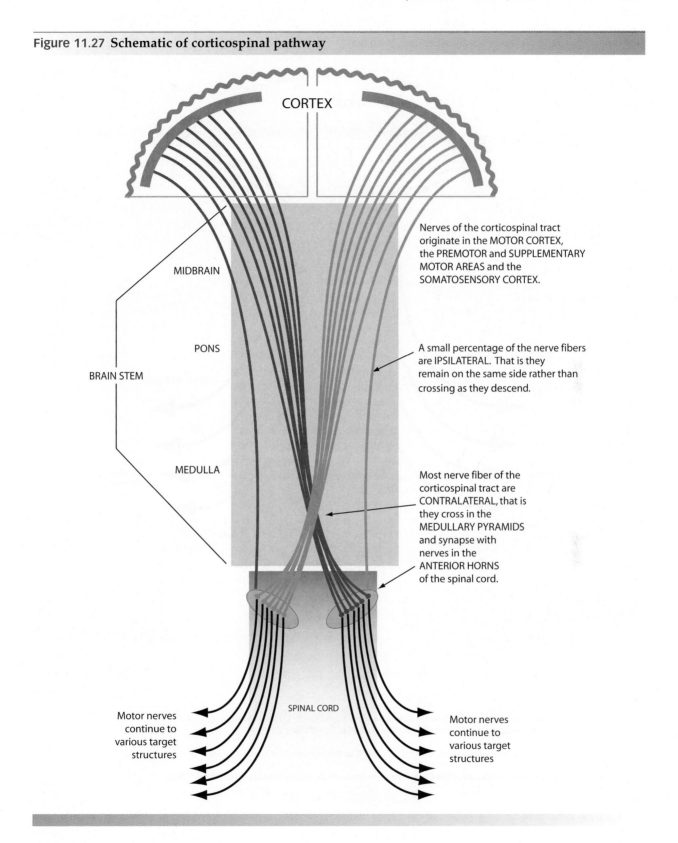

CORTEX

MIDBRAIN

PONS

BRAIN STEM

MEDULLA

SPINAL CORD

Nerves of the corticospinal tract originate in the MOTOR CORTEX, the PREMOTOR and SUPPLEMENTARY MOTOR AREAS and the SOMATOSENSORY CORTEX.

A small percentage of the nerve fibers are IPSILATERAL. That is they remain on the same side rather than crossing as they descend.

Most nerve fiber of the corticospinal tract are CONTRALATERAL, that is they cross in the MEDULLARY PYRAMIDS and synapse with nerves in the ANTERIOR HORNS of the spinal cord.

Motor nerves continue to various target structures

Motor nerves continue to various target structures

Figure 11.28 Schematic of corticonuclear pathway

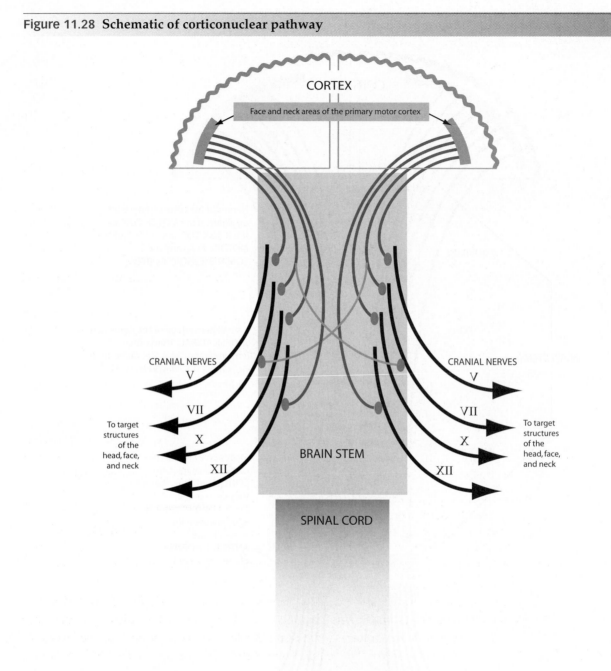

Nerves in the corticonuclear pathway originate in the face and neck areas of the motor cortex. They synapse in the brain stem with CRANIAL NERVES V, VII, X, and XII.

They synapse with the nerves on the SAME SIDE as the hemisphere in which they originate (IPSILATERAL).

An exception occurs in that CN VII fibers also cross over to the opposite side (CONTRALATERAL).

Motor Units

LMN fibers projecting from cranial and spinal motor neurons to voluntary muscles have axonic endings that synapse with muscle fibers. The synapse between an axon and the muscle fiber it innervates is called by several names, including neuromuscular junction, **myoneural junction**, or **motor end plate** (Figure 11.29).

The myoneural junction functions similarly to a nerve-to-nerve synapse. The vesicles of the presynaptic neuron contain the neurotransmitter acetylcholine (ACh), which acts in an excitatory fashion. When the vesicles are stimulated by an action potential, the acetylcholine is released into the synapse. This generates an EPSP, which causes the muscle fiber to contract. After a very short interval, the acetylcholine is inactivated. Inactivation occurs through several mechanisms. One mechanism works by degrading the chemical into its component parts via an enzyme called **acetylcholinesterase**. Once the ACh is broken down, it can no longer be recognized by the receptor sites, thus stopping its excitatory action. Another mechanism is called reuptake, in which the intact neurotransmitter is recycled back into the vesicles of the presynaptic neuron.

The way that muscles contract is essentially the same process as that by which nerves fire. Similar to neurons, which have a resting potential of around –70 mV, the inside of a muscle fiber at rest has negative charge of roughly –95 mV. When the ACh is released into the neuromuscular junction, sodium channels in the membrane surrounding the fiber are opened, allowing sodium ions to diffuse into the fiber. This has the effect of reducing the negative charge within the fiber and creates a small depolarization called an **end-plate potential (EPP)**. If the EPP reaches a critical threshold, an all-or-none action potential occurs and the muscle fiber contracts. Once the fiber has contracted, it is followed by a brief refractory period during which it is repolarized and returns to its original resting potential.

One motor neuron can innervate varying numbers of muscle fibers. A motor neuron with its associated muscle fibers is called a **motor unit**. The ratio of a motor neuron to the number of fibers it innervates is called the **innervation ratio**. Different structures have motor unit sizes that depend on the function and level of motor control of that structure. For example, large leg muscles that do not require very fine neuromuscular control, but generate a lot of muscular force, have motor units with large innervation ratios. One axon innervates many muscle fibers, around 600 to 1000 fibers per axon (Mihailoff & Haines, 2002). By contrast, smaller structures that do not generate much force and require fine levels of control, such as the laryngeal muscles, have much smaller motor units of 10 to 100 fibers per axon. How strongly a muscle contracts depends on the number of motor units that are activated.

There are three types of motor units, each associated with a different type of muscle fiber. Type S (slow) units are associated with dark red muscle fibers. These fibers do not generate much force but also do not fatigue easily. They are activated by small-diameter motor neurons that have slower conduction rates. These fibers are found in large numbers in muscles that are associated with maintaining posture. Postural muscles are called slow twitch muscles and can continue to contract for long periods of time. Type FF (fast fatigable) units are associated with light-colored larger fibers that generate large amounts of force for brief amounts of time. They are activated by large-diameter, fast-conducting nerves and dominate in muscles

Figure 11.29 Neuromuscular junction

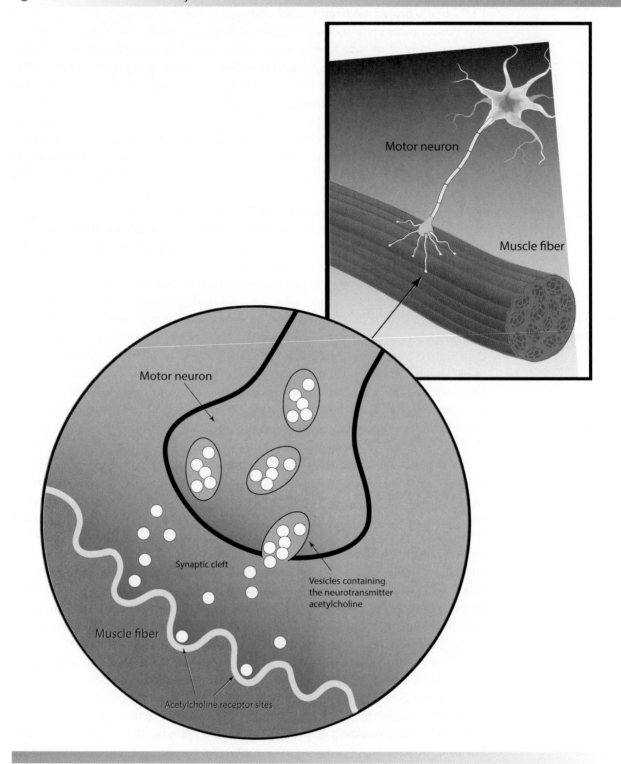

Motor neuron

Muscle fiber

Motor neuron

Synaptic cleft

Vesicles containing
the neurotransmitter
acetylcholine

Muscle fiber

Acetylcholine receptor sites

associated with rapid movements. Muscles innervated by FF units are referred to as fast twitch. Type FR (fatigue resistant) units share characteristics of the other two types. These muscles generate nearly but not quite as much force as fast twitch muscles but are more fatigue resistant and can therefore sustain contraction for longer periods than can fast twitch muscles. Motor units also differ in terms of size: S units are the smallest in terms of their cell bodies, FF units are the largest, and FR units fall in between. The size difference plays an important role in how the muscle force needed for smooth movement is regulated. As noted above, motor neurons fire and trigger an action potential when a critical voltage threshold is reached. Smaller neurons have a lower threshold than larger ones. Thus, the small S units are the first to fire when stimulated. As stimulation becomes more intense, they fire with increasing rapidity. This in turn causes the FR units to fire. Should stimulation continue to increase and FR units fire more rapidly, then FF units are recruited as well and add their force to the movement. This is called the size principle.

Principles of Motor Control

Becoming familiar with neural pathways and brain structures forms the basis for understanding some principles involved in motor control systems. These systems include feedback and feedforward control, efference copy, and motor equivalence.

Feedback and Feedforward

Feedback is an engineering term that refers to the process whereby the output of a system is returned to the input in order to influence the ensuing output. Systems can be thought of as being either closed loop or open loop. Closed-loop systems return the output back to the original input for purposes of comparison and correction. Open-loop systems do not use feedback to modify the output of the system. Speech production relies on both types of systems. In terms of speech production, feedback refers to any type of sensory information available to the speaker, such as auditory information, proprioceptive information, and tactile information. Feedback operates as a control system that allows an individual to detect and correct any errors in his or her speech production. Feedback channels, however, do not operate instantaneously, so that sometimes a speaker has already made an error before he or she becomes aware of it and is able to correct it. In speech production, auditory feedback is probably the most crucial type of information when a child is learning to speak his or her native language. This is clearly evident in the case of prelingually deaf children, who typically have great difficulty in acquiring the appropriate vocal tract positions to generate the phonemes of the language. Auditory feedback becomes less vital once the language has been learned, although there is some evidence that speakers who are deafened later in life may lose some degree of intelligibility due to the hearing loss and lack of auditory feedback. However, most normal speakers do not need a lot of auditory feedback in order to produce intelligible speech, probably because speech is a highly practiced motor skill.

Speech production also uses feedforward information. **Feedforward** refers to the process whereby output from one system becomes the input to another system. In terms of speech production, this means that, for example, sensory information from the jaw during the production of a particular phoneme may be input to other articulators, such as the lips and tongue, and modify the activity of these articulators. In this case, the original information from the jaw is not returned to the original source but acts to influence other articulators. Feedforward mechanisms act much more rapidly than feedback systems. This allows articulatory movements to be modified "online," resulting in a great deal of precision during speech production. Feedforward mechanisms have been demonstrated in experiments in which a speaker's articulators are perturbed unpredictably in some way as he or she is producing an utterance. It has been shown that, typically, the acoustic output is not affected, and the individual makes extremely rapid adjustments of the perturbed and unperturbed articulators (tens of milliseconds) in order to maintain the acoustic integrity of the utterance.

Sensory information is crucial for the motor activities of speech production. Sensory information obtained from proprioceptors, joint receptors, mechanoreceptors, and baroreceptors, as well as auditory, kinesthetic, and cutaneous information, provides important information about muscle systems during speech production (Abbs, 1996; Barlow, 1999). This information is used to regulate and adjust motor output and to coordinate muscular adjustments between articulators. Abbs (1996) noted that while particular motor goals are planned (i.e., specific phonemes or articulator movements), the specific patterns of muscle contractions and joint movements are programmed flexibly based on current sensory and motor information from articulatory, respiratory, and phonatory structures. This is in accordance with the concept of motor equivalence, first described in the early twentieth century. Motor equivalence refers to the ability of the motor system to achieve a particular movement goal or output with a great degree of variability in the individual components of the movement. Speech is a goal-oriented process of moving the articulators into the appropriate position for specific sounds. As long as the correct sound is achieved—that is, the acoustic output is maintained—the precise positioning of the articulators is not important. Experiments using a bite block to fix the mandible in position have shown that even with the jaw fixed, speakers are able to produce an acceptable vowel by slightly adjusting other articulators to compensate for the disruption in normal production. It is likely that feedforward and efference copy mechanisms are involved in making these extremely rapid compensations.

Efference Copy

Efference copy refers to the notion that when a neural motor command signal is sent to a muscle or structure, a second simultaneous "copy" of the signal is transmitted to various sensory systems as well, in order to prepare the sensory system for the anticipated consequences of the motor act (Barlow, 1999). We know that there are many sensory and motor pathways between the sensorimotor areas of the cortex, subcortical structures, and cerebellum. Nerve pathways from the cortex to the cerebellum provide the cerebellum with efference copy signals from the primary motor cortex as well as sensory feedback from the primary sensory cortex (Barlow, 1999). The cerebellum is then in a position to evaluate the ongoing movement and to correct any errors, and projects the new information back to the motor cortex (feedback) as well as to peripheral structures via various nerve pathways (feedforward).

Summary

The nervous system is divided into the central nervous system, which includes the brain and spinal cord, and the peripheral nervous system, which includes the cranial and spinal nerves.

Neurons are the basic building blocks of the nervous system, and consist of a cell body, dendrites, and an axon; glial cells perform many metabolic functions.

Neurons work through a complex electrochemical process by which an action potential is generated and transmitted to other neurons at the synapse.

The brain is contained within the meninges and is given buoyancy by the cerebrospinal fluid, which is manufactured in the ventricles and circulates around the brain and spinal cord.

The brain is divided into two hemispheres, connected by the corpus callosum.

The cortex of the brain is highly convoluted and is divided into frontal, parietal, temporal, occipital, and limbic lobes.

Within the white matter of the cerebrum are several subcortical structures, including the basal nuclei, thalamus, and hypothalamus.

The brain stem includes the midbrain, pons, and medulla, which connects to the spinal cord; cranial nerves have their points of origin in various regions of the brain stem.

The cerebellum is an important structure for coordinating different aspects of movement, such as direction, force, and speed.

The zone of language is currently conceptualized as a critical region among several overlapping and widely distributed neural networks in the brain.

Motor control systems involved in speech production include the motor cortical areas, as well as the upper and lower motor neurons; feedback and feedforward are important components of motor control.

REVIEW EXERCISES

1. Identify three types of glial cells and explain the difference between them and neurons in terms of structure and function.

2. Describe the process whereby neurons in a resting state are depolarized and repolarized when stimulated.

3. Identify and describe the areas of the cortex important in the understanding and comprehension of speech.

4. Explain how the subcortical areas and the cerebellum are involved in speech production.

5. Compare and contrast the cranial nerves important for speech and hearing in terms of their origins and effects.

6. Describe the differences and similarities between the corticospinal and corticonuclear nerve pathways.

7. Explain the concepts of feedback, feedforward, efference copy, and motor equivalence with regard to speech production.

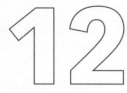
CLINICAL APPLICATION

Brain Imaging in the Evaluation and Treatment of Disorders of the Nervous System

STUDENT LEARNING OBJECTIVES

After reading this chapter you will

○ Identify techniques used to image brain structure.

○ Understand methods of imaging brain function.

○ Appreciate how brain imaging techniques are used to expand knowledge about stuttering.

○ Be familiar with ways in which brain imaging techniques have been used for diagnosis of neurological diseases such as Parkinson's disease and Alzheimer's disease.

○ Appreciate the value of brain imaging techniques in assessing treatment efficacy in certain neurological diseases.

The way in which the brain functions and the ways in which the brain can malfunction have long fascinated scientists and researchers as well as professionals who work with individuals with brain damage. Methods have been devised over past decades to try to access brain structure and function in order to understand and compare normal and abnormal neural working and to create treatment strategies to restore brain function or to compensate for the damage.

With the advent over the past few decades of sophisticated computerized technology, this objective has become much more attainable. Current brain imaging techniques allow fine details of brain structures to be visualized, manipulated, and quantified, providing the opportunity for unparalleled understanding of normal and abnormal brain function. These new techniques have also been applied to the study of normal and disordered human communication, allowing for confirmation or rejection of theories, expansion of models, and insight into the efficacy of various surgical, pharmacological, and behavioral treatment techniques.

Much of the available information about brain function and its relationship to human behavior, including communicative behavior, has come from individuals with various types of neurological disorders or injuries. For example, a lot of what is known about the function of cortical and subcortical areas such as Broca's area and the basal nuclei has been derived by examining the deficits in function of people who have suffered a stroke or other brain injury that affects a specific region. With current brain imaging techniques it has now become possible to evaluate normal function from brain-behavior data obtained from neurologically normal individuals. This is preferable, because information derived from individuals with brain damage is often complicated by factors such as age and time post-injury (Plante, 2001), as well as premorbid factors such as education level and socioeconomic status. In addition, relying on correlations between damaged areas and resulting behaviors does not take into account factors such as undamaged brain areas that may, at least partially, compensate for the lost function.

Current brain imaging techniques can be categorized on the basis of whether they depict brain structure (anatomy) or reflect brain function (physiology). They can also be classified in terms of the type of technology used. Brain structure is accessed by specialized X-rays and imaging techniques. Brain function is typically indicated indirectly by measuring electrical, biochemical, or physiologic characteristics of the nervous system (Watson & Freeman, 1997). This chapter will focus on the primary methods of imaging brain structure, including computerized tomography and magnetic resonance imaging; as well as the main techniques for evaluating function, including functional magnetic resonance imaging, positron emission tomography, single photon emission computerized tomography, transcranial magnetic stimulation, and quantitative electroencephalography. We will then explore how the use of these techniques has enhanced the understanding of communication disorders resulting from various neurological causes.

Techniques for Imaging Brain Structure

Computerized Tomography

Computerized tomography (CT) is an X-ray technique. Like conventional (planar) X-rays, CT is sensitive to the density of tissues, so X-rays are absorbed differently by the different parts of the body. The denser the tissue, the more radiation energy it absorbs, resulting in a lighter X-ray image. In X-ray images of the brain the skull appears white because bone absorbs the most X-rays. The cerebral ventricles or fluid-filled cavities in the brain absorb little radiation energy and appear black. Brain matter has intermediate density and appears gray.

The difference between planar X-rays and CT is that a CT image is constructed from numerous scans of the brain structure as the X-ray and the X-ray detectors rotate around the individual's head (Watson & Freeman, 1997). This results in many different angles at which the structure is scanned, and the resulting scans are combined by computer into a detailed three-dimensional image of cross sections of selected thicknesses of cortical and subcortical regions of the brain. Because of the ability to produce cross-sectional images of the bones and soft tissues of the body, CT scans are useful for examining injuries. Current CT scanners are able to image slices of the target structure very quickly (Haines, Raila, & Terrell, 2002).

In brain CT imaging, a series of X-ray beams are sent through the skull, and a device on the other side of the scanner records the different levels of density.

Contrast dyes maybe injected into a vein to allow detection of blockages or problems in the blood vessels. This is why a CT scan is often one of the first tests done to evaluate a patient who has suffered a stroke. Most ischemic strokes are less dense and appear darker than in the healthy brain, whereas the blood present in a hemorrhagic stroke is denser and appears white on the CT image.

Advantages of CT include the short (1 s per slice) imaging times and widespread availability of the technology. Because of its excellent differentiation between tissues of varying densities the technique allows detection of calcification and hemorrhage (Laughlin & Montanera, 1998). CT is typically used to diagnose tumors, cerebrovascular disease, head trauma, and cerebral atrophy (Watson & Freeman, 1997). The disadvantage, as with any other X-ray, is the radiation and resulting potential health risks to the patient.

Magnetic Resonance Imaging

Magnetic resonance imaging (MRI) is a noninvasive imaging technique that uses a magnetic field and radio waves to create detailed images of the organs and tissues. These images show the anatomy of the brain at high resolution and are used to diagnose a wide variety of brain disorders, including brain tumors, multiple sclerosis, and stroke. During the exam the patient lies on a narrow table, which slides into a large tunnel-shaped scanner. MRI takes advantage of the cellular basis of human tissue. One of the major components of tissue is water, and hydrogen atoms constitute one element of water molecules (H_2O). Over 70 percent of brain tissue is composed of water (Parry & Matthews, 2002). Hydrogen atoms behave like miniature magnets spinning around an axis at a certain frequency. They are normally aligned randomly rather than in specific patterns. During an MRI, the patient is exposed to a super-powerful magnet that temporarily aligns the water molecules in the body. A brief radiofrequency (RF) wave or pulse is then directed into the patient. When the frequencies of the RF pulse and the spinning hydrogen protons are close to each other, constructive interference (resonance) occurs, and the protons gain energy. When the radiofrequency wave is turned off, the hydrogen atoms gradually return to their original random alignments, a process called relaxation. As the molecules relax, they release energy in the form of radio waves, which are detected and amplified by a specialized receiver. Different tissues within the brain contain slightly different amounts of water. For example, neurons have higher concentration of water than myelin (Parry & Matthews, 2002). The differences in water and hydrogen content produce the contrasts between different tissues, based on the distribution of hydrogen atoms (Lauter, 1997). This result in radio signals with different amplitudes and different relaxation times. A computer transforms this information into images of the target structure.

A major advantage of MRI is that it does not use radiation and therefore poses no health risks. Because of this, MRI has been used extensively to study the brain not only in people with various disorders and diseases but also in healthy individuals. A large body of knowledge has been obtained of normal brain structures from infants to the very old. Another advantage of MRI is that it can distinguish fine differences between soft tissues such as gray and white matter, cerebrospinal fluid, and vascular structures. With this technique, it is also possible to detect differences between normal and abnormal tissue, such as the plaques that occur in multiple sclerosis. Because of the very high degree of spatial resolution that can be obtained with MRI (1 mm), it is even possible to identify individual cranial nerves and subcortical structures (Lauter, 1997). Thus, MRI is a valuable tool for diagnosis of many brain diseases and disorders. There are some disadvantages, however. Imaging times are longer for MRI than for CT, and the cost is higher. Some individuals are not able to undergo MRI because of the presence of metal devices in the body, such as aneurysm clips, pacemakers, or cochlear implants.

Techniques for Imaging Brain Function

Techniques for imaging brain function are based on blood flow within the brain, brain metabolism of oxygen and glucose, electrical properties of brain physiology, or some combination of these. Whatever technique is used, functional neuroimaging is based on the rationale that the performance of any task places specific information processing demands on the brain, and these demands are met through local changes in neural activity (Fiez, 2001). This results in changes to blood flow within the activated brain area, as well as to metabolism within that region. These changes can then be either directly or indirectly measured in various ways.

Functional Magnetic Resonance Imaging

Functional magnetic resonance imaging (fMRI) measures tiny metabolic changes that take place in an active part of the brain. The technique works by detecting changes in blood flow and oxygen levels that occur in response to neural activity. When an area of the brain becomes active it uses more oxygen and recruits blood to replace the depleted oxygen. fMRI scans produce detailed images of metabolic activity in distinct areas of the brain. This has been useful for showing the parts of the brain that are involved in a particular mental or cognitive process.

Like regular MRI, fMRI is an index of changes in the oxygen content of the blood in a particular brain area or region of interest (ROI). It can be used as such because of the way nerves function. Recall that after a neuron has fired, neurotransmitter is released into the synapse. Shortly thereafter, the neurotransmitter is either degraded or taken back into the pre synaptic neuron, a process that requires energy. The increased energy is provided by increased oxygen, with a corresponding increase in the local blood flow within the region. The increase in blood flow to a specific area is known as the **hemodynamic response**, and it is this response that is measured in fMRI. The response is correlated with different types of tasks and different brain regions that are activated during such tasks. Thus, fMRI is an indirect measure of brain function, since it is the hemodynamic response that is measured rather than the actual neuronal function.

A major advantage of fMRI is that it is a safe and noninvasive means of assessing how an individual's brain function changes over time or in different situations. This is valuable when evaluating effects of brain damage on various types of communicative activities. It is also an excellent diagnostic tool for neurological conditions and can be useful in assessing recovery patterns with and without treatment interventions. Another advantage is that both fMRI and conventional MRI scans can be obtained together in a single session. This allows both structural and functional components of neurological images to be compared, yielding a rich source of correlated information. In addition, fMRI instrumentation is widely available for medical use. A disadvantage of fMRI is that the scanning process is relatively slow, because it is based on the hemodynamic response that occurs around 450 msec after the nerve has fired (Lauter, 1997). Also, the scanner is noisy, which can interfere with stimuli that are presented auditorily during speech and language tasks.

Positron Emission Tomography

Positron emission tomography (PET) is a test that examines the brain's blood flow and metabolic activity. PET is based on identifying the distribution of an injected or inhaled radioactive substance called a **tracer**, combined with a chemical such as glucose, in a patient's brain. The tracer is eliminated from the individual's body within a relatively short period of approximately 6 to 24 hours. Commonly used tracers include oxygen, nitrogen, carbon, and fluorine. The amount of accumulation of the tracer in a particular brain area depends on the degree of blood flow, which is related to the amount of neural activity in that region (Raphael et al., 2007). Areas of the brain that are more active absorb more of the tracer; less active areas absorb less. An index of regional cerebral blood flow (rCBF) is produced with this technology.

The radioactive tracer gradually disintegrates and emits positrons, which are positively charged particles. The positrons collide with electrons, producing gamma rays that are detected and measured by computers. Cross-sectional areas of the brain are scanned from many directions, producing a three-dimensional representation of the scanned area. The PET scanner rotates around the patient, providing sequences of colored three-dimensional images. The image is interpreted in terms of degree of activity of the brain regions, represented by different colors. Areas that are red indicate high levels of activity; areas that appear purple or black reflect little or no activity. Activity levels in between are represented by colors in between red and purple.

PET scans are useful for detecting tissue abnormalities such as tumors and for assessing whether tumors are benign or malignant. This technology is helpful in determining whether a brain tumor can be surgically removed.

Current PET technology allows for a much faster scanning time than in previous years, with a time of 40 s to scan the entire brain (Lauter, 1997). However, scanning time depends on the type of tracer used. Radioactive isotopes that have a longer half-life require longer scan times. The shorter the scan time, the more conditions or activities are able to be performed within a single session.

An advantage of the PET technique is the ability to make comparisons within and between individuals in terms of cognitive-related changes in blood flow. It is also possible to superimpose PET scans on MRI scans, which allows greater anatomical accuracy in correlating brain structure with brain function. There are, however, several disadvantages. One is the radiation to which the individual is exposed, which is around three times that of a conventional chest X-ray. Others are its limited availability and the need to manufacture tracer substances (Plante, 2001). In addition, compared to CT and MRI, PET produces less detailed images of the structure because of its less fine spatial resolution. Compared to MRI resolution, which can be as fine as 1 mm, PET resolution is approximately 5 mm.

Single Photon Emission Computed Tomography

Single photon emission computed tomography (SPECT) is used to examine how blood flows through the veins and arteries in the brain. SPECT is based on similar principles to PET. The major difference is in the type of radioisotope that is used. In SPECT, the radioisotope creates single photons as the isotope decays rather than gamma rays, as in PET. These photons are then measured. Like PET scans, SPECT images can also be combined with CT or MRI, allowing the correlation of brain structure with brain function. The disadvantage of SPECT technology compared to PET is the higher radiation because of the isotopes with longer half-lives that must be used (Lauter, 1997). Both techniques, however, have been used in studies to determine differences in cognitive functioning based on differences in rCBF in groups of people with and without communication disorders.

Electroencephalography and Evoked Potentials

Electroencephalography (EEG) is a technique of recording the electrical potentials generated by the brain. EEG is used to detect abnormalities related to electrical activity in the brain. It tracks and records brain wave patterns, which are typically quite recognizable. Electrodes are positioned in various locations on the surface of the person's scalp, and the potentials are detected and amplified by specialized equipment. Current EEG techniques use computers to obtain and analyze the data and allow for accurate quantification of information. These techniques are known as qEEG (quantitative EEG), and their development and use has allowed a wider collection of information from several different brain regions simultaneously. The information from several different areas can be correlated to show the degree to which different brain regions coordinate their activity during a particular task (Lauter, 1997). Colored images are also obtained from qEEG, with different colors representing different levels of activity (Kent, 1997a). The brain electrical output is analyzed by means of a Fourier analysis, which produces a display of dominant frequencies occurring within the brain during different types of activities. There are four major frequencies of brain electrical activity: alpha, beta, delta, and theta. Alpha waves have a dominant frequency of 8 to 13 Hz and occur when an individual is very relaxed. Beta wave frequency is 13 Hz or higher and occurs when an individual is paying close attention to a task. Delta waves have a frequency of less than 4 Hz, which occurs during deep sleep. Theta wave frequency is 4 to 8 Hz, occurring when a person is feeling drowsy.

A particular category of qEEG technology is known as **evoked potentials** (EP), also called *event-related potentials* (ERP). These are brain electrical potentials that occur in response to some kind of stimulus, which may be tactile, visual, or auditory. Surface electrodes on the scalp are used to obtain and analyze the brain electrical activity occurring before, during, or after the person's response. The resulting waveform typically shows several peaks and valleys. These are labeled in terms of their polarity (positive or negative) and the time in milliseconds that elapsed between their occurrence and the initial stimulus.

Many behavioral studies have been done to show the relationship between the brain electrical activity, the task that the subject is performing, and the presumed cortical or subcortical area(s) involved in the activity. One of the most-studied EPs is the P300. This is a positive peak that occurs approximately 300 msec after an auditory or visual stimulus. The stimuli are presented in an "odd-ball" paradigm, in which a few rare or unfamiliar stimuli are randomly presented within a series of standard or familiar stimuli. The peak occurs only in response to the unfamiliar stimuli. This potential has been linked to the way in which individuals process, recognize, and identify important or different stimuli. Both the latency of the P300 in terms of the time it takes for the response to occur after the initial stimulus and the amplitude of the resulting response can be measured and provide important information. An increased latency suggests that the person takes longer to process the stimulus. The amplitude of the response has been shown to increase when the stimuli are unpredictable or highly significant to the subject. Thus, this potential is considered to be an index of mental alertness and cognitive activity.

Another evoked potential is the N400, this one occurring around 400 msec after the stimulus and with a negative polarity. This potential has been shown to be linked to semantic judgment. That is, it occurs when there is a mismatch between the meaning of a sentence and the use of a particular word that does not fit with the meaning. An example is, "She went swimming in the taxi."

The readiness potential (RP) signals an upcoming motor response. The RP is a negative potential that starts to occur around one second before an actual voluntary movement and continues through the beginning portion of the movement. This potential reaches its maximum amplitude just after the movement has started to occur and is believed to index cortical preparation for movement.

The advantage of EEG and EP techniques is that they allow the timing of brain events to be recorded and interpreted in relation to a specific stimulus. The disadvantage is that because the electrical brain signals are averaged, it is difficult to specify precisely which neural structures are participating in the cognitive activity.

Transcranial Magnetic Stimulation

Transcranial magnetic stimulation (TMS) is a technique that is based on inducing weak electric currents in the brain to cause neurons to fire. A coil of wire enclosed in plastic is placed next to the individual's skull and produces a magnetic field that creates the current. The current passes through the skull and activates nearby neurons, thus enabling circumscribed areas of cortex to be stimulated (Siebner, Peller, Takano, & Conrad, 2001). This technique is noninvasive and causes little, if any, discomfort to the person (George et al., 2003). The technique was originally introduced to investigate neurotransmission along the corticospinal tract, spinal roots, and peripheral nerves in humans (Rossini & Rossi, 2007). Over the past several years, TMS has been widely used to measure neuromuscular function in the evaluation and treatment of many neurological disorders such as stroke, Parkinson's disease, and multiple sclerosis. It is also used as a treatment technique in psychiatric disorders such as depression. Findings from TMS studies could be helpful in evaluating neurosurgical approaches like deep brain stimulation (George et al., 2003). TMS can also be used in conjunction with other brain imaging techniques such as EEG, MRI and fMRI, and PET. For example, the concurrent use of TMS and EEG has been reported as a promising approach to evaluate corticocortical connectivity and brain reactivity with high temporal resolution (Rossini & Rossi, 2007).

Siebner et al. (2001) noted that a combination of TMS and functional imaging can be useful in three principal ways. First, brain imaging before TMS is helpful in defining the accurate coil position over the specific cortical area under investigation. Second, imaging the brain during the TMS procedure may be useful for assessing cortical excitability and functional connectivity within the cerebrum. Third, brain imaging after treatment with TMS can show the therapeutic effects of the procedure.

Table 12.1 lists the advantages and disadvantages of techniques for imaging brain structure and function.

Table 12.1 Advantages and Disadvantages of Various Brain Imaging Techniques

Techniques that image brain structure

	Advantages	Disadvantages
CT	Provides detailed 3D image Differentiates between tissues of different densities Short imaging time Widely available	Possible health risks from radiation
MRI	Distinguishes fine differences between soft tissues Can be used to study disordered or normal structures High degree of spatial resolution No risk of radiation	Longer imaging times than CT Cannot be used with metal devices More costly than CT

Techniques that image brain function

	Advantages	Disadvantages
fMRI	Can assess how brain function changes over time or in different situations Safe and noninvasive Can be used in conjunction with MRI	Relatively slow scanning time Scanner is noisy
PET	Good for detecting tissue abnormalities Can compare cognitive related changes in blood flow within and between individuals Can superimpose PET scans on MRI scans	Spatial resolution less than MRI and CT Possible health risks from radiation Scanning time depends on tracer
SPECT	Similar to PET	Higher radiation than PET
qEEG	Excellent temporal resolution Used to index different aspects of cognitive function	Averaging of brain electrical signals prevents precise specification of underlying neural structures
TMS	Safe and non invasive Can be used to evaluate and treat selected neurological and psychiatric disorders	No reported disadvantages

Use of Brain Imaging Techniques in Communication Disorders

The brain imaging techniques discussed in the previous section have wide applicability to disorders involving speech, language, and hearing. The diagnostic evaluation of brain function in neurological disorders such as stroke, Parkinson's disease, Alzheimer's disease, multiple sclerosis, and others has been greatly enhanced by the ability to visualize damaged and undamaged neural structures. The efficacy of treatment techniques for a particular individual can be assessed over a period of time with these tools, and comparisons can be made between different types of therapeutic interventions, including surgical, pharmacological, and behavioral treatments.

We will begin with a discussion of brain imaging techniques that have been used to examine neural function in stuttering. Although stuttering is not an overt neurological disease, it has been believed for many decades that there is a neurological component to the disorder. We will then look at some of the findings that have been reported for overt neurological diseases such as Parkinson's disease, multiple sclerosis, and Alzheimer's disease.

Stuttering

Since the 1920s, researchers have suspected that the root cause of stuttering may be some kind of neurological dysfunction. Travis, in 1928, was the first to propose that hemispheric dominance for language in people who stutter (PWS) is different than for normally fluent speakers. Normal speech production is primarily under left hemisphere control. Travis and others suggested that PWS lack this lateralized control, and that it is the lack of clear-cut dominance that results in the stuttered output. Early EEG studies in the 1980s investigated alpha brain wave activity in PWS. These studies (e.g., Boberg, Yeudall, Schopplocher, & BoLassen, 1983; Moore, 1984; Moore, 1986; Moore & Lang, 1977 et al.) did report findings that were in agreement with the idea of nondominant hemisphere lateralization in PWS for verbal tasks. What was particularly interesting was that there were reports that after intensive stuttering therapy, the alpha activity normalized (e.g., Boberg et al., 1983).

More recent studies have used PET, SPECT, and qEEG to investigate brain function in PWS. For example, Finitzo, Pool, Devous, and Watson (1991), using qEEG, found a global reduction of EEG amplitude in the beta frequency range over the right posterior temporal and bi-occipital sites. The same group of researchers (Pool et al., 1991) performed a SPECT study of rCBF in people who do and do not stutter. PWS showed reductions in blood flow compared to age- and gender-matched controls in various brain regions of interest in each hemisphere. The subjects who stuttered underwent MRIs in order to rule out any vascular problems that might reduce the blood flow. The authors suggested that the reductions may reflect metabolic or functional anomalies that somehow contribute to the stuttering.

PET studies have confirmed differences in brain activation between PWS and fluent speakers, as well differences in PWS under various speaking conditions. Ingham, Fox, and Ingham (1994) assessed brain activation during solo and choral reading. Choral reading is known to be a fluency-enhancing condition for most people who stutter. The authors reported that the nonstuttering speakers showed bilateral (left > right) activation of the primary sensorimotor cortex during both conditions. The participants who stuttered showed increased neural activity during the solo reading condition in the supplementary motor area (left > right) and the superior portion of the premotor cortex (right > left). During the choral reading condition, however, the activation of these regions was either reduced or eliminated. In a later study, Ingham, Fox, and Ingham (1997) reported a variety of differences between normally fluent speakers and PWS. For normally fluent speakers, both solo and choral reading activated brain regions including supplementary motor area, superior lateral premotor cortex, primary motor cortex for mouth, Broca's area, and cerebellum. Activations were either in the left hemisphere or bilateral. However, when the PWS were disfluent in the solo reading condition, the supplementary motor area and the superior lateral premotor cortex were considerably more active than the controls. Further, the superior lateral premotor cortex was lateralized to the right in the PWS. Similarly, the primary motor cortex in the PWS was most strongly activated in the right hemisphere. Cerebellar activation was markedly more intense in the PWS than in the fluent speakers, for both solo and choral reading. The PWS also showed activations in brain areas not seen in the fluent speakers, including the insula, lateral thalamus, and globus pallidus. However, the group of PWS showed similar activations of Broca's area as did the control subjects. The authors noted that stuttering was characterized by extensive hyperactivity of the motor system, with right hemisphere lateralization of primary and extraprimary motor cortices. Stuttering speakers showed activation of primary auditory area during speech, and this was not the case for the nonstuttering speakers. Braun et al. (1997) noted that during language formulation tasks, fluent speakers showed markedly asymmetrical cerebral activity, which lateralized to the left hemisphere. This was not the case for speakers who stuttered. During periods of disfluency, the PWS failed to activate Wernicke's area as well as other areas that are believed to be important in the formulation and expression of spoken language. Similar findings have been reported by Kroll, DeNil, Kapur, and Houle (1997) and Wu et al. (1995).

Taken together, these reports have led to a suggestion that a complex network of neural structures involved in motor control does not function normally in PWS (Buchel & Sommer, 2004). One hypothesis for the proposed motor control deficit is that there is an excessive amount of dopamine within the CNS that reduces efficient functioning of the basal nuclei (Wu et al., 1997). However, it is not clear if the increased level of dopamine is a cause or an effect of the stuttering. Clinical implications can be taken from studies like these. If stuttering, at least in some individuals, is found to be due to excessive dopamine activity, then pharmacological treatments may be effective in eliminating or reducing the motor aspects of the disorder.

Stroke

Stroke, medically known as cerebrovascular accident (CVA), is the loss of brain functions resulting from a disruption of blood supply to the brain. This can be caused by a hemorrhage (bleed), a blockage such as an embolism, or an ischemia (lack of blood). When an area of the brain is deprived of blood it ceases to function and may result in paralysis of the limbs on one side of the body and/or aphasia, a loss of language. The extent to which the brain can functionally reorganize following stroke has important implications for the rehabilitation of aphasia. Rehabilitation requires information regarding the neurological and behavioral consequences of brain damage, as well as an understanding of the impact of treatment. Current research has emphasized the potential of fMRI to address some critical questions about the rehabilitation of stroke.

Matthews, Honey, and Bullmore (2006) suggested that fMRI may help clinical researchers overcome obstacles to rehabilitating neurologically based disorders, such as aphasia. For example, rehabilitation is often quite costly and it is difficult to identify those who would benefit most from treatment and which treatment protocol would be most efficacious. Matthews et al. (2006) asserted that patterns of brain activation, relatively early after a stroke, may indicate the potential for substantial behavioral recovery. Because fMRI may detect functional changes in the brain over time, longitudinal fMRI studies administered post stroke might help predict the optimal time to administer an intensive program of rehabilitation. Another problem in rehabilitation is the limited evidence that supports a meaningful outcome. Given the heterogeneity of both the population of people who have strokes and the pathology that causes it, it is difficult to systematically test the efficacy of certain clinical protocols. There are very few randomized clinical control trials documenting the behavioral benefits of specific treatment protocols for aphasia. According to Matthews et al. (2006), fMRI is sensitive to the changes following treatment because functional systems can be objectively assessed. fMRI therefore holds great potential for substantiating the outcomes of clinical intervention with neurological populations.

Parkinson's Disease

Parkinson's disease (PD) results from a loss of dopamine in the substantia nigra of the basal nuclei. The major characteristics of this disorder include bradykinesia (slowness of movement), rigidity, and tremor. Brain imaging techniques, primarily using PET, have provided a valuable means of diagnosing and treating this disease. Studies have investigated brain metabolism in patients with PD both while on and off their medications. Researchers have reported increased metabolism for these patients in the striatum and globus pallidus (Grafton, 2004). The increased activity is consistent with the loss of neural inhibition normally provided by the dopaminergic neurons within the substantia nigra. An fMRI study by Grafton (2004) focused on patients in early stages of PD. These individuals showed reduced activation in the supplementary motor area (SMA) and the contralateral motor cortex during a simple finger movement task. Grafton (2004) noted that individuals with PD may show compensation for the decreased activity in the SMA by recruiting the lateral premotor cortex to maintain the movement, a finding that was corroborated by an fMRI showing reduced SMA activation but increased activation of the lateral premotor cortex bilaterally. With L-Dopa medication, however, the hypoactivation in the SMA normalized.

Brain imaging has also been used to identify PD before clinical symptoms have appeared. Clinical symptoms typically only emerge after the loss of dopamine cells has reached a certain level. Thus, at the time of diagnosis there is likely to be considerable degeneration of the substantia nigra, although the actual symptoms shown by the patient may be very mild (Heissa & Hilkera, 2004). Brain imaging may provide a way of differentiating PD from other neurological disorders at the early stages, as well for measuring the progression and severity of the disease (Heissa & Hilkera, 2004). This is critically important for providing the most appropriate treatment. PET and SPECT are the preferred techniques to detect loss of neurotransmitter function, as well as brain metabolism and blood flow, in patients with PD. Heissa and Hilkera (2004) reported on a PET study that showed the progression of PD in individuals by determining the amount of tracer absorbed by basal nuclei structures. As the disease progressed, a decreasing amount of the tracer was absorbed, demonstrating the decreasing amount of activation in specific basal nuclei components. There was an average decrease per year in the amount of tracer of 8 percent in the striatum and the putamen and 4 percent in the caudate region. PET studies have also been used to demonstrate the effectiveness of different drug therapies as well as of human fetal cell transplantation.

Another avenue for examining changes in PD is via the use of EPs to determine cognitive changes that occur. Cognitive decline is a major feature of PD, with some patients experiencing increasing dementia over the progression of the disease. The P300 potential is a noninvasive way of indexing cognitive function. Prabhakar, Syal, and Srivastava (2000) compared individuals with and without early PD using the P300 "odd-ball" paradigm. Patients with PD did not have any overt clinical signs of dementia. These individuals were tested before starting pharmacological treatment, after 15 days of treatment, and after 3 and 6 months of treatment. The authors found that after the 6-month interval, the P300 response was significantly increased in latency in the PD patients, showing decrements in cognitive function, even though the motor symptoms had shown improvement with treatment.

Multiple Sclerosis

Multiple sclerosis (MS) is a progressive disease that affects both the upper and lower motor neurons, but that has a very variable progression in terms of its clinical symptoms. In this disease, there is a progressive loss of myelin, which hinders the proper conduction of nerve impulses. However, the loss of motor function does not necessarily correspond to the degree of the demyelinization (Miller, Grossman, Reingold, & McFarland, 1998). This means that MRI imaging of brain structures may not provide a totally satisfactory picture of the patient's neural function, although MRI does provide an objective and direct assessment of the structural changes that continue to occur in the course of the disease. Researchers at the Dartmouth Brain Imaging Laboratory used both MRI and fMRI to examine how the brains in people with MS reorganized in terms of motor ability and memory in response to the lesion load (i.e., the total volume of brain tissue affected by the demyelinization). They reported that the brain's neural circuitry does adapt to the damage, which may account for the lack of correspondence between degree of damage and clinical symptoms.

Several investigators have shown that a series of MRIs over a time period can help to predict which individuals with clinically isolated symptoms of MS will go on to develop the full-blown disease (e.g., Brex et al., 2001; Miller et al., 1998). This is important information in order to prescribe the most appropriate drug therapy, and researchers are using MRI to determine the effectiveness of certain medications on lesion load in MS.

Alzheimer's Disease

Alzheimer's disease (AD) is a progressive neurological disease with dementia as its major hallmark. Memory and cognitive abilities decline, and in the late stages of the disease, motor dysfunction also appears. Researchers at various brain imaging labs around the United States are working to find patients at high risk for AD even before they develop symptoms (Ullrich, 2004). For example, investigators at the Medical College of Wisconsin have used fMRI to find a risk marker for AD. The marker measures small changes in blood flow in brain areas such as the hippocampus, which, as noted in Chapter 11, is a region involved in memory. Researchers at the Dartmouth Brain Imaging Lab used fMRI to measure the effects of medication on memory. The investigators found that treatment that enhances acetylcholine function can improve memory in patients with mild cognitive impairments. Thus, fMRI studies can be an effective tool in diagnosing AD before the onset of severe symptoms. This is vitally important, because memory-enhancing drugs are most effective early on in the disease (Parry & Matthews, 2002).

Brain imaging has also been useful in determining the neural correlates of other symptoms in AD, such as apathy. Apathy is defined as a lack of motivation in behavior, cognition, and affect (Benoit, Clairet, Koulibaly, Darcourt, & Robert, 2004). Benoit et al. (2004) used SPECT to determine the correlation between apathy and neural function in patients with AD and found abnormal blood flow in the frontal cortex and the anterior cingulate area. The authors noted that the anterior cingulate is important in integrating behaviors that contribute to goal-directed behavior, including emotional, sensory, and vegetative aspects of the behavior.

As well as PET, SPECT, and fMRI, event-related potentials have been used extensively over the past two decades to investigate the cognitive deterioration in AD. In particular, there is a very large body of information based on the P300 potential. For example, Szelies, Mielke, Grond, and Heiss (2002) reported that P300 latency was correlated with the degree of severity of the disease, with longer latencies associated with more severe cognitive deficits. Olichney and Hillert (2004) noted that late potentials occurring after approximately 200 msec were abnormal in patients with AD, while earlier occurring potentials that are not dependent on cognitive processing were generally intact. They suggested that using the P300 paradigm can help to quantify the effects of drugs that improve attention, such as cholinesterase inhibitors. These drugs have been shown to improve cognitive function in Alzheimer's disease (AD) and other forms of dementia (Werber, Gandelman-Marton, Klein, & Rabey, 2003). However, as noted by Werber et al. (2003), the efficacy of such treatments has primarily been based on subjective assessment methods such as standardized neuropsychological tests. The authors assessed various pharmacological treatments with the cholinesterase inhibitors tacrine and donepezil (DPZ) before the initiation of treatment and after 26 weeks of treatment, with standardized assessment tests as well as the P300 potential. The latency of the potential improved considerably in conjunction with improvements on the standardized cognitive test. In a similar study, Katada et al. (2003) investigated the effects of donepezil taken daily for 6 months by patients with AD. P300 latency was reduced after the course of treatment, with a parallel improvement on a standardized test for cognitive function in AD. Thomas, Iacono, Bonanni, D'Andreamatteo, and Onofrj (2001) likewise evaluated cholinesterase inhibitors using the P300 potential. They compared patients treated with two types of cholinesterase inhibitors (donepezil and rivastigmine) versus those treated with doses of vitamin E. Those patients treated with either of the cholinesterase inhibitors showed increases in cognitive scores accompanied by decreases in P300 latencies; patients receiving vitamin E exhibited worsening cognitive deficits and longer P300 latencies. Taken together, these results suggest that P300 latency provides very useful information on the progression of AD, especially in the longitudinal follow-up of patients undergoing treatment with cholinesterase inhibitors. The P300 potential, however, does not appear to be sensitive to the specific degree of cognitive decline. Pokryszko-Dragan, Slotwinksi, and Podemski (2003) reported that while the mean latency of P300 was significantly prolonged in the entire group of patients with mild and moderate AD, the differences did not distinguish between individuals with mild impairment and those with moderate levels of cognitive deficit. Despite this one drawback, many studies have confirmed that prolonged latencies for P300 may be an accurate, noninvasive, and reliable marker for AD. This is invaluable in the diagnosis of AD because the latency of the potential is altered in cases of early AD, while overt cognitive degeneration is not yet apparent (Fernandez-Lastra, Morales-Rodriguez, & Penzol-Dias, 2001).

Summary

Current imaging techniques that depict brain structure include computerized tomography (CT) and magnetic resonance imaging (MRI).

Brain function can be imaged with functional MRI (fMRI), positron emission tomography (PET), single photon emission computed tomography (SPECT), transcranial magnetic stimulation (TMS), and quantitative electroencephalography (qEEG).

PET and SPECT studies demonstrate differences in neural function between people who stutter and normally fluent speakers.

PET studies have been used to identify Parkinson's disease before the appearance of clinical symptoms, as well as to show the progression of the disease.

The P300 potential has been used extensively in Alzheimer's disease as a marker of cognitive function.

REVIEW EXERCISES

1. Explain the importance of obtaining brain-behavior information from healthy individuals with normal brain function, as well as from individuals with neurological diseases or disorders.

2. Identify two advantages and two disadvantages for each of the brain imaging techniques discussed in the chapter.

3. Define *hemodynamic response* and discuss the role of the response in fMRI.

4. Discuss the relationship between PET, SPECT, and rCBF.

5. Identify the characteristics of the P300 potential that make it suitable for indexing cognitive function.

6. Discuss how the theory of cerebral lateralization in stuttering has been advanced by means of current brain imaging techniques.

7. Describe three ways in which diagnosis and treatment of various neurological disorders is enhanced by brain imaging techniques.

INTEGRATIVE CASE STUDY

① Mrs. Ginsberg

Background

Rose Ginsberg, an 83-year-old woman living in an assisted-care facility, has lately been complaining that she can't find her car keys, despite the fact that she has not been driving for the past 4 years. In addition, her daughter has noticed that she has a lot of difficulty finding words and has a hard time getting to the point of a conversation. Her daughter is concerned that her mother may be showing signs of dementia and has requested that her mother be referred for a neurological exam. Fortunately, the facility is affiliated with a nearby hospital known for its team approach to diagnosis and treatment of neurological disorders.

Clinical Observations

The diagnostic protocol at the center includes a neurological exam with brain imaging techniques as appropriate, a neuropsychological exam, and a speech and language evaluation. During the evaluation, Mrs. Ginsberg appears oriented to time and place. She is somewhat agitated but cooperates with all requests.

Brain Imaging

MRI testing fails to show any structural changes to the brain. The neurologist and neuropsychologist decide to perform an evoked potential test using the P300 potential. The test reveals that P300 latency is significantly lengthened, suggesting early stages of cognitive decline. The speech and language evaluation substantiate Mrs. Ginsberg's daughter's reports of significant word-finding difficulties, short-term memory loss, difficulty with topic maintenance, and circumlocution.

Clinical Questions

a. Do you think that a pharmacological approach to this patient might be appropriate? Why or why not?

b. What would be the role of the speech–language pathologist in Mrs. Ginsberg's case?

c. If the patient is ultimately diagnosed with Alzheimer's disease, what other brain imaging techniques (if any) might be useful to document the progression of the disease?

Models and Theories of Speech Production and Perception

STUDENT LEARNING OBJECTIVES

After reading this chapter you will

○ Appreciate the differences between theories and models.

○ Understand the concept of degrees of freedom in speech production.

○ Describe some important models and theories of speech production, such as target models, feedback and feedforward models, and action theory.

○ Identify the factors that influence the perception of speech, including the lack of correspondence between linguistic and acoustic units.

○ Appreciate the link between perception and production of speech.

○ Become familiar with the motor theory of speech perception.

Models and theories are tools that help one to understand and predict the behavior or functioning of a system or some part of a system. Once one understands the various parts of a system, how they are related to each other, and how the system works as a whole, it is possible to predict how the system will work in different situations. This knowledge can then be applied to understanding how the system or any of its parts breaks down under specific conditions, possibly leading to the development of procedures to repair the system.

The systems of speech production and perception are very complex and include many separate subsystems (respiration, phonation, articulation/resonance, audition, nervous system) that must work together in a coordinated fashion. Each of these systems is composed of many structures that must also cooperate to achieve the goals and targets of the system. For example, respiration is a system comprised of numerous bones, cartilages, muscles, and other structures that work in a coordinated manner to achieve the goal of inhaling and exhaling. The phonatory system consists of the larynx with all its cartilages, muscles, membranes, and true and false vocal folds, all acting to achieve the goal of voice production. And all the systems work together to achieve the final goal: the rapid, meaningful production and perception of speech sounds to encode and decode our thoughts, ideas, and feelings in a linguistically appropriate manner.

The speech production and perception systems can break down at any point within any of the subsystems. Because these systems and subsystems are so complex, it is necessary to have theories that integrate current knowledge about them; and to make models of the systems to test and extend our knowledge about how they work, how they break down, and how breakdowns can best be compensated for or repaired. The terms *theory* and *model* are often used interchangeably, but there are important differences between the two.

Models

A model is a simplification of a system or any of its parts. Models are constructed to represent the system in some way that can then be manipulated in a controlled manner. Modeling a system can be done in numerous ways, such as fashioning a physical or mechanical version of the system to be tested, using specimens for physiological modeling, or applying mathematical and computer algorithms to the system. An example of a mechanical model is a classic one developed by Georg von Békésy, who proposed a theory of hearing based on the traveling wave along the basilar membrane in the cochlea. In his model of the cochlea, a sheet of rubber of varying thickness levels simulated the basilar membrane and was placed in a tank of water representing the endolymph within the cochlea. Waves of different frequencies were introduced into the tank. As von Békésy's theory predicted, at high frequencies the thin part of the rubber sheet vibrated with the highest amplitude, and at low frequencies the thicker part of the sheet responded with the greatest amplitude of vibration. Thus, von Békésy's model of the traveling wave provided support for his theory of hearing.

Physiological models often use specimens taken from animal or human cadavers to determine how a particular structure responds under different conditions. For example, a current theory relating to phonation states that the hydration level of the vocal folds affects vocal fold tissue viscosity. Viscosity is proportional to phonation pressure threshold (PTP), the minimum subglottal pressure required to set the vocal folds into vibration. This theory has been the basis for clinical management of some laryngeal problems in which lack of hydration of the vocal folds has been the assumed cause of increased effort in initiating vibration. Based on this assumption, patients are encouraged to increase the humidification of their environments and to drink large amounts of water. Jiang, Ng, and Hanson (1999) used excised canine larynges to test the hydration theory. The larynges were mounted on a special holder and dehydrated with warm, dry air. Air was blown through the vocal folds, causing vibration and sound production to occur, and PTP was measured. Within about 5 minutes of dehydration, vibration and sound production stopped. The larynges were then immersed in a saline solution for 30 minutes, and PTP was determined again. PTP decreased after the rehydration, allowing sound production to occur with increased efficiency. These findings confirmed clinical impressions that hydration is critical in the physiology of normal phonation.

Mathematical and computer models are an effective means of explaining phenomena and testing theories. One such model deals with the way in which neurological, biomechanical, and aerodynamic factors interact to generate jitter in the human voice. Titze (1991) was interested in teasing out the effects of neurological sources on jitter, such as the number of motor units contributing to muscular contraction and the firing rate of the motor units. The application of mathematical models to the activity of the thyroarytenoid muscle allowed Titze to hold certain parameters of muscle function constant, vary other parameters in a systematic manner, and thus isolate the effects on the resulting jitter values. In this way, Titze demonstrated that around 0.2 to 1.2 percent of jitter in the human voice seems to result from neurological sources.

Theories

A theory is a statement about a particular phenomenon, incorporating the underlying principles and assumptions. A theory is a way of interpreting facts about the phenomenon in an integrated manner. Theories help to explain observed data and information and can be used to make predictions about events related to the phenomenon in question. Because theories are based on incoming information and new research, they are always subject to change.

Theories are not just interesting from a research point of view; they also help to institute changes in practice. These changes can have far-reaching effects in the clinical domain. For example, prior to the late 1970s, most clinicians and researchers in speech pathology believed that spasmodic dysphonia (SD) had a psychological origin. The belief was based on certain aspects of the disorder, such as its resistance to traditional voice therapy, its often close association with stressful periods in a person's life, and the fact that many people with this disorder had great difficulty in normal conversational speech but were able to sing, or whisper, or talk at a higher than normal pitch without trouble. Therefore, the treatment for this disorder was often focused on a combination of speech therapy and psychological counseling. However, in the late 1970s and 1980s, data started accumulating suggesting that the cause of spasmodic dysphonia is neurological in origin. Many different speech laboratories around the United States gathered experimental data about the neurological aspects of this disorder. By about the mid-1980s, the theory of causation changed from psychogenic to neurogenic. Based on a neurogenic theory of causation, current treatment techniques have a neurological, rather than a psychological, basis. For instance, injections of Botox are often prescribed, which affects the neuromuscular functioning of the vocal folds. Botox injection has been shown to be extremely effective in alleviating the symptoms of SD in most patients, whereas previous traditional voice and psychological treatments had not, in general, been successful. Thus, research and theory interact with each other to generate new research, new theories, and new practices.

Models and theories abound in trying to explain various aspects of speech production and perception. The following discussion will focus on a select number of classic and current models and theories that attempt to account for the processes involved in production and perception of speech.

Speech Production

Speech production is a remarkably complex motor activity in which the activation of numerous muscles involved in respiration, phonation, and articulation must be coordinated and integrated at extremely rapid rates. Many structures in the respiratory, phonatory, and articulatory systems can move in different ways, at different speeds, and in different combinations. For example, the lower lip and jaw can move in phase with each other (have the same relative timing) and in the same direction; out of phase with each other (different relative timing) but in the same direction; or in phase with each other but in opposite directions (Kent, 1997a). Each different potential muscular contraction of each muscle in each system constitutes what is known as a *degree of freedom*, so the total number of possible degrees of freedom is enormous. The speech motor system must somehow regulate all the muscular contractions of all the speech subsystems to ensure that the appropriate structures are moving rapidly and in the correct sequences to generate the target sounds and words. As an example, just to say the sentence "I'm leaving for work today at 8:00" involves inhaling the appropriate volume of air using the external intercostal muscles and the diaphragm to expand the thoracic cavity and lungs; ensuring the optimal chest-wall position for exhalation by recruiting the abdominal muscles; contracting and relaxing the intrinsic muscles of the larynx in order to generate vocal fold vibration for the voiced phonemes and cease vocal fold vibration for the voiceless phonemes while simultaneously regulating pitch and loudness; opening and closing the velopharyngeal passageway at appropriate points in the utterance; and coordinating all these aspects with the movements of the articulators to generate specific phonemes. Under normal circumstances, speakers achieve this seemingly daunting feat with unthinking ease.

In addition to the intrinsic factors noted above, sounds vary with the context in which they are produced and are influenced by the speaker's dialect, rate, stress patterns, and clarity of articulation. Further, coarticulation results in enormous variability in the production of a target sound. A given speech sound often can be produced in several different ways, and this variability in production is a central factor in speech motor regulation.

There are numerous models and/or theories that attempt to explain the processes involved in speech production, including target models, feedback/feedforward models, and action theory. Components of these models/theories tend to overlap.

Spatial and Articulatory Target Models

Target models describe speech production as a physical specification of a planned phonological unit such as a syllable or word (Tatham & Morton, 2011). Targets have been hypothesized to be either spatial (articulatory) or acoustic (auditory). Spatial models posit that there is an internalized map of the vocal tract in the brain that allows the speaker to move his or her articulators to specific regions within the vocal tract. The speaker can achieve the targets no matter from what position the articulator(s) begin(s) the movement. The fact that articulators must reach a particular position from different starting points is important, because it means that the movements of the articulator for a specific sound cannot be invariant, but must change depending on the starting point. For example, to achieve the velar target for the /k/ sound, the tongue would have to move in a different trajectory depending on the preceding vowel. The path of the tongue would vary depending on whether the preceding vowel was /a/ (low back), /u/ (high back), or /i/

(high front). Spatial models propose that a series of spatial targets are specified in advance by the speaker's brain, with feedback coming from the articulators back to the brain to regulate the fine movements and correct any errors.

In acoustic–auditory models the goal to be achieved is the acoustic output; the articulatory movements used to achieve the acoustic output may vary. Thus, a speaker may use different articulatory movements to achieve a particular speech sound, depending on factors such as the adjacent sounds, the speaker's rate of speech, and different patterns of stress.

Both articulatory and acoustic targets form the basis for a framework presented by Perkell, Matthies, Svirsky, and Jordan (1995) to explain the segmental (phonetic) aspects of speech production. In their framework, morphemes and words consist of sequences of segments, characterized by combinations of what the authors call *contrast-defining features*. These features form the input to the speech motor programming system and specify how the articulators are to be moved or positioned and/or what acoustic properties are to be achieved by these movements. The generation of a segment usually requires the coordination of movements of several articulators. In the case of a consonant, the segmental description specifies the major articulator (such as the lips, tongue blade, or tongue body) and its positioning, which forms a constriction in the vocal tract. Other features specify the action of secondary articulators (such as the glottis and velum). The movements of the secondary articulators must be coordinated with the timing of the primary articulation. The ultimate goals of the articulatory movements are acoustic patterns that will enable the listener to understand what is said. However, for the speaker's production mechanism, the goals are defined as regions in acoustic and articulatory space. For example, in the utterance /uku/, the acoustic goal for the /u/ may be a region in formant frequency space, and its articulatory goal may be information related to the configuration of the vocal tract. The /k/ has several acoustic goals, including a silent interval and a burst of aperiodic noise. The articulatory goals may be to have the tongue body produce a complete closure with adequate force in the velopalatal region and to build up enough intraoral air pressure to produce a noise burst at the moment of release. Perkell et al. (1995) noted that the features may be modified in terms of the sizes and locations of their regions in articulatory and acoustic space, depending on context and suprasegmental aspects. For instance, if the sequence /uku/ were embedded in a word, the target region of formant values for the /u/ might be reduced toward those of a more neutral vowel, and the force of contact for the /k/ might be less. Control of the relative timing of articulatory movements around the acoustic landmarks is programmed, in the model, by a mechanism that uses an internal model of relations among commands to the articulators, their movements, and the acoustic consequences of those movements. The internal model is acquired and maintained with the use of auditory and somatosensory feedback from the articulators (i.e., tactile and proprioceptive feedback). Once speech has been learned, however, auditory feedback is not used in the online, moment-to-moment control of articulatory movements. Somatosensory feedback probably is used online, moment to moment, but at lower levels in a hierarchically organized system of speech motor control. One important purpose of this hierarchical organization is to reduce the number of degrees of freedom that has to be controlled by higher levels.

Feedback and Feedforward Models

Feedback refers to the transfer of part of the output of a system back to the input to regulate and correct any errors in the output. In terms of voluntary movement, a motor activity is monitored while it is in process, and any deviations from the intended task are corrected based on sensory information derived from the task (Tourville, Reilly, & Guenther, 2008). There are four stages involved in feedback of motor control: In the first stage, a movement error is detected by comparing the intended sensory goal with actual somatosensory information about the movement; during the second stage, a neural command to correct the movement is generated; the third stage involves the transmission of the corrective command to the muscles; and contraction of the muscles to correct the movement comprises the fourth stage (Perkell, 2010). The somatosensory feedback includes information about touch, tissue contact, muscle length, rates of change of muscle length, muscle tension, and joint angle (Perkell, 2010). This information is transmitted by sensory nerve fibers from peripheral receptors in the vocal tract and larynx to the central nervous system. In terms of speech production, the output is the articulatory or acoustic signal. As an individual speaks, he or she hears the output through the auditory system, and also obtains information about the movements of the articulators through proprioceptive, kinesthetic, and tactile channels. For example, the output signal may be a specific movement or position of the tongue. Information about the movement is sent to the brain by the feedback loop, including feedback from sensory receptors for touch, position, and movement. The output sent to the brain is compared with the intended movement. If there is a discrepancy between the actual and intended movements, an error signal is generated and sent back to the periphery (i.e., the appropriate muscles) to correct the problem. The feedback operation takes place by means of a neural mechanism called the **gamma loop**. Gamma nerve fibers conduct nerve signals away from muscles toward the spinal cord, while alpha nerve fibers bring nerve signals to muscles. Gamma nerve fibers synapse within the spinal cord with alpha nerve fibers and do not proceed to higher brain centers. Because the operation is automatic, without any cognitive processing, the speed of feedback is enhanced (Tatham & Morton, 2011).

While feedback is clearly an important aspect of speech motor control, there are two major factors that suggest that feedback alone is not enough to control speech production. First, feedback channels tend to be relatively slow, whereas the movements involved in speech production are extremely rapid. By the time an articulatory or auditory error has been detected, the speaker will have already moved on to a different sound. Second, if speech were purely under feedback control, disruption of feedback channels should have a serious effect on speech production. Many experimenters have used different methods to interfere with normal feedback, such as the application of topical anesthesia to target articulators, nerve blocks, noise masking to prevent auditory feedback, and bite blocks of various sizes to immobilize the jaw. Most of these studies have shown that speech is minimally affected, if at all, by these types of disruptions. Normal speakers compensate extremely well for disruptions, and typically the compensation occurs almost instantaneously.

Whereas feedback models depend on a time delay during which the signals from the periphery (i.e., vocal tract) return to a central processor in the brain for comparison of the intended and the actual movements, feedforward signals make adjustments at the periphery so that the system is primed to move in an efficient, coordinated manner. Feedforward models assert that the performance of a motor task is based on previously learned commands, so the individual does not have to rely on sensory information during the task in order to make corrections (Tourville et al., 2008). Being able to predict the sensory consequences of speaking allows for the outcome of any articulatory action to be estimated and used before the actual sensory feedback becomes available (Christoffels, van de Ven, Waldorp, Formisano, & Schiller, 2011). This process depends on the interaction between the motor and sensory systems in which the prediction of sensory consequences of motor commands is compared to the actual sensory feedback, and mismatches between actual and predicted signals are neurally encoded (Christoffels et al., 2011). Feedforward is therefore a much faster process, which may help to explain why disruptions such as bite blocks do not have much of an effect on speech production.

It is likely that both feedback and feedforward are used in the control and regulation of speech production. Feedback control is used as the young child learns the correspondences between the acoustic and articulatory aspects of speech sounds, and relies on both auditory and somatosensory information to establish these links. Feedback control and regulation may also be used more in suprasegmental aspects of speech production such as intonation, vocal intensity, and speaking rate (Perkell, 2010). Once speech has fully developed, feedforward motor programs become habitual, and feedforward control becomes primary (Golfinopoulos et al., 2011; Perkell, 2010). However, feedback is available when necessary to correct and detect errors (Perkell, 2010). If errors persist over a number of repetitions, the corrective commands become incorporated into future feedforward commands. This is the mechanism by which feedforward commands are learned and refined (Perkell, 2010).

The DIVA Model

Both feedback and feedforward components are included in the Directions Into Velocities of Articulators (DIVA) model. This model is based on the relationships among sensory targets, brain activity, speech motor output, and the resulting auditory and somatosensory sensations (Perkell, 2010). DIVA allows for the quantification of the neuroanatomical interactions between cortical motor, somatosensory, and auditory brain regions that are active during speech (Guenther & Vladusich, 2009). Consequently, it is possible to directly compare the activity of model components in computer simulations of perturbed and unperturbed speech to speakers performing the same tasks during magnetic resonance imaging procedures (Tourville et al., 2008). Such comparisons have demonstrated strong correspondences between computer predictions and actual speaker responses to various perturbations to speech. The model has demonstrated that auditory goals are strongest during early learning of speech, and these goals actively shape the feedforward commands. Once the feedforward commands are available and a somatosensory target is learned, then the target itself becomes part of the process (Perkell, 2010). The somatosensory target represents the expected tactile and proprioceptive sensations associated with the sound (Guenther & Vladusich, 2009). During the initial development of speech motor control, command signals in the feedforward control loop are updated on each attempt by the child to produce the sound, using the auditory feedback from that attempt. This results in a more accurate feedforward command for the next attempt, and eventually the feedforward command by itself is sufficient to produce the sound in normal circumstances (Guenther & Vladusich, 2009). The model has also demonstrated that feedforward control appears to be predominantly regulated by the left hemisphere, while auditory feedback control is mainly controlled in the frontal areas of the right hemisphere (Tourville et al., 2008).

The DIVA model has been used to explain maintenance of or disruptions to speech motor control. For example, it can explain how postlingually deafened speakers typically maintain high levels of speech intelligibility despite the loss of auditory feedback. According to the model, the speaker maintains intelligibility because his or her feedforward system is intact, although some deterioration in the feedforward commands may occur (Perkell, 2010). The model also suggests how damage to motor areas in the left hemisphere (e.g., stroke) is more likely to disrupt stored feedforward speech motor commands and hinder the production of fluent speech (Tourville et al., 2008). This is commonly seen in individuals with Broca's aphasia. Stuttering is another area that may be at least partly explained by the model. It has been hypothesized that people who stutter may have poor feedforward control for speech and therefore tend to rely excessively on the slower auditory feedback system (Max, Guenther, Gracco, Ghosh, & Wallace, 2004).

Action Theory

Action theory is a goal-oriented theory of motor activity based on the notion of **coordinative structures**. Coordinative structures refer to groups of muscles that link up together to perform a particular task. The linkages between muscles are not fixed: A muscle might be grouped with a particular set of muscles to achieve one particular goal, and with a different set of muscles in a different coordinative structure to achieve a different goal. A central feature of the theory is that for any specific motor task, the motor cortex does not specify the individual muscles involved in the activity but rather issues gross instructions (Tatham & Morton, 2011). Based on the instructions an appropriate coordinative structure is selected, comprising a set of muscles that form an integrated unit focused on achieving the specified activity. The different muscular responses in a coordinative structure can be adjusted to meet the requirements of a particular task under different conditions. For example, the lip and jaw muscles function as a coordinative unit in bilabial closure. Typically, the lip and jaw muscles cooperate to close the lips. However, if the person has a bite block clamped between his or her teeth to immobilize the lower jaw, the upper and lower lips can compensate by increasing the force or extent of their movement. If the lips cannot move for some reason, the jaw by itself can bring the lips together. This theory allows for a great deal of flexibility in the organizational linkages between muscles and structures.

Speech Perception

Speech perception is an active cognitive process in which the listener recognizes and interprets incoming acoustic signals (Tatham & Morton, 2011). Perception depends on many factors, including the listener's ability to recognize the phonemes, syllables, and prosodic patterns of his or her language; the individual's knowledge of the phonological, syntactic, semantic, and pragmatic features of his or her language; and the person's ability to detect and interpret the emotional content of a message (Tatham & Morton, 2011). The clarity of the signal and the context of the activity also influence how speech is perceived. A further layer of complexity is that although the output of speech is a continuously varying waveform, the linguistic elements that make up speech are produced in a serial order. The order is important for meaning: Although the phonemes /k/, /t/, and /æ/ are used in the words *cat*, *tack*, and *act*, the order in which they are produced determines how the word will be perceived and recognized. Linguistically, speech is a sequence of elements. The question is precisely which elements are serialized. The elements could be specific features of a sound (e.g., voicing or nasality), phonemes, syllables, parts of syllables, or other larger or smaller elements.

Speech perception is not based on a linear correspondence between the acoustic speech signal and the linguistic phonemic units that are perceived by an individual (Goldstein, Pouplier, Chen, Saltzman, & Byrd, 2007; Tatham & Morton, 2011). One reason for the lack of correspondence is that acoustic characteristics of a given phoneme vary depending on context. The /k/ in /ku/, for example, will have somewhat different acoustic features than the /k/ in /ki/. The same has been shown to be true for the /d/ in /di/ versus /du/. A rising F_2 transition in /di/ and a falling one in /du/ both serve as acoustic cues for /d/.

Another example of the role of context in the recognition of specific phonemes is the frequency of stop bursts. Depending on context, burst frequency signals different places of articulation. Research has shown that when a burst is centered at 1440 Hz it is heard as /pi/ before /i/ and /u/, but as /k/ before /a/. Also, because of coarticulation, information is present about the acoustic properties of a specific phoneme, as well as the phonemes that precede and follow it. Consequently, although one perceives speech as a series of separate and distinct phonemes and words, the acoustic boundaries between phonemes are blurred. Listeners, thus, must somehow transform a continuously varying acoustic wave into categories of separate sounds, syllables, words, and connected speech. Decoding a spoken message involves the analysis of various-sized components of the signal, including acoustic, phonetic, phonological, lexical, suprasegmental, syntactic, and semantic components. Listeners have been shown to be flexible in the strategies they use to process auditory information based on the information available to them in the signal and the information available from their store of linguistic knowledge (Nygaard & Pisoni, 1995). Speakers seem to plan their utterances as a string of segments, while listeners try to use all available cues within the signal to decode the acoustic signal into a sequence of appropriate linguistic labels (Tatham & Morton, 2011).

Much research effort has been expended on the question of the basic unit of perception. Do listeners perceive acoustic–phonetic features, allophones, phonemes, syllables, or larger units of speech? This question remains an issue, although each of these units has some evidence in its support. It may be that individuals rely more on one kind of unit than another depending on the situation and context of the speech to be perceived. For example, in a quiet listening environment with no competing noise such as background party noise or work-related noise, listeners may pay more attention to smaller units and rely less on the syllabic structure of speech to perceive meaningful information. In a noisy situation, the person may be forced to process at a higher level of linguistic information to supplement and facilitate acoustic–phonetic recognition.

A listener's stage of development may play a role in how he or she processes acoustic information. There is evidence that infants and young children may process auditory information using larger units such as syllables, whereas older children and adults may rely more on smaller units such as phonemes. Children appear to go through a developmental weighting shift, in which their perceptual strategies change with increasing linguistic experience (Nittrouer, 1996a). Very young children seem to focus more on syllables to process speech information, because with their limited lexicons they do not need to process auditory information at a more detailed level. As the child's lexicon increases, so too does the need for more detailed acoustic–phonetic representation of words to discriminate between the greater number of similar words in the child's memory.

Nittrouer (1996a) suggested that mature language users appear to weight the various components of the signal in ways that they know will lead to correct decisions about phoneme identity, that is, by focusing on the spectral characteristics of the sound wave. Young children focus more on formant transitions between syllables to divide the acoustic signal into syllabic units. As the child matures, he or she begins to weight the more static and more detailed components of the signal more heavily.

Another factor that is central to the issue of speech perception is the link between the production and perception of speech. A substantial amount of recent research has demonstrated that the motor system can modify how a listener perceives specific auditory cues (e.g., Sato et al., 2011; Watkins, Strafella, & Paus, 2003); conversely, perception can influence the production of sounds. This notion will be discussed more fully in the following section on motor theory.

Motor Theory

An early and still very influential theory of speech perception is the motor theory, developed at the Haskins Laboratory at Yale University in the 1950s. Motor theory is an active theory that stresses the link between perception and production of speech. In essence, according to this theory, an individual perceives speech because he or she produces speech. Because listeners have experience in producing speech sounds themselves, they are aware, at some level, of the relationship between movements of the articulators, vocal tract configurations, and the acoustic consequences of articulator movements and positions.

The older version of motor theory assumes that speech perception is unique, relying on a special processor located somewhere in the brain to decode speech. Another assumption of the older version is that there are unchanging, invariant motor commands in the form of neural signals to the articulators to produce the same phoneme in different phonetic contexts. Research, however, does not support many of the assumptions of the original motor theory. For instance, Peter Eimas and colleagues (e.g., Eimas, Miller, & Jusczyk, 1987) carried out research demonstrating that prelingual infants up to about 10 months of age are able to discriminate not only the phonemes of their ambient language, but the phonetic contrasts between most of the sounds in most of the world's languages. Clearly, infants do not have experience in producing phonemes and are not aware of how phonemes are produced by the articulators. The fact that infants are not able to produce the sounds that they can perceive contradicts the basic tenet of motor theory.

The motor theory has recently been revised. In the revised theory the acoustic signal is thought to be perceived in terms of articulatory gestures that individuals are innately able to perceive, such as tongue backing and lip rounding. The listener does not, however, perceive the actual movements but an abstract articulatory plan (called a **gesture**) that controls the vocal tract movements (Hawkins, 1999b). Hawkins (1999b) defined a gesture as one of a family of movement patterns that all achieve the same goal, such as a particular constriction in the vocal tract (e.g., bilabial closure). Gestures for speech can be thought of as the basic units of speech production, which control and coordinate the cooperative activity of the articulators. The gestures are neuromotor commands that are specific to speech. They are phonetic in character, invariant, and accessible only in the specialized phonetic module in the brain. The theory proposes that listeners somehow retrieve the intended gesture for the underlying phoneme from the variable acoustic signal by compensating for the effects of coarticulation.

In recent years, evidence has been accumulating that supports some of the features of motor theory. For example, anatomical and functional connections have been discovered between the speech perception and production systems, which allow the motor system to be accessed online during the speech perception process (Schwartz, Basirat, Ménard, & Sato, 2010). It has been shown that information is transmitted in both directions between the sensory and motor regions of the brain, and between brain areas that underlie production of speech in the anterior regions and perception of speech in the posterior regions (D'Ausilio, Craighero, & Fadiga, 2010; Watkins, Strafella, & Paus, 2003). Watkins et al. (2003) reported that when individuals either listened to speech or visually observed speech-related lip movements, the motor units involved with the motor aspects of speech production demonstrated enhanced excitability. This was particularly apparent in the left hemisphere.

The discovery of a class of neurons called *mirror neurons* has helped to explain the link between speech perception and production. Mirror neurons provide the neuroanatomical link between perception and production by matching observed actions to corresponding areas of the observer's motor cortex, including the primary motor cortex, premotor cortex, and supplementary motor area (Scott,

McGettigan, & Eisner, 2009; Tremblay & Small, 2011). These neurons fire during both execution and observation of actions (Iacoboni, 2008; Tremblay & Small, 2011). In terms of speech, the same neural circuits are activated during both perception and production of a syllable or word (Scott et al., 2009; Tremblay & Small, 2011). This co-activation has been corroborated by brain imaging studies, which indicate that the primary motor cortex including portions of Broca's area demonstrate mirror system properties (Callan, Callan, Gamez, Sato, & Kawato, 2010). Results of brain imaging experiments have shown that when an individual sees or hears presented syllables and words, areas in the motor cortex are activated in addition to areas in the temporal lobe associated with hearing and understanding (D'Ausilio, Craighero, & Fadiga, 2010). Schwartz et al. (2010) reported that brain areas involved in the planning and execution of speech gestures (i.e., left inferior frontal gyrus, ventral premotor, and primary motor cortices) and areas involved in proprioception related to mouth movements (i.e., somatosensory cortex) are activated during auditory, visual, and/or auditory/visual speech perception. Thus, speech perception appears to be based on the integration of sensory and motor information that involves both superior temporal and premotor cortex (Iacoboni, 2008).

Not only does evidence suggest a strong connection between motor activity and perception, but the motor response is stronger when the recorded muscle and the presented speech stimulus involve the same articulator (Sato, Buccino, Gentilucci, & Cattaneo, 2010; Yuen, Davis, Brysbaert, & Rastle, 2010). D'Ausilio et al. (2009) used transcranial magnetic stimulation while subjects heard labial or alveolar phonemes. Reportedly, participants' recognition of phonemes was faster when the corresponding brain region regulating the articulator involved in the sound was stimulated; perception was slower when the articulator region and the sound were not concordant. Scott et al. (2009) reported that speech sounds with different places of articulation (e.g., /p/ and /t/) differentially activated the motor areas that are associated with different articulators, resulting in differential patterns of motor cortex response to /p/ and /t/. Studies by D'Ausilio et al. (2009), Devlin and Aydelott (2008), and Meister et al. (2007) have also shown that the activation of the motor system during speech perception is involved in discriminating specific phonemes.

The relationship between production and perception may be stronger when there is some kind of interference with the perceptual task. This was demonstrated by D'Ausilio, Bufalari, Salmas, and Fadiga (2011), who compared the performance of subjects discriminating between syllables in a noisy (masking noise) and non-noisy context. Their results suggested that the motor cortex may play a more significant role in speech perception when the stimuli are degraded or under adverse listening conditions, and that the contribution of the motor system may be to improve perception in noisy situations. The fact that high levels of speech perception ability are present in individuals with acquired damage or complete deactivation of the motor speech system, in healthy infants who have not yet acquired speech, and in nonhuman animals supports this position (e.g., Hickok, Costanzo, Capasso, & Miceli, 2011).

Summary

A theory is a statement about a particular phenomenon, incorporating underlying principles, facts, and assumptions.

Theories change based on incoming research and effect practice.

A model is a simplification of a system that can be manipulated in a controlled manner.

Models can be mechanical, physiological, mathematical, or computer based.

Numerous theories of speech production have been proposed, including target models, feedback and feedforward models, action theory, and others.

Target models describe speech as a series of either spatial or acoustic–auditory targets that a speaker attempts to achieve.

Feedback is used to detect and correct errors in speech output; feedforward signals are used to make articulatory adjustments online.

Coordinative structures refer to flexible groupings of muscles that may change depending on the particular speech output goal.

Motor theory emphasizes the link between speech production and speech perception in terms of articulatory gestures that individuals are innately able to perceive.

Mirror neurons have been proposed to act as the neuroanatomical linkage between speech perception and production.

REVIEW EXERCISES

1. Differentiate between models and theories and give an example of each to illustrate your points.

2. Explain what is meant by the problem of degrees of freedom and give an example from an area of speech production.

3. List the critical elements in Perkell's articulatory and acoustic target framework of speech production.

4. Describe the DIVA model. Do you think this model provides a convincing explanation of speech production? Why or why not?

5. Explain why the lack of acoustic and linguistic correspondence is a major issue in speech perception.

6. Elaborate on the main aspects of motor theory, including the recent discovery of mirror neurons.

Glossary

Absolute refractory period Brief period following an action potential during which the nerve cannot fire, no matter how strong the stimulation.

Absorption Damping of a wave.

Accelerated speech Speech that sounds excessively rapid, often occurring in Parkinson's disease.

Accessory muscles of respiration Muscles of the rib cage, back, and neck that may contribute to respiration depending on bodily demands.

Acetylcholinesterase Enzyme that degrades the neurotransmitter acetylcholine into its component chemicals.

Acoustic-admittance meter See *tympanometer*.

Acoustic reflex Middle ear reflex that attenuates intense sounds of 80 dB or more; also called the *stapedial reflex*.

Acoustic resonator Air-filled container in which the air is forced to vibrate in response to another vibration.

Action potential (AP) Wave of depolarization that travels along the length of an axon.

Additive noise Noise in the vocal signal; also called *spectral noise.*

Adductor spasmodic dysphonia Neurological voice disorder characterized by vocal fold spasms.

Admittance Measure of how easily energy is transmitted through a system, measured in siemens in the modern metric system (formerly milliohms).

Afferent Sensory nerve that transmits information from sensory receptors toward the central nervous system.

Alveolar ducts Openings of the respiratory bronchioles leading into an alveolus.

Alveolar pressure Pressure of the air within the alveoli of the lungs.

Alveolar ridge Anterior portion of the hard palate formed by the alveolar processes of the maxilla.

Alveoli Microscopic thin-walled structures within the lungs filled with air.

Amplitude Amount of displacement of an object from its rest position.

Amplitude perturbation Cycle-to-cycle variability in vocal fold amplitude; also called *shimmer*.

Amygdala Structure of the limbic system involved in learning and memory.

Amyotrophic lateral sclerosis Progressive neurological disease affecting all voluntary muscles.

Anterior commissure Location on the thyroid cartilage forming the anterior attachment of the vocal folds.

Anterior corticospinal tract Motor nerve pathway formed by the fibers of the corticospinal tract that do not decussate at the medulla but that synapse ipsilaterally with neurons in the anterior horns of the spinal cord.

Anticipatory coarticulation The modification of a sound by the preceding sound.

Antiformant See *antiresonance*.

Antiresonance Type of acoustic filtering that results in frequencies within a bandwidth being attenuated rather than amplified; on a spectrogram, looks like a very weak formant.

Aperiodic Without a period. An aperiodic wave is a wave in which cycles do not take the same amount of time to occur.

Aphonia Complete absence of voice.

Aponeurosis Broad, flat sheet of tendon.

Applied (or driving) frequency Frequency that acts as an input to a resonator.

Apraxia Difficulty sequencing articulatory movements for speech.

Arachnoid mater Middle layer of the meninges.

Articulatory overshoot Situation in which articulators make contact with excessive force.

Articulatory undershoot Situation in which articulators fail to achieve the appropriate articulatory target.

Aryepiglottic folds Folds of connective tissue and muscle fibers running from the sides of the epiglottis to the apex of the arytenoid cartilages.

Arytenoid adduction Surgical technique to rotate the arytenoid cartilages to improve glottal closure.

Arytenoid cartilages Paired cartilages of the larynx that form a joint with the cricoid cartilage.

Aspiration Noise generated by turbulence as air moves through the glottis.

Association nuclei Thalamic nuclei that receive and transmit nerve impulses to and from broad cortical areas.

Astrocytes Most common type of glial cell in the nervous system, with projections that connect to blood capillaries and transport nutrients from the blood to the nerve cell.

Attenuation rate Rate, in decibels per octave, at which a resonator's amplitude of response is attenuated. Also known as *roll-off rate*, *rejection rate*, and *slope*.

Audibility Refers to whether a specific speech cue is presented at a level that a hearing-impaired person can hear.

Audiogram Graph that represents an individual's hearing thresholds at selected frequencies.

Auditory area Graph that represents the limits of human hearing in terms of frequency and amplitude.

Axon Projection off the cell body that transmits impulses away from the cell body.

Backward coarticulation An upcoming sound influencing the preceding sound.

Band-pass filter Resonator that transmits acoustic energy in a range of frequencies between an upper and a lower cutoff frequency.

Band-stop filter Resonator that attenuates frequencies within a certain range.

Bandwidth Range of frequencies that a resonator will transmit.

Basilar membrane Base of the cochlear duct; basal portion nearest the tympanic membrane is narrow and stiff, with the membrane becoming wider and more compliant toward the apical portion farthest from the tympanic membrane.

Bernoulli principle Aerodynamic law which states that air flowing through a constriction increases in velocity and decreases in pressure.

Biphasic closure Type of vocal fold closing pattern commonly seen in pulse register; characterized by partial closure, followed by opening, and then full closure.

Botox injection Procedure in which minute amounts of botulinum toxin are injected into the vocal folds to alleviate spasms.

Boyle's law Law which states that a volume varies inversely with pressure, given a constant temperature.

Bradykinesia Difficulty and/or slowness in initiating movements.

Breath group Utterance produced on one exhalation.

Breathiness Vocal quality that sounds aspirated due to air loss and turbulence at the glottis.

Broadly tuned Resonator that transmits a wide range of frequencies.

Bronchi Structures that branch off the trachea and enter the lungs; part of the lower respiratory system.

Bronchial tree Part of the respiratory system that includes the trachea, bronchi, and bronchioles.

Bronchioles Smallest subdivisions of the bronchial system.

Brownian motion Random high-speed movement of molecules due to their inherent energy.

Carryover coarticulation A preceding sound in an utterance modifies an ensuing sound; also called *left-to-right coarticulation*.

Cartilaginous glottis Posterior two-fifths of the glottis; bounded by vocal processes.

Caudate nucleus Part of the basal nuclei.

Center frequency Same as natural, or resonant, frequency.

Central sulcus Groove on the cortex that divides the brain into anterior and posterior portions.

Central tendon Flat sheet of tendon in the center portion of the diaphragm.

Cerebellar peduncles Three nerve pathways (inferior, middle, superior) connecting the cerebellum to the brain stem and thalamus.

Cerebral peduncles Large bundles of nerve pathways in the midbrain that form a continuation of the internal capsule.

Cerebrospinal fluid (CSF) Clear fluid within the subarachnoid space that circulates around the brain and spinal cord.

Cerumen Waxy substance produced in the external auditory meatus.

CGS system Metric measurement in which c = centimeters, g = grams, and s = seconds.

Chest wall shape Positioning of the chest wall for speech production.

Chest wall system Part of the respiratory system that includes the rib cage, abdomen, and diaphragm.

Choroid plexus cells Specialized cells within the ventricles that produce cerebrospinal fluid.

Cilia Tiny hairlike projections within parts of the respiratory system, such as the trachea and nasal cavities, that help to filter the incoming air.

Circle of Willis A roughly circular-shaped configuration of arteries that provide blood to the brain; made up of the internal carotid and vertebral arteries as well as branches of these vessels.

Clavicular breathing Breathing pattern in which the shoulders are raised on inspiration, producing strain in the neck and laryngeal areas.

Closed quotient (CQ) EGG measure based on the ratio of the closed phase of the duty cycle to the period of the entire cycle.

Closed-to-open ratio (C/O ratio) EGG measure based on the difference in time between the closing and opening phases of the duty cycle, divided by the duration of the closed phase.

Coarticulation Overlapping of articulatory movements in time so that acoustic characteristics of adjacent sounds influence each other.

Cochlea Snail-shaped spiral canal housing the nerve receptors for hearing.

Cochlear duct Structure that divides the cochlea along most of its length; also called the *cochlear partition*.

Cognates Pairs of sounds with the same manner and place of articulation but differing in voicing.

Complex sound Sound with two or more frequencies.

Compliance The ease with which a body can be displaced or deformed.

Compression Area of positive pressure.

Conductive hearing loss Hearing loss caused by problems in the transmission of sound to the inner ear.

Consonant-to-vowel amplitude ratio Relationship of the amplitude of a consonant to the adjacent vowel.

Constructive interference Waves that combine and increase the amplitude of the resulting wave.

Contact index (CI) EGG measure based on the ratio of the difference in time between closing and opening phases, divided by the duration of the closed phase.

Contact quotient See *closed quotient*.

Continuous spectrum Spectrum that depicts aperiodic sound with an envelope that connects all the frequencies in the sound.

Coordinative structures Functional linkages between muscles working in synergy to achieve an objective.

Corner vowels Vowels produced with the tongue as far as possible from the neutral tongue position; represent the limits of vowel articulation.

Corniculate cartilages Paired cartilages located at the apex of the arytenoid cartilages.

Corona radiata Large mass of myelinated nerve fibers from many different brain areas that diverge and flare out in a fan shape as they travel toward the cerebral cortex.

Corpus callosum Thick band of white matter nerve pathways connecting the right and left hemispheres of the brain.

Cover–body model Model of the vocal folds that describes their layered structure and different levels of stiffness.

Cricoarytenoid joints Joints involved in adduction and abduction of the vocal folds.

Cricoid cartilage Unpaired ring of cartilage forming the inferior portion of the larynx.

Cricopharyngeus muscle Muscle located at the inferior border of the pharynx.

Cricothyroid (CT) Intrinsic muscle of the larynx composed of oblique and erect parts; elongates and tenses the vocal folds.

Cricothyroid joints Joints involved in lengthening and shortening the vocal folds to regulate F_0.

Cricotracheal membrane Sheet of membrane that connect the cricoid cartilage to the trachea.

Crossover Perceptual boundary between two sounds on an acoustic continuum; related to categorical perception.

Cuneiform cartilages Small elastic cartilages embedded in the aryepiglottic folds.

Cutoff frequency Frequency at which a resonant system is unresponsive.

Cycles per second Number of cycles of vibration occurring in one second, equivalent to frequency.

Damping Decrease in amplitude.

Dead air Small amount of air not involved in oxygen–carbon dioxide exchange.

Decibel (dB) scale A logarithmic ratio scale that compares the amplitude and/or intensity of a target sound to a standard reference sound.

Deep brain stimulation (DBS) Surgical technique designed to reduce rigidity and tremors resulting from neurological disorders.

Dendrites Projections from the nerve cell body that transmit impulses toward the cell body.

Density Mass of a substance, a material, or an object per unit of volume.

Depolarization Brief reversal of electrical charge within a neuron, going from negative (270 mV) to positive (30 mV).

Destructive interference Waves that combine and decrease the amplitude of the resulting wave.

Developmental dyslexia Disorder in which a person's reading ability is significantly lower than what would be predicted on the basis of age and intellectual ability.

Diaphragm Muscle that makes up the floor of the thoracic cavity and is instrumental in respiration.

Diffraction Change in direction of a wave as it travels around an obstacle.

Diplophonia Perception of two simultaneous pitches in a person's voice.

Direct (pyramidal) system Motor system comprising the corticospinal and corticonuclear nerve tracts; involved in the control of fine, skilled voluntary movements.

Distocclusion Condition in which the mandible is retracted due to abnormal occlusion.

Dopamine Inhibitory neurotransmitter deficient in Parkinson's disease.

Dorsal horns Posterior portion of the gray matter of the spinal cord made up of nerve cell bodies that receive sensory information.

Driving pressure Difference between high- and low-pressure areas that causes air to flow between these areas.

Dura mater Outermost layer of the meninges; made up of periosteal and meningeal parts.

Duration Length of time a speech sound lasts.

Duty cycle Phases of a vocal fold vibratory cycle, including closing, closed, opening, and open.

Dyne Unit of measure of force and pressure.

Dysarthria Term for a group of speech production disorders in which the speech musculature is weak, paralyzed, or uncoordinated.

Dysphonia Any kind of vocal dysfunction resulting in a deviant-sounding voice.

Dyspnea Subjective sensation of difficulty and/or discomfort during breathing.

Efferent Motor nerve that transmits information from the nervous system to muscles and glands.

Elasticity Restoring force that brings an object back to its original size, shape, or position after having been displaced or deformed.

Electroglottography (EGG) Method of evaluating vocal fold function based on the difference between electrical conductivity of tissue and air; also called *laryngography.*

End-expiratory level (EEL) Endpoint of a normal quiet exhalation, equal to resting expiratory level.

End-plate potential (EPP) Small graded depolarization of a muscle fiber.

Endolymph Fluid within the membranous canal of the cochlea.

Endotracheal intubation Process in which a breathing tube is inserted into the trachea through the larynx.

Envelope Line that connects the frequencies of a complex sound represented on a spectrum.

Epiglottis Unpaired cartilage of the larynx involved in swallowing.

Epithelium Type of tissue that lines the inner surfaces of the respiratory system.

erg Measure of energy in the CGS system.

Esophageal speech Speech produced by vibrating the superior portion of the esophagus.

Evoked potentials Also called *event-related potentials*; brain electrical activity that occurs in response to a controlled stimulus.

Excitatory post synaptic potential (EPSP) Occurs when the threshold of the post synaptic neuron is lowered, making it easier for the neuron to fire.

Expiratory reserve volume (ERV) Amount of air that can be exhaled below tidal volume.

External auditory meatus Channel leading from the pinna to the tympanic membrane; also known as the *ear canal.*

Extrapyramidal system Collective term for a multisynaptic series of nerve pathways in the central nervous system running from the cerebral cortex and making synaptic connection in the basal nuclei and cerebellum before synapsing with spinal and brain stem motor nuclei.

Extrinsic muscles Muscles that have one attachment within a given structure (e.g., tongue, larynx) and one outside the structure.

$F_0F_1F_2$ **strategy** Type of signal-processing strategy used in a cochlear implant, based on estimates of F_1 and F_2 frequencies, at a rate based on the F_0 of the signal or on a random rate around the F_0.

F_0**SPL profile** Graph that plots phonational frequency range against dynamic range; also called *voice range profile* or *phonetogram.*

F_1 **cutback** Delay of F_1 relative to the beginning of the F_2 transition.

False vocal folds Also called *ventricular vocal folds*; they lie parallel and superior to true vocal folds.

Falsetto register A range of very high F_0 with a thin, breathy quality; also called *loft.*

Fasciculi Nerve pathways formed by long association fibers linking different cortical regions.

Feedback Transfer of part of the output of a system back to the input to correct any errors in the output.

Feedforward Signals that make adjustments at the periphery of a system to prime the system.

Fetal cell transplantation (FCT) Surgical treatment for Parkinson's disease, designed to replenish missing dopamine.

Final common pathway Term for the cranial and spinal nerves that supply motor innervation to all the muscles in the body.

Final consonant deletion Phonological process in which the final consonant of a word is omitted.

Fixed channel strategy Type of signal processing strategy used in a cochlear implant, in which the acoustic signal is divided into 4 to 12 frequency bands, and energy in all the bands is transmitted at each cycle.

Flocculonodular lobe Lobe of the cerebellum.

Flow Movement of a particular volume of air during an interval of time.

Flow volume loop (FVL) Graph of respiratory function showing velocity of airflow on the vertical axis and volume of air inspired/expired on the horizontal axis.

Formant Resonance of the vocal tract; a frequency area of acoustic energy in vowels and other resonant sounds.

Formant trajectory Frequency path that a formant follows across an entire segment, such as a vowel.

Formant transition Shift in formant frequency.

Fourier analysis Mathematical procedure to identify the individual sinusoids in a complex sound.

Frequency Rate of vibration of an object.

Frequency perturbation Cycle-to-cycle variability in vocal frequency; also called *jitter*.

Frication Characteristic noise present in fricative sounds.

Fronting Phonological process in which a sound with a more anterior place of articulation is substituted for one with a more posterior place of articulation.

Functional residual capacity Amount of air in the lungs and airways at the end of a normal quiet exhalation.

Fundamental frequency (F_0) Lowest frequency of a complex periodic sound.

Funiculi Myelinated sensory and motor pathways bundled into large tracts in the spinal cord.

Gamma loop Synapse within the spinal cord between gamma nerve fibers conducting nerve signals away from muscles and alpha nerve fibers bringing nerve signals to muscles.

Genioglossus muscle Extrinsic tongue muscle; retracts the tongue or draws it [tongue] forward.

Gestures A family of movement patterns that achieve the same articulatory/acoustic goal.

Glial cells Term for different types of connective tissues in the nervous system.

Globus pallidus Part of the basal nuclei.

Glossometry Technique used to visualize tongue position within the oral cavity using light-emitting diode photo sensors mounted on a pseudopalate.

Glottal spectrum Spectrum of the laryngeal tone before it is modified in the vocal tract.

Glottis Space between the true vocal folds.

Golgi apparatus Microscopic organelle within cell cytoplasm that secretes proteins and sugars.

Gyri Raised surfaces on the cortex of the brain.

Half-power points Points corresponding to the upper and lower cutoff frequencies of a resonator. Also called *3 dB down points*.

Half-wave resonator Tube open at both ends; only one half of a wave fits in the resonator at any one time.

Harmonic content Relationship between the frequencies in a sound and their respective amplitudes; spectral composition of a sound.

Harmonic frequencies Frequencies above F_0 in a complex periodic sound.

Harmonic spacing Distance between harmonic frequencies in a complex sound.

Harmonics-to-noise ratio Measure, in dB, of the ratio of harmonic energy to noise energy in the voice.

Helicotrema Point of communication between the scala vestibuli and scala tympani at the end of the cochlear duct.

Hemodynamic response Increase in local brain blood flow in response to a particular cognitive task.

Hertz (Hz) Unit of measurement of frequency.

Heteronym Noun–verb pair in which the two words are contrasted by stress, with a noun receiving stress on the first syllable and a verb receiving stress on the second syllable.

High-pass filter Resonator that transmits acoustic energy above a specific lower cutoff frequency.

Hippocampus Structure of the limbic system; involved in learning and memory.

Hoarseness Vocal quality combining breathy plus rough characteristics.

Homunculus Caricature representing the differing amounts of neural tissue devoted to motor and sensory representations of different body structures.

Hyoglossus muscle Extrinsic tongue muscle; pulls the sides of the tongue downward.

Hyoid bone Bone from which the larynx is suspended; also forms the attachment for the tongue.

Hyothyroid membrane Sheet of membrane that connects the thyroid cartilage to the hyoid bone.

Hyperadducted Vocal folds adducted with excessive medial compression.

Hypernasality Distortion of an oral sound due to excessive nasal resonance.

Hypoadducted Vocal folds adducted with insufficient medial compression.

Hyponasality Distortion of a nasal sound due to insufficient nasal resonance.

Hypoventilation Inadequate ventilation resulting in reduced oxygen and increased concentrations of carbon dioxide in the bloodstream.

Identification tasks Procedures in which listeners transcribe what a speaker says.

Immittance Measure of how easily a system can be set into vibration by a driving force; includes the admittance and impedance of a system.

Immittance audiometry Method for diagnosing middle ear problems based on immittance.

Impedance Measure of the opposition of a system to a flow of energy through it, measured in ohms.

Impedance mismatch Difference in impedance between two mediums.

Incident wave Sound wave generated by a vibrating object.

Incus One of the ossicles of the middle ear; also called the *anvil.*

Indirect (extrapyramidal) system Multisynaptic motor system comprising nerve pathways that synapse with subcortical and cerebellar neurons before synapsing with motor neurons in the brain stem and spinal cord.

Inertia Tendency of matter to remain at rest or in motion unless acted on by an outside force.

Inferior colliculi Two masses of gray matter in the midbrain that project to the medial geniculate nucleus of the thalamus and are involved in auditory processing.

Inferior labial frenulum Small flap of tissue connecting the inner surface of the lower lip to the midline of the mandible.

Inferior longitudinal muscle Intrinsic tongue muscle; pulls tip downward, retracts the tongue.

Infrahyoid muscles Extrinsic muscles of larynx; depress the larynx.

Inhibitory post synaptic potential (IPSP) Occurs when the threshold of the postsynaptic neuron is raised, making it more difficult for the neuron to fire.

Innervation ratio Ratio of a motor neuron to the number of muscle fibers it innervates.

Inspiratory capacity Amount of air that can be inhaled from end-expiratory level; combination of TV plus IRV.

Inspiratory reserve volume (IRV) Amount of air that can be inhaled above tidal volume.

Interarytenoid (IA) Intrinsic muscle of the larynx composed of transverse and oblique fibers; adducts the vocal folds.

Intercostal muscles Made up of internal and external sets of muscles running between the ribs on both sides.

Interference Combining of waves in terms of areas of high and low pressure.

Intermaxillary suture Immovable joint between the palatine processes of the maxilla.

Intermediate zone Region in the spinal cord where the ventral and dorsal horns join.

Internal capsule Large mass of myelinated nerve fibers including corticothalamic, thalamocortical, corticonuclear, and corticospinal fibers.

International System of Units (SI) Modernized international metric system that uses seven base units including length, mass, time, electric current, thermodynamic temperature, amount of substance, and luminous intensity.

Interneurons Neurons that connect to each other over short or long distances; most numerous type of neurons in the human nervous system.

Intonation Variation of F_0 over an utterance.

Intrapleural pressure Pressure within the pleural space between the lungs and thorax.

Ion Atom or group of atoms that carry a positive or negative electrical charge due to gaining or losing an electron.

Jitter Cycle-to-cycle variability in frequency of vocal fold vibration; also called *frequency perturbation*.

joule (J) Measure of energy in the MKS system.

Labial valve Valve of the vocal tract formed by the lips.

Lamina propria Sheet of mucous membrane surrounding the body of the vocal folds; has superficial, intermediate, and deep layers.

Laminar flow Flow of air in which molecules move in a parallel manner at the same speed.

Laryngeal valve Valve of the vocal tract formed by the true vocal folds.

Laryngeal ventricle Space between the true and false vocal folds.

Laryngectomy Surgical removal of all or part of the larynx, usually due to cancer.

Laryngography More commonly called *electroglottography*; method of evaluating vocal fold function based on electrical conduction.

Laryngopharyngeal reflux Reflux from the stomach that enters the pharyngeal area and comes into contact with the posterior larynx.

Laryngopharynx Portion of the pharynx behind the larynx.

Laryngospasms Involuntary spasms of the vocal folds.

Lateral corticospinal tract Motor nerve pathway also called pyramidal tract; originates in the sensorimotor cortex; most fibers decussate at the medulla and then synapse with neurons in the anterior horns of the spinal cord.

Lateral cricoarytenoid (LCA) Intrinsic muscle of the larynx; adducts the vocal folds.

Lateral fissure Deep groove on the cortical surface of the brain that divides the brain into superior and inferior regions.

Lateral geniculate body Thalamic nucleus that processes visual information and relays it to the visual cortex.

Lateral vestibulospinal tract Motor nerve pathway that originates in the vestibular nuclei in the medulla and synapses with anterior horn spinal motor neurons.

Left-to-right coarticulation A preceding sound in an utterances influences an upcoming sound.

Levator veli palatini Muscle that forms a slinglike arrangement and elevates the velum.

Limbic system Made up of the limbic lobe, hippocampus, amygdala, mamillary bodies, and some thalamic nuclei; involved in emotional, sexual, and visceral functions.

Line spectrum Graph in which the frequencies in a complex periodic sound are depicted as vertical lines. The height of the line indicates the amplitude of the component frequency.

Linear scale Scale in which successive units increase by the same amount.

Linearized magnetometer Instrument used to measure movements of the chest wall.

Lingual frenulum Band of connective tissue joining the inferior portion of the tongue to the mandible.

Lingual valve Valve of the vocal tract formed by the tongue and other structures within the vocal tract.

Logarithmic scale Scale in which successive units increase by increasing amounts.

Logogen A neural processing device assumed to be associated with each word in a person's vocabulary.

Longitudinal cerebral fissure Deep groove on the cortex of the brain that divides the brain into two hemispheres.

Longitudinal phase difference Timing difference between the anterior and posterior portions of the vocal folds as they open and close during vibration.

Low-pass filter Resonator that transmits acoustic energy below a specific upper cutoff frequency.

Lower cutoff frequency (F_1) Frequency below F_c at which there is a 3 dB lower amplitude of response than at F_c.

Lower motor neuron (LMN) Comprised of cranial and spinal nerve cell bodies and their axons that connect with voluntary muscles.

Lower respiratory system Part of the respiratory system that includes the trachea, bronchial tubes, and lungs.

Lumen Interior of a tube such as the trachea or larynx.

Lx wave Waveform generated by electroglottography, with time on the horizontal axis and voltage on the vertical axis.

m-of-n strategy Type of signal-processing strategy used in a cochlear implant in which n equals the overall number of frequency bands represented in the acoustic signal, and m represents a smaller number of channels with the highest energy peaks in a particular processing cycle.

Mainstem bronchi Primary bronchi entering the lungs.

Malleus One of the ossicles of the middle ear; also called the *hammer*.

Malocclusion Problem in upper and/or lower dental arch relationships.

Manner of articulation Way in which the articulators relate to each other to regulate the flow of air through the vocal tract.

Manometer Instrument used to measure static pressures in cm H_2O.

Manubrium Long section of the malleus, attaching to the tympanic membrane.

Maximum phonational frequency range (MPFR) Complete range of frequencies that an individual can produce.

Mechanical resonator Resonator that does not contain a body of air.

Medial compression Force exerted by the LCA and IA muscles to bring the vocal folds to midline.

Medial geniculate body Thalamic nucleus that processes auditory information and relays it to the auditory cortex.

Medialization thyroplasty Surgical technique to position vocal folds closer together and reduce glottal insufficiency.

Median sulcus Divides the tongue into right and left sides.

Mel Unit of pitch on a psychophysical scale.

Membranous glottis Anterior three-fifths of the glottis; bounded by vocal ligament.

Meninges Three layers of connective tissues and the spaces between them that form a protective covering for the brain and spinal cord.

Mesiocclusion Condition in which the mandible protrudes too far forward due to abnormal occlusion.

Microbar Measurement of dynes per centimeter squared. 1 microbar = 1 dyne/cm^2.

Microglia Type of glial cells in the nervous system that destroy harmful organisms.

Micrognathia Occlusal problem in which the mandible is small in relation to the maxilla.

Mitochondria Microscopic organelle within cell cytoplasm involved in cell respiration and energy production.

Mixed hearing loss Combination of conductive and sensorineural hearing loss.

MKS system Metric system in which M = meters, K = kilograms, S = seconds.

Modal register Most commonly used register for normal conversational speech, encompassing the midrange of F_0.

Monophthongs Vowels produced with a relatively constant tongue position and unchanging resonance.

Motor end-plate See *neuromuscular junction*.

Motor unit A motor neuron with the associated muscle fibers that it innervates.

MPEAK strategy Type of signal-processing strategy used in a cochlear implant, in which electrodes representing F_1 and F_2 are stimulated, as well as two or three other electrodes representing the higher formant regions.

Mucosal wave Undulating wavelike motion of the vocal folds during vibration, particularly evident in the cover.

Multiphasic closure Pattern of vocal fold vibration in which there are numerous partial openings and closings prior to complete closure.

Muscular hydrostat A muscular organ without a cartilaginous or bony skeleton; derives support through selective muscular contraction.

Muscular process Projection of arytenoid cartilage to which various intrinsic laryngeal muscles attach.

Musculus uvuli Muscle on the nasal surface of the velum; helps to raise the velum.

Myoelastic–aerodynamic theory of phonation Theory that explains vocal fold vibration in terms of muscular, elastic recoil and aerodynamic forces.

Myoneural junction See *neuromuscular junction*.

Narrowband spectrogram Shows the fundamental frequency and individual harmonics in a sound.

Narrowly tuned See *sharply tuned*.

Nasal conchae Three small bones (inferior, middle, superior) that form the sides of the nose.

Nasal formant High-intensity, low-frequency formant present in nasal sounds.

Nasal murmur Extra resonances present in nasal sounds due to the coupling of the oral and nasal cavities.

Nasal septum Cartilaginous and bony plate that separates the nasal cavities.

Nasopharynx Portion of the pharynx behind the nasal cavities.

Natural frequency Frequency at which an object vibrates freely; also called *resonant frequency*.

Negative pressure Pressure lower than atmospheric pressure.

Neocortex Type of cortical tissue that is greatly expanded in humans compared to other primates.

Neoglottis Vibrating element following laryngectomy, usually formed by the pharyngoesophageal segment.

Neuromuscular junction Synapse between an axon and the muscle fiber it innervates; also known as *myoneural junction* or *motor end-plate*.

Neurotransmission Communication between neurons accomplished by the movement of chemicals or electrical signals across a synapse.

Neutrocclusion Normal occlusal relationship between upper and lower dental arches.

newton (N) Unit of measure of force in the modernized metric system.

Nissl bodies Microscopic organelle within cell cytoplasm that synthesizes proteins.

Nodes of Ranvier Breaks in the myelin sheath around an axon that serve to increase the nerve's rate of impulse conduction.

Obstruent Type of sound made by obstructing or constricting the flow of air through the vocal tract.

Occlusion Relationship between the upper and lower dental arches and the positioning of individual teeth.

Octave A doubling or halving of frequency.

Offglide End point of a diphthong.

Ohm Unit of electrical resistance.

Oligodendrocytes Glial cells that form myelin sheaths around nerves in the central nervous system.

Onglide Starting point for the first vowel in a diphthong.

Open quotient EGG measure that reflects the duration of the opening of the glottis in relation to the entire vibratory cycle.

Optimum pitch Range of pitches used by an individual that are produced with minimum vocal effort.

Optopalatography Technique that measures the intensity of light reflected from the surface of the tongue and the location and amount of pressure of the contact.

Orbicularis oris Circular muscle of the lips.

Organ of Corti Sensory nerve receptor for hearing, consisting of rows of inner and outer hair cells.

Oropharynx Portion of the pharynx behind the oral cavity.

Oscillation Back-and-forth movement of an object.

Ossicles Series of three small connecting bones in the middle ear.

Otitis media Middle ear infection.

Otitis media with effusion Buildup of fluid in the middle ear, caused by infection.

Otoacoustic emissions Low-intensity sounds originating in the cochlea and transmitted to the external auditory meatus; can be spontaneous or evoked.

Otosclerosis Formation of spongy bone around the stapes that prevents it from being set into vibration.

Palatal aponeurosis Broad, flat sheet of tendon that attaches the velum to the hard palate.

Palatine bones Bones of the skull that form the posterior one-quarter of the hard palate.

Palatine processes Projections of the maxilla that form the anterior three-quarters of the hard palate.

Palatoglossus Muscle that forms anterior faucial pillars; depresses the velum or elevates the tongue.

Palatometry Technique for displaying articulatory contacts using electrodes mounted on a pseudopalate.

Palatopharyngeus Muscles that form the posterior faucial pillars and narrow the pharyngeal cavity.

Parallel distributed processing models Computer models that simulate the neural processing of the human brain.

Paresis Slight or partial paralysis.

Parietal pleura Membrane that lines the inner surface of the thoracic cavity.

Pascal (P) Unit of measure of pressure in the modernized metric system.

Passband Acoustic resonator that transmits frequencies between the upper and lower cutoff frequencies.

Pattern Playback (PP) Instrument that converts visual patterns into sounds.

Perceptual magnet effect Notion that individuals are able to identify prototypical examples of a vowel better than nonprototypical examples.

Perilymph Fluid between the bony canal and the membranous canals of the cochlea.

Period Amount of time consumed by each cycle in a wave.

Periodic Wave in which each cycle takes the same amount of time to occur.

Pharyngeal constrictors Muscles that consist of inferior, middle, and superior fibers; they constrict the pharynx during swallowing.

Pharyngo esophageal segment Ring of muscle formed by the cricopharyngeus that separates the lower pharynx from the upper esophagus.

Phase Relative timing of compressions and rarefactions of waves.

Phon Unit of loudness on a psychophysical scale.

Phonation threshold pressure (PTP) Minimum amount of P_s needed to set the vocal folds into vibration.

Phonological processes Strategies used to simplify the motoric complexity of phonetic segments.

Pia mater Innermost layer of the meninges; closely follows the convolutions of the brain.

Pinna External portion of the ear, on either side of the head.

Pitch sigma Frequency variability, in semitones, in a person's voice.

Place of articulation Location in the vocal tract where articulators contact or approximate each other.

Plethysmograph Instrument used to measure changes in the cross-sectional areas of the chest wall.

Pleural fluid Fluid within the pleural space, having a negative pressure.

Pleural linkage The mechanism by which the lungs and thoracic cavity are linked together to function as a unit.

Pleural space Small potential space between the parietal and visceral pleurae.

Pneumotachometer Instrument used to measure airflows during respiration.

Pneumothorax Collapse of a lung due to penetration of the pleural lining.

Positive pressure Pressure higher than atmospheric pressure.

Postcentral gyrus Region immediately posterior to the central sulcus containing the primary somatosensory areas.

Posterior cricoarytenoid (PCA) Intrinsic muscle of larynx; abducts the vocal folds.

Precentral gyrus Region immediately anterior to the central sulcus containing the primary motor cortex.

Prephonatory chest wall movements Positioning of the chest wall that facilitates the generation of pressures for speech production.

Presbylaryngis Term used to characterize the aging of the laryngeal mechanism.

Presbyphonia Term for the vocal changes resulting from the aging process.

Pressure Force that acts perpendicularly on a surface.

Probe tip Device inserted in the external auditory meatus to measure immittance of the middle ear.

Pseudopalate Thin acrylic plate custom-designed to cover a person's hard palate and upper teeth.

Pulmonary function testing (PFT) Term that covers a variety of tests designed to assess the amount of air an individual is able to inhale and exhale, as well as how efficiently the person moves air into and out of the lungs.

Pulmonary system Part of the respiratory system that includes the lungs and airways.

Pulse register A range of very low F_0 with a creaky quality; also called *glottal fry, vocal fry, creaky voice.*

Pure tone Sound with only one frequency.

Putamen Part of the basal nuclei.

Pyramidal system Collective term for the corticospinal and corticonuclear (corticobulbar) pathways of the central nervous system from the cerebral cortex that synapse directly onto spinal and brain stem motor nuclei.

Quality Acoustically, the relationship between the harmonic frequencies and their amplitudes in a complex sound; perceptually, the tone or timbre of a sound.

Quarter-wave resonator Resonator that is open at one end and closed at the other; lowest resonant frequency has a wavelength four times the length of the resonator.

Radiation characteristic Effect that occurs when the sound traveling through the vocal tract is radiated beyond the mouth into the atmosphere, with the mouth acting like a high-pass filter.

Rarefaction Area of negative pressure.

Ratio scale Scale that describes relationships between quantities.

Recoil forces Forces generated when structures are restored to their original positions after being displaced.

Reflection A wave's collision with a surface and traveling back toward the source.

Refraction Change in the direction a wave is traveling due to a local difference in temperature.

Register Perceptually distinct region of vocal quality that can be maintained over a range of F_0.

Rejection rate See *attenuation rate*.

Relative refractory period Brief period following the absolute refractory period during which the nerve can only fire with stronger than normal stimulation.

Relaxation pressures Air pressures generated by the recoil forces of the respiratory system.

Relay nuclei Thalamic nuclei that receive and transmit nerve impulses to and from specific cortical areas.

Release burst Burst of aperiodic sound following the silent gap in a stop sound.

Repolarization Reversal of voltage in a neuron from positive back to negative.

Residual volume Volume of air remaining in the lungs after a maximum exhalation that cannot be voluntarily expelled.

Resonance (or filter) curve Graph that displays the frequency response of a resonant system. Also known as *transfer function*.

Resonant frequency Frequency at which an object vibrates, depending on its physical characteristics; also called *natural frequency*.

Resonator Object that vibrates in response to another vibration; can be mechanical or acoustic.

Respiratory bronchioles Subdivisions of the terminal bronchioles.

Respiratory kinematic analysis Methods of estimating lung volumes from rib cage and abdominal movements.

Resting expiratory level State of equilibrium in the respiratory system when P_{alv} equals P_{atmos}.

Resting membrane potential (RMP) Electrical voltage across the nerve cell membrane at rest with a negative charge of 270 mV within the cell and a positive electrical charge in the extracellular fluid, resulting in polarization.

Reticular activating system Part of the reticular formation in the brain stem that controls alertness and consciousness.

Reticular formation Diffuse network of nuclei that forms the core of the brain stem.

Reverberation Process of generating a sound that lasts slightly longer due to interaction of incident and reflected waves.

Rhotic sounds Sounds that have /r/ coloring, seen acoustically in a characteristic lowering of F_3.

Right-to-left coarticulation An upcoming sound in an utterance influences the preceding sound.

Rise time Time it takes for the amplitude envelope or spectrum of a sound to reach its highest value.

Roll-off rate See *attenuation rate*.

Roughness Vocal quality that sounds raspy and low pitched due to aperiodic vocal fold vibration.

Round window Opening between the scala tympani and the middle ear, covered with membrane.

Rubrospinal tract Motor nerve pathway that originates in the red nucleus of the midbrain and synapses contralaterally with neurons in the anterior horns of the spinal cord.

Scaling procedures Procedure in which listeners rate an individual's overall speech intelligibility.

Schwann cells Glial cells that form myelin sheaths around nerves in the peripheral nervous system.

Secondary bronchus Subdivision of the mainstem bronchi, supplying the lobes of the lungs.

Self-sustaining oscillator Vibratory system in which vibration continues without an external force needing to be applied for each cycle.

Sensorineural hearing loss Hearing loss due to disease or damage to the inner ear or auditory nerve.

Sharply tuned Resonator that transmits a narrow range of frequencies; also called *narrowly tuned.*

Shimmer Cycle-to-cycle variability in amplitude of the vocal fold vibration; also called *amplitude perturbation.*

Shunt resonator Closed branch leading off a resonator; also called *side-branch resonator.*

Sibilants Fricatives characterized by intense high-frequency energy.

Side-branch resonator Closed branch leading off a resonator; also called *shunt resonator.*

Siemens Units of electrical conductance; also called *millimhos.*

Silent gap Time on a spectrogram of a stop sound during which no sound is seen because pressure is building up.

Simple harmonic motion A smooth back-and-forth movement with a characteristic pattern of acceleration through the rest position and deceleration at the endpoints of the movement.

Sinusoid Pure tone with a sinusoidal shape on a waveform.

Slope See *attenuation rate.*

Slope index Measure of a formant transition based on the duration and frequency extent of the transition. Measured in hertz per millisecond (Hz/msec).

Soma Cell body of a neuron; composed of cytoplasm and nucleus.

Somatotopic organization Organization of motor control according to body structure.

Sonorants Class of sounds that are always voiced; airflow is neither completely laminar nor turbulent.

Source-filter theory Theory that describes how the vocal tract filters glottal sound waves to generate different vowels.

Spasmodic dysphonia Voice disorder characterized by laryngeal spasms.

Spatial summation Process by which nerve impulses reach the cell body or dendrites at slightly different locations and add together.

Specific language impairment (SLI) Disorder in which children show a significant problem with language, in the face of normal hearing, normal nonverbal intelligence, and no known neurological problems.

Spectral noise Additive noise in the glottal spectrum.

Spectrum Graph with frequency on the horizontal axis and amplitude on the vertical axis; line spectrum represents periodic sounds, continuous spectrum represents aperiodic sounds.

Speed quotient EGG measure based on the ratio of opening-phase duration to closing-phase duration in the vibratory cycle.

Spinocerebellar tract Sensory nerve pathway from the spinal cord to the cerebellum that transmits information about pain, temperature, touch, and proprioception.

Spinothalamic tract Sensory nerve pathway from the spinal cord to the thalamus that transmits information about pain, temperature, and touch.

Spirometer Instrument that measures lung volumes; can be wet or dry.

Spreading activation models Computer models that simulate the neural processing of the human brain. Also called *parallel distributed processing.*

Standard reference sound Sound with an amplitude of 20 µPa and intensity of 10^{-12} W/m².

Standing wave Wave in which areas of positive and negative pressures occur at the same time and in the same location; gives the appearance of being stationary rather than traveling through the medium.

Stapedius Muscle in the middle ear; involved in the acoustic reflex.

Stapes One of the ossicles of the middle ear; also called the *stirrup.*

Stereocilia Hair like projections extending from the inner and outer hair cells of the inner ear.

Stiffness Resistance of a structure to being displaced or deformed.

Stress Emphasis placed on a syllable or word by increasing pitch, intensity, and/or duration.

Striatum Part of the basal nuclei comprised of the caudate and putamen.

Stridents Fricatives characterized by intense high-frequency energy.

Stridor Wheezing sound that occurs during breathing; can be inspiratory, expiratory, or both.

Styloglossus muscle Extrinsic tongue muscle; elevates and retracts the tongue.

Subarachnoid space Space between the arachnoid mater and the pia mater; filled with cerebrospinal fluid.

Subdural space Space between the dura mater and the arachnoid mater.

Subsonic Frequencies below the range of human hearing.

Substantia nigra Part of the basal nuclei involved in the production of dopamine.

Sulci Shallow depressions on the cortex of the brain.

Superior colliculi Two masses of gray matter in the midbrain that project to the lateral geniculate nucleus of the thalamus and are involved in visual processing.

Superior labial frenulum Small flap of tissue connecting the inner surface of the upper lip to the midline of the alveolar region.

Superior longitudinal muscle Intrinsic tongue muscle; elevates the tip.

Supersonic Frequencies above the range of human hearing.

Suprahyoid muscles Extrinsic muscles of larynx; elevate the larynx.

Suprasegmental characteristics F_0, intensity, and duration changes that occur over a sequence of phonemes, syllables, words, or sentences; they signal linguistic and extralinguistic meanings.

Suprathreshold discriminability Ability of an individual with hearing loss to recognize a sound when it is presented at an audible level.

Suprathreshold level Level at which a hearing-impaired person can hear a specific speech signal.

Surfactant Substance that keeps alveoli inflated by lowering the surface tension of the alveolar walls.

Synapse Gap between neurons where communication between nerves takes place; may be axo-axonal, axo-somatic, or axo-dendritic.

Synergy Functional linkages between muscles working to achieve a specific movement goal.

Target undershoot Failure of articulators to reach the intended vowel target, resulting in a reduction in F_1/F_2 vowel space.

Tectorial membrane Gel-like membrane forming the roof of the organ of Corti.

Temporal gap In pulse register, a brief interval during which no acoustic energy is present.

Temporal processing problem Difficulty processing the rapid changes in frequency and intensity that are characteristic of speech.

Temporal summation Process by which nerve impulses reach the cell body within a very short time of each other and add together.

Tensor tympani Muscle of the middle ear, involved in auditory tube function.

Tensor veli palatini Muscle of the velum that opens the auditory tube.

Terminal branches Also known as *telodendria*; the endpoint of an axon.

Terminal bronchioles Subdivisions of the tertiary bronchi.

Terminal buttons Small sacs on the terminal branches of an axon filled with neurotransmitter molecules.

Tertiary bronchi Subdivisions of the secondary bronchi, supplying the segments of the lungs.

Thoracic cavity Chest cavity bounded by the ribs, sternum, vertebral column, and diaphragm, in which the lungs are housed.

3 dB down points See *half-power points*.

Threshold of hearing Sound that a pair of normal human ears can detect 50 percent of the time under ideal listening conditions.

Threshold of pain Intensity level of 130 dB, which causes a sensation of pain in the ears.

Thyroarytenoid muscle Body of the vocal folds.

Thyroid cartilage Largest cartilage of the larynx; unpaired.

Tidal volume (TV) Volume of air breathed in and out during a cycle of respiration.

Tonotopic organization Spatial organization of a structure (e.g., basilar membrane) in terms of frequency distribution.

Torque A twisting, rotary force.

Torus tubarius Bulge in the lateral pharyngeal wall caused by the enlargement of cartilage where the auditory tube opens into the pharynx.

Total laryngectomy Surgical procedure in which the entire larynx is removed, usually due to cancer.

Total lung capacity (TLC) Total amount of air that the lungs are capable of holding, including residual volume.

Tracer Radioactive substance used in emission tomography.

Trachea Membranocartilaginous tube inferior to the larynx; part of the lower respiratory system.

Transducer Device that converts energy from one form to another.

Transfer function See *resonance curve*.

Transglottal pressure Pressure difference across the vocal folds, between tracheal pressure and supraglottal pressure.

Transpulmonary pressure Difference between the pressure inside the lungs and the intrapleural pressure.

Transverse muscle Intrinsic tongue muscle; pulls edges toward midline.

Transverse palatine suture Suture between the palatine bones and palatine processes.

True vocal folds Multilayered structures attached to anterior commissure anteriorly and vocal processes posteriorly; vibrating element of the larynx.

Turbulent flow Irregular flow with random variations in pressure.

Tympanic membrane Eardrum.

Tympanogram Graph of the immittance of the middle ear.

Tympanometer Instrument that measures and displays the immittance of the middle ear.

Umbo Tip of the conical surface of the tympanic membrane.

Upper cutoff frequency (F_u) Frequency above F_c at which there is a 3 dB less amplitude of response than at F_c.

Upper motor neuron (UMN) Comprised of nerve cells bodies and their axons arising from various cortical areas and projecting to the brain stem and spinal cord.

Upper respiratory system Part of the respiratory system that includes the pharynx and the oral and nasal cavities.

Variable resonator Resonator whose frequency response changes as the resonator changes its shape.

Velopharyngeal passage Portion of the pharynx between the posterior margins of the oral and nasal cavities.

Velopharyngeal valve Valve of the vocal tract formed by the velum and posterior portion of the pharynx.

Velum Soft palate.

Ventral anterior (VA) and ventral lateral (VL) nuclei Thalamic nuclei that receive input from the basal nuclei and cerebellum and project to the motor areas of the cerebral cortex.

Ventral horns Anterior portion of the gray matter of the spinal cord made up of nerve cell bodies that project fibers to skeletal muscles.

Vermis Midline portion of the cerebellum that connects the two cerebellar hemispheres.

Vertical muscle Intrinsic tongue muscle; pulls the tongue downward.

Vertical partial laryngectomy (VPL) Surgical procedure in which a portion of the larynx is removed.

Vertical phase difference Timing difference between the inferior and superior borders of the vocal folds as they open and close during vibration.

Vestibular membrane Roof of the cochlear duct.

Visceral pleura Membrane covering the outer surface of each lung.

Vital capacity Maximum amount of air that can be exhaled after a maximum inhalation.

Vocal ligament Portion of the vocal folds consisting of intermediate and deep layers of the lamina propria.

Vocal process Projection of the arytenoid cartilage to which the vocal folds attach.

Voice bar Band of low-frequency energy sometimes seen on a spectrogram of a voiced stop or fricative, reflecting vocal fold vibration.

Voice onset time (VOT) In a stop consonant, time between the release burst to the beginning of vocal fold vibration for the following vowel.

Voicing Vibration of the vocal folds during phonation.

Volume Amount of space occupied by something in three dimensions.

Volume velocity Rate of flow.

Vowel quadrilateral Diagram representing the tongue positions of height and advancement for vowels.

Vowel reduction Neutralization of a vowel so its formants look more like a schwa.

Watt (W) Measure of power.

Waveform Graph with time on the horizontal axis and amplitude on the vertical axis.

Wave front Outermost area of the sound wave propagating spherically through the air.

Wavelength Distance covered by one complete cycle of a wave.

Wet spirometer Instrument that measures lung volumes and capacities.

White noise Aperiodic sound that has its energy distributed fairly evenly throughout the spectrum.

Wideband spectrogram Shows the formant structure of sounds and the filtering function of the vocal tract.

References

Abbs, J. H. (1996). Mechanisms of speech motor execution and control. In N. J. Lass (Ed.), *Principles of experimental phonetics* (pp. 93–111). St. Louis: Mosby.

Adler, R. K., Hirsch, S., & Mordaunt, M. (2006). *Voice and communication therapy for the transgender/transsexual client: A comprehensive clinical guide.* San Diego, CA: Plural Publishing, Inc.

Adler-Bock, M., Bernhardt, B. M., Gick, B., & Bacsfalvi, P. (2007). The use of ultrasound in remediation of North American English /r/ in 2 adolescents. *American Journal of Speech–Language Pathology, 16,* 128–139.

Aerainer, R., & Klingholz, F. (1993). Quantitative evaluation of phonetograms in the case of functional dysphonia. *Journal of Voice, 7,* 136–141.

Al Bawab, Z., Turicchia, L., Stern, R. M., & Raj, B. (2009). Deriving vocal tract shapes from electromagnetic articulograph data via geometric adaption and matching. www.cs.cmu.edu/~robust/Papers/is2009_ZiadAlBawabEtAl.pdf.

Alberti, P. W. R., & Jerger, J. F. (1971). Probe-tone frequency and the diagnostic value of tympanometry. *Archives of Otolaryngology, 99,* 206–210.

Altman, K. W., Simpson, C. B., Amin, M. R., Abaza, M., Balkissoon, R., & Casiano, R. R. (2002). Cough and paradoxical vocal fold motion. *Otolaryngology-Head and Neck Surgery, 127,* 501–511.

American National Standard Specifications for Audiometers, ANSI S3.6 – 1969. American National Standards Institute, New York.

American Thoracic Society (1998). Dyspnea: Mechanisms, assessment, and management: A consensus statement.

Andrianopoulos, M. V., Gallivan, G., J., & Gallivan, K. H. (2000). PVCM, PVCD, EPL, and irritable larynx syndrome: What are we talking about and how do we treat it? *Journal of Voice, 14,* 607–618.

Ansel, B. M., & Kent, R. D. (1992). Acoustic–phonetic contrasts and intelligibility in the dysarthria associated with mixed cerebral palsy. *Journal of Speech and Hearing Research, 35,* 296–308.

Appleton, S. L., Adams, R. J., Wilson, D. H., Taylor, A. W., & Ruffin, R. E. (2005). Spirometric criteria for asthma: Adding further evidence to the debate. *Journal of Allergy and Clinical Immunology, 116,* 976–982.

Arias, M. R., Ramón, J. L., Campos, M., & Cervantes, J. J. (2000). Acoustic analysis of the voice in phonatory fistuloplasty after total laryngectomy. *Otolaryngology-Head and Neck Surgery, 122,* 743–747.

Awan, S. N., & Frenkel, M. L. (1994). Improvements in estimating the harmonics-to-noise ratio of the voice. *Journal of Voice, 8,* 255–262.

Awan, S. N., & Mueller, P. R. (1996). Speaking fundamental frequency characteristics of white, African American, and Hispanic kindergartners. *Journal of Speech and Hearing Research, 39,* 573–577.

Bailey, E. F., & Hoit, J. D. (2002). Speaking and breathing in high respiratory drive. *Journal of Speech, Language, and Hearing Research, 45,* 89–99.

Baken, R. J. (1992). Electroglottography. *Journal of Voice, 6,* 98–110.

Baken, R. J. (1996). *Clinical measurement of speech and voice.* San Diego, CA: Singular.

Baken, R. (2005). An overview of laryngeal function for voice production. In R. Sataloff, *Professional voice: The science and art of clinical care, 3rd ed.* (pp. 237–256). San Diego, CA: Plural Publishing, Inc.

Baken, R. J., & Orlikoff, R. F. (2000). *Clinical measurement of speech and voice* (2nd ed.). San Diego, CA: Singular Thomson Learning.

Baken, R., & Cavallo, S. (1981). Prephonatory chest wall posturing. *Folia Phoniatrica et Logopedica, 33,* 193–202.

Baker, K. K., Ramig, L. O., Johnson, A. B., & Freed, C. R. (1997). Preliminary voice and speech analysis following fetal dopamine transplants in 5 individuals with Parkinson disease. *Journal of Speech and Hearing Research, 40,* 615–626.

Baker, S., Davenport, P., & Sapienza, C. (2005). Examination of strength training and detraining effects in expiratory muscles. *Journal of Speech, Language, and Hearing Research, 48,* 1325–1333.

Balter, M. S., Adams, S. C., & Chapman, K. R. (2001). Inhaled beclomethasone dipropionate improves acoustic measures of voice in patients with asthma. *Chest, 120,* 1829–1834.

Barlow, S. M. (1999). *Handbook of clinical speech physiology.* San Diego, CA: Singular.

Bartle, C. J., Goozee, J. V., Scott, D., Murdoch, B. E., & Kuruvilla, M. (2006). EMA assessment of tongue-jaw co-ordination during speech in dysarthria following traumatic brain injury. *Brain Injury, 20,* 529–545.

Bartle-Meyer, C. J., Murdoch, B. E., & Goozee, J. V. (2009). An electropalatographic investigation of lingua-palatal contact in participants with acquired apraxia of speech: A quantitative and qualitative analysis. *Clinical Linguistics and Phonetics, 23,* 688–716.

Bass, H. (1973). The flow volume loop: Normal standards and abnormalities in chronic obstructive pulmonary disease. *Chest, 63,* 171–176.

Baudonck, N., D'haeseleer, E., Dhooge, I., & Van Lierde, K. (2011). Objective vocal quality in children using cochlear implants: A multiparameter approach. *Journal of Voice, 25,* 683–691.

Baylor, C. R., Yorkston, K. M., Eadie, T. L., Strand, E. A., & Duffy, J. (2006). A systematic review of outcome measurement in unilateral vocal fold paralysis. *Journal of Medical Speech–Language Pathology, 14,* xxvii–lvii.

Behrman, A., & Orlikoff, R. F. (1997). Instrumentation in voice assessment and treatment: What's the use? *American Journal of Speech Language Pathology, 6,* 9–16.

Belafsky, P. C., Postma, G. M., & Koufman, J. A. (2001). Validity and reliability of the reflux finding score (RFS). *Laryngoscope, 111,* 1313–1317.

Belafsky, P. C., Postma, G. M., & Koufman, J. A. (2002). Validity and reliability of the reflux symptom index (RSI). *Journal of Voice, 16,* 274–277.

Benabid, A. L. (2003). Deep brain stimulation for Parkinson's disease. *Current Opinion in Neurobiology, 13,* 696–706.

Benjamin, B. (1981). Frequency variability in the aged voice. *Journal of Gerontology, 36,* 722–726.

Bennett, S. (1983). A 3–year longitudinal study of school-aged children's F_0s. *Journal of Speech and Hearing Research, 26,* 137–142.

Benoit, M., Clairet, S., Koulibaly, P. M., Darcourt, J., & Robert, P. H. (2004). Brain perfusion correlates of the Apathy Inventory dimensions of Alzheimer's disease. *International Journal of Geriatric Psychiatry, 19,* 864–869.

Benson, B. E., Baredes, S., Schwartz, R. A., & Kumar, M. (2006). Stridor. http://emedicine.medscape.com/article/995267-diagnosis.

Bernhardt, B., Bacsfalvi, P., Gick, B., Radanov, B. A., & Williams, R. (2005). Exploring the use of electropalatography and ultrasound in speech habilitation. *Journal of Speech–Language Pathology and Audiology, 29,* 169–182.

Bernhardt, B., Gick, B., Bacsfalvi, P., & Adler-Bock, M. (2005). Ultrasound in speech therapy with adolescents and adults. *Clinical Linguistics and Phonetics, 19,* 605–617.

Bernhardt, B., Gick, B., Bacsfalvi, P., & Ashdown, J. (2003). Speech habilitation of hard of hearing adolescents using electropalatography and ultrasound as evaluated by trained listeners. *Clinical Linguistics and Phonetics, 17,* 199–216.

Bernhardt, M. B., Bacsfalvi, P., Adler-Bock, M., Shimizu, R., Cheney, A., Giesbrecht, N., O'Connell, M., Sirianni, J., & Radanov, B. (2008). Ultrasound as visual feedback in speech habilitation: Exploring consultative use in rural British Columbia, Canada. *Clinical Linguistics and Phonetics, 22*, 149–162.

Bernstein, L. E., & Stark, R. E. (1985). Speech perception development in language-impaired children: A 4-year follow-up study. *Journal of Speech and Hearing Disorders, 50*, 21–30.

Bertino, G., Bellomo, A., Miana, C., Ferrero, F., & Staffieri, A. (1996). Spectrographic differences between tracheal-esophageal and esophageal voice. *Folia Phoniatrica et Logopedica, 48*, 255–261.

Bhandari, A., Izdebski, K., Huang, C., & Yan, Y. (2012). Comparative analysis of normal voice characteristics using simultaneous electroglottography and high speed digital imaging. *Biomedical Signal Processing and Control, 7*, 20–26.

Bielamowicz, S., Kapoor, R., Schwartz, J., & Stager, S. V. (2004). Relationship among glottal area, static supraglottic compression, and laryngeal function studies in unilateral vocal fold paresis and paralysis. *Journal of Voice, 18*, 138–145.

Bien, S., Okla, S., van As-Brooks, C. J., & Ackerstaff, A. H. (2010). The effect of a heat and moisture exchanger (Provox HME) on pulmonary protection after total laryngectomy: A randomized controlled study. *European Archives of Otorhinolaryngology, 267*, 429–435.

Biever, D. M., & Bless, D. M. (1989). Vibratory characteristics of the vocal folds in young adult and geriatric women. *Journal of Voice, 3*, 120–131.

Binder, J. R., Frost, J. A., Hammeke, T. A., Cox, R. W., Rao, S. M., & Prieto, T. (1997). Human brain language areas identified by functional magnetic resonance imaging. *Society for Neuroscience, 17*, 353–362.

Birnbaum, H. G., Ivanova, J. I., Yu, A. P., Hsieh, M., Seal, B., Emani, S., Rosiello, R., & Colice, G. L. (2009). Asthma severity categorization using a claims-based algorithm or pulmonary function testing. *Journal of Asthma, 46*, 67–72.

Bishop, D. V. M., Bishop, S. J., Bright, P., James, C., Delaney, T., & Tallal, P. (1999). Different origin of auditory and phonological processing problems in children with language impairment: Evidence from a twin study. *Journal of Speech, Language, and Hearing Research, 42*, 155–168.

Blager F. B. (2006). Vocal cord dysfunction. *Perspectives on Voice and Voice Disorders, 16*, 7–10.

Blomgren, M., Chen, Y., Ng, M., & Gilbert, H. (1998). Acoustic, aerodynamic, physiologic, and perceptual properties of modal and vocal fry registers. *Journal of the Acoustical Society of America, 103*, 2649–2658.

Blumin, J. H., & Merati, A. (2008). Laryngeal reinnervation with nerve-nerve anastomosis versus laryngeal framework surgery alone: A comparison of safety. *Otolaryngology-Head and Neck Surgery, 138*, 217–220.

Boberg, E., Yeudall, L., Schopplocher, D., & BoLassen, P. (1983). The effects of an intensive behavioral program on the distribution of EEG alpha power in stutterers during the processing of verbal and visuospatial information. *Journal of Fluency Disorders, 8*, 245–263.

Boliek, C. A. (1997). *Respiratory function in voice and speech disorders: Clinical implications.* Paper presented at the annual convention of the American Speech–Language–Hearing Association, Boston.

Boliek, C. A., Hixon, T. J., Watson, P. J., & Jones, P. B. (2009). Refinement of speech breathing in healthy 4- to 6-year-old children. *Journal of Speech, Language, and Hearing Research, 52*, 990–1007.

Boliek, C. A., Hixon, T. J., Watson, P. J., & Morgan, W. J. (1996). Vocalization and breathing during the first year of life. *Journal of Voice, 10*, 1–22.

Boliek, C. A., Hixon, T. J., Watson, P. J., & Morgan, W. J. (1997). Vocalization and breathing during the second and third years of life. *Journal of Voice, 11*, 373–390.

Boothroyd, A. (1978). Speech perception and sensorineural hearing loss. In M. Ross & T. G. Giolas (Eds.),

Auditory management of hearing-impaired children: Principles and prerequisites for intervention (pp. 44–68). Baltimore: University Park Press.

Bortolini, U., Zmarich, C., Fior, R., & Bonifacio, S. (1995). Word-initial voicing in the production of stops in normal and preterm Italian infants. *International Journal of Pediatric Otorhinolaryngology, 31*, 191–206.

Braun, A. R., Varga, M., Stager, S., Schulz, G., Selbie, S., Maisog, J. M., Carson, R. E., & Ludlow, C. L. (1997). A typical lateralization of hemispheral activity in developmental stuttering: An $H_2 15$ O positron emission tomography study. In W. Hulstijn, H. F. M. Peters, & P. H. H. M. Van Lieshout (Eds.), *Speech production: Motor control, brain research and fluency disorders* (pp. 279–292). Amsterdam: Elsevier.

Brex, P. A., Miszkiel, K. A., Riordan, J. I., Plant, G. T., Moseley, I. F., Thompson, A. J., & Miller, D. H. (2001). Assessing the risk of early multiple sclerosis in patients with clinically isolated syndromes: The role of a follow-up MRI. *Journal of Neurology, Neurosurgery and Psychiatry, 70*, 390–393.

Bright, K. E. (1997). Spontaneous otoacoustic emissions. In M. S. Robinette & T. J. Glattke (Eds.), *Otoacoustic emissions: Clinical applications* (pp. 46–62). New York: Thieme.

Brockmann, M., Drinnan, M. J., Storck, C., & Carding, P. N. (2011). Reliable jitter and shimmer measurements in voice clinics: The relevance of vowel, gender, vocal intensity, and fundamental frequency effects in a typical clinical task. *Journal of Voice, 25*, 44–53.

Brockmann, M., Storck, C., Carding, P. N., & Drinnan, M. J. (2008). Voice loudness and gender effects on jitter and shimmer in healthy adults. *Journal of Speech, Language, and Hearing Research, 51*, 1152–1160.

Broen, P. A., Strange, W., Doyle, S. S., & Heller, J. H. (1983). Perception and production of approximant contrasts by normal and articulation-delayed preschool children. *Journal of Speech and Hearing Research, 26*, 601–608.

Brown, M., Perry, A., Cheesman, A. D., & Pring, T. (2000). Pitch change in male-to-female transsexuals: Has phonosurgery a role to play? *International Journal of Language and Communication Disorders, 35*, 129–136.

Brown, W. S., Jr., Morris, R. J., & Murry, T. (1996). Comfortable effort level revisited. *Journal of Voice, 10*, 299–305.

Brown, W. S. Jr., Morris, R. J., Hollien, H,, & Howell, E. (1991). Speaking fundamental frequency characteristics as a function of age and professional singing. *Journal of Voice, 5*, 310–315.

Buchel, C., & Sommer, M. (2004). What causes stuttering? *PLOS Biology, 2*, e46.

Buddiga, P. (2010). Vocal cord dysfunction: Differential diagnosis and workup. http://emedicine.medscape.com/article/137782-diagnosis.

Bunton, K. (2005). Patterns of lung volume use during an extemporaneous speech task in persons with Parkinson disease. *Journal of Communication Disorders, 38*, 331–348.

Bunton, K., & Weismer, G. (2001). The relationship between perception and acoustics for a high-low vowel contrast produced by speakers with dysarthria. *Journal of Speech, Language, and Hearing Research, 46*, 1215–1228.

Buser, P., & Imbert, M. (1992). *Audition.* Cambridge, MA: MIT Press.

Calandruccio, L., Fitzgerald, T. S., & Prieve, B. A. (2006). Normative multifrequency tympanometry in infants and toddlers. *Journal of the American Academy of Audiology, 17*, 470–480.

Callan, D., Callan, A., Gamez, M., Sato, M.-A., & Kawato, M. (2010). Premotor cortex mediates perceptual performance. *NeuroImage, 51*, 844–858.

Campisi, P., Low, A. J., Papsin, B. C., Mount, R. J., & Harrison, R. V. (2006). Multidimensional voice program analysis in profoundly deaf children: Quantifying frequency and amplitude control. *Perceptual and Motor Skills, 103*, 40–50.

Carding, P. N., Steen, I. N., Webb, A., Mackenzie, K., Deary, I. J., & Wilson, J. A. (2004). The reliability and sensitivity to change of acoustic measures of voice quality. *Clinical Otolaryngology, 29*, 538–544.

Carney, A. E., & Moeller, M. P. (1998). Treatment efficacy: Hearing loss in children. *Journal of Speech, Language, and Hearing Research, 41*, S61–S84.

Carroll, T. L., Wu, Y.-H. E., McRay, M., & Gherson, S. (2012). Frame by frame analysis of glottic insufficiency using laryngovideostroboscopy. *Journal of Voice, 26*, 220–225.

Carter, P., & Edwards, S. (2004). EPG therapy for children with long-standing speech disorders: Predictions and outcomes. *Clinical Linguistics and Phonetics, 18*, 359–372.

Caruso, A. J., & Klasner Burton, E. (1987). Temporal acoustic measures of dysarthria associated with amyotrophic lateral sclerosis. *Journal of Speech and Hearing Research, 30*, 80–87.

Cerny, F. J., Panzarella, K. J., & Stathopoulos, E. (1997). Expiratory muscle conditioning in hypotonic children with low vocal intensity levels. *Journal of Medical Speech–Language Pathology, 5*, 141–152.

Chen, Y., Robb, M. P., & Gilbert, H. R. (2002). Electroglottographic evaluation of gender and vowel effects during modal and vocal fry phonation. *Journal of Speech, Language, and Hearing Research, 45*, 821–829.

Cheng, H. Y., Murdoch, B. E., Goozee, J. V., & Scott, D. (2007a). Electropalatographic assessment of tongue-to-palate contact patterns and variability in children, adolescents, and adults. *Journal of Speech, Language, and Hearing Research, 50*, 375–392.

Cheng, H. Y., Murdoch, B. E., Goozee, J. V., & Scott, D. (2007b). Physiologic development of tongue-jaw coordination from childhood to adulthood. *Journal of Speech, Language, and Hearing Research, 50*, 352–360.

Chernobelsky, S. (2002). The use of electroglottography in the treatment of deaf adolescents with puberphonia. *Logopedics, Phoniatrics, Vocology, 27*, 63–65.

Chiang, W. C., Goh, A., Tang, J. P. L., & Chay, O. M. (2008). Paradoxical vocal cord dysfunction: When a wheeze is not asthma. *Singapore Medical Journal, 49*, 110–112.

Childers, D. G. (1991). Assessment of the acoustics of voice production. In *Proceedings of a conference on assessment of speech and voice production: Research and clinical applications* (pp. 63–83). Bethesda, MD: U. S. Department of Health and Human Services.

Cho, T., & Ladefoged, P. (1999). Variation and universals in VOT: Evidence from 18 languages. *Journal of Phonetics, 27*, 207–229.

Choi, H.-S., Chung, S. M., Lim, J.-Y., & Kim, H. S. (2008). Increasing the closed quotient improves voice quality after type I thyroplasty in patients with unilateral vocal cord paralysis: Analysis using SPEAD program. *Journal of Voice, 22*, 751–755.

Christoffels, I. K., van de Ven, V., Waldorp, L. J., Formisano, E., & Schiller, N. O. (2011). The sensory consequences of speaking: Parametric neural cancellation during speech in auditory cortex. *PLOS ONE, 6*, e18307.

Christopher, K. L., & Morris, M. J. (2010). Vocal cord dysfunction, paradoxic vocal fold motion, or laryngomalacia? Our understanding requires an interdisciplinary approach. *Otolaryngology Clinics of North America, 43*, 43–66.

Clayman, C. B. (Ed.). (1995). *The human body: An illustrated guide to its structure, function, and disorders*. New York: Dorling Kindersley.

Cohn, J. R., Sataloff, R. T., & Branton, C. (2001). Response of asthma-related voice dysfunction to allergen immunotherapy: A case report of confirmation by methacholine challenge. *Journal of Voice, 15*, 558–560.

Cole, J., Kim, H., Choi, H., & Hasegawa-Johnson, M. (2007). Prosodic effects on acoustic cues to stop voicing and place of articulation: Evidence from radio news speech. *Journal of Phonetics, 35,* 180–209.

Coleman, R. F., Mabis, J. H., & Hinson, J. K. (1977). Fundamental frequency–sound pressure level profiles of adult male and female voices. *Journal of Speech and Hearing Research, 20,* 197–204.

Colletti, V. (1977). Multifrequency tympanometry. *Audiology, 16,* 278–287.

Colton, R. H., Woo, P., Brewer, D. W., Griffin, B., & Casper, J. (1995). Stroboscopic signs associated with benign lesions of the vocal folds. *Journal of Voice, 9,* 312–325.

Colton, R., & Casper, J. K. (1996). *Understanding voice problems: A physiological perspective for diagnosis and treatment* (2nd ed.). Baltimore, MD: Williams & Wilkins.

Connaghan, K. P., Moore, C. A., & Higashakawa, M. (2004). Respiratory kinematics during vocalization and nonspeech respiration in children from 9 to 48 months. *Journal of Speech, Language, and Hearing Research, 47,* 70–84.

Connor, C. M., Hieber, S., Arts, H. A., & Zwolan, T. A. (2000). Speech, vocabulary, and the education of children using cochlear implants: Oral or total communication? *Journal of Speech, Language, and Hearing Research, 43,* 1185–1204.

Cooper, H. (1991). Training and rehabilitation for cochlear implant users. In H. Cooper (Ed.), *Cochlear implants: A practical guide* (pp. 219–239). San Diego, CA: Singular.

Corbett, J. J., Haines, D. E., & Ard, M. D. (2002). The ventricles, choroid plexus, and cerebrospinal fluid. In D. E. Haines (Ed.), *Fundamental neuroscience* (2nd ed.). New York: Churchill Livingstone.

Cousineau, M., Demany, L., Meyer, B., & Pressnitzer, D. (2010). What breaks a melody: Perceiving F0 and intensity sequences with a cochlear implant. *Hearing Research, 269,* 34–41.

Culpepper, N. B. (1997). Neonatal screening via evoked otoacoustic emissions. In M. S. Robinette & T. J. Glattke (Eds.), *Otoacoustic emissions: Clinical applications* (pp. 233–270). New York: Thieme.

Dagenais, P. A. (1995). Electropalatography in the treatment of articulation/phonological disorders. *Journal of Communication Disorders, 28,* 303–329.

D'Ausilio, A., Bufalari, I., Salmas, P, Busan, P., & Fadiga, L. (2011). Vocal pitch discrimination in the motor system. *Brain & Language, 118,* 9–14.

D'Ausilio, A., Bufalari, I., Salmas, P., & Fadiga, L. (2012). The role of the motor system in discriminating normal and degraded speech sounds. *Cortex, 48,* 882–887.

D'Ausilio, A., Craighero, L., & Fadiga, L. (2012). The contribution of the frontal lobe to the perception of speech. *Journal of Neurolinguistics, 25,* 328–335.

D'Ausilio, A., Pulvermüller, F., Salmas, P., Bufalari, I., Begliomini, C., & Fadiga, L. (2009). The motor somatotopy of speech perception. *Current Biology, 19,* 381–385.

D'haeseleer, E., Depypere, H., Claeys, S., Wuyts, F. L., Baudonck, N., & Van Lierde, K. M. (2011). Vocal characteristics of middle-aged premenopausal women. *Journal of Voice, 25,* 360–366.

Darley, F. L., Aronson, A. E., & Brown, J. R. (1975). *Motor speech disorders.* Philadelphia: W. B. Saunders Company.

Davis, L. F. (1987). Respiration and phonation in cerebral palsy: A developmental model. *Seminars in Speech and Language, 8,* 101–106.

Davis, P. J., Zhang, S. P., Winkworth, A., & Bandler, R. (1996). Neural control of vocalization: Respiratory and emotional influences. *Journal of Voice, 10,* 23–38.

De Bodt, M. S., Huici M. E. H.-D., & Van De Heyning, P. H. (2002). Intelligibility as a linear combination of dimensions in dysarthric speech. *Journal of Communication Disorders, 35,* 283–292.

Decker, T. N. (1990). *Instrumentation: An introduction for students in the speech and hearing sciences.* New York: Longman.

Dedivitis, R. A., Sertorio, C. B., & Pfuetzenreiter, E. G. (2009). Videokymographic analysis of patients after frontolateral laryngectomy with sternohyoid muscle flap reconstruction. *Acta Otorhinolaryngologica Italica, 29,* 144–150.

Dehqan, A., & Scherer, R. C. (2011). Objective voice analysis of boys with profound hearing loss. *Journal of Voice, 25,* 61–65.

Dehqan, A., Ansari H., & Bakhtiar, M. (2010). Objective voice analysis of Iranian speakers with normal voices. *Journal of Voice, 24,* 161–167.

De Letter, M., Santens, P., De Bodt, M., Van Maele, G., Van Borsel, J., & Boon, P. (2007). The effect of levodopa on respiration and word intelligibility in people with advanced Parkinson's disease. *Clinical Neurology and Neurosurgery, 109,* 495–500.

Deliyski, D. (2007). Clinical feasibility of high-speed videoendoscopy. *Perspectives of Voice and Voice Disorders, 17 (1),* 12–16.

Deliyski, D. D., Evans, M. K., & Shaw, H. S. (2005). Influence of data acquisition environment on accuracy of acoustic voice quality measurements. *Journal of Voice, 19,* 176–186.

Deliyski, D. D., Petrushev, P. P., Bonilha, H. S., Gerlach, T. T., Martin-Harris, B., & Hillman, R. E. (2008). Clinical implementation of laryngeal high-speed videoendoscopy: Challenges and evolution. *Folia Phoniatrica et Logopedica, 60,* 33–44.

Deliyski, D. D., Shaw, H. S., & Evans, M. K. (2005). Adverse effects of environmental noise on acoustic voice quality measurements. *Journal of Voice, 19,* 15–28.

Deliyski, D., D., & Hillman, R. E. (2010). State of the art laryngeal imaging: Research and clinical implications. *Current Opinion in Otolaryngology-Head and Neck Surgery, 18,* 147–152.

De Pandis, M. F., Starace, A., Stefanelli, F., Marruzzo, P., Meoli, I., De Simone, G., Prati, R., & Stocchi, F. (2002). Modification of respiratory function parameters in patients with severe Parkinson's disease. *Neurological Sciences, 23,* S69–S70.

De Peuter, S., Van Diest, I., Lemaigre, V., Verleden, G., Demedts, M., & Van den Bergh, O. (2004). Dyspnea: The role of psychological processes. *Clinical Psychology Review, 24,* 557–581.

de Pinto, O., & Hollien, H. (1982). Speaking fundamental frequency characteristics of Australian women: Then and now. *Journal of Phonetics, 10,* 367–375.

Denes, P. B., & Pinson, E. N. (1993). *The speech chain: The physics and biology of spoken language* (2nd ed.). New York: W. H. Freeman.

Denny, D. (2004). Changing models of transsexualism. In U. Leli & J. Drescher (Eds.), *Transgender subjectives: A clinician's guide* (pp. 25–40). Binghamton, NY: Haworth.

Devlin, J. T., & Aydelott, J. (2008). Speech perception: Motoric contributions versus the Motor Theory. *Current Biology, 19,* R198–R200.

DeVries, S. M., & Newell Decker, T. (1992). Otoacoustic emissions: Overview of measurement methodologies. *Seminars in Hearing, 13,* 15–22.

Dickson, D. R., & Maue-Dickson, W. (1982). *Anatomical and physiological bases of speech.* Austin, TX: Pro-Ed.

Docherty, G. J. (1992). *The timing of voicing in British English obstruents.* New York: Fortis.

Dogan, M., Midi, I., Yazici, M. A., Kocak, I., Günal, D., & Sehitoglu, M. A. (2007). Objective and subjective evaluation of voice quality in multiple sclerosis. *Journal of Voice, 21,* 735–740.

Doherty, E. T., & Shipp, T. (1988). Tape recorder effects on jitter and shimmer extraction. *Journal of Speech and Hearing Research, 31,* 485–490.

Dorinsky, P. M., Edwards, L. D., Yancey, S. W., & Rickard, K. A. (2001). Use of changes in symptoms to predict changes in lung function in assessing the response to asthma therapy. *Clinical Therapeutics, 23*, 701–714.

Dorman, M. F. (2000). Speech perception by adults. In S. B. Waltzman & N. L. Cohen (Eds.), *Cochlear implants* (pp. 317–329). New York: Thieme.

Doshi, D. R., & Weinberger, M. M. (2006). Long-term outcome of vocal cord dysfunction. *Annals of Allergy, Asthma, & Immunology, 96*, 794–799.

Drewek, R., Garber, E., Stanclik, S., Simpson, P., Nugent, M., & Gershan, W. (2009). The FEF25–75 and its decline as a predictor of methacholine responsiveness in children. *Journal of Asthma, 46*, 375–381.

Dromey, C., Ramig, L. O., & Johnson, A. B. (1995). Phonatory and articulatory changes associated with increased vocal intensity in Parkinson's disease: A case study. *Journal of Speech and Hearing Research, 38*, 751–764.

Dubno, J., Dirks, D., & Schaefer, A. (1987). Effects of hearing loss on utilization of short-duration spectral cues in stop consonant recognition. *Journal of the Acoustical Society of America, 81*, 1940–1947.

Dull, C. E., Metcalfe, H. C., & Williams, J. E. (1960). *Modern physics*. New York: Holt, Rinehart and Winston.

Durrant, J. D., & Lovrinic, J. H. (1995). *Bases of hearing science* (3rd ed.). Baltimore, MD: Williams & Wilkins.

Dworkin, J. P. (1991). *Motor speech disorders: A treatment guide*. St. Louis, MO: Mosby Year Book.

Earnest, M. M., & Max, L. (2003). En route to the three-deimensional registration and analysis of speech movements: Instrumental techniques for the study of articulatory kinematics. *Contemporary Issues in Communication Science and Disorders, 30*, 5–25.

Echternach, M., Dippold, S., Sundberg, J., Arndt, S., Zander, M. F., & Richter, B. (2010). High-speed imaging and electroglottography measurements of the open quotient in untrained male voices' register transitions. *Journal of Voice, 24*, 644–650.

Echternach, M., Sundberg, J., Zander, M. F., & Richter, B. (2011). Perturbation measurements in untrained male voices' transitions from modal to falsetto register. *Journal of Voice, 25*, 663–669.

Eguchi, S., & Hirsh, L. J. (1969). Development of speech sounds in children. *Acta Otolaryngologica Supplement, 257*, 1–51.

Eid, N., Yandell, B., Howell, L., Eddy, M., & Sheikh, S. (2000). Can peak expiratory flow predict airflow obstruction in children with asthma? *Pediatrics, 105*, 354–358.

Eimas, P. D., Miller, J. L., & Jusczyk, P. W. (1987). On infant speech perception and the acquisition of language. In S. Harnad (Ed.), *Categorical perception: The groundwork of cognition* (pp. 161–195). Cambridge, UK: Cambridge University Press.

Eisen, A. H., & Ferrand, C. T. (1995). *Disfluencies in college age students with LLD, college age students who stutter, and normally speaking college age students*. Paper presented at the Annual Convention of the American Speech–Language–Hearing Association.

Elliott, L. L., & Hammer, M. A. (1993). Fine-grained auditory discrimination: Factor structures. *Journal of Speech and Hearing Research, 36*, 396–409.

Erber, N. P. (1975). Auditory-visual perception of speech. *Journal of Speech and Hearing Disorders, 40*, 481–492.

Ertmer, D. J. (2001). Emergence of a vowel system in a young cochlear implant recipient. *Journal of Speech, Language, and Hearing Research, 44*, 803–813.

Ertmer, D. J., & Stark, R. E. (1995). Eliciting prespeech vocalizations in a young child with profound hearing loss: Usefulness of real-time spectrographic speech displays. *American Journal of Speech–Language Pathology, 4*, 33–38.

Ertmer, D. J., Stark, R. E., & Karlan, G. R. (1996). Real-time spectrographic displays in vowel production training with children who have profound hearing loss. *American Journal of Speech–Language Pathology, 5*, 4–16.

Eskenazi, L., Childers, D. G., & Hicks, D. M. (1990). Acoustic correlates of vocal quality. *Journal of Speech and Hearing Research, 33,* 298–306.

Evans, M. K., & Deliyski, D. D. (2007). Acoustic voice analysis of prelingually deaf adults before and after cochlear implantation. *Journal of Voice, 21,* 669–682.

Fant, G. (1960). *Acoustic theory of speech production.* The Hague, Netherlands: Mouton.

Ferguson, S. H., & Kewley-Port, D. (2002). Vowel intelligibility in clear and conversational speech for normal-hearing and hearing impaired listeners. *Journal of the Acoustical Society of America, 112,* 259–271.

Ferguson, S. H., & Kewley-Port, D. (2007). Talker differences in clear and conversational speech: Acoustic characteristics of vowels. *Journal of Speech, Language, and Hearing Research, 50,* 1241–1255.

Fernandez-Lastra, A., Morales-Rodriguez, M., & Penzol-Diaz, J. (2001). Neurophysiological study and use of P300 evoked potentials for investigation in the diagnosis and of follow-up of patients with Alzheimer's disease. *Revistade Neurologia, 6,* 525–528.

Ferrand, C. T. (1995). Effects of practice with and without knowledge of results on jitter and shimmer levels in normally speaking women. *Journal of Voice, 9,* 419–423.

Ferrand, C. T. (2000). Harmonics-to-noise ratios in prepubescent girls and boys. *Journal of Voice, 14,* 9–14.

Ferrand, C. T. (2002). Harmonics-to-noise ratios: An index of vocal aging. *Journal of Voice, 16,* 480–487.

Ferrand, C. T. (2012). *Voice disorders: Scope of theory and practice.* Boston, MA: Pearson Education, Inc.

Ferrand, C. T., & Bloom, R. L. (1996). Gender differences in children's intonational patterns. *Journal of Voice, 10,* 284–291.

Fiez, J. A. (2001). Neuroimaging studies of speech: An overview of techniques and methodological approaches. *Journal of Communication Disorders, 34,* 445–454.

Finitzo, T., Pool, K. D., Devous, M. D., Sr., & Watson, B. C. (1991). Cortical dysfunction in developmental stutterers. In H. F. M. Peters, W. Hulstijn, & C. W. Starkweather (Eds.), *Speech motor control and stuttering* (pp. 251–262). Amsterdam: Elsevier.

Firoozi, F., Lemière, C., Beauchesne, M.-F., Forget, A., & Blais, L. (2007). Development and validation of database indexes of asthma severity and control. *Thorax, 62,* 581–587.

Fisher, K. V., Scherer, R. C., Guo, C. G., & Owen, A. S. (1996). Longitudinal phonatory characteristics after botulinum toxin type A injection. *Journal of Speech and Hearing Research, 39,* 968–980.

Fisher, K. V., Scherer, R. C., Swank, P. R., Giddens, C., & Patten, D. (1999). Electroglottographic tracking of phonatory response to Botox. *Journal of Voice, 13,* 203–218.

Fitch, J. (1990). Consistency of fundamental frequency and perturbation in repeated phonations of sustained vowels, reading, and connected speech. *Journal of Speech and Hearing Disorders, 55,* 360–363.

Fletcher, H. (1953). *Speech and hearing in communication.* Princeton, NJ: Van Nostrand Co.

Fletcher, S. G., Dagenais, P. A., & Crotz-Crosby, P. (1991a). Teaching consonants to profoundly hearing-impaired speakers using palatometry. *Journal of Speech and Hearing Research, 34,* 929–942.

Fletcher, S. G., Dagenais, P. A., & Crotz-Crosby, P. (1991b). Teaching vowels to profoundly hearing-impaired speakers using glossometry. *Journal of Speech and Hearing Research, 34,* 943–956.

Forrest, K., Weismer, G., Hodge, M., Dinnsen, D. A., & Elbert, M. (1990). Statistical analysis of word-initial /k/ and /t/ produced by normal and phonologically disordered children. *Clinical Linguistics and Phonetics, 4,* 327–340.

Fox, R. A., & Nissen, S. L. (2005). Sex-related acoustic changes in voiceless English fricatives. *Journal of Speech, Language, and Hearing Research, 48*, 753–765.

French, N. R., & Steinberg, J. C. (1947). Factors governing the intelligibility of speech sounds. *Journal of the Acoustical Society of America, 19*, 90–119.

Frieda, E. M., Walley, A. C., Flege, J. E., & Sloane, M. E. (2000). Adults' perception and production of the English vowel /i/. *Journal of Speech, Language, and Hearing Research, 43*, 129–143.

Fryauf-Bertschy, H., Tyler, R. S., Kelsay, D. M. R., Gantz, B. J., & Woodworth, G. G. (1997). Cochlear implant use by prelingually deafened children: The influences of age at implant and length of device use. *Journal of Speech, Language, and Hearing Research, 40*, 183–199.

Gamboa, J., Jimenez-Jimenez, F. J., Nieto, A., Montojo, J., Orti-Pareja, M., Molina, J. A., Garcia-Albea, E., & Cobeta, I. (1997). Acoustic voice analysis in patients with Parkinson's disease treated with dopaminergic drugs. *Journal of Voice, 11*, 314–320.

Gantz, B. J., & Turner, C. (2004). Combining acoustic and electrical speech processing: Iowa/Nucleus hybrid implant. *Acta Oto-laryngologica, 124*, 344–347.

Garcia, J. V., Rovira, J. M. V., & Sanvicens, L. G. (2010). The influence of the auditory prosthesis type on deaf children's voice quality. *International Journal of Pediatric Otorhinolaryngology, 74*, 843–848.

Garcia, M. J. V., Cobeta, I., Martin, G., Alonso-Navarro, H., & Jimenez-Jimenez, F. J. (2011). Acoustic analysis of voice in Huntington's Disease patients. *Journal of Voice, 25*, 208–217.

Gelfand, S. A. (1997). *Essentials of audiology.* New York: Thieme.

Gelfer, M. P., & Mikos, V. A. (2005). The relative contributions of speaking fundamental frequency and formant frequencies to gender identification based on isolated vowels. *Journal of Voice, 19*, 544–554.

Gelfer, M. P., & Schofield, K. J. (2000). Comparison of acoustic and perceptual measures of voice in male-to-female transsexuals perceived as female versus those perceived as male. *Journal of Voice, 14*, 22–33.

George, M. S., Nahas, Z., Lisanby, S. M. H., Schlaepfer, T., Kozel, F. A., & Greenberg, B. D. (2003). Transcranial magnetic stimulation. *Neurosurgery Clinics of North America, 14*, 283–301.

Gfeller, K., Witt, S., Adamek, M., Mehr, M., Rogers, J., Stordahl, J., & Ringgenberg, S. (2002). Effects of training on timbre recognition and appraisal by postlingually deafened cochlear implant recipients. *Journal of the American Academy of Audiology, 13*, 132–145.

Giannoni, C., Sulek, M., Friedman, E. M., & Duncan, N. O. (1998). Gastroesophageal reflux association with laryngomalacia: A prospective study. *International Journal of Pediatric Otorhinolaryngology, 43*, 11–20.

Gibbon, F. E. (2004). Abnormal patterns of tongue-palate contact in the speech of individuals with cleft palate. *Clinical Linguistics and Phonetics, 18*, 285–311.

Gibbon, F. E., Ellis, L., & Crampin, L. (2004). Articulatory placement for /t/, /d/, /k/, and /g/ targets in school age children with speech disorders associated with cleft palate. *Clinical Linguistics and Phonetics, 18*, 391–404.

Gibbon, F. E., & Paterson, L. (2006). A survey of speech and language therapists' views on electropalatography therapy outcomes in Scotland. *Child Language Teaching and Therapy, 22*, 275–292.

Gibbon, F. E., & Wood, S. E. (2003). Using electropalatography to diagnose and treat articulation disorders associated with mild cerebral palsy: A case study. *Clinical Linguistics and Phonetics, 17*, 365–374.

Gildea, T. R., & McCarthy, K. (2010). Pulmonary function testing. www.clevelandclinicmeded.com/medicalpubs/diseasemanagement/pulmonary/pulmoary-function-test.

Gill, F. B. (1995). *Ornithology* (2nd ed.). New York: W. H. Freeman.

Glasberg, B. R., & Moore, B. C. J. (1986). Auditory filter shapes in subjects with unilateral and bilateral cochlear impairments. *Journal of the Acoustical Society of America, 79*, 1020–1033.

Glaze, L. E., Bless, D. M., Milenkovic, P., & Susser, R. D. (1988). Acoustic characteristics of children's voice. *Journal of Voice, 2*, 312–319.

Goberman, A. M., & Blomgren, M. (2008). Fundamental frequency change during offset and onset of voicing in individuals with Parkinson disease. *Journal of Voice, 22*, 178–191.

Goberman, A., M., & Elmer, L. M. (2005). Acoustic analysis of clear versus conversational speech in individuals with Parkinson's disease. *Journal of Communication Disorders, 38*, 215–230.

Gold, W. M. (2005). Pulmonary function testing. In R. J. Mason, J. Murray, V. C. Broaddus, & J. Nadel (Eds.), *Textbook of respiratory medicine* (3rd ed.). Philadelphia, PA: Saunders Elsevier.

Golding-Kushner, K. J. (1997). Cleft lip and palate, craniofacial anomalies, and velopharyngeal insufficiency. In C. T. Ferrand & R. L. Bloom (Eds.), *Introduction to organic and neurogenic disorders of communication: Current scope of practice* (pp. 193–228). Boston: Allyn and Bacon.

Goldstein, L., Pouplier, M., Chen, L., Saltzman, E., & Byrd, D. (2007). Dynamic action units slip in speech production errors. *Cognition, 103*, 386–412.

Golfinopoulos, E., Tourville, J. A., Bohland, J. W., Ghosh, S, S., Nieto-Castanon, A., & Guenther, F. H. (2011). fMRI investigation of unexpected somatosensory feedback perturbation during speech. *NeuroImage, 55*, 1324–1338.

Golub, J. S., Chen, P.-H., Otto, K. J., Hapner, E., & Johns III, M. M. (2006). Prevalence of perceived dysphonia in a geriatric population. *Journal of the American Geriatrics Society, 54*, 1736–1739.

Goozee, J., V., Murdoch, B. M., Theodoros, D. G., & Stokes, P. D. (2000). Kinematic analysis of tongue movements in dysarthria following traumatic brain injury using electromagnetic articulography. *Brain Injury, 14*, 153–174.

Gotham-Rowan, M. M., & Laures-Gore, J. (2006). Acoustic-perceptual correlates of voice quality in elderly men and women. *Journal of Communication Disorders, 39*, 171–184.

Gracely, R. (2001). Dyspnea and pain: Similarities and contrasts between two very unpleasant sensations. *American Pain Society Bulletin, 11* (available from www.scribd.com/doc/93570544/dyspneu).

Grafton, S. T. (2004). Contributions of functional imaging to understanding parkinsonian symptoms. *Current Opinion in Neurobiology, 14*, 715–719.

Grandas, N. F., Jain, N. B., Denckla, J. B., Brown, R., Tun, C. G., Gallagher, M. E., & Garshick, E. (2005). Dyspnea during daily activities in chronic spinal cord injury. *Archives of Physical and Medical Rehabilitation, 86*, 1631–1635.

Grant, K. W., Walden, B. E., & Seitz, P. F. (1998). Auditory–visual speech recognition by hearing-impaired subjects: Consonant recognition, sentence recognition, and auditory–visual integration. *Journal of the Acoustical Society of America, 103*, 2677–2690.

Green, J. R., & Wang, Y.-T. (2003). Tongue-surface movement patterns during speech and swallowing. *Journal of the Acoustical Society of America, 113*, 2820–2833.

Greenberg, S. (1996). Auditory processing of speech. In N. J. Lass (Ed.), *Principles of experimental phonetics*. St. Louis, MO: C. V. Mosby.

Gregory, N. D., Chandran, S., Lurie, D., & Sataloff, R. T. (2012). Voice disorders in the elderly. *Journal of Voice, 26*, 254–258.

Groenen, P., Crul, T., Maassen, B., & van Bon, W. (1996). Perception of voicing cues by children with early otitis media with and without language impairment. *Journal of Speech and Hearing Research, 39*, 43–54.

Grossman, P., Wilhelm, F. H., & Brutsche, M. (2010). Accuracy of ventilatory measurement employing ambulatory inductive plethysmography during tasks of everyday life. *Biological Psychology, 84*, 121–128.

Grosvald, M. (2009). Interspeaker variation in the extent and perception of long-distance vowel-vowel coarticulation. *Journal of Phonetics, 37*, 173–188.

Guenther, F. H., & Vladusich, T. (2012). A neural theory of speech acquisition and production. *Journal of Neurolinguistics, 25*, 408–422.

Gugatschka, M., Kiesler, K., Obermayer-Pietsch, B., Schoekler, B., Schmid, C., Groselj-Strele, A., & Friedrich, G. (2010). Sex hormones and the elderly male voice. *Journal of Voice, 24*, 369–373.

Gurevich-Uvena, J., Parker, J. M., Fitzpatrick, T. M., Makashav, M. J., Perello, M. M., Blair, E. A., & Solomon, N. P. (2010). Medical comorbidities for paradoxical vocal fold motion (vocal cord dysfunction) in the military population. *Journal of Voice, 24*, 728–731

Hagoort, P., & van Turennout, M. (1997). The electrophysiology of speaking: Possibilities of event-related potential research on speech production. In W. Hulstijn, H. F. M. Peters, & P. H. H. M. Van Lieshout (Eds.), *Speech production: Motor control, brain research and fluency disorders* (pp. 351–361). Amsterdam: Elsevier.

Haines, D. E., & Mihailoff, G. A. (2002). The medulla oblongata. In D. E. Haines (Ed.), *Fundamental neuroscience* (2nd ed.). New York: Churchill Livingstone.

Haines, D. E., Mihailoff, G. A., & Yezierski, R. P. (2002). The spinal cord. In D. E. Haines (Ed.), *Fundamental neuroscience* (2nd ed.). New York: Churchill Livingstone.

Haines, D. E., Raila, F. A., & Terrell, A. C. (2002). Orientation to structure and imaging of the central nervous system. In D. E. Haines (Ed.), *Fundamental neuroscience* (2nd ed.). New York: Churchill Livingstone.

Hall, K. D., & Yairi, E. (1992). Fundamental frequency, jitter, and shimmer in preschoolers who stutter. *Journal of Speech and Hearing Research, 35*, 1002–1008.

Hapner, E., & Johns, M. M. (2007). Recognizing and understanding the limitations of laryngeal videostroboscopy. *Perspectives on Voice and Voice Disorders, 17(1)*, 3–7.

Hardcastle, W. (1976). *Physiology of speech production.* London: Academic Press.

Hardy, S. G. P., Chronister, R. B., & Parent, A. D. (2002). The hypothalamus. In D. E. Haines (Ed.), *Fundamental neuroscience* (2nd ed.). New York: Churchill Livingstone.

Harel, B., Cannizzaro, M., & Snyder, P. J. (2004). Variability in fundamental frequency during speech in prodromal and incipient Parkinson's disease: A longitudinal case study. *Brain and Cognition, 56*, 24–29.

Harmes, S., Daniloff, R. G., Hoffman, P. R., Lewis, J., Kramer, M. B., & Absher, R. (1984). Temporal and articulatory control of fricative articulation by speakers with Broca's aphasia. *Journal of Phonetics, 12*, 367–385.

Harnsberger, J. D., Brown, W. S. Jr., Shrivastav, R., & Rothman, H. (2010). Noise and tremor in the perception of vocal aging in males. *Journal of Voice, 24*, 523–530.

Harnsberger, J. D., Shrivastav, R., Brown, W. S., Rothman, H., & Hollien, H. (2008). Speaking rate and fundamental frequency as speech cues to perceived age. *Journal of Voice, 22*, 58–69.

Harrison, M., Roush, J., & Wallace, J. (2003). Trends in age of identification and intervention in infants with hearing loss. *Ear and Hearing, 24*, 89–95.

Hartelius, L., Nord, L., & Buder, E. H. (1995). Acoustic analysis of dysarthria associated with multiple sclerosis. *Clinical Linguistics and Phonetics, 9*, 95–120.

Hartinger, M., Tripoliti, E., Hardcastle, W. J., & Limousin, P. (2011). Effects of medication and subthalamic nucleus deep brain stimulation on tongue movements in speakers with Parkinson's disease using electropalatography: A pilot study. *Clinical Linguistics and Phonetics, 25*, 210–230.

Hartl, D. M., Hans, S., Crevier-Buchman, L., Vaissière, J., & Brasnu, D. F. (2009). Long-term acoustic comparison of thyroplasty versus autologous fat injection. *Annals of Otology, Rhinology, & Laryngology, 118*, 827–832.

Hassan, S. M., Malki, K. H., Mesallam, T. A., Farahat, M., Bukhari, M., & Murry, T. (2011). The effect of cochlear implantation and post-operative rehabilitation on acoustic voice analysis in post-lingual hearing impaired adults. *European Archives of Otorhinolaryngology, 268*, 1437–1442.

Hawkins, S. (1999a). Auditory capacities and phonological development: Animal, baby, and foreign listeners. In J. M. Pickett (Ed.), *The acoustics of speech communication: Fundamentals, speech perception theory, and technology* (pp. 183–197). Boston: Allyn and Bacon.

Hawkins, S. (1999b). Looking for invariant correlates of linguistic units: Two classical theories of speech perception. In J. M. Pickett (Ed.), *The acoustics of speech communication: Fundamentals, speech perception theory, and technology* (pp. 198–231). Boston: Allyn and Bacon.

Hawkins, S. (1999c). Reevaluating assumptions about speech perception: Interactive and integrative theories. In J. M. Pickett (Ed.), *The acoustics of speech communication: Fundamentals, speech perception theory, and technology* (pp. 232–288). Boston: Allyn and Bacon.

Hedrick, M. (1997). Effect of acoustic cues on labeling fricatives and affricates. *Journal of Speech, Language, and Hearing Research, 40*, 925–938.

Hedrick, M. S., & Carney, A. E. (1997). Effect of relative amplitude and formant transitions on perception of place of articulation by adult listeners with cochlear implants. *Journal of Speech, Language, and Hearing Research, 40*, 1445–1457.

Heissa, W. D., & Hilkera, R. (2004). The sensitivity of 18-fluorodopa positron emission tomography and magnetic resonance imaging in Parkinson's disease. *European Journal of Neurology, 11*, 5–12.

Heman-Ackah, Y., & Batory, M. (2003). Determining the etiology of mild vocal fold hypomobility. *Journal of Voice, 17*, 579–588.

Herbst, C., & Ternström, S. (2006). A comparison of different methods to measure the EGG contact quotient. *Logopedics, Phoniatrics, Vocology, 31*, 126–138.

Hickok, G., Costanzo, M., Capasso, R., & Miceli, G. (2011). The role of Broca's area in speech perception: Evidence from aphasia revisited. *Brain & Language, 119*, 214–220.

Hickok, G., Houde, J., & Rong, F. (2011). Sensorimotor integration in speech processing: Computational basis and neural organization. *Neuron Perspective, 69*, 407–422.

Hicks, M., Brugman, S. M., & Katial, R. (2008). Vocal cord dysfunction/paradoxical vocal fold motion. *Primary Care and Clinical Office Practice, 35*, 81–103.

Higgins, M. B., & Saxman, J. H. (1991). A comparison of selected phonatory behaviors of healthy aged and young adults. *Journal of Speech and Hearing Research, 34*, 1000–1010.

Hiki, S., & Itoh, H. (1986). Influence of palatal shape on lingual articulation. *Speech Communication, 5*, 141–158.

Hillenbrand, J., & Houde, R. A. (1996). Acoustic correlates of breathy vocal quality: Dysphonic voices and continuous speech. *Journal of Speech and Hearing Research, 39*, 311–321.

Hirschberg, J. (1999). Dysphonia in infants. *International Journal of Pediatric Otorhinolaryngology, 49 (suppl 1)*, S293–S296.

Hixon, T. J., Goldman, M., & Mead, J. (1973). Kinematics of the chest wall during speech production: Volume displacements of the ribcage, abdomen, and lung. *Journal of Speech and Hearing Research, 16*, 78–115.

Hixon, T. J., & Hoit, J. D. (2005). *Evaluation and management of speech breathing disorders*. Tucson, AZ: Redington Brown.

Hixon, T. J., Weismer, G., & Hoit, J. D. (2008). *Preclinical speech science: Anatomy, physiology, acoustics, perception.* San Diego, CA: Plural Publishing, Inc.

Hixon, T., Hawley, J., & Wilson, K. (1982). An around-the-house device for the clinical determination of respiratory driving pressure: A note on making simple even simpler. *Journal of Speech and Hearing Disorders, 47,* 413–415.

Hocevar-Boltezar, I., Vatovec, J., Gros, A., & Zargi, M. (2005). The influence of cochlear implantation on some voice parameters. *International Journal of Pediatric Otorhinolaryngology, 69*, 1635–1640.

Hoffman, P. R., Daniloff, R. G., Bengoa, D., & Schuckers, G. H. (1985). Misarticulating and normally articulating children's identification and discrimination of synthetic [r] and [w]. *Journal of Speech and Hearing Disorders, 50*, 46–53.

Hofman, P., & van Opstal, J. (2003). Binaural weighting of pinna cues in human sound localization. *Experimental Brain Research, 148*, 458–470.

Hoit, J. D. (1995). Influence of body position on breathing and its implications for the evaluation and treatment of speech and voice disorders. *Journal of Voice, 9*, 341–347.

Hoit, J. D., & Hixon, T. J. (1987). Age and speech breathing. *Journal of Speech and Hearing Research, 30*, 351–366.

Hoit, J. D., Banzett, R. B., Brown, R., & Loring, S. H. (1990). Speech breathing in individuals with cervical spinal cord injury. *Journal of Speech and Hearing Research, 33*, 798–807.

Hoit, J. D., Hixon, T. J., Watson, P. J., & Morgan, W. J. (1990). Speech breathing in children and adolescents. *Journal of Speech and Hearing Research, 33*, 51–69.

Hoit, J. D., Lansing, R. W., & Perona, K. E. (2007). Speaking-related dyspnea in healthy adults. *Journal of Speech, Language, and Hearing Research, 50*, 361–374.

Hoit, J. D., Shea, S. A., & Banzett, R. B. (1994). Speech production during mechanical ventilation in tracheostomized individuals. *Journal of Speech and Hearing Research, 37*, 53–63.

Holinger, L. D. (1998). Evaluation of stridor and wheezing. www.childsdoc.org/spring98/stridor/stridor.asp.

Holler, T., Campisi, P., Allegro, J., Chadha, N., K., Harrison, R. V., Papsin, B., & Gordon, K. (2010). Abnormal voicing in children using cochlear implants. *Archives of Otolaryngology-Head and Neck Surgery, 136*, 17–21.

Hollien, H. (1974). On vocal registers. *Journal of Phonetics, 2*, 125–143.

Hollien, H., & Shipp, T. (1972). Speaking fundamental frequency and chronologic age in males. *Journal of Speech and Hearing Research, 15*, 150–160.

Holmberg, E. B., Oates, J., Dacakis, G., & Grant, C. (2010). Phonetograms, aerodynamic measurements, self-evaluations, and auditory perceptual ratings of male-to-female transsexual voice. *Journal of Voice, 24*, 511–522.

Holmes, P. W., Lau, K. K., Crossett, M., Low, C., Buchanan, D., Hamilton, G. S., & Bardin, P. G. (2009). Diagnosis of vocal cord dysfunction in asthma with high resolution dynamic volume computerized tomography of the larynx. *Respirology, 14*, 1106–1113.

Holte, L., Margolis, R., & Cavanaugh, R. (1991). Developmental changes in multifrequency tympanograms. *Audiology, 30*, 1–24.

Honjo, I., & Isshiki, N. (1980). Laryngoscopic and voice characteristics of aged persons. *Archives of Otolaryngology, 106*, 149–150.

Horga, D., & Liker, M. (2006). Voice and pronunciation of cochlear implant speakers. *Clinical Linguistics and Phonetics, 20*, 211–217.

Horii, Y., & Fuller, B. F. (1990). Selected acoustic characteristics of voices before intubation and after extubation. *Journal of Speech and Hearing Research, 33,* 505–510.

Howard, S. (2004). Compensatory articulatory behaviours in adolescents with cleft palate: Comparing the perceptual and instrumental evidence. *Clinical Linguistics and Phonetics, 18,* 313–340.

Huber, J. E. (2008). Effects of utterance length and vocal loudness on speech breathing in older adults. *Respiratory Physiology and Neurobiology, 164,* 323–330.

Huber, J. E., & Darling, M. (2011). Effect of Parkinson's disease on the production of structured and unstructured speaking tasks: Respiratory physiologic and linguistic considerations. *Journal of Speech, Language, and Hearing Research, 54,* 33–46.

Huber, J. E., & Spruill III, J. (2008). Age-related changes to speech breathing with increased vocal loudness. *Journal of Speech, Language, and Hearing Research, 51,* 651–668.

Huber, J. E., Stathopoulos, E. T., Ramig, L. O., & Lancaster, S. L. (2000). Respiratory function and variability in individuals with Parkinson disease: Pre- and post-Lee Silverman Voice Therapy. *Journal of Medical Speech–Language Pathology, 11,* 185–201.

Hunter, L. L., & Margolis, R. H. (1992). Multifrequency tympanometry: Current clinical application. *American Journal of Audiology, 1,* 33–43.

Hustad, K. G. (2006). A closer look at transcription intelligibility for speakers with dysarthria: Evaluation of scoring paradigms and linguistic errors made by listeners. *American Journal of Speech–Language Pathology, 15,* 266–277.

Hutchins, J. B., Naftel, J. P., & Ard, M. D. (2002). The cell biology of neurons and glia. In D. E. Haines (Ed.), *Fundamental neuroscience* (2nd ed.). New York: Churchill Livingstone.

Iacoboni, M. (2008). The role of premotor cortex in speech perception: Evidence from fMRI and rTMS. *Journal of Physiology, 102,* 31–34.

Ihre, E., Zetterstrom, O., Ihre, E., & Hammarberg, B. (2004). Voice problems as side effects of inhaled corticosteroids in asthma patients—A prevalence study. *Journal of Voice, 18,* 403–414.

Ingham, R. J., Fox, P. T., & Ingham, J. C. (1994). Brain image investigation of the speech of stutterers and nonstutterers. *ASHA, 36,* 188.

Ingham, R. J., Fox, P. T., & Ingham, J. C. (1997). A H215O positron emission tomography study on adults who stutter: Findings and implications. In W. Hulstijn, H. F. M. Peters, & P. H. H. M. Van Lieshout (Eds.), *Speech production: Motor control, brain research and fluency disorders* (pp. 293–305). Amsterdam: Elsevier.

Inwald, E. C., Döllinger, M., Schuster, M., Eysholdt, U., & Bohr, C. (2011). Multiparametric analysis of vocal fold vibrations in healthy and disordered voices in high-speed imaging. *Journal of Voice, 25,* 576–590.

Iskarous, K. (2003). Task dynamics of the tongue. In S. Palethorpe & M. Tabain (Eds.), *Proceedings of the 6th International Seminar on Speech Production* (pp. 107–112). Sydney: Macquarie University.

Iwarsson, J., & Sundberg, J. (1999). Breathing behaviors during speech in healthy females and patients with vocal fold nodules. *Logopedics, Phoniatrics, Vocology, 24,* 154–169.

Jallon, J. F., & Berthommier, F. (2009). A semi-automatic method for extracting vocal tract movements from x-ray films. *Speech Communication, 51,* 97–115.

Jenkins, H. A., Cherniack, R., Szefler, S. J., Covar, R., Gelfand, E. W., & Spahn, J. D. (2003). A comparison of the clinical characteristics of children and adults with severe asthma. *Chest, 124,* 1318–1324.

Jerger, J. (1970). Clinical experience with impedance audiometry. *Archives of Otolaryngology, 92,* 311–324.

Jerger, J. F., & Stach, B. (1994). Hearing disorders. In F. D. Minifie (Ed.), *Introduction to communication sciences and disorders* (pp. 603–672). San Diego, CA: Singular.

Jerger, J., Harford, E., Clemis, J., & Alford, B. (1974). The acoustic reflex in eighth nerve disorders. *Archives of Otolaryngology, 99*, 409–413.

Jiang, J., Ng, J., & Hanson, D. (1999). The effects of rehydration on phonation in excised canine larynges. *Journal of Voice, 13*, 51–59.

Jines, N., & Drummond, S. (2006, November). *The diagnosis of vocal cord dysfunction: A case study.* Presented at the annual convention of the American Speech–Language–Hearing Association, Miami, FL.

Joglar, J. A., Nguyen, C., Garst, D. M., & Katz, W. F. (2009). Safety of electromagnetic articulography in patients with pacemakers and implantable cardioverter-defibrillators. *Journal of Speech, Language, and Hearing Research, 52*, 1082–1087.

Jotz, G. P., Cervantes, O., Abrahão, M., Settanni, F. A. P., & de Angelis, E. C. (2002). Noise-to-harmonics ratio as an acoustic measure of voice disorders in boys. *Journal of Voice, 16*, 28–31.

Kahane, J. C. (1982). Growth of the human prepubertal and pubertal larynx. *Journal of Speech and Hearing Research, 25*, 446–455.

Kalliakosta, G., Mandros, C., & Tzelepis, G. E. (2007). Chest wall motion during speech production in patients with advanced ankylosing spondylitis. *Journal of Speech, Language, and Hearing Research, 50*, 109–118.

Kamen, R. S., & Watson, B. C. (1991). Effects of long-term tracheostomy on spectral characteristics of vowel production. *Journal of Speech and Hearing Research, 34*, 1057–1065.

Kanaparthi, L. K., Lessnau, K.-D., & Sharma, S. (2012). Restrictive lung disease. http://emedicine.medscape.com/article/301760-overview.

Kaszuba, S. M., & Garrett, C. G. (2007). Strobovideolaryngoscopy and laboratory voice evaluation. *Otolaryngology Clinics of North America, 40*, 991–1001.

Katada, E., Sato, K., Sawaki, A., Dohi, Y., Ueda, R., & Ojika, K. (2003). Long-term effects of donepezil on P300 auditory event-related potentials in patients with Alzheimer's disease. *Journal of Geriatric Psychiatry and Neurology, 16*, 39–43.

Katz, W. F., Bharadwaj, S. V., & Carstens, B. (1999). Electromagnetic articulography treatment for an adult with Broca's aphasia and apraxia of speech. *Journal of Speech, Language, and Hearing Research, 42*, 1355–1366.

Katz, W. F., Bharadwaj, S. V., & Stettler, M. P. (2006). Influences of electromagnetic articulography sensors on speech production by healthy adults and individuals with aphasia and apraxia. *Journal of Speech, Language, and Hearing Disorders, 49*, 645–660.

Katz, W. F., Garst, D. M., Carter, G. S., McNeil, M. R., Fossett, T. R., Doyle, P. J., & Szuminsky, N. J. (2007). Treatment of an individual with aphasia and apraxia of speech using EMA visually-augmented feedback. *Brain and Language, 103*, 8–249.

Kazi, R., Kalagalingam, J., Venkitaraman, R., Prasad, V., Clarke, P., Nutting, C. M., Rhys-Evans, P., & Harrington, K. J. (2009). Electroglottographic and perceptual evaluation of tracheoesophageal speech. *Journal of Voice, 23*, 247–254.

Kazi, R., Singh, A., Al-Mutairy, A., De Cordova, J., O'Leary, L., Nutting, C., Clarke, P., Rhys-Evans, P., & Harrington, K. (2008). Electroglottographic analysis of valved speech following total laryngectomy. *Logopedics, Phoniatrics, Vocology, 33*, 12–21.

Kazi, R., Venkitaraman, R., Johnson, C., Prasad, V., Clarke, P., Newbold, K., Rhys-Evans, P., Nutting, C., & Harrington, K. (2008b). Prospective, longitudinal electroglottographic study of voice recovery following accelerated hypofractionated radiotherapy for T1/T2 larynx cancer. *Radiotherapy and Oncology, 87*, 230–236.

Kazi, R., Venkitaraman, R., Johnson, C., Prasad, V., Clarke, P., Rhys-Evans, P., Nutting, C. M., & Harrington, K. J. (2008a). Electroglottographic comparison of voice outcomes in patients with advanced laryngopharyngeal cancer treated by chemoradiotherapy or total laryngectomy. *International Journal of Radiation Oncology, Biology & Physiology, 70*, 344–352.

Keating, D., Turrell, G., & Ozanne, A. (2001). Childhood speech disorders: Reported prevalence, comorbidity and socioeconomic profile. *Journal of Paediatrics and Child Health, 37*, 431–436.

Kei, J., Allison-Levick, J., Dockray, J., Harrys, R., Kirkegard, C., Wong, J., Maurer, M., Hegarty, J., Young, J., & Tudehope, D. (2003). High-frequency (1000 Hz) tympanometry in normal neonates. *Journal of the American Academy of Audiology, 14*, 20–28.

Kelley, R. T., Colton, R. H., Casper, J., Paseman, A., & Brewer, D. (2011). Evaluation of stroboscopic signs. *Journal of Voice, 25*, 490–495.

Kelly, S., Main, A., Manley, G., & McLean, C. (2000). Electropalatography and the Linguagraph system. *Medical Engineering & Physics, 22*, 47–58.

Kempster, G. B., Kistler, D. J., & Hillenbrand, J. (1991). Multidimensional scaling analysis of dysphonia in two speaker groups. *Journal of Speech and Hearing Research, 34*, 534–543.

Kennedy, C. R., McCann, D. C., Campbell, M. J., Law, C. M., Mullee, M., Petrou, S., Watkin, P., Worsfold, S., Yuen, H. M., & Stevenson, J. (2006). Language ability after early detection of permanent childhood hearing impairment. *New England Journal of Medicine, 354*, 2131–2141.

Kent, J. F., Kent, R. D., Rosenbek, J. C., Weismer, G., Martine, R., Sufit, R., & Brooks, B. R. (1992). Quantitative description of the dysarthria in women with amyotrophic lateral sclerosis. *Journal of Speech and Hearing Research, 35*, 723–733.

Kent, R. D. (1994). *Reference manual for communicative sciences and disorders: Speech and language.* Austin, TX: Pro-Ed.

Kent, R. D. (1997a). Speech motor models and developments in neurophysiological science: New perspectives. In W. Hulstijn, H. F. M. Peters, & P. H. H. M. van Lieshout (Eds.), *Speech production: Motor control, brain research and fluency disorders* (pp. 13–36). Amsterdam: Elsevier.

Kent, R. D. (1997b). *The speech sciences.* San Diego, CA: Singular.

Kent, R. D., Dembowski, J., & Lass, N. J. (1996). The acoustic characteristics of American English. In N. J. Lass (Ed.), *Principles of experimental phonetics* (pp. 185–225). St. Louis, MO: C. V. Mosby.

Kent, R. D., Kent, J. F., Weismer, G., Sufit, R. L., Brooks, B. R., & Rosenbek, J. C. (1989). Relationships between speech intelligibility and the slope of second-formant transitions in dysarthric subjects. *Clinical Linguistics and Phonetics, 3*, 347–358.

Kent, R., & Netsell, R. (1975). A case study of an ataxic dysarthric: Cineradiographic and spectrographic observations. *Journal of Speech and Hearing Disorders, 40*, 115–134.

Kent, R. D., Netsell, R., & Bauer, L. L. (1975). Cineradiography assessment of articulatory mobility in the dysarthrias. *Journal of Speech and Hearing Disorders, 40*, 467–480.

Kent, R. D., & Read, C. (1992). *The acoustic analysis of speech.* San Diego, CA: Singular.

Kent, R. D., Sufit, R. L., Rosenbek, J. C., Kent, J. F., Weismer, G., Martin, R. E., & Brooks, B. R. (1991). Speech deterioration in amyotrophic lateral sclerosis: A case study. *Journal of Speech and Hearing Research, 34*, 1269–1275.

Kessinger, R. H., & Blumstein, S. E. (1997). Effects of speaking rate on voice-onset time in Thai, French, and English. *Journal of Phonetics, 25*, 143–168.

Kim, H. S., Moon, J. W., Chung, S. M., & Lee, J. H. (2011). A short-term investigation of dysphonia in asthmatic patients using inhaled budesonide. *Journal of Voice, 25*, 88–93.

Kim, Y., Kent, R. D., & Weismer, G. (2011). An acoustic study of the relationships among neurologic disease, dysarthria type, and severity of dysarthria. *Journal of Speech, Language, and Hearing Research, 54*, 417–429.

Kim, Y., Weismer, G., Kent, R. D., & Duffy, J. R. (2009). Statistical models of F2 slope in relation to severity of dysarthria. *Folia Phoniatrica et Logopaedica, 61*, 329–335.

Kimura, M., Imagawa, H., Nito, T., Sakakibara, K.-I., Chan, R. W., & Tayama, N. (2010). Arytenoid adduction for correcting vocal fold asymmetry: High-speed imaging. *Annals of Otology, Rhinology, & Laryngology, 119*, 439–446.

Kimura, M., Nito, T., Imagawa, H., Tayama, N., & Chan, R. W. (2008). Collagen injection as a supplement to arytenoid adduction for vocal fold paralysis. *Annals of Otology, Rhinology, and Laryngology, 117*, 430–436.

Klatt, D. (1975). Voice onset time, frication, and aspiration in word-initial consonant clusters. *Journal of Speech and Hearing Research, 18*, 686–706.

Klatt, D., & Klatt, L. C. (1990). Analysis, synthesis, and perception of voice quality variations among male and female talkers. *Journal of the Acoustic Society of America, 87*, 820–857.

Kleinow, J., Smith, A., & Ramig, L. O. (2001). Speech motor stability in IPD: Effects of rate and loudness manipulations. *Journal of Speech, Language, and Hearing Research, 44*, 1041–1051.

Klocke, R. A. (2006). Dead space: Simplicity to complexity. *Journal of Applied Physiology, 100*, 1–2.

Kochanski, G., Grabe, E., Coleman, J., & Rosner, B. (2005). Loudness predicts prominence: Fundamental frequency lends little. *Journal of the Acoustical Society of America, 118*, 1038–1054.

Konstantopoulos, L., Vikelis, M., Seikel, J. A., & Mitsikostas, D.-D. (2010). The existence of phonatory instability in multiple sclerosis: An acoustic and electroglottographic study. *Neurological Science, 31*, 259–268.

Kosch, P. C., & Stark, A. R. (1984). Dynamic maintenance of end expiratory lung volume in full term infants. *Journal of Applied Physiology, 57*, 1126–1133.

Koufman, J. A., & Block, C. (2008). Differential diagnosis of paradoxical vocal fold movement. *American Journal of Speech–Language Pathology, 17*, 327–334.

Krausert, C. R., Olszewski, A., E., Taylor, L. N., McMurray, J. S., Dailey, S. H., & Jiang, J. J. (2011). Mucosal wave measurement and visualization techniques. *Journal of Voice, 25*, 395–405.

Kroll, R. M., De Nil, L. F., Kapur, S., & Houle, S. (1997). A positron emission tomography investigation of post-treatment brain activation in stutterers. In W. Hulstijn, H. F. M. Peters, & P. H. H. M. Van Lieshout (Eds.), *Speech production: Motor control, brain research and fluency disorders* (pp. 307–319). Amsterdam: Elsevier.

Kuehn, D. P., & Tomblin, J. B. (1977). A cineradiographic investigation of children's w/r substitutions. *Journal of Speech and Hearing Disorders, 42*, 462–473.

Kuhl, P. K. (1991). Perception, cognition, and the ontogenetic and phylogenetic emergence of human speech. In S. E. Brauth, W. S. Hall, & R. J. Dooling (Eds.), *Plasticity of development* (pp. 73–106). Cambridge, MA: The MIT Press.

Kuhl, P. K., & Meltzoff, A. N. (1996). Infant vocalizations in response to speech: Vocal imitation and developmental change. *Journal of the Acoustical Society of America, 100*, 2425–2438.

Kuhl, P. K., Andruski, J. E., Chistovich, I. A., Kozhevnikova, E. V., Ryskina, V. L., Stolyarova, E. I., Sunberg, U., & Lacerda, F. (1997). Cross-language analysis of phonetic units in language addressed to infants. *Science, 277*, 684–686.

Kühn-Inacker, H., Shehata-Dieler, W., Müller, J., & Helms, J. (2004). Bilateral cochlear implants: A way to optimize auditory perception abilities in deaf children? *International Journal of Pediatric Otorhinolaryngology, 68*, 1257–1266.

Kunisue, K., Fukushima, K., Nagayasu, A., & Nishizaki, K. (2006). Longitudinal formant analysis after cochlear implantation in school-aged children. *International Journal of Pediatric Otorhinolaryngology, 70*, 2033–2042.

Kuruvilla, M., Murdoch, B., & Goozee, J. (2007). Electromagnetic articulography assessment of articulatory function in adults with dysarthria following traumatic brain injury. *Brain Injury, 21*, 601–613.

Lai-Fook, S. J. (2004). Pleural mechanics and fluid exchange. *Physiological Reviews, 84*, 385–410.

Lamarche, A., Ternström, S., & Pabon, P. (2010). The singer's voice range profile: Female professional opera soloists. *Journal of Voice, 24*, 410–426.

Lan, M.-C., Hsu, Y.-B., Chang, S.-Y., Huang, J.-L., Tai, S.-K., Chien, C.-H., & Chu, P.-Y. (2010). Office-based treatment of vocal fold polyp with flexible laryngovideostroboscopic surgery. *Journal of Otolaryngology-Head & Neck Surgery, 39*, 90–95.

Lane, H., Perkell, J., Svirsky, M., & Webster, J. (1991). Changes in speech breathing following cochlear implant in postlingually deafened adults. *Journal of Speech and Hearing Research, 34*, 526–533.

Langmore, S. E., & Lehman, M. E. (1994). Physiologic deficits in the orofacial system underlying dysarthria in amyotrophic lateral sclerosis. *Journal of Speech and Hearing Research, 37*, 28–37.

Lansing, R. W., Im, B. S.-H., Thwing, J. I., Legezda, A. T. R., & Banzett, R. B. (2005). The perception of respiratory work and effort can be independent of the perception of air hunger. *American Journal of Respiratory and Critical Care Medicine, 162*, 1690–1696.

Lau, D. P. C., Zhang, E. Z., Wong, S. M., Lee, G., & Chan, Y. H. (2010). Correlating voice handicap index and quantitative videostroboscopy following injection laryngoplasty for unilateral vocal fold paralysis. *Otolaryngology-Head and Neck Surgery, 143*, 190–197.

Laughlin, S., & Montanera, W. (1998). Central nervous system imaging: When is CT more appropriate than MRI? *Postgraduate Medicine, 104*, 73–90.

Lauter, J. L. (1997). Noninvasive brain imaging in speech motor control and stuttering: Choices and challenges. In W. Hulstijn, H. F. M. Peters, & P. H. H. M. Van Lieshout (Eds.), *Speech production: Motor control, brain research and fluency disorders* (pp. 233–257). Amsterdam: Elsevier.

LeDorze, G., Ouellette, L., & Ryalls, J. (1994). Intonation and speech rate in dysarthric speech. *Journal of Communication Disorders, 27*, 1–18.

Lee, E.-K., & Son, Y.-I. (2005). Muscle tension dysphonia in children: Voice characteristics and outcome of voice therapy. *International Journal of Pediatric Otorhinolaryngology, 69*, 911–917.

Lee, W. T., Milstein, C., Hicks, D., Akst, L. M., & Esclamado, R. M. (2007). Results of ansa to recurrent laryngeal nerve reinnervation. *Otolaryngology-Head and Neck Surgery, 136*, 450–454.

Lenden, J. M., & Flipsen, P. Jr. (2007). Prosody and voice characteristics of children with cochlear implants. *Journal of Communication Disorders, 40*, 66–81.

Leonard, L. B., McGregor, K. K., & Allen, G. D. (1992). Grammatical morphology and speech perception in children with specific language impairment. *Journal of Speech and Hearing Research, 35*, 1076–1085.

Leung, A. K. C., & Cho, H. (1999). Diagnosis of stridor in children. *American Family Physician, 60* (available from www.aafp.org/afp/991115ap/2289.html).

Li, F., Edwards, J., & Beckman, M. E. (2009). Contrast and covert contrast: The phonetic development of voiceless sibilant fricatives in English and Japanese toddlers. *Journal of Phonetics, 37*, 111–124.

Lieberman, P. (1967). *Intonation, perception, and language.* Cambridge, MA: MIT Press.

Liker, M., Mildner, V., & Sindija, B. (2007). Acoustic analysis of the speech of children with cochlear implants: A longitudinal study. *Clinical Linguistics and Phonetics, 21*, 1–11.

Lim, J.-Y., Choi, J.-N., Kim, K.-M., & Choi, H.-S. (2006). Voice analysis of patients with diverse types of Reinke's edema and clinical use of electroglottographic measurements. *Acta Oto-Laryngologica, 126*, 62–69.

Linville, S. E. (2004, October 19). The aging voice. *The ASHA Leader*.

Linville, S. E., & Fisher, H. B. (1985). Acoustic characteristics of perceived versus actual vocal age in controlled phonation by adult females. *Journal of the Acoustical Society of America, 78*, 40–48.

Liotti, M., Brannan, S., Egan, G., Shade, R., Madden, L., Abplanalp, B., Robillard, R., Lancaster, J., Zamarripa, F. E., Fox, P. T., & Denton, D. (2001). Brain responses associated with consciousness of breathlessness (air hunger). *PNAS, 98*, 2035–2040.

Lisker, L., & Abrahamson, A. (1967). Some effects of context on voice onset time in English stops. *Language and Speech, 10*, 1–28.

Little, M. A., Costello, D. A. E., & Harries, M. L. (2011). Objective dysphonia quantification in vocal fold paralysis: Comparing nonlinear with classical measures. *Journal of Voice, 25*, 21–31.

Lofqvist, A., & Gracco, V. L. (2002). Control of oral closure in lingual stop consonant production. *Journal of the Acoustical Society of America, 111*, 2811–2827.

Logemann, J. A., Fisher, H. B., Boshes, B., & Blonsky, E. R. (1978). Frequency and cooccurrence of vocal tract dysfunctions in the speech of a large sample of Parkinson patients. *Journal of Speech and Hearing Disorders, 43*, 47–57.

Loizou, P. C. (1998). Introduction to cochlear implants. *IEEE Signal Processing Magazine*, 101–130.

Loizou, P. C. (2006). Speech processing in vocoder-centric cochlear implants. In A. R. Møller (Ed.), *Cochlear and brainstem implants. Advances in otorhinolaryngology* (vol. 64; pp. 1–10). Basel, Switzerland: Karger.

Lorenz, R., Esclamado, R. M., Teker, A. M., Strome, M., Scharpf, J., Hicks, D., Milstein, C., & Lee, W. T. (2008). Ansa cervicalis-to-recurrent laryngeal nerve anastomosis for unilateral vocal fold paralysis: Experience of a single institution. *Annals of Otology, Rhinology, & Laryngology, 117*, 40–45.

Lotto, A. J., Hickok, G. S., & Holt, L. L. (2008). Reflections on mirror neurons and speech perception. *Trends in Cognitive Sciences, 13*, 110–114.

Lowell, S. Y., Barkmeier-Kraemer, J. M., Hoit, J. D., & Story, B. H. (2008). Respiratory and laryngeal function during spontaneous speaking in teachers with voice disorders. *Journal of Speech, Language, and Hearing Research, 51*, 333–349.

Lynch, J. C. (2002). The cerebral cortex. In D. E. Haines (Ed.), *Fundamental neuroscience* (2nd ed.; pp. 505–520). New York: Churchill Livingstone.

Ma, E. P.-M., & Love, A. L. (2010). Electroglottographic evaluation of age and gender effects during sustained phonation and connected speech. *Journal of Voice, 24*, 146–152.

Ma, T. P. (2002). The basal nuclei. In D. E. Haines (Ed.), *Fundamental neuroscience* (2nd ed.) (pp. 487–503). New York: Churchill Livingstone.

Maassen, B., & Povel, D.-J. (1985). The effect of segmental and suprasegmental corrections on the intelligibility of deaf speech. *Journal of the Acoustical Society of America, 78*, 877–886.

Mandulak, K. C., Haley, K. L., Zajac, D., & Ohde, R. N. (2009). *Distinction in production of voiceless sibilant fricatives in child speakers.* Paper presented at the annual convention of the American Speech–Language–Hearing Association, New Orleans, LA.

Manfredi, C., Bocchi, L., Bianchi, S., Migali, N., & Cantarella, G. (2006). Objective vocal fold vibration assessment from videokymographic images. *Biomedical Signal Processing and Control, 1*, 129–136.

Manfredi, C., Bocchi, L., Cantarella, G., & Peretti, G. (2012). Videokymographic image processing: Objective parameters and user-friendly interface. *Biomedical Signal Processing and Control, 7*, 192–195.

Manfredi, C., Giordano, A., Schoentgen, J., Fraj, S., Bocchi, L., & Dejonckere, P. H., (2012). Perturbation measurements in highly irregular voice signals: Performances/validity of analysis software tools. *Biomedical Signal Processing and Control, 7*, 409–416.

Manifold, J. A. Y., & Murdoch, B. E. (1993). Speech breathing in young adults: Effect of body type. *Journal of Speech and Hearing Research, 36*, 657–671.

Margolis, R. H., Bass-Ringdahl, S., Hanks, W. D., Holte, L., & Zapala, D. A. (2003). Tympanometry in newborn infants—1kHz norms. *Journal of the American Academy of Audiology, 14*, 383–392.

Martin, D., Fitch, J., & Wolfe, V. (1995). Pathologic voice type and the acoustic predictions of severity. *Journal of Speech and Hearing Research, 38*, 765–771.

Maryn, Y., Corthals, P., De Bodt, M., Van Cauwenberge, P., & Deliyski, D. (2009). Perturbation measures of voice: A comparative study between Multi-Dimensional Voice Program and Praat. *Folia Phoniatrica et Logopedica, 61*, 217–226.

Massery, M. (1991). Chest development as a component of normal motor development: Implications for pediatric physical therapists. *Pediatric Physical Therapy, 3*, 3–8.

Mate, M. A., Cobeta, I., Jimenez-Jimenez, F. J., & Figueiras, R. (2012). Digital voice analysis in patients with advanced Parkinson's disease undergoing deep brain stimulation therapy. *Journal of Voice, 26*, 496–501.

Mathieson, L. (2001). *Greene and Mathieson's The voice and its disorders, 6th ed*. Philadelphia, PA: Whurr Publishers.

Mathieson, L., Hirani, S. P., Epstein, R., Baken, R. J., Wood, G., & Rubin, J. S. (2009). Laryngeal manual therapy: A preliminary study to examine its treatment effects in the management of muscle tension dysphonia. *Journal of Voice, 23*, 353–366.

Matthews, P. M., Honey, G. D., & Bullmore, E. T. (2006). Applications of fMRI in translational medicine and clinical practice. *Nature Reviews/Neuroscience, 7*, 732–744.

Max, L., & Gracco, V. L. (2005). Coordination of oral and laryngeal movements in the perceptually fluent speech of adults who stutter. *Journal of Speech, Language, and Hearing Research, 48*, 524–542.

Max, L., Guenther, F. H., Gracco, V. L., Ghosh, S., S., & Wallace, M. E. (2004). Unstable or insufficiently activated internal models and feedback-biased motor control as sources of dysfluency: A theoretical model of stuttering. *Contemporary Issues in Communication Sciences and Disorders, 31*, 105–122.

McAllister, A., Sederholm, E., Sundberg, J., & Gramming, P. (1994). Relations between voice range profiles and physiological and perceptual voice characteristics in ten-year-old children. *Journal of Voice, 8*, 230–239.

McAnally, K. I., Hansen, P. C., Cornelissen, P. L., & Stein, J. F. (1997). Effect of time and frequency manipulation on syllable perception in developmental dyslexics. *Journal of Speech, Language, and Hearing Research, 40*, 912–924.

McAuliffe, M., & Ward, E. (2006). The use of electropalatography in the assessment and treatment of acquired motor speech disorders in adults: Current knowledge and future directions. *NeuroRehabilitation, 21*, 189–203.

McAuliffe, M. J., Ward, E. C., & Murdoch, B. E. (2006). Speech production in Parkinson's disease: II. Acoustic and electropalatographic investigation of sentence, word, and segment durations. *Clinical Linguistics and Phonetics, 20*, 19–33.

McCarthy, K., & Dweik, R. A. (2010). Pulmonary function testing. http://emedicine.medscape.com/article/303239-overview.

McFarland, D. H., & Smith, A. (1992). Effects of vocal task and respiratory phase on prephonatory chest-wall movements. *Journal of Speech and Hearing Research, 35,* 971–982.

McGlone R. E., & Shipp, T. (1971). Some physiologic correlates of vocal fry phonation. *Journal of Speech and Hearing Research, 14,* 769–775.

McKinney, J. (1994). *The diagnosis and correction of vocal faults.* Genovex Music Group.

McNeil, M. R., Fossett, T. R. D., Katz, W. F., Garst, D., Carter, G., Szuminsky, N., & Doyle, P. J. (2007). Effects of on-line kinematic feedback treatment for apraxia of speech. *Brain and Language, 103,* 8–249.

McNeil, M. R., Katz, W. F., Fossett, T. R. D., Garst, D. M., Szuminsky, N. J., Carter, G., & Lim, K. Y. (2010). Effects of online augmented kinematic and perceptual feedback on treatment of speech movements in apraxia of speech. *Folia Phoniatrica et Logopaedica, 62,* 127–133.

Mehanna, R., & Jankovic, J. (2009). Treatment of dysautonomia associated with Parkinson's disease. *Parkinsonism and Related Disorders, 15* (Suppl. 3), S224–232.

Mehanna, R., & Jankovic, J. (2010). Respiratory problems in neurologic movement disorders. *Parkinsonism and Related Disorders, 16,* 628–638.

Mehta, D. D., Deliyski, D. D., Quatieri, T. F., & Hillman, R. E. (2011). Automated measurement of vocal fold vibratory asymmetry from high-speed videoendoscopy recordings. *Journal of Speech, Language, and Hearing Research, 54,* 47–54.

Mehta, D. D., Deliyski, D. D., Zeitels, S. M., Quatieri, T. F., & Hillman, R. E. (2010). Voice production mechanisms following phonosurgical treatment of early glottic cancer. *Annals of Otology, Rhinology, & Laryngology, 119,* 1–9.

Meister, I. G., Wilson, S. M., Deblieck, C., Wu, A. D., & Iacoboni, M. (2007). The essential role of premotor cortex in speech perception. *Current Biology, 17,* 1692–1696.

Melcon, M., Hoit, J., & Hixon, T. (1989). Age and laryngeal airway resistance during vowel production. *Journal of Speech and Hearing Disorders, 54,* 282–286.

Mendes, A. P., Brown, W. S., Sapienza, C., & Rothman, H. B. (2006). Effects of vocal training on respiratory kinematics during singing tasks. *Folia Phoniatrica et Logopaedica, 58,* 363–377.

Mendoza, E., Valencia, N., Munoz, J., & Trujillo, H. (1996). Differences in voice quality between men and women: Use of the long-term average spectrum (LTAS). *Journal of Voice, 10,* 59–66.

Metz, D. E., & Schiavetti, N. (1995). Speech breathing processes of deaf and hearing-impaired persons. In F. Bell-Berti & L. J. Raphael (Eds.), *Producing speech: Contemporary issues.* [*For Katherine Safford Harris*] (pp. 187–198). New York: American Institute of Physics.

Metz, D. E., Schiavetti, N., Samar, V. J., & Sitler, R. W. (1990). Acoustic dimensions of hearing-impaired speakers' intelligibility: Segmental and suprasegmental characteristics. *Journal of Speech and Hearing Research, 33,* 476–487.

Meyers, T. A., Swirsky, M. A., Kirk, K. I., & Miyamoto, R. T. (1998). Improvements in speech perception by children with profound prelingual hearing loss: Effects of device, communication mode, and chronological age. *Journal of Speech, Language, and Hearing Research, 41,* 846–858.

Miccio, A. W., & Ingrisano, D. R. (2000). The acquisition of fricatives and affricates: Evidence from a disordered phonological system. *American Journal of Speech–Language Pathology, 9,* 214–229.

Michelsson, K., & Michelsson, O. (1999). Phonation in the newborn: Infant cry. *International Journal of Pediatric Otorhinolaryngology (suppl. 1),* S297–S301.

Michi, K. -I., Yamashita, Y., Imai, S., Suzuki, N., & Yoshida, H. (1993). Role of visual feedback treatment for defective /s/ sounds in patients with cleft palate. *Journal of Speech and Hearing Research, 36,* 277–285.

Midi, I., Dogan, M., Koseoglu, M., Can, G., Sehitoglu, M. A., & Gunal, D. I. (2008). Voice abnormalities and their relation with motor dysfunction in Parkinson's disease. *Acta Neurological Scandinavia, 117*, 26–34.

Mihailoff, G. A., & Haines, D. E. (2002). Motor system II: Corticofugal systems and the control of movement. In D. E. Haines (Ed.), *Fundamental neuroscience* (2nd ed.) (pp. 878–894). New York: Churchill Livingstone.

Miller, D. H., Grossman, R. I., Reingold, S. C., & McFarland, H. F. (1998). The role of magnetic resonance techniques in understanding and managing multiple sclerosis. *Brain, 121*, 3–24.

Miller, M. G., Weiler, J. M., Baker, B., Collins, J., & D'Alonzo, G. (2005). National Athletic Trainers Association position statement: Management of asthma in athletes. *Journal of Athletic Trainers, 40*, 224–245.

Milstein, C. F., & Watson, P. J. (2004). The effects of lung volume initiation on speech: A perceptual study. *Journal of Voice, 18*, 38–45.

Milstein, C., Qi, Y., & Hillman, R. (2000, June). *Laryngeal function associated with changes in lung volume during voice and speech production in normal speaking women.* Paper presented at the Voice Foundation 29th annual symposium, Philadelphia.

Mirasola, K. L., Braun, N., Blumin, J. H., Kerschner, J. E., & Merati, A. L. (2008). Self-reported voice-related quality of life in adolescents with paradoxical vocal fold dysfunction. *Journal of Voice, 22*, 373–378.

Mitchell, H. L., Hoit, J. D., & Watson, P. J. (1996). Cognitive–linguistic demands and speech breathing. *Journal of Speech and Hearing Research, 39*, 93–104.

Modarresi, G., Sussman, H., Lindblom, B., & Burlingame, E. (2004). An acoustic analysis of the bidirectionality of coarticulation in VCV utterances. *Journal of Phonetics, 32*, 291–312.

Moeller, M. P. (2000). Early intervention and language development in children who are deaf and hard of hearing. *Pediatrics, 106*, 46–51.

Molt, L. F. (1997). Event-related cortical potentials preceding phonation in stutterers and normal speakers: A preliminary report. In W. Hulstijn, H. F. M. Peters, & P. H. H. M. Van Lieshout (Eds.), *Speech production: Motor control, brain research and fluency disorders* (pp. 363–369). Amsterdam: Elsevier.

Monsen, R. B. (1979). Acoustic qualities of phonation in young hearing-impaired children. *Journal of Speech and Hearing Research, 22*, 270–288.

Moore, W. H., Jr. (1984). Hemispheric alpha asymmetries during an electromyographic biofeedback procedure for stuttering: A single-subject experimental design. *Journal of Fluency Disorders, 9*, 143–162.

Moore, W. H., Jr. (1986). Hemispheric alpha asymmetries of stutterers and nonstutterers for the recall and recognition of words and connected reading passages: Some relationships to severity of stuttering. *Journal of Fluency Disorders, 11*, 71–89.

Moore, W. H., & Lang, M. K. (1977). Alpha asymmetry over the right and left hemispheres of stutterers and control subjects preceding massed oral readings: A preliminary investigation. *Perceptual and Motor Skills, 44*, 223–230.

Mora, R., Jankowska, B., Guastini, L., Santomauro, V., Dellepiane, M., Crippa, B., & Salami, A. (2010). Computerized voice therapy in hypofunctional dysphonia. *Journal of Otolaryngology-Head & Neck Surgery, 39*, 615–621.

Morgan, E. E., & Rastatter, M. (1986). Variability of voice fundamental frequency in elderly female speakers. *Perceptual and Motor Skills, 63*, 215–218.

Morris, M. J. (2006). Vocal cord dysfunction: Etiologies and treatment. *Clinical and Pulmonary Medicine, 13*, 73–86.

Morris, M. J., & Christopher, K. L. (2010). Diagnostic criteria for the classification of vocal cord dysfunction. *Chest, 138*, 1213–1223.

Morris, M. J., Deal, L. E., & Bean, D. R. (1999). Vocal cord dysfunction in patients with exertional dyspnea. *Chest, 116*, 1676–1682.

Morris, M. J., Perkins, P. .J, & Allan, P. F. (2006). Vocal cord dysfunction: Etiologies and treatment. *Clinical Pulmonary Medicine, 13*, 73–86.

Morris, R. J. (1997). Speaking fundamental frequency characteristics of 8- through 10-year-old white and African-American boys. *Journal of Communication Disorders, 30*, 101–116.

Morris, R. J., McCrea, C. R., & Herring, K. D. (2008). Voice onset time differences between adult males and females: Isolated syllables. *Journal of Phonetics, 36*, 308–317.

Morrison, M., Rammage, L., & Emami, A. J. (1999). The irritable larynx syndrome. *Journal of Voice, 13*, 447–455.

Mortensen, M., & Woo, P. (2008). High-speed imaging used to detect vocal fold paresis: A case report. *Annals of Otology, Rhinology, & Laryngology, 117*, 684–687.

Motta, G., Cesari, U., Iengo, M., & Motta, G. (1990). Clinical application of electroglottography. *Folia Phoniatrica et Logopedica, 42*, 111–117.

Mu, L., & Sanders, I. (2010). Human tongue neuroanatomy: Nerve supply and motor endplates. *Clinical Anatomy, 23*, 777–791.

Murdoch, B. E., & Goozee, J. V. (2003). EMA analysis of tongue function in children with dysarthria following traumatic brain injury. *Brain Injury, 17*, 79–93.

Murdoch, B. E., Chenery, H. J., Stokes, P. D., & Hardcastle, W. J. (1991). Respiratory kinematics in speakers with cerebellar disease. *Journal of Speech and Hearing Research, 34*, 768–780.

Murphy, T. D., & Ren, C. L. (2009). Congenital stridor. Emedicine.

Murray, D. M., & Lawler, P. G. (1998). All that wheezes is not asthma: Paradoxical vocal cord movement presenting as severe acute asthma requiring ventilatory support. *Anesthesia, 53*, 1006–1011.

Murry, T., Cukier-Blaj, S., Kelleher, A., & Malki, K. H. (2011). Laryngeal and respiratory patterns in patients with paradoxical vocal fold motion. *Respiratory Medicine, 105*, 1891–1895.

Murry, T., Tabaee, A., Owezarzak, V., & Aviv, J. E. (2006). Respiratory retraining therapy and management of laryngopharyngeal reflux in the treatment of patients with cough and paradoxical vocal fold movement disorder. *Annals of Otology, Rhinology & Laryngology, 115*, 754–758.

Nair, G. (1999). *Voice-tradition and technology: A state-of-the-art studio.* San Diego, CA: Singular.

Napadow, V. J., Chen, Q., Wedeen, V. J., & Gilbert, R. J. (1999). Intramural mechanics of the human tongue in association with physiological deformations. *Journal of Biomechanics, 32*, 1–12.

Netsell, R., & Hixon, T. J. (1992). Inspiratory checking in therapy for individuals with speech breathing dysfunction (abstract). *ASHA, 34*, 152.

Newman, K. B., Mason, U. G. III, & Schmaling, K. B. (1995). Clinical features of vocal cord dysfunction. *American Journal of Respiratory Critical Care Medicine, 152*, 1382–1386.

Nguyen, D. D., & Kenny, D. T. (2009). Impact of muscle tension dysphonia on tonal pitch target implementation in Vietnamese female teachers. *Journal of Voice, 23*, 690–698.

Nielson, D. W., Heldt, G. P., & Tooley, W. H. (1990). Stridor and gastroesophageal reflux in infants. *Pediatrics, 85*, 1034–1039.

Nissen, S., L., & Fox, R. A. (2005). Acoustic and spectral characteristics of young children's fricative productions: A developmental perspective. *Journal of the Acoustical Society of America, 118*, 2570–2578.

Nittrouer, S. (1996a). Discriminability and perceptual weighting of some acoustic cues to speech perception by 3-year-olds. *Journal of Speech and Hearing Research, 39*, 278–297.

Nittrouer, S. (1996b). The relation between speech perception and phonemic awareness: Evidence from low-SES children and children with chronic OM. *Journal of Speech and Hearing Research, 39*, 1059–1070.

Nittrouer, S. (1999). Do temporal processing deficits cause phonological processing problems? *Journal of Speech, Language, and Hearing Research, 42*, 925–942.

Nittrouer, S., Studdert-Kennedy, M., & Neely, S. T. (1996). How children learn to organize their speech gestures: Further evidence from fricative-vowel syllables. *Journal of Speech and Hearing Research, 39*, 379–389.

Nolte, J. (2002). *The human brain: An introduction to its functional anatomy.* Philadelphia: Mosby.

Norton, S. J. (1992). Cochlear function and otoacoustic emissions. *Seminars in Hearing, 13*, 1–14.

Noyes, B. E., & Kemp, J. S. (2007). Vocal cord dysfunction in children. *Paediatric Respiratory Reviews, 8*, 155–163.

Nygaard, L. C., & Pisoni, D. B. (1995). Speech perception: New directions in research and theory. In J. L. Miller & P. D. Eimas (Eds.), *Speech, language, and communication* (pp. 69–76). New York: Academic Press.

Ochs, M. T., Humes, L. E., Ohde, R. N., & Grantham, D. W. (1989). Frequency discrimination ability and stop-consonant identification in normally hearing and hearing-impaired subjects. *Journal of Speech and Hearing Research, 32*, 133–142.

Ochs, M., Nyengaard, J. R., Jung, A., Knudsen, L., Voigt, M., Wahlers, T., Richter, J., & Gundersen, H. J. G. (2004). The number of alveoli in the human lung. *American Journal of Respiratory and Critical Care Medicine, 169*, 1120–1124.

Oguz, H., Tarhan, E., Korkmaz, M., Yilmaz, U., Safak, M. A., Demirci, M., & Ozluoglu, L. N. (2007). Acoustic analysis findings in objective laryngopharyngeal reflux patients. *Journal of Voice, 21*, 203–210.

Olichney, J. M., & Hillert, D. G. (2004). Clinical applications of cognitive event-related potentials in Alzheimer's disease. *Physical and Medical Rehabilitation Clinic of North America, 15*, 205–233.

Olsen, W. O., Noffsinger, D., & Kurdziel, S. (1975). Acoustic reflex and reflex decay: Occurrence in patients with cochlear and eighth nerve lesions. *Archives of Otolaryngology, 101*, 622–625.

Orlikoff, R. F. (1990). The relationship of age and cardiovascular health to certain acoustic characteristics of male voices. *Journal of Speech and Hearing Research, 33*, 450–457.

Orlikoff, R. F. (1991). Assessment of the dynamics of vocal fold contact from the electroglottogram: Data from normal male subjects. *Journal of Speech and Hearing Research, 34*, 1066–1072.

Orlikoff, R. F., Kraus, D. H., Harrison, L. B., Ho, M. L., & Gartner, C. J. (1997). Vocal fundamental frequency measures as a reflection of tumor response to chemotherapy in patients with advanced laryngeal cancer. *Journal of Voice, 11*, 33–39.

Pabon, J. P. H., & Plomp, R. (1988). Automatic phonetogram recording supplemented with acoustical voice quality parameters. *Journal of Speech and Hearing Research, 31*, 710–722.

Palmer, D., Dietsch, A., & Searl, J. (2012). Endoscopic and stroboscopic presentation of the larynx in male-to-female transsexual persons. *Journal of Voice 26*, 117–126.

Pantelemidou, V., Herman, R., & Thomas, J. (2003). Efficacy of speech intervention using electropalatography with a cochlear implant user. *Clinical Linguistics and Phonetics, 17*, 383–392.

Papastamelos, C., Panitch, H. B., England, S. E., & Allen, J. L. (1995). Developmental changes in chest wall compliance in infancy and early childhood. *Journal of Applied Physiology, 78*, 179–184.

Parker, A. J. (2008). Aspects of transgender laryngeal surgery. *Sexologies, 17*, 277–282.

Parry, A., & Matthews, P. M. (2002). *Functional magnetic resonance imaging (fMRI): A "window" into the brain.* Centre for Functional Magnetic Resonance Imaging of the Brain, Department of Clinical Neurology, University of Oxford. www.fmrib.ox.ac.uk/fmri_intro/fmri_intro.htm.

Parsons, J. P., Benninger, C., Hawley, M. P., Philips, G., Forrest, L. A., & Mastronarde, J. G. (2010). Vocal cord dysfunction: Beyond severe asthma. *Respiratory Medicine, 104,* 504–509.

Patel, A. C., Van Natta, M. L., Tonascia, J., Wise, R. A., & Strunk, R. C. (2008). Effects of time, albuterol, and budesonide on the shape of the flow-volume loop in children with asthma. *Journal of Allergy and Clinical Immunology, 122,* 781–787.

Patel, N. J., Jorgensen, C., Kuhn, J., & Merati, A. L. (2004). Concurrent laryngeal abnormalities in patients with paradoxical vocal fold dysfunction. *Otolaryngology-Head and Neck Surgery, 130,* 686–689.

Patel, R. R., Liu, L., Galatsanos, N., & Bless, D. M. (2011). Differential vibratory characteristics of adductor spasmodic dysphonia and muscle tension dysphonia on high-speed digital imaging. *Annals of Otology, Rhinology, & Laryngology, 120,* 21–32.

Patel, R., & Grigos, M. I. (2006). Acoustic characterization of the question-statement contrast in 4, 7 and 11 year old children. *Speech Communication, 48,* 1308–1318.

Patel, R., Dailey, S., & Bless, D. (2008). Comparison of high-speed digital imaging with stroboscopy for laryngeal imaging of glottal disorders. *Annals of Otology, Rhinology, & Laryngology, 117,* 413–424.

Pederson, M. F., Moller, S., Krabbe, S., Bennett, P., & Svenstrup, B. (1990). Fundamental voice frequency in female puberty measured with electroglottography during continuous speech as a secondary sex characteristic: A comparison between voice, pubertal stages, oestrogens, and androgens. *Journal of Pediatric Otorhinolaryngology, 20,* 16–23.

Pegoraro-Krook, M. I. (1988). Speaking fundamental frequency characteristics of normal Swedish subjects obtained by glottal frequency analysis. *Folia Phoniatrica et Logopedica, 40,* 82–90.

Peng, S.-C., Tomblin, J. B., Spencer, L. J., & Hurtig, R. R. (2007). Imitative production of rising speech intonation in pediatric cochlear implant recipients. *Journal of Speech, Language, and Hearing Research, 50,* 1210–1227.

Penner, M. J., & Zhang, T. (1997). Prevalence of spontaneous otoacoustic emissions in adults revisited. *Hearing Research, 103,* 28–34.

Perkell, J. S. (2012). Movement goals and feedback and feedforward control mechanisms in speech production. *Journal of Neurolinguistics 25,* 382–407.

Perkell, J. S., Matthies, M. L., Svirsky, M. A., & Jordan, M. I. (1995). Goal-based speech motor control: A theoretical framework and some preliminary data. *Journal of Phonetics, 23,* 23–35.

Perouse, R., & Coulombeau, B. (2010). Electrolaryngographic analysis in the diagnosis and phonosurgical treatment of benign laryngeal pathologies. *Logopedics, Phoniatrics, Vocology, 35,* 90–97.

Peterson, G., & Barney, H. (1952). Control methods used in a study of the vowels. *Journal of the Acoustical Society of America, 24,* 175–184.

Pick, G., Evans, E. F., & Wilson, J. P. (1977). Frequency resolution in patients with hearing loss of cochlear origin. In Evans E. F. & Wilson, J. P. (Eds.), *Psychophysics and Physiology of Hearing.* London: Academic Press.

Pickett, J. M. (1999). *The acoustics of speech communication: Fundamentals, speech perception theory, and technology.* Boston: Allyn and Bacon.

Pickles, J. O. (1988). *Introduction to the physiology of hearing* (2nd ed.). London: Academic Press.

Plag, I., Kunter, G., & Schramm, M. (2011). Acoustic correlates of primary and secondary stress in North American English. *Journal of Phonetics, 39,* 362–374.

Plante, E. (2001). Neuroimaging in communication sciences and disorders. *Journal of Communication Disorders, 34*, 441–443.

Poburka, B. J. (1999). A new stroboscopy rating form. *Journal of Voice, 13*, 403–413.

Poissant, S. F., Peters, K. A., & Robb, M. P. (2006). Acoustic and perceptual appraisal of speech production in pediatric cochlear implant users. *International Journal of Pediatric Otorhinolaryngology, 70*, 1195–1203.

Pokryszko-Dragan, A., Slotwinski, K., & Podemski, R. (2003). Modality-specific changes in P300 parameters in patients with dementia of the Alzheimer type. *Medical Science Monitor, 9*, 130–134.

Pontes, P., Brasolotto, A., & Behlau, M. (2005). Glottic characteristics and voice complaint in the elderly. *Journal of Voice, 19*, 84–94.

Ponton, C. W., Moore, J. K., & Eggermont, J. J. (1996). Auditory brain stem response generation by parallel pathways: Differential maturation of axonal conduction time and synaptic transmission. *Ear & Hearing, 17*, 402–410.

Pool, K. D., Devous, M. D., Sr., Freeman, F. J., Watson, B. C., & Finitzo, T. (1991). Regional cerebral blood flow in developmental stutterers. *Archives of Neurology, 48*, 509–512.

Porter, R. J., Hogue, D. M., & Tobey, E. A. (1995). Dynamic analysis of speech and nonspeech respiration. In F. Bell-Berti & L. J. Raphael (Eds.), *Producing speech: Contemporary issues. [For Katherine Safford Harris]* (pp. 169–185). New York: American Institute of Physics.

Prabhakar, S., Syal, P., & Srivastava, T. (2000). P300 in newly diagnosed non-dementing Parkinson's disease: Effect of dopaminergic drugs. *Neurology India, 48*, 239–242.

Prakup, B. (2012). Acoustic measures of the voices of older singers and nonsingers. *Journal of Voice, 26*, 341–350.

Prieve, B. A. (1992). Otoacoustic emissions in infants and children: Basic characteristics and clinical application. *Seminars in Hearing, 13*, 37–52.

Pruthi, T., & Espy-Wilson, C. A. (2004). Acoustic parameters for automatic detection of nasal manner. *Speech Communication, 43*, 225–239.

Puts, D. A., Hodges, C. R., Cardenas, R. A., & Gaulin, S. J. C. (2007). Men's' voices as dominance signals: Vocal fundamental and formant frequencies influence dominance attributions among men. *Evolution and Human Behavior, 28*, 340–344.

Qian-Jie, F., Galvin, J., Xiaosong, W., & Nogaki, G. (2005). Moderate auditory training can improve speech performance of adult cochlear implant patients. *Acoustics Research Letters Online, 6*, 106–111.

Raaymakers, E. M. J. A., & Crul, T. A. (1988). Perception and production of the final /s/-ts/ contrast in Dutch by misarticulating children. *Journal of Speech and Hearing Disorders, 53*, 262–270.

Raj, A., Gupta, B., Chowdhury, A., & Chadha, S. (2010). A study of voice changes in various phases of menstrual cycle and in postmenopausal women. *Journal of Voice, 24*, 363–368.

Ramig, L. O. (1992). The role of phonation in speech intelligibility: A review and preliminary data from patients with Parkinson's disease. In R. D. Kent (Ed.), *Intelligibility in speech disorders: Theory, measurement and management* (pp. 119–156). Amsterdam: John Benjamin.

Ramig, L. O., & Dromey, C. (1996). Aerodynamic mechanisms underlying treatment-related changes in vocal intensity in patients with Parkinson disease. *Journal of Speech and Hearing Research, 39*, 798–807.

Ramig, L. O., Countryman, S., Thompson, L. L., & Horii, Y. (1995). Comparison of two forms of intensive speech treatment for Parkinson's disease. *Journal of Speech and Hearing Research, 38*, 1232–1251.

Raphael, L. J., Borden, G. J., & Harris, K. S. (2007). *Speech science primer: Physiology, acoustics, and perception of speech* (5th ed.). Philadelphia: Lippincott Williams & Wilkins.

Rattenbury, H. J., Carding, P. N., & Finn, P. (2004). Evaluating the effectiveness and efficiency of voice therapy using transnasal flexible laryngoscopy: A randomized controlled trial. *Journal of Voice, 18,* 522–533.

Reilly, K. J., & Moore, C. A. (2009). Respiratory movement patterns during vocalizations at 7 and 11 months of age. *Journal of Speech, Language, and Hearing Research, 52,* 223–239.

Reubold, U., Harrington, J., & Kleber, F. (2010). Vocal aging effects on F0 and the first formant: A longitudinal analysis in adult speakers. *Speech Communication, 52,* 638–651.

Riede, T., & Zuberbühler, K. (2003). Pulse register phonation in Diana monkey alarm calls. *Journal of the Acoustical Society of America, 113,* 2919–2926.

Rihkanen, H., Leinonen, L., Hiltunen, T., & Kangas, J. (1994). Spectral pattern recognition of improved voice quality. *Journal of Voice, 8,* 320–326.

Robb, M. P., Crowell, D. H., & Dunn-Rankin, P. (2007). Cry analysis in infants resuscitated for apnea of infancy. *International Journal of Pediatric Otorhinolaryngology, 71,* 1117–1123.

Robb, M., & Saxman, J. (1985). Developmental trends in vocal fundamental frequency of young children. *Journal of Speech and Hearing Research, 28,* 420–429.

Robinette, M. S. (1992). Clinical observations with transient evoked otoacoustic emissions with adults. *Seminars in Hearing, 13,* 23–36.

Roland, N. J., Bhalla, R. K., & Earis, J. (2004). The local side effects of inhaled corticosteroids. *Chest, 126,* 213–219.

Rosen, K. M., Goozee, J. V., & Murdoch, B. E. (2008). Examining the effects of multiple sclerosis on speech production: Does phonetic structure matter? *Journal of Communication Disorders, 41,* 49–69.

Rosen, K. M., Kent, R. D., Delaney, A. L., & Duffy, J. R. (2006). Parametric quantitative acoustic analysis of conversation produced by dysarthric and HC speakers. *Journal of Speech, Language, and Hearing Research, 49,* 395–411.

Rosen, S., & Howell, P. (1991). *Signals and systems for speech and hearing.* New York: Academic Press.

Rosner, B. S., Lopez-Bascuas, L. E., Garcia-Albea, J. E., & Fahey, R. P. (2000). Voice-onset times for Castilian Spanish initial stops. *Journal of Phonetics, 28,* 217–224.

Ross, M., Brackett, D., & Maxon, A. B. (1991). *Assessment and management of mainstreamed hearing-impaired children.* Austin, TX: Pro-Ed.

Rossini, P. M., & Rossi, S. (2007). Transcranial magnetic stimulation: Diagnostic, therapeutic, and research potential. *Neurology, 68,* 484–488.

Roubeau, B., Henrich, N., & Castellengo, M. (2009). Laryngeal vibratory mechanisms: The notion of vocal register revisited. *Journal of Voice, 23,* 425–438.

Rowlett, R. (2000). How many? A dictionary of units of measurement. University of North Carolina at Chapel Hill. www.unc.edu/~rowlett/units/sipm.html.

Roy, N., Bless, D. M., Heisey, D., & Ford, C. N. (1997). Manual circumlaryngeal therapy for functional dysphonia: An evaluation of short- and long-term treatment outcomes. *Journal of Voice, 11,* 321–331.

Roy, N., Nissen, S. L., Dromey, C., & Sapir, S. (2009). Articulatory changes in muscle tension dysphonia: Evidence of vowel space expansion following manual circumlaryngeal therapy. *Journal of Communication Disorders, 42,* 124–135.

Rubin, A. D., Praneetvatakul, V., Heman-Ackah, Y., Moyer, C. A., Mandel, S., & Sataloff, R. T. (2005). Repetitive phonatory tasks for identifying vocal fold paresis. *Journal of Voice, 19,* 679–686.

Russell, A., Penny, L., & Pemberton, C. (1995). Speaking fundamental frequency changes over time in women: A longitudinal study. *Journal of Speech and Hearing Research, 38,* 101–109.

Russell, B. A., Cerny, F. J., & Stathopoulos, E. T. (1998). Effects of varied vocal intensity on ventilation and energy expenditure in women and men. *Journal of Speech, Language, and Hearing Research, 41,* 239–248.

Russell, N. K., & Stathopoulos, E. (1988). Lung volume changes in children and adults during speech production. *Journal of Speech and Hearing Research, 31,* 146–155.

Rvachew, S., & Jamieson, D. G. (1989). Perception of voiceless fricatives by children with a functional articulation disorder. *Journal of Speech and Hearing Disorders, 54,* 193–208.

Ryalls, J., Baum, S., & Larouche, A. (1991). Spectral characteristics for place of articulation in the speech of young normal, moderately and profoundly hearing-impaired French Canadians. *Clinical Linguistics and Phonetics, 3,* 165–179.

Saigusa, H., Saigusa, M., Aino, I., Iwasaki, C., Li, L., & Niimi, S. (2006). M-mode color Doppler ultrasonic imaging of vertical tongue movement during articulatory movement. *Journal of Voice, 20,* 38–45.

Saito, K., Kimura, M., Imagawa, H., Nito, T., Tayama, N., & Shiotani, A. (2010). High-speed digital imaging of the neoglottis after supracricoid laryngectomy with cricohyoidoepiglottopexy. *Otolaryngology-Head and Neck Surgery, 142,* 598–604.

Sakakura, K., Chikamatsu, K., Toyoda, M., Kaai, M., Yasuoka, Y., & Furuya, N. (2008). Congenital laryngeal anomalies presenting as chronic stridor: A retrospective study of 55 patients. *Auris Nasus Larynx, 35,* 527–533.

Salomão, G. L., & Sundberg, J. (2009). What do male singers mean by modal and falsetto register? An investigation of the glottal voice source. *Logopedics, Phoniatrics, Vocology, 34,* 73–83.

Sammeth, C. A., Dorman, M. F., & Stearns, C. J. (1999). The role of consonant–vowel amplitude ratio in the recognition of voiceless stop consonants by listeners with hearing impairment. *Journal of Speech, Language, and Hearing Research, 42,* 42–55.

Sanuki, T., Yumoto, E., Minoda, R., & Kodama, N. (2010). Effects of type II thyroplasty on adductor spasmodic dysphonia. *Otolaryngology-Head and Neck Surgery, 142,* 540–546.

Sapienza, C. M., & Stathopoulos, E. T. (1994). Respiratory and laryngeal measures of children and women with bilateral vocal fold nodules. *Journal of Speech and Hearing Research, 37,* 1229–1243.

Sapienza, C. M., & Stathopoulos, E. T. (1995). Speech task effects on acoustic and aerodynamic measures of women with vocal nodules. *Journal of Voice, 9,* 413–418.

Sapienza, C. M., Stathopoulos, E. T., & Brown, W. S. (1997). Speech breathing during reading in women with vocal nodules. *Journal of Voice, 11,* 195–201.

Sapir, S. (2007). *Vowel Articulation Index as a robust acoustic index of dysarthric vowel articulation: Evidence from the speech of individuals with and without idiopathic Parkinson's disease.* Presented at the annual conference of the Israeli Association of Physical and Rehabilitation Medicine.

Sapir, S., Ramig, L. O., Spielman, J., L., & Fox, C. (2010). Formant centralization ratio: A proposal for a new acoustic measure of dysarthric speech. *Journal of Speech, Language, and Hearing Research, 53,* 114–125.

Sataloff, R. T., Castell, D. O., Katz, P. O., & Sataloff, D. M. (2006). *Reflux laryngitis and related disorders, 3rd ed.* San Diego, CA: Plural Publishing, Inc.

Sato, M., Buccino, G., Gentilucci, M., & Cattaneo, L. (2010). On the tip of the tongue: Modulation of the primary motor cortex during audiovisual speech perception. *Speech Communication, 52,* 533–541.

Sato, M., Grabski, K., Glenberg, A. M., Brisebois, A., Basirat, A., Ménard, L., & Cattaneo, L. (2011). Articulatory bias in speech categorization: Evidence from use-induced motor plasticity. *Cortex, 47,* 1001–1003.

Saunders, J. (2005). Asthma. In H. A. Boushey, P. B. Corry, J. V. Fahey, E. G. Burchard, & P. G. Wood (Eds.), *Mason, Murray and Nadell's textbook of respiratory medicine* (4th ed.). New York: Elsevier.

Schaeffer, N. (2007). Speech breathing behavior and vocal fold function in dysphonic participants before and after therapy during connected speech: Preliminary observations. *Contemporary Issues in Communication Science and Disorders, 34,* 61–72.

Schaeffer, N., Cavallo, S. A., Wall, M., & Diakow, C. (2002). Speech breathing behavior in normal and moderately to severely dysphonic subjects during connected speech. *Journal of Medical Speech–Language Pathology, 10,* 1–18.

Schneider, B., & Bigenzahn, W. (2003). Influence of glottal closure configuration on vocal efficacy in young normal-speaking women. *Journal of Voice, 17,* 468–480.

Schwartz, J.-L., Basirat, A., Ménard, L., & Sato, M. (2012). The Perception-for-Action Control Theory (PACT): A perceptuo-motor theory of speech perception. *Journal of Neurolinguistics, 25,* 336–354.

Scott, S. K., McGettigan, C., & Eisner, F. (2009). A little more conversation, a little less action – candidate roles for the motor cortex in speech perception. *Nature Reviews/Neuroscience, 10,* 295–302.

Sebel, P., Stoddart, D. M., Waldhorn, R. E., Waldmann, C. S., & Whitfield, P. (1987). *Respiration: The breath of life.* New York: Torstar Books.

Seccombe, L. M., Giddings, H. L., Rogers, P. G., Corbett, A. J., Hayes, M. W., Peters, M. J., & Veitch, E. M. (2011). Abnormal ventilatory control in Parkinson's disease: Further evidence for non-motor dysfunction. *Respiratory Physiology & Neurology, 179,* 300–304.

Seddoh, S. A. K., Robin, D. A., Sim, H. -S., Hageman, C., Moon, J. B., & Folkins, J. W. (1996). Speech timing in apraxia of speech versus conduction aphasia. *Journal of Speech and Hearing Research, 39,* 590–603.

Seifert, E., Oswald, M., Bruns, U., Vischer, M., Kompis, M., & Haeusler, R. (2002). Changes of voice and articulation in children with cochlear implants. *International Journal of Pediatric Otorhinolaryngology, 66,* 115–123.

Seikel, J. A., Drumright, D. G., & Seikel, P. (2004). *Essentials of anatomy and physiology for communication disorders.* Clifton Park, NY: Thomson Delmar Learning.

Seikel, J. A., King, D. W., & Drumright, D. G. (1997). *Anatomy and physiology for speech and language.* San Diego, CA: Singular.

Selby, J. C., Gilbert, H. R., & Lerman, J. W. (2003). Perceptual and acoustic evaluation of individuals with laryngopharyngeal reflux pre- and post-treatment. *Journal of Voice, 17,* 557–570.

Shanks, J. E., Lilly, D. J., Margolis, R. H., Wiley, T. L., & Wilson, R. H. (1988). Tympanometry. *Journal of Speech and Hearing Disorders, 53,* 354–377.

Shinn, P., & Blumstein, S. E. (1983). Phonetic disintegration in aphasia: Acoustic analysis of spectral characteristics for place of articulation. *Brain and Language, 20,* 90–114.

Siebner, H. R., Peller, M., Takano, B., & Conrad, B. (2001). New insights into brain function by combination of transcranial magnetic stimulation and functional brain mapping. *Nervenarzt, 72,* 320–326.

Siemons-Lühring, D. I., Moerman, M., Martens, J.-P., Deuster, D., Müller, F., & Dejonckere, P. (2009). Spasmodic dysphonia, perceptual and acoustic analysis: Presenting new diagnostic tools. *European Archives of Otorhinolaryngology, 266,* 1915–1922.

Silbergleit, A. K., Johnson, A. F., & Jacobson, B. H. (1997). Acoustic analysis of voice in individuals with amyotrophic lateral sclerosis and perceptually normal voice quality. *Journal of Voice, 11,* 222–231.

Silman, S., & Gelfand, S. A. (1981). The relationship between magnitude of hearing loss and acoustic reflex threshold levels. *Journal of Speech and Hearing Disorders, 46,* 312–316.

Silman, S., & Silverstein, C. A. (1991). *Auditory diagnosis: Principles and applications.* San Diego, CA: Academic Press.

Silverman, E. P., Garvan, C., Shrivastav, R., & Sapienza, C. M. (2012). Combined modality treatment of adductor spasmodic dysphonia. *Journal of Voice, 26,* 77–86.

Silverman, E. P., Sapienza, C. M., Saleem, A., Carmichael, C., Davenport, P. W., Hoffman-Ruddy, B., & Okun, M. S. (2006). Tutorial on maximum inspiratory and expiratory mouth pressures in individuals with idiopathic Parkinson disease (IPD) and the preliminary results of an expiratory muscle strength training program. *NeuroRehabilitation, 21,* 71–79.

Singh, A., Kazi, R., De Cordova, J., Nutting, C. M., Clarke, P., Harrington, K. J., & Rhys-Evans, P. (2008). Multidimensional assessment of voice after vertical partial laryngectomy: A comparison with normal and total laryngectomy voice. *Journal of Voice, 22,* 740–745.

Sivasankar, M., & Fisher, K. V. (2002). Oral breathing increases P_{th} and vocal effort by superficial drying of vocal fold mucosa. *Journal of Voice, 16,* 172–181.

Skodda, S., Visser, W., & Schlegel, U. (2011). Vowel articulation in Parkinson's disease. *Journal of Voice, 25,* 467–472.

Skodda, S., Visser, W., & Schlegel, U. (2012). Acoustical analysis of speech in progressive supranuclear palsy. *Journal of Voice, 25,* 725–731.

Slavin, D. C., & Ferrand, C. T. (1995). Factor analysis of proficient esophageal speech: Toward a multidimensional model. *Journal of Speech and Hearing Research, 38,* 1224–1231.

Smith, A., & Denny, M. (1990). High frequency oscillations as indicators of neural control mechanisms in human respiration, mastication, and speech. *Journal of Neurophysiology, 63,* 745–758.

Smith, M. E., Roy, N., & Stoddard, K. (2008). Ansa-RLN reinnervation for unilateral vocal fold paralysis in adolescents and young adults. *International Journal of Pediatric Otorhinolaryngology, 72,* 1311–1316.

Smitheran, R., & Hixon, T. J. (1981). A clinical method for estimating laryngeal airway resistance during vowel production. *Journal of Speech and Hearing Disorders, 46,* 138–147.

Smits, I., Ceuppens, P., & De Bodt, M. S. (2005). A comparative study of acoustic voice measurements by means of Dr. Speech and Computerized Speech Lab. *Journal of Voice, 19,* 187–196.

Sodersten, M., & Lindestad, P-A. (1990). Glottal closure and perceived breathiness during phonation in normally speaking subjects. *Journal of Speech and Hearing Research, 33,* 601–611.

Sokoloff, A. J. (2000). Localization and contractile properties of intrinsic longitudinal motor units of the rat tongue. *Journal of Neurophysiology, 84,* 827–835.

Solomon, N. P., & Charron, S. (1998). Speech breathing in able-bodied children and children with cerebral palsy: A review of the literature and implications for clinical intervention. *American Journal of Speech Language Pathology, 7,* 61–78.

Solomon, N. P., & DiMattia, M. S. (2000). Effects of a vocally fatiguing task and systemic hydration on phonation threshold pressure. *Journal of Voice, 14,* 341–362.

Solomon, N. P., & Hixon, T. J. (1993). Speech breathing in Parkinson's disease. *Journal of Speech and Hearing Research, 36,* 294–310.

Sorenson, D. N. (1989). A F_0 investigation of children ages 6–10 years old. *Journal of Communication Disorders, 22,* 115–123.

Speaks, C. E. (1992). *Introduction to sound: Acoustics for the hearing and speech sciences.* New York: Chapman and Hall.

Sperry, E. E., & Klich, R. J. (1992). Speech breathing in senescent and younger women during oral reading. *Journal of Speech and Hearing Research, 35,* 1246–1255.

Speyer, R., Wieneke, G. H., & Dejonckere, P. H. (2004). Documentation of progress in voice therapy: Perceptual, acoustic, and laryngostroboscopic findings pretherapy and posttherapy. *Journal of Voice, 18,* 325–340.

Speyer, R., Wieneke, G. H., van Wijck-Warnaar, I., & Dejonckere, P. H. (2003). Effects of voice therapy on the voice range profiles of dysphonic patients. *Journal of Voice, 17,* 544–556.

Spielman, J., Mahler, L., Halpern, A., Gilley, P., Klepits-kaya, O., & Ramig, L. (2011). Intensive voice treatment (LSVT-LOUD) for Parkinson's disease following deep brain stimulation of the subthalamic nucleus. *Journal of Communication Disorders, 44,* 688–700.

Sprague, B. H., Wiley, T. L., & Goldstein, R. (1985). Tympanometric and acoustic-reflex studies in neonates. *Journal of Speech and Hearing Research, 28,* 265–272.

Stanton, A. E., Sellars, C., MacKenzie, K., McConnachie, A., & Bucknall, C. E. (2009). Perceived vocal morbidity in a problem asthma clinic. *The Journal of Laryngology and Otology, 123,* 96–102.

Stark, R. E., & Heinz, J. M. (1996a). Perception of stop consonants in children with expressive and receptive–expressive language impairments. *Journal of Speech and Hearing Research, 39,* 676–686.

Stark, R. E., & Heinz, J. M. (1996b). Vowel perception in children with and without language impairment. *Journal of Speech and Hearing Research, 39,* 860–869.

Stathopoulos, E. T. (1986). The relationship between intraoral air pressure and vocal intensity in children and adults. *Journal of Speech and Hearing Research, 29,* 71–74.

Stathopoulos, E. T. (1997). *Respiratory function in voice and speech disorders: Clinical implications.* Paper presented at the American Speech–Language–Hearing Association annual convention, Boston.

Stathopoulos, E. T., & Sapienza, C. M. (1993). Respiratory and laryngeal function of women and men during vocal intensity variation. *Journal of Speech and Hearing Research, 36,* 64–75.

Stathopoulos, E. T., & Sapienza, C. M. (1997). Developmental changes in laryngeal and respiratory function with variations in sound pressure level. *Journal of Speech, Language, and Hearing Research, 40,* 595–614.

Stathopoulos, E. T., & Weismer, G. (1985). Oral airflow and air pressure during speech production: A comparative study of children, youths, and adults. *Folia Phoniatrica et Logopedica, 37,* 152–159.

Stathopoulos, E. T., Hoit, J. D., Hixon, T. J., Watson, P. J., & Solomon, N. P. (1991). Respiratory and laryngeal function during whispering. *Journal of Speech and Hearing Research, 34,* 761–767.

Stelmach, I., Grzelewski, T., Bobrowska-Korzeniowska, M., Stelmach, P., & Kuna, P. (2007). A randomized, double-blind trial of the effect of anti-asthma treatment on lung function in children with asthma. *Pulmonary Pharmacology & Therapeutics, 20,* 691–700.

Stemple, J. C. (1997). *Respiratory function in voice and speech disorders: Clinical implications.* Paper presented at the annual convention of the American Speech–Language–Hearing Association, Boston.

Stepp, E. L., Brown, R., Tun, C. G., Gagnon, D. R., Jain, N. B., & Garshick, E. (2008). Determinants of lung volumes in chronic spinal cord injury. *Archives of Physical Medicine Rehabilitation, 89,* 1499–1506.

Stevens, K. N., & Blumstein, S. E. (1978). Invariant cues for place of articulation in stop consonants. *Journal of the Acoustical Society of America, 64,* 1358–1368.

Stone, M. (2005). A guide to analyzing tongue motion from ultrasound images. *Clinical Linguistics & Phonetics, 19,* 455–501.

Stone, M., Parthasarathy, V., Iskarous, K., NessAiver, M., & Prince, J. (2003). Tissue strains and tongue shapes: Combining tMRI and ultrasound. *Proceedings of the 15th International Congress of Phonetic Sciences.* Barcelona, Spain. August 3–9, 2003. Universitat Auto'noma de Barcelona.

Strand, E. A., Buder, E. H., Yorkston, K. M., & Olson Ramig, L. (1994). Differential phonatory characteristics of four women with amyotrophic lateral sclerosis. *Journal of Voice, 8,* 327–339.

Strange, W. (1999). Perception of vowels: Dynamic consistency. In J. M. Pickett (Ed.), *The acoustics of speech communication: Fundamentals, speech perception theory, and technology* (pp. 153–165). Boston: Allyn and Bacon.

Subtelny, J. D., Worth, J. H., & Sakuda, M. (1966). Intraoral pressure and rate of flow during speech. *Journal of Speech and Hearing Research, 9,* 498–518.

Subtelny, J., Li, W., Whitehead, R., & Subtelny, J. D. (1975). Cephalometric and cineradiographic study of deviant resonance in hearing-impaired speakers. *Journal of Speech and Hearing Disorders, 54,* 249–263.

Sulter, A. M., Schutte, H. K., & Miller, D. G. (1995). Differences in phonetogram features between male and female subjects with and without vocal training. *Journal of Voice, 9,* 363–377.

Summers, W. V., & Leek, M. R. (1992). The role of spectral and temporal cues in vowel identification by listeners with impaired hearing. *Journal of Speech and Hearing Research, 35,* 1189–1199.

Suskind, D. L., Zeringue, G. P. III, Kluka, E. A., Udall, J., & Liu, D. C. (2001). Gastroesophageal reflux and pediatric otolaryngologic disease: The role of antireflux surgery. *Archives of Otolaryngology-Head and Neck Surgery, 127,* 511–514.

Švec, J., G., Šram, F., & Schutte, H. K. (2007). Videokymography in voice disorders: What to look for? *Annals of Otology, Rhinology, & Laryngology, 116,* 172–180.

Szelies, B., Mielke, R., Grond, M., & Heiss, W. D. (2002). P300 in Alzheimer's disease: Relationship to dementia severity and glucose metabolism. *Neuropsychobiology, 46,* 49–56.

Takano, S., & Honda, K. (2007). An MRI analysis of the extrinsic tongue muscles during vowel production. *Speech Communication, 49,* 49–58.

Takano, S., Kimura, M., Nito, T., Imagawa, H., Sakakibara, K.-I., & Tayama, N. (2010). Clinical analysis of presbylarynx-vocal fold atrophy in elderly individuals. *Auris Nasus Larynx, 37,* 461–464.

Takemoto, H. (2001). Morphological analyses of the human tongue musculature for three-dimensional modeling. *Journal of Speech, Language, and Hearing Research, 44,* 95–107.

Tallal, P., Miller, S. L., Bedi, G., Byma, G., Wang, X., Nagarajan, S. S., Schreiner, C., Jenkins, W. M., & Merzenich, M. M. (1996). Language comprehension in language-learning impaired children improved with acoustically modified speech. *Science, 271,* 81–84.

Talmadeg, C. L., Long, G. R., Murphy, W. J., & Tubis, A. (1993). New off-line method for detecting spontaneous otoacoustic emissions in human subjects. *Hearing Research, 71,* 170–182.

Tamplin, J., Brazzale, D. J., Pretto, J. J., Ruehland, W. R., Buttifant, M., Brown, D. J., & Berlowitz, D. J. (2011). Assessment of breathing patterns and respiratory muscle recruitment during singing and speech in quadriplegia. *Archives of Physical and Medical Rehabilitation, 92,* 250–256.

Tanner, K., Sauder, C., Thibeault, S. L., Dromey, C., & Smith, M. E. (2010). Vocal fold bowing in elderly male monozygotic twins: A case study. *Journal of Voice, 24,* 470–476.

Tantisira, K. G., Fuhlbrigge, A., L., Tonascia, J., Van Natta, M., Zeiger, R. S., Strunk, R. C., Szefler, S. J., & Weiss, S. T. (2006). Bronchodilation and bronchoconstriction: Predictors of future lung function in childhood asthma. *Journal of Allergy and Clinical Immunology, 117,* 1264–1271.

Tashjian, D. B., Tirabassi, M. V., Moriarty, K. P., & Salva, P. S. (2002). Laparoscopic Nissen fundoplication for reactive airway disease. *Journal of Pediatric Surgery, 37,* 1021–1023.

Tatham, M., & Morton, K. (2011). *A guide to speech production and perception.* Edinburgh University Press.

Taylor, B. N., & Thompson, A. (2008). *The International System of Units (SI)*. U. S. Department of Commerce, NIST Special Publication 330.

Thomas, A., Iacono, D., Bonanni, L., D'Andreamatteo, L., & Onofrj, M. (2001). Donepezil, rivastigmine, and vitamin E in Alzheimer disease: A combined P300 event-related potentials/neuropsychologic evaluation over 6 months. *Clinical Neuropharmacology, 24*, 31–42.

Thornton, J. (2008). Working with the transgender voice: The role of the speech and language therapist. *Sexologies, 17*, 271–276.

Tigges, M., Wittenberg, T., Mergell, P., & Eysholdt, U. (1999). Imaging of vocal fold vibration by digital multiplane kymography. *Computerized Medical Imaging and Graphics, 23*, 323–330.

Titze, I. R. (1991). A model for neurologic sources of aperiodicity in vocal fold vibration. *Journal of Speech and Hearing Research, 34*, 460–472.

Titze, I. R. (1994). *Principles of voice production*. Englewood Cliffs, NJ: Prentice Hall.

Titze, I. R. (1995). *Workshop on acoustic voice analysis: Summary statement*. Iowa City, IA: National Center for Voice and Speech.

Titze, I. R., & Liang, H. (1993). Comparison of F0 extraction methods for high-precision voice perturbation measurements. *Journal of Speech and Hearing Research, 36*, 1120–1133.

Tjaden, K., & Turner, G. S. (1997). Spectral properties of fricatives in amyotrophic lateral sclerosis. *Journal of Speech and Hearing Research, 40*, 1358–1372.

Tjaden, K., & Wilding, G. (2004). Rate and loudness manipulations in dysarthria: Acoustic and perceptual findings. *Journal of Speech, Language, and Hearing Research, 47*, 766–783.

Tjoa, T. (2011). Throat anatomy. http://emedicine.medscape.com/article/1899345-overview#aw2aab6b3.

Tourville, J. A., Reilly, K. J., & Guenther, F. H. (2008). Neural mechanisms underlying auditory feedback control of speech. *NeuroImage, 39*, 1429–1443.

Tremblay, P., & Small, S. L. (2011). On the context-dependent nature of the contribution of the ventral premotor cortex to speech perception. *NeuroImage, 57*, 1561–1571.

Treole, K., Trudeau, M. D., & Forrest, L. A. (1999). Endoscopic and stroboscopic description of adults with paradoxical vocal fold dysfunction. *Journal of Voice, 13*, 143–152.

Trépanier, L. L., Kumar, R., Lozano, A. M., Lang, A. E., & Saint-Cyr, J. A. (2000). Neuropsychological outcome of GPi pallidotomy and GPi or STN deep brain stimulation in Parkinson's disease. *Brain and Cognition, 42*, 324–347.

Trullinger, R. W., & Emanuel, F. W. (1983). Airflow characteristics of stop-plosive consonant productions of normal-speaking children. *Journal of Speech and Hearing Research, 26*, 202–208.

Turley, R., & Cohen, S. (2009). Impact of voice and swallowing problems in the elderly. *Otolaryngology— Head and Neck Surgery, 140*, 33–36.

Turner, C. W., Chi, S. L., & Flock, S. (1999). Limiting spectral resolution in speech for listeners with sensorineural hearing loss. *Journal of Speech, Language, and Hearing Research, 42*, 773–784.

Turner, G. S., Tjaden, K., & Weismer, G. (1995). The influence of speaking rate on vowel space and speech intelligibility for individuals with amyotrophic lateral sclerosis. *Journal of Speech and Hearing Research, 38*, 1001–1013.

Tye-Murray, N. (1987). Effects of vowel context on the articulatory closure postures of deaf speakers. *Journal of Speech and Hearing Research, 30*, 99–104.

Tye-Murray, N. (1991). The establishment of open articulatory postures by deaf and hearing talkers. *Journal of Speech and Hearing Research, 34*, 453–459.

Tyler, A. A., Figurski, G. R., & Langsdale, T. (1993). Relationships between acoustically determined knowledge of stop place and voicing contrasts and phonological treatment progress. *Journal of Speech and Hearing Research, 36,* 746–759.

Ubrig, M. T., Goffi-Gomez, M. V. S., Weber, R., Menezes, M. H. M., Nemr, N. K., Tsuji, D. H., & Tsuji, R. K. (2011). Voice analysis of postlingually deaf adults pre- and postcochlear implantation. *Journal of Voice, 25,* 692–699.

Ullrich, D. (2004). Imaging research seeks early detection of Alzheimer's risk. *MCW Health News.* http:// healthlink.mcw.edu.

Uloza, V., Saferis, V., & Uloziene, I. (2005). Perceptual and acoustic assessment of voice pathology and the efficacy of endolaryngeal phonomicrosurgery. *Journal of Voice, 19,* 138–145.

Valálik, I., Smehók, G., Bognár, L., & Csókay, A. (2011). Voice acoustic changes during bilateral subthalamic stimulation in patients with Parkinson's disease. *Clinical Neurology and Neurosurgery, 113,* 188–195.

Van As-Brooks, C. J., Koopmans-van Beinum, F. J., Pols, L. C. W., & Hilgers, F. J. M. (2006). Acoustic signal typing for evaluation of voice quality in tracheoesophageal speech. *Journal of Voice, 20,* 355–368.

Van Camp, K. J., Creten, W. L., Van de Heyning, P. H., & Vanpeperstraete, P. M. (1983). Optimizing tympanometric variables for detecting middle ear traumas. *Scandinavian Audiology Supplement, 17,* 7–10.

Van den Berg, J. (1958). Myo-elastic aerodynamic theory of voice production. *Journal of Speech and Hearing Research, 1,* 227–244.

Van Houtte, E., Van Lierde, K., & Claeys, S. (2011). Pathophysiology and treatment of muscle tension dysphonia: A review of the current knowledge. *Journal of Voice, 25,* 202–207.

Van Nuffelen, G., Middag, C., De Bodt, M., & Martens, J.-P. (2009). Speech technology-based assessment of phoneme intelligibility in dysarthria. *International Journal of Language and Communication Disorders, 44,* 716–730.

Vashani, K., Murugesh, M., Hattiangadi, G., Gore, G., Keer, V., Ramesh, V. S., Sandur, V., & Bhatia, S. (2010). Effectiveness of voice therapy in reflux-related voice disorders. *Diseases of the Esophagus, 23,* 27–32.

Ventura, S., M., R., Freitas, D., R., S., & Tavares, J., M., R., S. (2011). Toward dynamic magnetic resonance imaging of the vocal tract during speech production. *Journal of Voice, 25,* 511–518.

Vercueil, L., Linard, J. P., Wuyam, B., Pollak, P., & Benchetrit, G. (1999). Breathing pattern in patients with Parkinson's disease. *Respiration Physiology, 118,* 163–172.

Verdonck-de Leeuw, I. M., Festen, J. M., & Mahieu, H. F. (2001). Deviant vocal fold vibration as observed during videokymography: The effect on voice quality. *Journal of Voice, 15,* 313–322.

Vertigan, A. E., Theodoros, D. G., Winkworth, A. L., & Gibson, P. G. (2008). Acoustic and electroglottographic voice characteristics in chronic cough and paradoxical vocal fold movement. *Folia Phoniatrica et Logopedica, 60,* 210–216.

Vlahakis, N. E., Patel, M. A., Maragos, N. E., & Beck, K. C. (2002). Diagnosis of vocal cord dysfunction: The utility of spirometry and plethysmography. *Chest, 122,* 2246–2249.

Vogel, A. P., & Maruff, P. (2008). Comparison of voice acquisition methodologies in speech research. *Behavior Research Methods, 40,* 982–987.

Vorperian, H. K., & Kent, R. D. (2007). Vowel acoustic space development in children: A synthesis of acoustic and anatomic data. *Journal of Speech, Language, and Hearing Research, 50,* 1510–1545.

Wake, M., Hughes, E. K., Poulakis, Z., Collins, C., & Rickards, F. W. (2004). Outcomes of children with mild-profound congenital hearing loss at 7 to 8 years: A population study. *Ear and Hearing, 25,* 1–8.

Walden, B. E., Busacco, D. A., & Montgomery, A. A. (1993). Benefit from visual cues in auditory-visual speech recognition by middle-aged and elderly persons. *Journal of Speech and Hearing Research, 36,* 431–436.

Waldstein, R. S., & Baum, S. R. (1991). Anticipatory coarticulation in the speech of profoundly hearing-impaired and normally hearing children. *Journal of Speech and Hearing Research, 34,* 1276–1285.

Walker, M., & Messing, B. (November, 2006). *Stroboscopic interpretation: Inter-rater reliability among professionals.* Paper presented at the annual meeting of the American Speech-Language-Hearing Asssociation, Miami.

Watkins, K. E., Strafella, A. P., & Paus, T. (2003). Seeing and hearing speech excites the motor system involved in speech production. *Neuropsychologia, 41,* 989–994.

Watson, B. C., & Freeman, F. J. (1997). Brain imaging contributions. In R. F. Curlee & G. M. Siegel (Eds.), *Nature and treatment of stuttering: New directions* (pp. 143–166). Boston: Allyn and Bacon.

Watson, B. U., & Miller, T. K. (1993). Auditory perception, phonological processing, and reading ability/disability. *Journal of Speech and Hearing Research, 36,* 850–863.

Watson, M. A., King, C. S., Holley, A. B., Greenburg, D. L., & Mikita, J. A. (2009). Clinical and lung function variables associated with vocal cord dysfunction. *Respiratory Care, 54,* 467–473.

Watson, P. (1997). *Respiratory function in voice and speech disorders: Clinical implications.* Paper presented at the annual convention of the American Speech–Language–Hearing Association, Boston.

Watson, P., & Hixon, T. (1985). Respiratory kinematics in classical (opera) singers. *Journal of Speech and Hearing Research, 28,* 104–122.

Watson, P., Hixon, T., Stathopoulos, E., & Sullivan, D. (1990). Respiratory kinematics in female classical singers. *Journal of Voice, 4,* 120–128.

Webster, D. B. (1999). *Neuroscience of communication* (2nd ed.). San Diego, CA: Singular.

Weinberg, B., & Bennett, S. (1971). Speaker sex recognition of five and six-year old children's voices. *Journal of the Acoustical Society of America, 50,* 1210–1213.

Weismer, G., & Laures, J. S. (2002). Direct magnitude estimates of speech intelligibility in dysarthria: Effects of a chosen standard. *Journal of Speech, Language, and Hearing Research, 45,* 421–433.

Weismer, G., Martin, R., Kent, R. D., & Kent, J. F. (1992). Formant trajectory characteristics of males with amyotrophic lateral sclerosis. *Journal of the Acoustical Society of America, 91,* 1085–1098.

Weismer, G., Yunusova, Y., & Westbury, J. (2003). Interarticulator coordination in dysarthria: An x-ray microbeam study. *Journal of Speech, Language, and Hearing Research, 46,* 1247–1261.

Werber, E. A., Gandelman-Marton, R., Klein, C., & Rabey, J. M. (2003). The clinical use of P300 event related potentials for the evaluation of cholinesterase inhibitors treatment in demented patients. *Journal of Neural Transmission, 110,* 659–669.

Wermke, K., & Robb, M. P. (2010). Fundamental frequency of neonatal crying: Does body size matter? *Journal of Voice, 24,* 388–394.

Werth, K., Voigt, D., Döllinger, M., Eysholdt, U., & Lohscheller, J. (2010). Clinical value of acoustic voice measures: A retrospective study. *European Archives of Otorhinolaryngology, 267,* 1261–1271.

West, J. B. (2005). *Respiratory physiology: The essentials.* Hagerstown, MD: Lippincott Williams & Wilkins.

Whalen, D. H., Levitt, A. G., & Goldstein, L. M. (2007). VOT in the babbling of French-and English-learning infants. *Journal of Phonetics, 35,* 341–352.

Wheat, M. C., & Hudson, A. I. (1988). Spontaneous speaking fundamental frequency of 6-year-old black children. *Journal of Speech and Hearing Research, 31,* 723–725.

White, K. R. (2003). The current status of EHDI programs in the United States. *Mental Retardation and Developmental Disabilities Research Reviews, 9*, 79–88.

Whitehead, R. L. (1983). Some respiratory and aerodynamic patterns in the speech of the hearing impaired. In I. Hochberg, H. Levitt, & M. J. Osberger (Eds.), *Speech of the hearing impaired* (pp. 97–116). Baltimore, MD: University Park Press.

Whiteside, S. P., Dobbin, R., & Henry, L. (2003). Patterns of variability in voice onset time: A developmental study of motor speech skills in humans. *Neuroscience Letters, 347*, 29–32.

Whiteside, S. P., Grobler, S., Windsor, F., & Varley, R. (2010). An acoustic study of vowels and coarticulation as a function of utterance type: A case of acquired apraxia of speech. *Journal of Neurolinguistics, 23*, 145–161.

Williams, M., Purdy, S., & Barber, C. (1995). High frequency probe tone tympanometry in infants with middle ear effusion. *Australian Journal of Otolaryngology, 2*, 169–173.

Williamson, I. J., Matusiewicz, S. P., Brown, P. H., Greening, A. P., & Crompton, G. K. (1995). Frequency of voice problems and cough in patients using pressurized aerosol inhaled steroid preparations. *European Respiratory Journal, 8*, 590–592.

Winkworth, A. L., Davis, P. J., Adams, R. D., & Ellis, E. (1995). Breathing patterns during spontaneous speech. *Journal of Speech and Hearing Research, 38*, 124–144.

Witt, J. D., Fisher, J. R. K. O., Guenette, J. A., Cheong, K. A., Wilson, B. J., & Sheel, A. W. (2006). Measurement of exercise ventilation by a portable respiratory inductive plethysmograph. *Respiratory Physiology & Neurobiology, 154*, 389–395.

Wolfe, V. I., & Ratusnik, D. L. (1988). Acoustic and perceptual measurements of roughness influencing judgments of pitch. *Journal of Speech and Hearing Disorders, 53*, 15–22.

Wolfe, V. I., Ratusnik, D. L., Smith, F. H., & Northrop, G. (1990). Intonation and fundamental frequency in male-to-female transsexuals. *Journal of Speech and Hearing Disorders, 55*, 43–50.

Wolk, L., Abdelli-Beruh, N. B., & Slavin, D. (2012). Habitual use of vocal fry in young adult female speakers. *Journal of Voice, 26*, 111–116.

Workinger, M. S., & Kent, R. D. (1991). Perceptual analysis of the dysarthrias in children with athetoid and spastic cerebral palsy. In C. A. Moore, K. M. Yorkson, & D. R. Beukelman (Eds.), *Dysarthria and apraxia of speech: Perspectives on management* (pp. 109–126). Baltimore, MD: Paul H. Brookes.

Wu, J. C., Maguire, G., Riley, G., Fallon, J., LaCasse, L., Chin, S., Klein, E., Tang, C., Cadwell, S., & Lotenberg, S. (1995). A positron emission tomography [18F]deoxyglucose study of developmental stuttering. *Neurology Report, 6*, 501–505.

Wu, J. C., Maguire, G., Riley, G., Lee, A., Keator, D., Tang, C., Fallon, J., & Najafi, A. (1997). Increased dopamine activity associated with stuttering. *Clinical Neuroscience and Neuropsychology, 8*, 767–770.

Xie, Y., Zhang, Y., Zheng, Z., Liu, Z., Zhuang, P., Li, Y., & Wang, X. (2011). Changes in speech characters of patients with Parkinson's disease after bilateral subthalamic nucleus stimulation. *Journal of Voice, 25*, 751–758.

Xu, Y., & Son, X. (2002). Maximum speed of pitch change and how it may relate to speech. *Journal of the Acoustic Society of America, 111*, 1399–1413.

Xue, S. A., & Deliyski, D. (2001). Effects of aging on selected acoustic voice parameters: Preliminary normative data and educational implications. *Educational Gerontology, 27*, 159–168.

Yelken K, Gultekin E, Guven M, Eyibilen A, & Aladag, I. (2010). Impairment of voice quality in paradoxical vocal fold motion dysfunction. *Journal of Voice, 24*, 724–727.

Yoshinaga-Itano, C. (2003). Early intervention after universal neonatal hearing screening: Impact on outcomes. *Mental Retardation and Developmental Disabilities Research Reviews, 9,* 252–266.

Yoshinaga-Itano, C., Sedey, A. L., Coulter, D. K., & Mehl, A. L. (1998). Langauge of early- and later-identified children with hearing loss. *Pediatrics, 102,* 1161–1171.

Youmans, S. R., & Stierwalt, J. A. G. (2006). Measures of tongue function related to normal swallowing. *Dysphagia, 21,* 102–111.

Yuen, I., Davis, M. H., Brysbaert, M., & Rastle, K. (2010). Activation of articulatory information in speech perception. *PNAS, 107,* 592–597.

Yumoto, E., Gould, W. J., & Baer, T. (1982). Harmonics-to-noise ratio as an index of the degree of hoarseness. *Journal of the Acoustical Society of America, 71,* 1544–1550.

Yunusova, Y., Green, J. R., & Mefferd, A. (2009). Accuracy assessment for AG500, electromagnetic articulograph. *Journal of Speech, Language, and Hearing Research, 52,* 547–555.

Zagólski, O. (2009). Electroglottography in elderly patients with vocal fold palsy. *Journal of Voice, 23,* 567–571.

Zagólski, O., & Carlson, E. (2002). Electroglottographic measurements of glottal function in vocal fold paralysis in women. *Clinical Otolaryngology, 27,* 246–253.

Zemlin, W. R. (1998). *Speech and hearing science: Anatomy and physiology* (4th ed.). Boston: Allyn and Bacon.

Zeng, F.-G., & Turner, C. W. (1990). Recognition of voiceless fricatives by normal and hearing-impaired subjects. *Journal of Speech and Hearing Research, 33,* 440–449.

Zhang, Y., Jiang, J. J., Biazzo, L., & Jorgensen, M. (2005). Perturbation and nonlinear dynamic analyses of voices from patients with unilateral laryngeal paralysis. *Journal of Voice, 19,* 519–528.

Zharkova N., & Hewlett, N. (2009). Measuring lingual coarticulation from midsagittal tongue contours: Description and example calculations using English /t/ and /a/. *Journal of Phonetics, 37,* 248–256.

Ziegler, W., & von Cramon, D. (1983). Vowel distortion in traumatic dysarthria: A formant study. *Phonetica, 40,* 63–78.

Ziegler, W., Hoole, P., Hartmann, E., & von Cramon, D. (1988). Accelerated speech in dysarthria after acquired brain injury: Acoustic correlates. *British Journal of Disorders of Communication, 23,* 215–228.

Zimmerman, G. (1980). Articulatory dynamics of fluent utterances of stutterers and nonstutterers. *Journal of Speech and Hearing Research, 23,* 95–107.

Zoumalan, R., Maddalozzo, J., & Holinger, L. D. (2007). Etiology of stridor in infants. *Annals of Otology, Rhinology, & Laryngology, 116,* 329–334.

Zuur, J. K., Muller, S. H., Vincent, A., Sinaasappel, M., de Jongh, F. H. C., & Hilgers, F. J. M. (2009). The influence of a heat and moisture exchanger on tracheal climate in a cold environment. *Medical Engineering & Physics, 31,* 852–857.

Index

Note: In this index, *t* after the page number refers to a table and *f* refers to a figure.